Yellow Fever

ALSO BY S.L. KOTAR AND J.E. GESSLER
AND FROM McFARLAND

Cholera: A Worldwide History (2014)

Smallpox: A History (2013)

The Rise of the American Circus, 1716–1899 (2011)

Ballooning: A History, 1782–1900 (2011)

*The Steamboat Era: A History of Fulton's Folly
on American Rivers, 1807–1860* (2009)

Yellow Fever
A Worldwide History

S.L. Kotar *and* J.E. Gessler

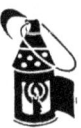

McFarland & Company, Inc., Publishers
Jefferson, North Carolina

LIBRARY OF CONGRESS CATALOGUING-IN-PUBLICATION DATA

Names: Kotar, S. L., author. | Gessler, J. E., co-author.
Title: Yellow fever : a worldwide history / S.L. Kotar and J.E. Gessler.
Description: Jefferson, North Carolina : McFarland & Company, Inc.,
Publishers, 2017. | Includes bibliographical references and index.
Identifiers: LCCN 2016058972 | ISBN 9780786479191 (softcover : alkaline paper) ∞
Subjects: LCSH: Yellow fever—History. | Epidemics—History. | Tropical
medicine—History. | World health—History.
Classification: LCC RA644.Y4 K68 2017 | DDC 614.5/41—dc23
LC record available at https://lccn.loc.gov/2016058972

BRITISH LIBRARY CATALOGUING DATA ARE AVAILABLE

**ISBN (print) 978-0-7864-7919-1
ISBN (ebook) 978-1-4766-2628-4**

© 2017 S.L. Kotar. All rights reserved

*No part of this book may be reproduced or transmitted in any form
or by any means, electronic or mechanical, including photocopying
or recording, or by any information storage and retrieval system,
without permission in writing from the publisher.*

Front cover image of patients in yellow fever hospital,
Havana, Cuba, 1899 (Library of Congress)

Printed in the United States of America

*McFarland & Company, Inc., Publishers
Box 611, Jefferson, North Carolina 28640
www.mcfarlandpub.com*

To the Old Friend, always,
and to everyone on the Island

Acknowledgment

The authors gratefully acknowledge the dedication, support and hard work done by Amy Christine Zimmerman, without whose help this book could never have been completed.

Table of Contents

Acknowledgment vi
Preface 1

1. Yellow Fever: A Perspective 5
2. The Early Colonial Period 11
3. A Question of Quarantine 31
4. The American Plague 44
5. "Particulars of the Plague in Philadelphia" 56
6. Most Unhappy Consequences 68
7. The Controversies of Yellow Fever Continue to Rage 76
8. The "Great Epidemic" of 1798 87
9. Is Yellow Fever More Deadly Than the Plague? 103
10. The Repository of Knowledge 118
11. Daily Mortality Is Now More Considerable 128
12. The Baneful Effects of Yellow Fever 138
13. Corpses Still Animated: Yellow Fever, 1820–1829 150
14. "All the evils which hell may contain" 169
15. The "Dead Book" 182
16. New Orleans: A City of Desolation 194
17. "To the manor born" 205
18. The "Quarantine War" and the "Quarantine Armada" 215
19. Deluge of Yellow Fever in the South and Worldwide Epidemics 223
20. The American Un-Civil War Period, 1860–1866 239
21. Holding On Until the Other Jack (Frost) Says "Enough!" 248
22. I Am "writing from the city of the dead" 254
23. Quarantine and Avarice, 1870–1873 267

24. "Falling Like Leaves"	283
25. "The grim monster still on his pathway": The Outbreaks of 1878	293
26. "We are almost entirely ignorant"	305
27. Mosquitoes and Germ Theories	318
28. Panama and Nicaragua: Two Canals, Two Views	330
29. Cuba and the "Patriotic Disease"	340
30. After War: Science and Sanitation	354
31. Into the 20th Century	365
32. Panama!	370
33. "America to Slay the World's Disease Germs"	378
34. Taking Steps Against a Deadly Enemy	393
Glossary	397
Chapter Notes	407
Bibliography	423
Index	433

Preface

In developed nations of the 21st century the horrors of yellow fever are difficult to fathom. When considering the disease, images of the Panama Canal with infected mosquitoes buzzing around the heads of imported laborers probably comes to mind. Symptomology is likely vague: headaches, yellowness and fever would be the most common. It evokes shock to discover the staggering death tolls, in spite of the horrific "cures," and horror to realize yellow fever was used as a form of biological warfare as early as the Civil War. Worse, it challenges the imagination to comprehend that yellow fever not only exists today in a deadly form but also presents complex health care problems to those poverty-stricken countries prone to the disease. But it is not only the people of Africa and South America who are threatened. Yellow fever exists today as a viable biological weapon and, potentially worse, viral fevers of the same class threaten the health of the world. Open a newspaper or scan the Internet and you are likely to find headlines capable of turning your blood cold. On November 30, 2015, for instance, in the *St. Louis Post-Dispatch,* one article began this way "Brazil links dengue-like virus to birth defects in babies." This is living history that has the potential to reawaken and augment old horrors by making them new again.

The authors hope that by allowing readers to absorb words written by those who lived through these terrible times their agony can resonate as keenly today as it did hundreds of years ago and lead to a better understanding of the obstacles before us. Two contrasting views, both written by physicians in the first two decades of the nineteenth century, serve to illustrate the state of the medical practitioner and the patient, a state that has not appreciably changed since at least the 1500s:

> When the vital energy sinks, it cannot be again revived; the benumbing poison of the contagion destroys it. The body of the patient then exhales miasmata, not perceptible to the senses, which attaches it to the bedding, clothes, furniture, and even the walls of the apartment, which then become capable of infecting individuals, more or less promptly....[1]

> All the violence of disease now rushed in upon me, hurrying on towards rapid destruction. The light was intolerable, and the pulsations of the head and eyes were most excruciating—conveying a sensation as if three or four hooks were fastened into the globe of each eye, and some person, standing behind me, was dragging them forcibly from their orbits back into the head, the cerebrum being, at the same time, detached from its membranes, and leaping about violently within the cranium. A wearying pain occupied my back and limbs, and in particular the calves of my legs, feeling as if dogs were gnawing down to the bones, while a tormenting restlessness possessed my whole frame, and totally prevented the slightest approach to ease or quiet. The skin was burning, and conveyed a pangent sensation when touched: the pulse was quickened but not very full; the tongue was white and parched, with excessive thirst and constant dryness of the mouth, lips, and teeth.[2]

Yellow fever was well-known in Africa, South and Central America, the Caribbean and Mexico but it also adversely affected the southern latitudes of the United States. The disease was not exclusively limited to warm climates, however. In the early years of the United States it touched as far north as Boston, while striking Philadelphia (then the capital of the new nation) with plague-like ferocity that touched the lives of many of the Founding Fathers, as well as affected the reputation of America's most famous physician, Dr. Benjamin Rush.

No authority of the times could explain the cause, much less offer proof of whether the disease was imported or of local origin. No method existed to make a definitive diagnosis, and treatments were varied, horrific and unsuccessful. The subject of quarantine became more of a political battle than a medical concern, evoking bitter, sometimes violent reactions from frightened people. African Americans were erroneously thought to be immune from the disease and were employed as nurses to treat the sick. Businessmen raged against restrictions on imported and exported goods that reduced their profit margins while, as always, more savvy entrepreneurs found ways to make a "killing" in the markets.

Complicating matters was the dissemination of information that either lessened or augmented national fears. For example, yellow fever came calling at New Orleans early in 1853. On Friday, July 22, Charity Hospital admitted 27 patients and discharged 44, while registering 48 deaths, 43 attributed to that dreaded malady. For the last week of July, as the *New Orleans Delta* was opining the disease was "worse than ever before," the Charity reported 130 deaths.

As *Delta* newspapers were transported across the country by land and steamboat, exchange editors in other cities lifted articles and statistics, either publishing them verbatim or, more commonly, editing them as space dictated. If the reader were fortunate, appended to the beginning would be a nonspecific acknowledgment of source, such as, "New Orleans papers of Sunday have been received." (Unfortunately, of course, the original source was not cited nor was the specific date. As the transfer of information was often delayed, "Sunday" might refer to one, two or even three weeks earlier.) In tracing the convoluted trail, the *Zanesville (OH) Courier* published the correct number of deaths (130) on July 30, 1853, having copied the statistics from a Philadelphia paper of the 29th. The editor of a Baltimore paper, however, either misread the number or a typesetter made a mistake in setting copy, as other exchanges garnering data from its July 30 issue listed mortality as being 190. Other than inadvertently adding 60 to the death toll, the paragraph from the Baltimore paper was identical. As the telegraph became the standard for transmitting information, timeliness was improved but the probability of human error remained constant.

One thing historians take away from decades of research is the often depressing realization that people never change. When two or more opposing views are held, the concept of compromise becomes more theoretical than actual, whether the subject to be debated arose in the 17th century or the 21st century. Every side of the debate held to its own tenets, believing they *must* be right and the other side wrong. When the subject is a disease that has the potential to destroy thousands of lives during the course of an epidemic, quarrels tend to follow two paths: vitriolic accusation—with the occasional biting sarcasm—and violence.

Citing the oft-expressed lament, "When doctors disagree, who can be trusted?" average citizens—those most directly affected by the menace of impending doom—are left to their own resources. With direct observation as the first tool, reliance on religion and superstition follow as humanity struggles to comprehend the physical and moral causes of the seemingly incomprehensible presence of plague, a term used generically to describe everything from the Black Death to yellow fever.

In the case of the latter, three questions dominated the centuries: nosology, or the name and identification of the disease as a specific entity; treatment of the symptoms and ultimately a cure; and a determination of its origin, which led directly into the economically charged issue of quarantine. All three issues were inextricably linked but as no answers were immediately forthcoming they tended to be addressed separately, adding to the confusion and uncertainty.

Lacking modern methods, early practitioners were forced to rely on primitive methods of identification. Complicating matters, the symptoms of yellow fever were often vague and easily confused with other diseases. Between the 1600s and the early 1900s, it was classified as a nondescript fever, a malarial disease or a digestive disorder and was thought to arise from miasma, certain conditions in the atmosphere or even alcoholism. As the science of sanitation developed (most notably practiced by Union general Benjamin Butler in New Orleans during the Civil War when yellow fever cases were extremely low), scientists hoped they had found a preventative if not a cure. When epidemics recurred in cities considered to be most healthful, however, researchers looked elsewhere, suggesting everything from boiling to freezing, the cremation of bodies, and, most often, strict quarantine of passengers and baggage. Because no two cities, states or national governments could agree on universal terms and conditions, results were often erratic and unsatisfactory.

Although as varied as methods of prevention, cures were far less successful. The *Crown Point (IN) Register* of October 24, 1878, spoke for nearly everyone when it announced, "It is not especially credible to the condition of medical science in this country that, after the terrible losses we have endured from yellow fever, the doctors should be utterly at a loss how to treat it; and it is not going too far to say that the doctors kill more than the fever does." Another newspaper echoed the sentiment by noting. "The New Orleans *Times* abandons all hopes of ever understanding yellow fever and its treatment. The doctors are also in the same fix. The *Times* says: 'It seems quite out of the question that the doctors will ever afford us the smallest relief....' Now that this point is settled, we needn't worry with the doctors any longer."[3]

One of the most interesting aspects of historical research, and a subject paramount to us in compiling this data, is uncovering small bits of humor and trivia that instill the human element into dates and events. On the subject of prevention, it was commonly believed (without comprehending why) that higher elevations were a safe place to go when yellow fever struck. The observation was actually correct because mosquitoes (then the unknown carrier) do not fly beyond a certain height. One fellow in the 1800s took this concept to heart when he declared that the way to protect from the disease was to build a fence around your property. On the face of it, the assertion sounds laughable. How could a wooden fence serve as protection against yellow fever? But knowing today what that gentleman didn't know then—that mosquitoes always fly in a straight line and don't have the ability to solve the problem of merely flying a foot or two higher to get over the fence—they merely turn around and go back the way they came. Barring the incidental insect blown over the obstacle by the wind, this solution was probably more effective than most of the other outlandish ideas suggested over the course of several centuries.

It is not surprising that war and economics played the ultimate roles in unraveling the mysteries of yellow fever. The disastrous attempt by the French to construct the Panama Canal (of which it was written, "Every great engineering feat ever accomplished has cost more or less in human life, but nothing in history, so far as our knowledge extends, compares to the death roll already reported from Panama"),[4] the Cuban revolutions against Spain, the Spanish-American War and finally the United States' determination to finish the Panama Canal, added an urgency to the problem that ultimately settled the cause and transmission of yellow fever and the subsequent acceptance of inoculation.

Nor is it surprising that credit for these momentous discoveries was unevenly and perhaps unfairly distributed. The idea of mosquitoes as the carrier had been demonstrated for decades before the well-publicized breakthroughs after the Spanish-American War and American intervention in Panama. Trial-and-error human tests with inoculation had been successfully, if not scientifically proven, and scientific papers presented in various countries detailed numerous theories and experiments. The result, still evolving, is that it required the hearts, minds and lives of innumerable dedicated scientists to bring us to the point we are today. Whether their names are lost or obscured by history, they were all heroes in a cause to better the human condition. The authors of their combined histories humbly salute them.

CHAPTER 1

Yellow Fever: A Perspective

As the contagion of the plague is moſt subtile and inviſible, and often makes dreadful ravage; ſo it behoves mankind to uſe all proper precautions in preventing the ſpreading of that deſtructive peſt; which the principle of ſelf preſervation ſtrongly excites us to, and in doing of which we may expect the concurrence of the divine bleſſing on our well-meant endeavours.[1]

Yellow fever, so named from the jaundice observed in victims, is an acute viral hemorrhagic disease contracted from the bite of a female mosquito. The only known hosts of the virus are primates and the *Aedes* and *Heamogogus* species of mosquitos that include *Aedes aegypt,* the so-called yellow fever mosquito and *Aedes albopictus,* the "tiger" mosquito. The disease, known variously as "yellow jack" (short for "yellow jacket"), "yellow plague," "Yellow Rainer," "Bronze John," "dock fever," "ship fever" (also associated with typhus), "stranger's fever," "American plague"[2] or simply the catch-all "plague," gained prominence in historical records during the 1500s but that is misleading. Symptoms of yellow fever, although thoroughly described in the medical and popular print of the time, were nonspecific, leading to confusion over precise diagnosis. Even today clinical diagnosis begins with a medical history of the victim's exposure to infected areas and ends only by advanced laboratory identification. It is therefore impossible, at present, to state with certainty the time of its first appearance.

Mainstream research has described the origin of yellow fever as likely occurring in Africa and spreading through the Americas via the slave trade during the 16th century. The first Western-documented description of yellow fever in the New World appeared in 1647. In 1885, a study published by the *New York Sun* reported the commonly held theory that "the dread scourge is the direct result of the slave traffic, having been unknown in America till brought by the accursed trade. The African disease, intensified by the filthy habits of human cargoes, came first to this port [Vera Cruz, Mexico] and elsewhere on the continent with a slave ship in 1699, and in like manner was transferred to all the West Indies. When the negro insurrection in San Domingo drove the white population into exile, the emigrants carried the contagion to all the cities of the United States, even away up in the interior of Massachusetts." The article added that yellow fever was believed to have been introduced into Rio de Janeiro via the African slave trade and from there was transported to the upper wards of New Orleans. Simultaneously, the Crescent City was infected from ships from Cuba where passengers had contracted "vomito" at Havanna.

While such historical accounts augmented the theory, fresh compotation of data drawing on new sources offers the possibility that the actual origin of the disease may have been Central or South America. Pre-Colombian text, written in the Mayan language, can be interpreted as indicating epidemic yellow fever had occurred in that region before 1492. Richard Ligon's 1657 text, *A True and Exact History of the Island of Barbadoes*, mentions the disease broke out in early September 1747 and before the end of the month "the living were scarcely able to bury the dead." Other studies suggest yellow fever may have appeared in West Africa only between 1760 and 1770,[3] while the first European text describing what was likely yellow fever in coastal West Africa dates only from 1764 (Sierra Leone) and 1778 (Senegal).[4] W.C. Gorges, an expert on tropical diseases who was intimately involved in medical affairs during preconstruction of the Panama Canal, also believed that yellow fever originated in South and Central America.[5]

Yellow fever today is endemic in 44 countries in sub-Saharan Africa and Latin America. In Africa, an estimated 508 million people in 31 countries are at risk; in Latin America 13 countries are affected, with Bolivia, Brazil, Colombia, Ecuador and Peru being the most susceptible, effecting a combined population of over 900 million people. Although the disease has never been reported in Asia, the region remains at risk due to increasingly favorable conditions. Historically, yellow fever epidemics have occurred in North America and Europe, most notably England, Ireland, France, Italy, Spain and Portugal, and, while not endemic, the disease can occur virtually anywhere from imported cases.

Yellow fever is an arbovirus of the *flavivirus* genus. The transmission cycle is primarily dependent on the female mosquito (males do not carry the virus). After the two-winged insect sucks the blood of a primate in the first three or four days of the victim's fever, the virus from the blood passes into the *aegypti*'s stomach. During the next twelve days, if the concentration is high enough, the virions may infect the epithelial cells and reproduce before being passed into the blood system of the mosquito (haemocoel). From there, the virus enters the salivary glands and is injected into the victim the next time the mosquito feeds. The *aegypti* feeds every three days and is capable of infecting a different primate with each meal for the duration of her life, which typically lasts until frost strikes. In this manner, the insect transmits yellow fever from monkey to monkey, from monkey to human and from human to human. It is also significant to note that recent findings indicate the likelihood of transvarial and transstadial transmission from a female mosquito to her eggs and then larvae, allowing for the continuance of the disease even when there are no adults.[6] This transmission of yellow fever without an identified host likely explains isolated outbreaks in previously yellow fever-free areas.

Yellow Fever Virus

Group	IV
Order	Unassigned
Family	*Flaviviridae*
Genus	*Flavivirus*
Species	Yellow fever virus

The genus *Flavivirus* includes a group of viruses spread by mosquitoes, including West Nile, dengue and Japanese encephalitis. Compared to other viruses, yellow fever is not considered one of the more powerful diseases in that it cannot exist outside the body for more than a few hours, is not spread through the air or by contact and does not mutate as readily as other viruses. Its greatest asset to survival is in its choice of vector— the seemingly ever-present mosquito.

The yellow fever virus is round with 20 smooth sides that protect the single strand of RNA. The coating is composed of proteins that attract human cells. Once in contact, the process of receptor-mediated endocytosis begins. Once healthy cells surround the virus, it uses the cell's internal composition to replicate the viral proteins and RNA until the new particles burst through the cell. Duplicated millions of times, the host body fills with the virus. This explains why viruses resist treatment by antibiotics: any drug that had the capacity to destroy it would also destroy the cell. The characteristic "fever" in yellow fever is the result of the body attempting to kill off the virus invasion.[7]

In studying yellow fever, three classifications of mosquito are made: domestic (those bred around houses); wild (those bred in the jungle), and semidomestic (those bred in both habitats).

Transmission of Yellow Fever

Sylvatic (jungle) yellow fever: In tropical rainforests, monkeys are infected by wild mosquitoes that pass the disease to other monkeys by feeding on them. When humans enter the rain forests, they are bitten by infected mosquitoes and may contract the disease.

Intermediate (savannah) yellow fever: In humid or semi-humid sections of Africa, small-scale epidemics occur when semidomestic mosquitoes infect both monkeys and humans. This is the most common type of outbreak in Africa and can lead to major epidemics when the disease is carried into more populated areas where there are domestic mosquitoes and unvaccinated people. Different mosquitoes of the genus *Aedes* are involved.

Urban yellow fever: Large epidemics occur when infected people introduce the virus into highly populated areas with large numbers of *Aedes* mosquitoes and nonimmune people.[8]

In the African urban cycle, only the *Aedes africanus* mosquito is involved. Also capable of transmitting other diseases such as dengue and chikungunya, the urban cycle is responsible for all major outbreaks of yellow fever in Africa. Except for an outbreak of yellow fever in Bolivia in 1999, the urban cycle no longer exists in South America. The sylvatic cycle involving the *Aedes africanus* (Africa) and mosquitoes of the genus *Haemogogus* and *Sabethes* (South America) serve as vectors (transmitters). Lower primates are the most affected, although the animals are mostly asymptomatic. In South America the sylvatic cycle is presently the only way humans infect one another, explaining the low incidence of yellow fever on the continent. Humans infected in the jungle transport the virus to cities, where the *Aedes aegypti* serves as the vector. The seemingly impossible task of eliminating the *Aedes aegypti* mosquito makes eradication of yellow fever a distant dream.[9]

Symptomology of Yellow Fever

Once an individual is bitten by an infected mosquito the virus incubates in the body for 3 to 6 days. Symptoms of yellow fever include arrhythmia (characterized as "irregular heartbeats"), bleeding that may progress to hemorrhage, coma, decreased urine output, delirium, fever, headache, jaundice (yellow eyes and skin), muscle aches, red eyes, face and tongue, seizures, vomited stomach contents and occasionally blood.[10]

The three stages of the disease are categorized as "Stage 1," or the infectious stage, where the victim suffers mild symptoms that briefly ease after 3–4 days. "Stage 2," or the remission stage, occurs when the fever and other symptoms go away. At this point most people recover but after 24 hours 15 percent of patients take a turn for the worse. "Stage

3," or the intoxication stage, includes major organ failure (heart, liver, kidneys), bleeding disorders, seizures, coma and death. Half of those entering the toxic stage die within 10 to 14 days. The remainder recover without significant organ damage. Persons of all ages are susceptible to the disease, but the elderly are more likely to suffer severe symptoms.[11]

Like cholera, the great killer of the 19th century, yellow fever cases have increased rather than decreased over the past several decades. This is attributed to declining immunity to infection, deforestation, urbanization, population migration and climate change. Presently, an estimated 200,000 cases are confirmed each year, resulting in the tragic and preventable deaths of 30,000 individuals.

Historic Identification of Yellow Fever

When discussing yellow fever it is important to keep in mind that until advanced laboratory tests were developed in the 20th century yellow fever was a clinical diagnosis. Without clearly defined symptoms such as those characterizing smallpox (and even then there were heated arguments in the 19th century over a definitive diagnosis), local doctors were forced to rely on the patient's oral history and their own eyes. The situation further complicated by the fact that the cause of yellow fever was not positively established until the 1890s, practitioners relied on their experience and personal penchants for how to identify and treat the disease.

Through the 1840s yellow fever was classified under the vague distinction of *febris continua*, or a continued fever. In the nosology of the times, this was a division of the order *Febres*, in the class *Pyrexiae* of Dr. William Cullen's authoritative text, *Synopsis of Methodical Nosology*, 1792.

Febris Continua

Continued fevers have no intermission, but exacerbations come on usually twice in one day. The genera of continued fevers are:

(1) *Synocha*, or inflammatory fever, known by increased heat; pulse frequent, strong and hard; urine high-coloured; senses not much impaired.

(2) *Typhus*, or putrid-tending fever, which is contagious, and is characterized by moderate heat; quick, weak and small pulse; senses not much impaired, and great prostration of strength. This genus has two species; *Typhus petechialis*, attended with petechiae; and *Typhus icterodes*, or yellow fever.[12]

Typhus *icterodes* was described as "typhus with symptoms of jaundice." The word "petechia" came from the Italian *petechio*, meaning a flea bite, because the spots resembled the bites of fleas. In general practice, the word meant a red or purple spot that resembled a flea bite.[13] Grouping yellow fever with typhus further complicated the problem of a correct diagnosis, although it is easy to see why this was done. The following is an 1842 description, taken from the *Lexicon Medicum; or Medical Dictionary*:

Typhus: A species of continued fever, characterized by great debility, a tendency in the fluids to putrefaction and the ordinary symptoms of fever. It is to be readily distinguished from the inflammatory by the smallness of the pulse, and the sudden and great debility which ensues on its first attack; and, in its more advanced stage, by the petechiae, or purple spots, which come out in various parts of the body, and the foetid stools which are discharged; and it may be distinguished from a nervous fever by the great violence of all its symptoms on it first coming on.

The most general cause that gives rise to this disease is contagion, applied either immediately from the body of a person laboring under it, or conveyed in clothes, or merchandise, &c; but it may be occasioned by the effluvia arising from either animal or vegetable substances in a decayed or putrid state; and, hence it is that in low and marshy countries it is apt to be prevalent when intense and sultry heat quickly succeeds any great inundation. A want of proper cleanliness and confined air are likewise causes of this fever; hence it prevails in hospitals, jails, camps, and on board of ships, especially when such places are much crowded, and the strictest attention is not paid to a free ventilation and due cleanliness. A close state of the atmosphere with damp weather, is likewise apt to give rise to putrid fever.

On the first coming of this disease, the person is seized with languor, dejection of spirits, amazing depression and loss of muscular strength, universal weariness and soreness, pains in the head, back, and extremities, and rigors; the eyes appear full, heavy, yellowish, and often a little inflamed; the temporal arteries throb violently, the tongue is dry and parched, respiration is commonly laborious and interrupted with deep sighing; the breath is hot and offensive, the urine is crude and pale, the body is costive, and the pulse is usually quick, small, and hard, and now and then fluttering and unequal. Sometimes a great heat, load and pain are felt at the pit of the stomach, and a vomiting of bilious matter ensues.

As the disease advances, the pulse increases in frequency (beating often from 100 to 130 in a minute); there is a vast debility, and great heat and dryness in the skin, oppression at the breast, with anxiety, sighing, and moaning; the thirst is greatly increased; the tongue, mouth, lips and teeth are covered over with a brown or black tenacious fur; the speech is inarticulate and scarcely intelligible; the patient mutters much, and delirium ensues. The fever continuing to increase still more in violence, symptoms of putrefaction show themselves; the breath becomes highly offensive; the urine deposits a black and foetid sediment; the stools are dark, offensive, and pass off insensibly; haemorrhages issue from the gums, nostrils, mouth and other parts of the body; livid spots of petechiae appear on the surface; the pulse intermits and sinks; the extremities grow cold; hiccoughs ensue and death at last closes the tragic scene.

When this fever does not terminate fatally, it generally begins, in cold climates, to diminish about the commencement of the third week, and goes off gradually towards the end of the fourth, without any very evident crisis; but in warm climates it seldom continues above a week or ten days, if so long.... The appearances usually perceived on dissection, are inflammations of the brain and viscera, but more particularly of the stomach and intestines, which are now and then found in a gangrenous state.

This vivid definition touches on the major symptoms of yellow fever, including jaundice, fever and hemorrhage. The fact yellow fever occasioned vomiting also caused early physicians to classify it as a bilious disease, a distinction that would garner great attention throughout the centuries.

Although it is tempting to think that Dr. Robert Hooper, author of the *Lexicon,* and his contemporaries were on the right path when they attributed the cause of typhus and yellow fever to miasma (the poisoned air from swamps and decaying matter, incidentally where mosquitoes bred) and a want of personal cleanliness, these causes were vague and often cited in diseases ranging from cholera to tuberculosis.

Prevention and Treatment of Yellow Fever

As noted above, eradication of yellow fever would require the total elimination of the disease-carrying vectors, a monumental and perhaps undesirable task. Therefore, prevention remains the priority in lowering case numbers. Simple and cost-effective measures include draining swamps and wet areas where mosquitoes breed in urban areas, avoiding areas where mosquitoes are abundant and distribution of mosquito nets.

At present there is no known therapy or drug regimen for the disease. Therefore, in conjunction with simple preventative measures, vaccination is the greatest tool in the

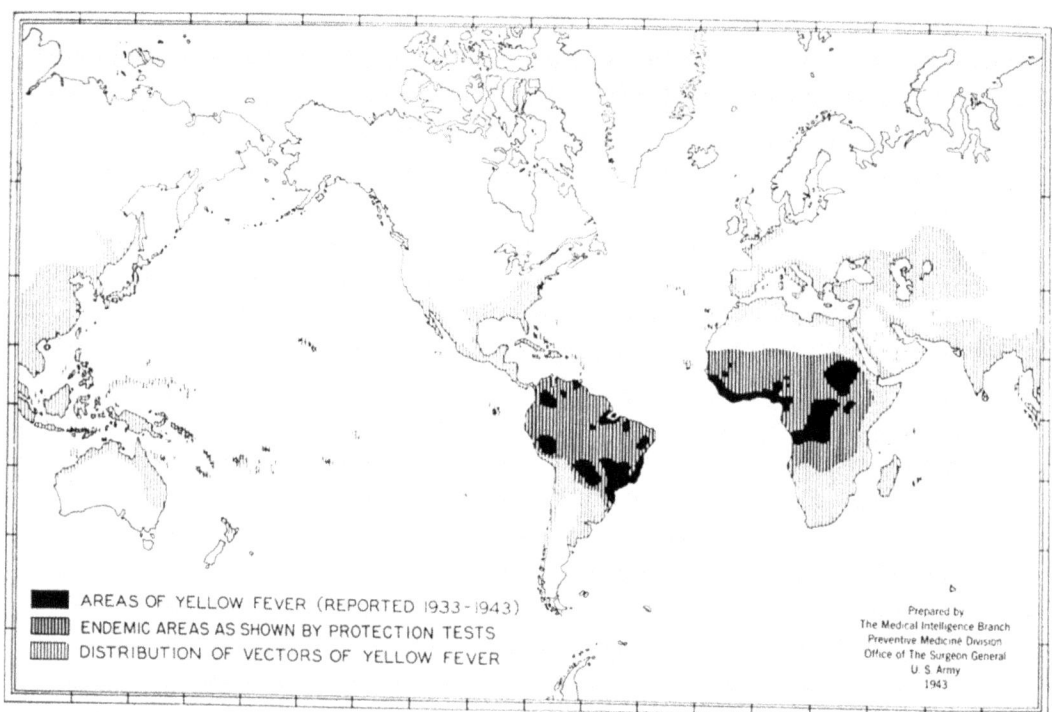

United States Army world map, 1943, showing yellow fever areas of contagion (courtesy National Library of Medicine).

arsenal against yellow fever. A safe and effective vaccine has been in use since the middle of the 20th century but to immunize all people at risk is a worldwide effort. That it must be achieved was underscored by a 2013 World Health Organization bulletin that concluded "a single dose of vaccination is sufficient to confer life-long immunity against yellow fever disease."[14]

Chapter 2

The Early Colonial Period

By the "John," Capt. Paul, from St. Kitt's, we hear, that the Small Pox and Yellow Fever rage in a cruel Manner in that Island, and sweep off great Numbers of the Whites; and to aggravate their Afflictions, they are in perpetual Apprehension of the Negroes Insurrection.[1]

As early as the 1630s Barbados was a major source of trade with England, prompting numerous British subjects to immigrate to the island. In the decade that followed, Dutch seafarers raiding the West African coast seeking gold, ivory and palm oil quickly realized the profit to be gained by human trafficking and added slaves to their cargoes. Joined by the Portuguese, Spanish and British, captains found ready markets in the West Indies region, particularly Barbados. Whether transmitted by human carriers or mosquitoes hatched from previously laid eggs in the moist, warm holds of wooden ships, by 1647 a major epidemic affecting white residents occurred at Barbados.

Once an individual contracted and survived yellow fever, as was true of smallpox, they were conferred lifelong protection against further attacks. Many Africans, exposed to the disease in childhood, likely suffered only minor symptoms, never realizing they had passed through a potentially fatal fever. Europeans, who had never been exposed to the disease in their native countries and therefore had no acquired immunity, fell ill and died. Without understanding the cause and effect of the malady, people observed that those of dark complexion appeared to be unaffected and inferred that they possessed a natural immunity. This erroneous assumption, carried into the 20th century, would later prove disastrous during yellow fever epidemics when slaves were employed in caring for the sick and burying the dead. Far removed from their homeland and in successive generations unexposed to yellow fever as children, they fell victim to it in horrific numbers.

On a wider scale, infected crews returning home carried yellow fever into Portugal, Spain, Great Britain, France, Germany, The Netherlands and the eastern colonies of what would become the United States. Only Asia, which provided an ideal climate and housed the yellow fever mosquito, remained free from contagion. The explanation may be as simple as the fact that Asian countries were never involved in the African slave trade.

During 1648 and 1649 outbreaks of yellow fever were reported in St. Kitts, Guadeloupe and Cuba. The earliest epidemic reported in the Americas occurred in Yucatan in 1648, the disease likely spread by traders and buccaneer ships that carried mosquitoes or crews infected from the 1647 Barbados epidemic. While small outbreaks of yellow fever might have occurred throughout the Caribbean in the intervening years, the next definitive epidemic appeared in Brazil in 1685.

It would not be long before war lent a hand in the spread of disease. In 1688 William of Orange invaded England with 14,000 troops to prevent the formation of an Anglo-French alliance against the United Provinces. The unpopular Roman Catholic King James II lost his throne and fled to France on December 23, 1688. The accession of William and Mary to the British monarchy on February 13, 1689, brought about an abrupt change of foreign policy toward France, precipitating the first of the French and Indian Wars, known as the "War of the League of Augsburg" (1688–1697) and referred to as "King William's War" in the colonies.

In 1690 a French warship departed Bangkok and put in at Recife, South Africa, where it appears yellow fever contagion was brought aboard. Arriving at Martinique, the fever spread ashore where it was called the *mal de Siam*. For the next decade yellow fever spread extensively through the Caribbean, "with the epidemiological characteristics of a newly introduced disease among a previously unexposed population," indicating significant incidence of yellow fever had been absent from the Antilles for some period.[2]

Hostilities reached North America in 1690. Within several months, Schenectady, New York, was burned by the French and the Indians; British colonial forces subsequently attacked Port Royal, Nova Scotia and Quebec. Yellow fever became a precipitating factor in 1693 when an English fleet under Sir Francis Wheeler sailed for the Caribbean for the purpose of working with the colonists in Barbados and Antigua in an attack on Martinique. When his crew fell ill and Wheeler encountered stiff French resistance, he altered plans, sailing for Boston to aid the British colonists in an attack on French forces in Canada. Sickness continued to plague the fleet and by the time the ships reached the Massachusetts Bay Colony over half the contingent had died, many from yellow fever. Warned of the situation, the colonial governor attempted to quarantine the troops but without success; by July, disease had spread to the city, killing several. Wheeler's subsequent departure for England and the return of cold weather in the fall ended the threat. A yellow fever outbreak was recorded in Boston in 1693 but was the last to occur during this conflict. The first of the French and Indian Wars ended with the Treaty of Ryswick (September 30, 1697), returning Acadia to France and restoring the status quo in the colonies.

The next known outbreak of yellow fever north of the West Indies struck Philadelphia and Charles Town (Charleston), South Carolina, in 1699. (Some accounts indicate yellow fever struck New York City in 1668 but these appear to be based solely on Noah Webster's 1799 book, *A Brief History of Epidemics and Pestilential Disease*. In the language of the day, Webster described an "autumnal bilious fever in its infectious form" that terrified the city in 1668. As the threat of yellow fever importation from the Caribbean was known and feared and as the disease was considered by medical men to be of a bilious nature, Webster either assumed or relied on contemporary reports to name yellow fever as the source.) Whatever its true cause, so many New Yorkers died within a short period that Governor Dongan ordered a day of fast and penance to appease God, as he was "punishing this land for its sins." There are no authenticated medical records to prove the diagnosis of yellow fever, however, and it is unlikely to have been the causative agent.[3]

The second of the French and Indian Wars (known as the "War of Spanish Succession" and by the name "Queen Anne's War" in the colonies) occurred from 1702 to 1713. Yellow fever may have actually reached New York, in July 1702, where it was believed to have been imported from St. Thomas.[4] It became known as the "Great Sickness," and by September 17 the city was so infected the governor, council and state supreme court were

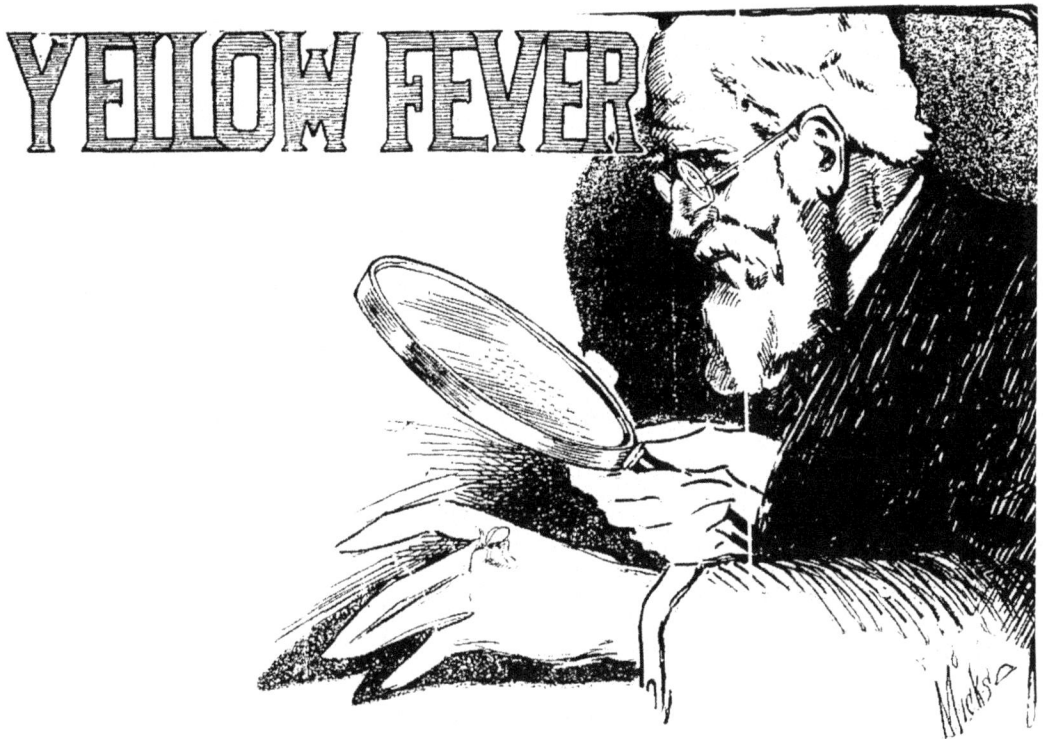

A scientist examines a yellow fever–carrying mosquito that he allows to bite him. Without doubt, the discoveries made on the transmission of this deadly disease were the result of numerous scientists putting their lives on the line for the greater good of humanity (*Syracuse* [New York] *Herald*, October 13, 1907).

forced to abandon their offices and temporarily move to Jamaica, Long Island. In what had already become standard procedure in England when malignant distempers of this type struck, a proclamation requiring the quick burial of victims was issued and a weekly day of fast and humiliation appointed.

If the plague were yellow fever, late summer temperatures must have remained high, and moist conditions and stagnant, open water were readily available to enable mosquitoes to breed. By September 27 Mr. Cornbury reported to the Lords of Trade: "[I]n ten weeks time, sickness has swept away upwards of five hundred people of all ages and sexes. Some men of note and amongst the rest Capt. Stapleton dyed two days ago, he was Commander of her Majesty Ship Jersey and brought me into this Province."[5]

"Some men of note" included Brandt Schuyler, the alderman from the south ward. The former mayor, Thomas Noell, lay dying, and most of the aldermen and assistants were also stricken or had abandoned the city for the country in an attempt to flee the "pestilential distemper."[6] Three days later, at the request of Mr. Vesey, George Keith, a.m., a missionary from the Society for Propagating the Gospel, preached "at the Weekly Fast, which was appointed by the government, by reason of the great mortality that was then at New York, where above Five Hundred died in the Space of a few weeks; and that very Week, about Seventy died."[7]

The first record of yellow fever on the lower Mississippi appeared at Biloxi, 90 miles from New Orleans, in 1702. At the time, the settlement was a French military post founded by Iberville in 1699. Three years later the disease was reported at Mobile.[8] Sporadic outbreaks in the West Indies led to the importation of yellow fever into Charles town, where a probable epidemic occurred in 1706.

Queen Anne's War was ended by the Treaty of Utrecht. France ceded the Hudson Bay territory, Newfoundland and Nova Scotia to Great Britain and agreed to a British protectorate over the Iroquois Indians. After the war yellow fever outbreaks were again reported in Charles Town in 1728 and 1732.

Interspersed between the second and third French and Indian Wars was the "War of Jenkins' Ear," 1739–1742, which later merged into the War of Austrian Succession. It started when Robert Jenkins, captain of the ship *Rebecca*, claimed guards under orders from a Spanish commander severed his ear in 1731 and told him to take it to his king, George II. Jenkins exhibited his ear in the House of Commons, inflaming public opinion against the Spanish. Prime Minister Robert Walpole declared war on October 23, 1739. Continental fighting between Spanish forces occurred in Florida, South Carolina and Georgia, but the most notable conflict was seen when a British expedition mounted in Jamaica attacked Cartagena, the main port of the Spanish colony in Colombia. The assault ended in disaster due to poor military judgment, the severity of the climate and disabling tropical diseases. The result of the war was inconclusive.[9] Troop transfers and ships coming to the North American colonies during these troubled times were likely responsible for introducing yellow fever into Charles Town in 1739, Philadelphia in 1741 and New Haven, Connecticut, in 1742.[10]

War news and the subsequent disruption of trade became a topic of considerable interest in Great Britain. Newspaper accounts began appearing on a regular basis apprising those back home of the situation. Two reports, the first from London (1739) and the second from Dublin (1740), give a picture of typical notices concerning the prevalence of disease:

> By a Ship arriv'd from St. Kit's we have Advice, that at the Leeward Islands there are great Prospects of plentiful Crops; and that at Back-Stair Island the Yellow Fever and Small-Pox have carry'd off 500 Persons in two Months; the former of Which is much abated, but the latter still rages all over the Island.[11]
>
> And from the Island of St. Christopher's we learn, that the Yellow Fever, which Was very rife in that Island about a Year ago, is again broke out, and carries off Number of People.[12]

Closer to home, a 1743 report from Limerick informed readers that a "bomb-ketch" (sailing vessel) had been driven into Shottery Island, about 8–10 leagues above the River Shannon, in great distress. She belonged to Admiral Vernon's squadron and had lost most of her crew to yellow fever.[13]

"They either kill or cure"

Yellow fever appeared in Virginia in 1737, 1741 and 1742. One of the physicians directly involved was John Mitchell, M.D., a Fellow of the Royal Society of London. Mitchell transcribed his experiences, thoughts and conclusions into a folio he later sent to Benjamin Franklin. In his text, Mitchell observed that the symptoms suffered by those in Virginia were "much the same as those observed by [Dr. Warren] in the malignant fever of Barbadoes." The first appearance was a "pain in the head and back and about the stomach, succeeded by grievous anxieties and oppression about the praecordia. And in general this distemper may be defined to be, a pestilential fever proceeding from a *contagious miasma sui generis,* which inflames the stomach and adjacent viscera, obstructs the biliary ducts, and dissolves the adipose humours; to which generally succeeds an effusion of a bilious or other yellow humour upon the external or internal surface of the body, unless prevented by some means or other."

On autopsy, he discovered that "the blood vessels in general seemed very empty of blood, even the vena cava and its branches; but the vena portae was full and distended as usual; the blood seemed to be collected in the viscera; for upon cutting the lungs, or sound liver, or spleen, they bled freely." Further analysis revealed that "the serum made not above a sixth or eighth part of the whole, which was of a deep yellow or saffron colour.... On this every one who saw this blood was convinced that the distemper was what is generally called the yellow fever in America." This yellowness, Mitchell believed, seen also on the skin and eyes, was not, as commonly was held, "a salutary effort of nature to get rid of her oppression" but was, rather, "the most threatening symptom which appears in the whole disease," indicating an inflamed liver from a stoppage of bile through the common duct.

"This distemper is remarkably contagious," Mitchell deduced, stemming from the fact that in Virginia where people lived "in separate and distinct plantations, consisting of numbers of servants and slaves," if one contracted the fever "there was little security for the rest, but removal." The fever spread slower than measles or smallpox, but it raged more violently in the spring and from Christmas to Whitsuntide. Changes in the seasons put a stop to the disease. In the West Indies, where there were no such vicissitudes of weather, the only way to stop transmission was through purification of infected places or removal of the sick. The most common prophylactic resorted to was the common alexipharmic method with snake-root drams, which he "knew to prove ineffectual." Instead, he recommended 6–8 ounces of blood taken from the arm. "Some fell into large sweats or plentiful breathings, soon after bleeding; by which their disorders went off; but those that did not sweat, and their complaints continued, took a vomit of ipecacuanha soon after bleeding, and the night after the vomit fell into the like sweats, by the plentiful use of tepid diluents and warm covering. After these applications, the distemper never formed itself, as it ever did when these complaints were neglected."

Powerful words, yet Mitchell mitigated them almost immediately: "We cannot always perhaps expect such good effects from it." On the subject of emetics, he decided, "They either kill or cure." Ultimately, he concluded large evacuations should be used to avoid inflammation of the viscera, stressing that "contagious, malignant fevers proceed from a venomous miasma received *ab extra;* which, like all other poisons, ought to be discharged as soon as possible." He ultimately expressed the unorthodox belief "the body is not to be strengthened, but [cured] by removing what weakens and oppresses it.... On this account an ill-timed scrupulousness about the weakness of the body is often of bad consequence in these urging circumstances, for it is that which seems chiefly to make evacuations necessary, which nature ever attempts, after the humours are fit to be expelled, but is not able to accomplish, for the most part, in this disease." In other words, the mistake lay in attempting to strengthen the body when it should actually be made weaker by extreme evacuations to rid the body of poisons and thus clear the way toward healing.[14]

Mitchell's quote—"They either kill or cure," taken from Celsus's observation on bleeding in apoplexy—was to take on greater meaning during the yellow fever epidemic at Philadelphia in 1793, when his work, having passed from the hands of Benjamin Franklin to Dr. Benjamin Rush, became the inspiration for a radical new treatment.

The French and Indian Wars

Letters from New York dated September 7, 1742, indicated yellow fever raged in so violent a manner "great Numbers daily die." The same letters advised that the populace of that province struck against Captain Ellis, commander of the *Gosport* man of war, and later went aboard ship and confined two lieutenants on account of their having been "very rigorous in pressing Men out of the Merchant Ships in that Harbour."[15] The epidemic may have lingered into 1743.

The third of the French and Indian Wars (known as the "War of the Austrian Succession" and by the name "King George's War" in the colonies) was fought from 1744 to 1748 when France, Prussia and Spain joined forces against England.

London newspapers, under the heading "Plantation News," updated readers on events in the colonies. A general gleaning from October 23, 1745, indicated that Captain La Favire had returned to port from the Bay of Honduras without any freight because the Spanish had taken control of the New River and threatened to take possession of the Old. Indians in New England had "rose on the Inhabitants" in Sheepscut, New England, killing several, and Captain Bibby had discovered a brigantine off Newfoundland "without any living Creature on board, except a Cat." Equally grim news came from Charles Town, South Carolina, where there had been for some time a "sickness in this Province, which has carried off great Numbers of People, particularly the new Inhabitants. The Sickness consists of the Black Vomit, and the Nervous and Yellow Fever."[16]

Although specifying three separate causes, according to standard medical practice, black vomit was not a disease but a symptom of yellow fever. Once a patient reached the stage of throwing up old (black) blood, there were few, if any documented cases of recovery. Because of its fatal implications, and in conjunction with early attempts at proving or disproving the contagion of yellow fever (a controversy holding wide medical, economic and political ramifications), great attention was paid to this emesis.

Reporting on the analysis of black vomit before the American Philosophical Society on June 20, 1800, Dr. Cathral stated that experiments on this singular morbid excretion revealed that it contained an acid that was not carbonic, phosphoric nor sulphuric and that it might be smelled, tasted and even swallowed without inducing yellow fever or even any sickness at all. He concluded it to be an altered secretion from the liver.

As a further means of discovery dependent on firsthand observation and personal trial, Dr. May of Philadelphia dropped black vomit matter into his eyes and never experienced inconvenience or sickness. Going a step further, Dr. Firth of Salem, New Jersey, published a "Dissertation on Malignant Fever" hoping to conclusively prove one way or the other whether yellow fever was contagious. He concluded it was not, using as one basis for his argument his experiments on black vomit. Firth's trials during the 1802–1803 yellow fever season included inoculating himself on the arm with matter just discharged from a moribund patient. His wound became slightly inflamed but after three days healed normally without the formation of pus. Subsequent experiments with inoculation on various other parts of his body produced the same result. To further prove his point, he exposed himself to the exhalations of the vomit while acted upon by the heat of an iron skillet and later swallowed, in pill form, the thick substance that remained after evaporation, again without effect.[17]

Nervous fever, or *febris nervosa,* was considered by Cullen to be a variety of *typhus mitior,* although other authorities considered it a distinct disease. Adding to the confusion of diagnosis, the symptoms of nervous fever were sufficiently vague: they began with a loss of appetite, increased heat and vertigo, leading to nausea, vomiting, great languor and pain in the head. As conditions worsened, the pulse quickened and the fever increased. Toward the seventh or eighth day, the patient became delirious and it was not until the 14th to 20th day that the fever broke.[18]

Further outbreaks of yellow fever were recorded in New York and Charles Town in 1745 and 1748 and in Philadelphia in 1747.[19] During the course of the war an expedition of New Englanders under Sir William Pepperrell, in cooperation with a fleet under Sir Peter Warren, captured Ft. Louisbourg on June 16, 1745, and Indian trader and commissary of New York for Indian Affairs William Johnson succeeded in setting the Iroquois on the warpath. French retaliatory raids subsequently burned Saratoga and Albany, New York. The Treaty of Aix-la-Chapelle, October 18, 1748, ended the War of the Austrian Succession, returning Fort Louisbourg to France and renewing Great Britain's privilege of transporting slaves to Spanish possessions in America.

Unfortunately, this would not end colonial struggles between England and France. As tensions worsened, colonial news once again filled British newspapers. A July 10, 1749, report from Boston indicated that two French men of war with eighty guns each and 10 transport, carrying the governor and troops to garrison Chebucto, Halifax, Nova Scotia, had arrived from France, while on the 21st of June Governor Cornwallis of Nova Scotia arrived on his majesty's ship *Sphinx*. Additionally, the French had recently at Louisbourg, Cape Breton Island, Nova Scotia, lost "a great number of Men on their Passage by the Small Pox, Yellow Fever, &c. and that our People arrived at Chebucto from England, lost only one Child in their Passage." On a slightly more uplifting note, the following sentence added, "We likewise hear, that French Rum and Molasses were so plenty at Louisbourg, that Rum was sold for Nine-pence per Gallon; and Molasses exceedingly cheap."

The last of the four French and Indian Wars (known in Europe as the "Seven Years' War") dragged on between 1754 and 1763, becoming the "great war for empire" between England and France. Not surprisingly, military updates dominated "plantation news" subheadings in British newspapers. In 1757, dated September 1 at Charles Town, South Carolina, the last advances from Providence on August 19 were "more favourable to us than our former Accounts from thence were." News garnered under a flag of truce from Port au Paix averred that the yellow fever "raged violently amongst the French on Hispaniola, and swept off Multitudes; by which Calamity, together with the Want of Provisions, their Fears of being attacked by Admiral Coates, and their Island being surrounded by English Privateers (so that no vessel could get into or dared to stir out of any of their Ports) they were reduced to the greatest Distress imaginable, and rendered (for the present) absolutely incapable of undertaking any Thing from that Quarter."[20]

In 1761 yellow fever was imported into Cuba, possibly from Vera Cruz. The following year it ran through British forces besieging Havana, where the disease made its way to Philadelphia.[21] The resultant plague of 1762 instilled terror into the city famed for its medical knowledge. As hundreds of its citizens were killed by the mysterious malady, questions piled upon one another: what was the deadly disease? where did it come from?

how could it be stopped? Answers in this time of crisis were not easy to come by. The spectre of West Indian yellow fever was raised when a trunk, belonging to a youth who had died of the disease at Barbados, was returned to his home city. When it was opened, the stench proved so great that everyone in the room sickened and several died. If the epidemic had spread from this incident it not only gave the malignant fever a name but implicated miasma as the cause.

Others were not as certain. In a story that might have been taken verbatim from the chronicles of cholera victims of the era, tales were told of how the frequency and severity of fevers were reduced after Dock Creek was paved and made a street. This pointed to a local origin of the distemper. Augmenting this theory was a local physician named Bond, who claimed the distemper originated locally, bore some connection to stagnant water and could be prevented by proper sanitation. For a cure he advocated the "sulphurous chalybeate waters" of Philadelphia, which he believed would strengthen digestion, counteract the heat of summer, dilute the thick, putrid bile and destroy "the effect of a hot, moist and putrid atmosphere."[22] The most famous of the chalybeate waters (containing nothing but iron in solution) resorted to for health and pleasure were at Stafford Springs, Connecticut, and Orange and Schooley's Mountain Springs, New Jersey. The Ballston and Saratoga waters of New York, although containing iron, were not ranked among the chalybeate, having other and more powerful ingredients in their composition.[23]

Eventually the Philadelphia contagion was traced to a West Indies ship recently arrived from Havana that had put into Sugar House Wharf, below South Street. A sick seaman had been brought ashore and clandestinely carried to the house of a man named Leadbutter, where he soon died and was secretly buried. Eventually, Leadbutter, his family and many others throughout the city perished. The proof was not absolute, however, and many remained skeptical. The most important question—that of a cure—remained elusive.[24]

An act of the Philadelphia Assembly, passed January 1774, addressed concerns that future infectious diseases might be brought into the city. Section 2 stated that no ship commander having on board more than 40 passengers and crew or "any person disordered with any infectious disease, or coming from any sickly port or place, shall bring his ship or vessel, or suffer or permit the same to be brought nearer to the city of Philadelphia, than the island called Little Mud Island, near the mouth of the river Schuylkill, nor shall land or bring on shore, nor cause or suffer to be landed or brought on shore, at any port or place within this province ... until he shall have obtained a licence or permit in writing." Section 3 added that if any ship had "any person disordered with any infectious disease, or coming from any sickly port or place is arrived at or near the Province Island," a physician appointed by the governor should be taken aboard who was to search the ship and inspect the passengers, requiring a list of how many persons died onboard and an account of the health and diseases of passengers and crew. The act also authorized the sum of one hundred pounds to be forfeited by the commander if he knowingly failed to make a true and just account.[25]

Interestingly, a review of Dr. Benjamin Rush's 1794 book, *An Account of the Bilious Remitting Yellow Fever, as It Appeared in the City of Philadelphia in the Year 1793*, noted the following: "The Yellow Fever has appeared in Philadelphia, and some other parts of America, in the summers of 1741 and 1762, but there are no intermediate periods mentioned of its existence; and of those periods we have no other records than of its irrefutable mortality; no medical facts whatever to guide the practitioner. The incorrect fragments, collected in the present publication, of those times, therefore, like the other authorities quoted from itinerant writers on West-India diseases, had better been omitted, because they are no better than *ignes fatui*, and may bewilder incautious readers."[26]

After the reduction of forces at the conclusion of the French and Indian Wars, ships returning to England brought yellow fever with them. Those arriving at Spithead from Louisburg were afflicted with that distemper as well as scurvy. James Lind, physician to the King's Hospital at Haslar, published "Two Papers on Fevers and Infection" (1763) in which he described yellow fever and a second species of intermittent fever. Symptoms included cough, copious expectoration and lancinating pains in the thorax. Some of those who recovered remained "dull of hearing," while others later died consumptive. Interestingly, Lind believed this infection was communicated by ships manned partly from jails.[27]

In another paper published by Dr. Lind in 1768, "Treatise on the Diseases Incidental to Europeans in Hot Climates," he argued the point that no matter how unhealthy a climate was there were always times of the year when life was safer than at others and the most obvious remedy was to move to a safer area during the sickly season and return during the healthy one. Expressing astonishment "at the absurdity of mankind in never thinking of this so simple and easy a method" of avoiding disease, he offered several examples to prove his point. One involved seamen returning to Portsmouth in 1765. For three months during the summer and autumn when epidemical sickness most prevailed, those living aboard ships that lay in Spithead harbor near the mud enjoyed perfect health and not one of them was sent to Haslar Hospital from any ship at Spithead.

His second example cited the yellow fever and black vomit sickness at Cadiz that depopulated the city. An officer and several crew off his majesty's ship *Tweed* went ashore and were seized with fever; those who were sent back to their ship recovered with no ill effects. A similar situation occurred in Admiral Broderick's squadron, which lay at anchor off the island of Sardinia. Those who remained shipbound retained perfect health, but those who slept on shore contracted a fatal fever.

Lastly, in 1765 a mortal fever prevailed at Pensacola, from which a regiment newly arrived during the sickly season lost 120 men as well as 11 out of 12 officers' wives. The companies on the men of war *Tartar* and *Prince Edward*, lying one mile distant from shore, maintained their health, as did those living outside the fort. Those who suffered most were billeted inside barracks sheltered from the sea breezes by the walls of the fort and subjected to sultry and unhealthy air. Soldiers who contracted the fever and were returned to their ships quickly recovered, "or, at least, by this change of air, the fever being divested of its most mortal symptoms, soon assumed the form of an intermittent." Lind did add, however, that those who live on ships were not always exempt from diseases of the adjacent country. The reverse was often the case, whether from unavoidable accidents or "ignorance almost unpardonable."[28]

The West Indies

To underscore the very real danger of yellow fever, a letter dated July 20, 1751, from Jamaica indicated that the disease had been prevalent on the island for five weeks. A second account reported that the same "distemper" had visited several ships in the harbor and that nine seamen in one day were carried on shore at Kingston to be buried.

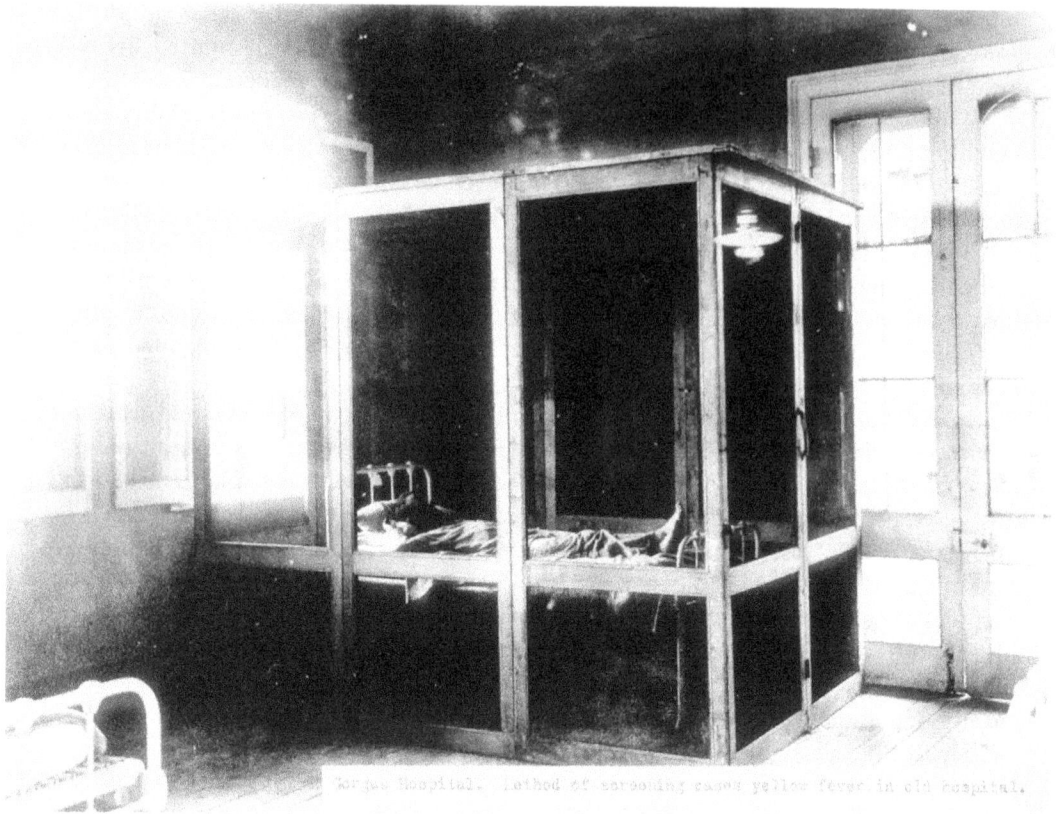

A heart-rending photograph of a yellow fever victim segregated from other patients and lying in a screened bed at Gorgas Hospital, Ancon, Canal Zone (courtesy National Library of Medicine).

By 1765 little had been accomplished to diminish the severity of yellow fever. Advances from St. Anne's, Jamaica, dated August 5, 1765, reported "another misfortune, the yellow fever and sickness had raged more severely this season than for some years passed, by which great numbers had been carried off." Of importance, the letter also warned that the sugar crop had been greatly diminished by bad weather and variable winds and that the rainy season immediately following had considerably hurt the cotton and pimento crops.[29]

Where there is disease there must be a cure. Failing that, the inevitable result is to resort to nostrums and notions. And where there are nostrums there are testimonials. By 1749, British newspapers were already filling with advertisements extoling the virtues of what today would be called over-the-counter self-help medicines. Many of these powders and elixirs were not new to the public but were given added value by including yellow fever to the seemingly endless list of ills they purportedly cured. On a more mercenary note, it never hurt to add that the mixtures were so reasonably priced even the least affluent could afford to purchase them.

In the September 7–9, 1749, edition of the *Whitehall Evening-Post; or, London Intelligencer,* Samuel Yeats certified the truth of his statement that on his passage from Barbados in September of that year, he was "taken by a most violent (called at Barbadoes the Yellow) Fever, which occasioned me to bleed at the Mouth, Ears, Nose and Eyes, to that violent Degree, that I was given over by all about me for Death; and having about Half a Bottle of your Balsam of Life on board my Ship (the Kendal Merchant of Lancaster) by pouring a few Drops into my Ears and Nose, and at the same Time taking some inwardly, it entirely stopt the Bleeding, and by continuing to take the Remainder of the Bottle, I was restored to Admiration; but having no more Balsam of Life on board, I had a Relapse a few Days after my Arrival." He added that two of his servants were taken with the same disorder. One took the Balsam and recovered; the other, who did not take it, died.

If sweet herbs, oils and perhaps some alcohol were not to one's taste, John Martin Morland, master and part owner of the ship *The Owners Goodwill*, of George Town Winyaw, South Carolina, testified that in February 1750 he sold to Mr. Beard, collector, "two Papers of SAMUEL MAJOR'S *Imperial Phoenix Snuff*, which cured him of great Pain and Disorder in the Head, with an Ague and Yellow Fever." Furthermore, the wife of Mr. William Shackford, vintner, "was cured of the Yellow Fever, which had made her also Blind, so that she could not walk for Nine Months, by two Papers of the Snuff." However, it required three papers of snuff to cure Captain William Brown, who had "for several Months a Deafness in both Ears, and the Yellow Fever." For those interested, the snuff was sold by Samuel Major within Bishopsgate for one shilling a paper, while the Royal Patent Medicinal Snuff was sold at the same place for two shillings and six-pence a paper.[30]

The "*Excellent* British Fever Pill" promised a cure for fevers, agues and all internal inflammations" and was "excellent for the Yellow Fever, common in the West Indies." Priced at 2s a box, the promoter added that the pills were "now recommended with a real Desire of publick Good, and that the Poor may partake of its Usefulness, as well as the Rich, it is sold at so reasonable a Price as 1s. 6d the Pot, with a printed Bill of Directions."[31]

Patent medicines were not the only commercial endeavor that appeared in the wake of this new and suddenly important disease. By 1750 numerous books appeared on the scene providing information on diseases of the West Indies while, in some cases, incidentally promoting personal nostrums. Dale Ingram, surgeon and "man-midwife," published *A Critical Enquiry into the Rise and Progress of the Yellow Fever in the West Indies*, "wherein are explained the Nature of Contagion, the Reasons of the Periodical Appearance of this, and other Infectious Distempers, in particular Climates and Countries, from whence is deduced a rational Method of Cure."[32]

Other books of the 1750s included *The Civil and Natural History of Jamaica*, a work published by subscription by Pat. Browne, MD, that included a chapter titled "A Regular History of the Yellow Fever, with an Account of Its Cause and Nature, and the Best Methods to Prevent or Alleviate Its Most Destructive Symptoms" (1754). Another work by Dale Ingram, *An Historical Account of the Several Plagues That Have Appeared in the World Since the Year 1346* (1754), included "a peculiar Account of the Yellow Fever, showing its periodical Appearance to be similar to the Plague." *A Dissertation on Fevers and Inflammatory Distempers* by R. James, MD, appeared in 1755. To this was added *An Account of the Success with Which the Fever Powder Has Been Given in the Small Pox, Yellow Fever, Slow Fever, and Rheumatism*, which was apparently prepared as a "professional pamphlet" to promote the sale of "Dr. James's Fever Powder," which sold for 2s 6d, with allowances for those who "buy it for charitable Uses, or to sell again." In a separate ad the same year, Dr. James promoted his "Powder for Fevers" by remarking that it was a most effectual remedy for "slow and latent Fevers, which are generally mistaken for Vapours and Hysterics."

Dr. James's "fever powders" became one of the most successful empirical remedies on the market and were extremely popular in both the European and North American markets, through which he gained a very great reputation that lasted into the mid–1800s. It was felt the success of his fever powder was due in large measure to his free use of Peruvian bark, administered after he had "evacuated the *primae viae* by the use of his antimonial preparation that contained, at first, some combination of 'mercurials.'" James's published specification was to "take some antimony, calcine it with heat, adding a sufficient quantity of animal oil and salt, then boil it in melted nitre for a considerable time, then separate the powder from the nitre by dissolving it in water." Medical men of the time noted, however, that "the real recipe has been studiously concealed, and a false one published in its stead." After James died in 1776, Dr. Pearson of London determined the original powder consisted of a mixture of 57 percent oxyde (oxidized) antimony with 43 percent phosphate of lime. The British College, guided by Pearson's results, adopted this formula for producing an imitation.[33] For those with North American interests, "Essays and Observations, Physical and Literate," by a Society at Edinburgh, included "a description of the American Yellow Fever."[34]

For all the proposed treatments, the disease continued to be a source of anxiety and death in the West Indies. Between the months of June-September 1758, yellow fever raged so greatly in Kingston that 500 souls, many presumably coming from the ships in the harbor, departed life and were buried in the city. The following year reports from British Antigua in the Leeward Islands indicated the disease was "very mortal," especially among the seamen, and had spread into St. John's.[35]

The Profession of Physic Regarding Yellow Fever

In the course of investigating the cause of yellow fever a number of dedicated scientists sacrificed their lives for the greater good of humanity. These individuals were heroes in the true sense of the word. By exposing themselves to this deadly disease, they placed the welfare of humanity over their own safety. It is ironic, then, that the first two researchers claimed by yellow fever (albeit in a peripheral way) came amidst scandal and disgrace.

In 1752 a pamphlet entitled *Essays on the Bilious Fever: Containing the Different Opinions of Those Eminent Physicians John Williams and Parker Bennet, of Jamaica* appeared for sale at the cost of two shillings. Because it was published posthumously, the original Jamaican publisher and his British counterpart, T. Waller, Fleet Street, who reprinted it, added, "Which was the Cause of a DUEL, and terminated in the DEATH of Both." With that addendum the pamphlet could hardly fail to garner notice, if for nothing more than the salacious details of the "duel." The *London Monthly Review* of July 1, 1752, began its review as follows:

> As our climate is happily exempted from this fever, which rages in the *British* islands in *America*, the catastrophe these essays terminated in, *viz*, the death of both the authors, may probably excite the curiosity of the public more than the subject itself would. However, as our intercourse with these islands is very considerable, and a majority of our natives, on their first arrival there, are very liable to those it seizes, it may not be amiss to give a summary account, and even some judgment of those tracts.

The publisher, equally aware of the value added to the work by the death of its authors, added this:

> TO THE PUBLIC: An authentic account of the death of the unfortunate doctor *Williams* and doctor *Bennet* of *Kingston* in *Jamaica*, on the 29th of *December*, 1750, caus'd by the following Papers.
>
> After a great deal of ill language they proceeded to blows, which caused challenges and acceptance, and the morning after doctor *Bennet* went arm'd with his sword and a brace of pistols to doctor *Williams's* door very early, and knocked him up; *Williams* saw from his window who it was, and what he had to expect; upon which he loaded his pistols with *Goose*, or *Swan* shot; and slinging his drawn-sword by a ribband upon his wrist, came down, and opening the door, just sufficient to admit his hand with a pistol, poured a shot full into poor *Bennet's* breast, who had delivered his own arms to his boy, whilst he called *Williams* out; which when he had done, he continued to pursue *Bennet*, reeling to his boy, and wounded him with the other pistol in his knee. *Bennet* by this time had gained his sword only, which was fastened so strongly in the scabbard, that with all his endeavours he could not draw it. When *Williams* had fired his second pistol, *Bennet* turned upon him, thanked God he had the power to be reveng'd, and whilst he endeavoured to release his imprison'd weapon, begged of God to invigorate him a few moments; but *Williams* then gave him a mortal thrust under his right arm, which pierced the lungs on both sides; having done this he was turning to run for it, but that moment *Bennet* drew his sword, and made a pass at *Williams*, which entering under the right clavicle or collar bone, pierced the internal jugular vein, and finished its course in the shoulder blade, breaking off at the place of entrance; however, *Williams* run about ten or fifteen yards and then fell, suffocated with his blood, and never spoke more. The unfortunate *Bennet* survived him for about four hours, and then expired, in the most agonizing pains imaginable.

The pamphlet itself is almost as curious as the disharmony between the two parties. The first section, entitled "An Essay on the Bilious, or Yellow Fever of Jamaica," was written by Dr. Williams. In the preface he notes, "That the disease was sufficiently known, but little could be done for the patient, and that, in its greatest degree, this fever was generally incurable." He opened the text by presenting a historical perspective, tracing it back to the writing of Hippocrates and noting that symptomology between the past and present was probably to be attributed to "the difference of climate and the manner of living." Williams believed the yellow fever was brought on by "suddenly cooling the body and checking perspiration after hard exercise in the heat of the sun," adding that it was not limited to one season but appeared at all times in Jamaica.

After delineating those fevers occurring in the "Carribee Islands" and North America, he concluded, "So there cannot be a greater, tho' general mistake, than to imagine all yellow fevers of the same *genus*, and that they should all be treated in the same manner." The distinguishing symptoms of the malady he considered to be "fever, great anxiety, heat and pain at the *scrobiculum cordis*, proceeding from an obstruction of the bile and some degree of inflammation of the liver, which frequently causes a jaundice, bilious vomitings, or ejections, or both." He wrote, "Bleeding seems highly necessary in the beginning of this fever, not only in easing the pains and anxiety, which are a great part of the disease, but also in reducing the degree of heat, for as *Wainwright* observes, *The heat of an animal is in a compound proportion of its quantity of blood, and the celerity of its motions*. So that, by diminishing the quantity of blood, we lessen the heat and thirst, for fever of the thin parts will be dissipated, and consequently, by this, we reduce, in some degree, the fever." He later added "arteriotomy or cupping with scarifications seems to excel venaesection, for the following reason: those persons who die of ardent fevers, or acute disorders, have their arteries full and veins empty, on the contrary, those who die from slow fevers, or chronic disorders, have their veins full and arteries empty."

Williams believed "solutive purges and apozems" with manna seemed to be

LAMPLOUGH'S
PYRETIC SALINE.

An Effervescing and Tasteless Salt; most Invigorating, Vitalising, and Refreshing.

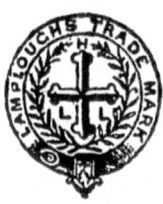 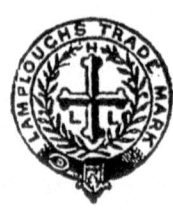

Gives Instant Relief in Headache, Sea or Bilious Sickness, Indigestion, Constipation, Lassitude, Low Spirits, Heartburn, Feverish Colds, and **prevents** and quickly cures the worst form of Typhus, Scarlet, Jungle, and other Fevers; Prickly Heat, Small-Pox, Measles, Eruptive or Skin Complaints, and various other Altered Conditions of the Blood.

The testimony of Medical Gentlemen and the Professional Press has been unqualified in praise of LAMPLOUGH'S PYRETIC SALINE, as possessing most important elements calculated to restore and maintain Health, with *Perfect Vigour of Body and Mind.*

Dr. Prout : " Unfolding germs of immense benefit to mankind."

Dr. Morgan : "It furnishes the blood with its lost saline constituents."

Dr. Turley : "I found it act as a specific, in my experience and family, in the worst form of scarlet fever, *no* other medicine being required."

Dr. W. Stevens : "Since its introduction the fatal West India Fevers are deprived of their terrors."

Dr. Sparkes : (Government Medical Inspector of Emigrants from the Port of London) writes : "I have great pleasure in bearing my cordial testimony to its efficacy in the treatment of many of the ordinary and chronic forms of Gastric Complaints and other forms of Febrile Dyspepsia."

Dr. J. W. Dowsing : "I used it in the treatment of forty-two cases of Yellow Fever, and I am happy to state I never lost a single case."

In Patent Glass-stoppered Bottles, 2s. 6d., 4s. 6d., 11s., *and* 21s. *each.*

LAMPLOUGH'S CONCENTRATED LIME-JUICE SYRUP.
A PERFECT LUXURY.

In Patent Glass-stoppered Bottles, 2s. *and* 4s. 6d. *each.*

H. LAMPLOUGH,
Consulting Chemist, 113, Holborn, London, E.C.

British citizens had a keen interest in yellow fever preventatives, as the nation held territories in the West Indies and trade was of vital importance. Yellow fever was considered a "white man's disease," and sailors working on vessels putting in at those ports frequently became victims. The testimony of captains and ship doctors were often sought from promoters of nostrums and remedies, always promising miraculous means of prevention and cures (*Brief: The Week's News*, London, August 13, 1880).

absolutely necessary in the beginning of yellow fever, for they cooled and eased the patient while moderating heat, thirst and anxiety. He recommended clysters and emollients and the use of acid medicines; he argued against blisters and suggested the patient be given a diluting and relaxing diet, warm baths and kept in large, open areas. The medical reviewer for the *Monthly Review* generally agreed with Williams's treatments except for his disinclination to use blisters and "vomits." The remainder of the pamphlet consisted of an epistle (which the reviewer called "wretched" poetry), the purpose of which seems to have been to direct accusations toward Bennet, and letters written for publication between Williams and Bennet by which they attempted to destroy the other's reputation. It is likely that sales of this work were predicated on interest evoked by the vitriolic and pedantic letters rather than the medical dissertations.

On a less sensational note, Dr. William Hillary's book (printed in Octavo, price five shillings), *Observations on the Changes of the Air, and the Concomitant Epidemical Diseases, in the Island of Barbadoes* (1759), detailed many known and speculative facts about the disease. Citing authentic accounts and "from the nature and symptoms of the disease," Hillary believed yellow, or putrid, bilious fever was indigenous to the West Indies and to those parts of the American continent lying within or near the tropics. In so stating, he refuted the opinion of Dr. Warren (a contemporary authority), who believed the fever was a native of Palestine, brought from there to Marseilles, where it spread to other islands of the West Indies around 1722. Hillary also rejected the notion of its being pestilential and contagious.

According to his arguments, drawn from "reason, from philosophy, and experience," he felt yellow fever most commonly seized foreigners to the climate, which explained why the French called it *la Fievre Matelotte*. Those arriving in Barbados from a colder or more temperate climate were particularly susceptible, the malady being exacerbated if they freely consumed vinous or spirituous liquors, performed hard labor or violent exercise, exposed themselves to the scorching rays of the sun or the heavy dews or damp air of the night. As described, it appeared at all times and in all seasons, with no difference other than that the symptoms were more acute and the fever higher in hot weather, raging with the utmost violence in hot, dry seasons preceded by moist warm weather.

In Dr. Hillary's experience, the patient was first seized with faintness, followed by a sickness at the stomach, generally a giddiness in the head and soon after that chills and horror (rarely a rigor or convulsive shuddering), which were soon followed by violent heat and high fever attended with acute darting pains in the head and back as well as a "flushing in the face, with an inflamed redness and burning heat in the eyes; great anxiety or apprehension about the precordia, with a train of direful symptoms." These last he considered the pathological symptoms of yellow fever, especially when accompanied with bilious yellow vomiting, great anxiety and frequent sighing.

The blood, he found, even at the first appearance of the disorder, was often exceedingly florid red, thin and rarified. When the patient fainted, Hillary continued, his skin turned yellow about the face and neck, recovering its natural color as the faintness went off. These symptoms continued until about the third day (sometimes not longer than the first or second) or in peculiar cases to the end of the fourth day: "The first shows the quick dissolution of the blood, and the great malignity of the disease, and the last the contrary; both are hastened or retarded by improper management, and other circumstances. This may be called the first stadium of the disease, which ends for the most part on the third day."

Towards the conclusion of the first stage, the pulse, which was quick, becomes low; the vomiting "grows porraceous and incessant and a comatose disposition with interrupted deliriums ensues. In some the thirst is great but in others not so much. The pulse continues low, often quick, with cold clammy sweats. The eyes, which were at first inflamed and red, then of a dusky color, turn yellow. This yellowness soon spreads itself around the mouth, eyes, temples, and neck and shortly after is diffused all over the body." Contrary to the opinion of others who held this to be an "encouraging prognostic," Hillary stated it commonly proved a mortal symptom, indicating "a great colliquation and dissolution of the blood, and a gangrenescent state of the fluids."

The author did admit that the yellow diffusion "of bile over the surface of the body" sometimes proved critical but added that it did not appear before the eighth or ninth day when coma and other "bad symptoms began to abate, the yellowness increasing as they decreased." When it appeared early, it was "not only symptomatical, as it arises from the colliquated, putrid, dissolved, and gangrenescent state of the blood, but it too frequently ushers in the last and fatal symptoms of the disease," including deep coma, profuse hemorrhages from different parts of the body, delirium, and laborious and interrupted respiration, coldness of the entire body, convulsions and death. Thus," he finished, "from the first appearance of the symptomatical yellowness, the patient may be said to be in the last stage of the disease, at whatever time it comes on."

Livid spots were often reported on yellow fever victims, especially about the praecordia, accompanied by gangrene in other parts of the body. Death soon followed. After death, the body appeared much fuller of the "large livid blackish and mortified spots" around the praecordia and the region of the lower belly. Upon dissection, the gall bladder and biliary ducts were found to be turgid and filled with a putrid dark bile; the liver, stomach and parts adjoining were covered with blackish mortified spots." The whole corpse soon putrefied "and could be kept but a few hours above ground." Hillary determined, therefore, "that a bilious putrefying diathesis is introduced into the blood, and all the circulating fluids." He further held that, contrary to Dr. Warren, bile had a principal share in exciting this fever and the putrid state of the blood. His indications and intentions of cure were as follows:

(1) To moderate the too great and rapid motion of the fluids, and abate the heat and violence of the fever in the two first days of the disease, with all possible expedition and safety.

(2) To evacuate and carry out of the body that putrid bile, and those unfound humours as early in the distemper as may be.

(3) To stop the putrescent disposition of the fluids, and prevent gangrene, by suitable antiseptics.

To answer the first intention (and contrary to other authorities) Hillary prescribed bleeding on the first appearance of the fever in a quantity proportional to the violence of the symptoms and the constitution and circumstances of the patient: "Between 12 to 20 ounces of blood is to be taken and if the pulse rose, repeated phlebotomy the second but seldom the third day, performed with utmost caution." Bleeding left the patient's blood "in a dissolved state, and the pulse so low, that diminishing the momentum of the blood" further would hasten mortification and death.

While Hillary acknowledged that the great stomach irritation and continual vomiting indicated use of an emetic, he found that even the most gentle doses so violently stimulated and inflamed the coats of the stomach that he strictly forbade their use. Instead, he brought large draughts of water into the sick room, sometimes adding simple oxymel or a light infusion of green tea "to carry off the putrid humours and assist nature." After the patient had "puked" between seven to nine times, he gave *Extract Thebaic. Gr. J. vel jfs.* (opium extract: the use of opium as a medicine can be traced back to Diagoras, a near contemporary of Hippocrates, and was probably used even earlier),[36] forbidding the patient to eat or drink for two hours after. By this method "all symptoms were moderated, the patient refreshed, and a truce obtained from the incessant vomiting." This laid the foundation for other medicines such as cooling juleps or other antiphlogistic and antiseptic medicines.

By 1785 Dr. Gilbert Blane noted that there was "a certain medium [method] in giving opium," for an "under dose" would produce disturbance instead of rest, and when given in large quantities, it threw the body into convulsions which terminated in death. The best method, as suggested by Dr. Warren, was to use small quantities and administer it frequently. He added that the liquid form was preferable to the solid, as the effects would sooner be seen and a better judgment formed "on how far it is proper to push it."[37]

Experienced physicians of the late 1700s suggested that the use of nitre or any of its preparations was contraindicated from the fact that it was rarely tolerated by the stomach, while saline draughts (highly regarded antimetics) were thought to weaken the patient. However, their use was dependent upon circumstances. If given in the early stages, the *mistura antimetica* was prescribed for different types of icterical and inflammatory disorders. When considering acid juleps, the saline draught, composed of salt of wormwood, lemon juice and simple cinnamon water, was also useful.

If the bowels were constipated, a gentle clyster was given before the administration of an opiate. After the effects of the *thebaic extract* ceased, a gentle antiphlogistic and antiseptic purge was administered. If, however, the patient was seized with a purging after vomiting, a mild dose of toasted rhubarb followed by an antiseptic anodyne often

> **WAR WITH SPAIN.**
>
> Are you ready? You are probably aware that the air of Cuba is foul with miasma, yellow fever germs and all sorts of other germs. You who expect to be called upon by the president to fight for the honor of this great nation must see to it that your blood is in perfect condition. You must begin now and take Sassafras Tea. You know that sassafras tea will fortify your system against those "pesky germs." **Spencer, the North Side Druggist,** has just gotten in a supply of fresh bark. Begin immediately.

The use of tea as a preventative and curative of any number of illnesses was common throughout Europe and the United States throughout the 16th through 19th centuries. Taken internally, applied externally or used to ward off "germs," many miraculous qualities were attributed to it (*Iola* [Kansas] *Register*, February 26, 1898).

resulted in success. (Although it was considered irregular to practice purging in other fevers, doing so was found to be beneficial in yellow fever victims.) When a painful burning heat in the hypochonders or about the praecordia occurred, a gentle dose of manna and tamarinds seldom failed to carry off the pain and heat by a discharge of the putrid bilious matter that excited them: "On or after the third day when the pulse sinks and coma appears and a yellowness is diffused over the skin, attention turns to sustaining the *vis vitae* by increasing the momentum of the circulating fluids." This was done by liberally plying antiseptics and making every attempt to stop the growing putrefaction. Unfortunately, the *Peruvian bark*, the medicine most likely to effect this purpose, can in no form be kept in the stomach. The best medicine at this point became the *rad. serpent. Virginiana*. Should this fail to raise the pulse, the quantity of snake-root and saffron were to be increased or the *vinum croceum,* the *contectio cardiaca* or similar warm medicine given "till a glowing heat is diffused over the whole body." If the fever increased, it was to be moderated by cooling juleps and antiseptics but never by volatile alkaline salts or spirits, "which dissolve and increase the putrescent state of the fluids."

Running contrary to the standard medical practice of the day, Hillary noted that vesicatories (blisters: used to increase and strengthen the pulse) were common practice in almost every case of dysentery and inflammatory fever, and he argued that they damaged the skin and should never be used. Pertaining to diet, he advised it be thin, light and of small quantity.[38]

Dr. Lind, of King's Hospital, London, believed that as soon as the first symptoms of shivering and sickness at the stomach appeared in a case of yellow fever, a gentle vomit should be induced, which often "entirely prevented the fever." After loose stools developed from either an emetic or clysters, the patient was put to bed and given a "sweating and quieting draught, containing 5 grains of salt of hartshorn, and from 15 to 20 drops of Thebaic tincture." At other times, 5 grains of camphire with large drafts of vinegar whey was administered every four hours. If fever remained after administration of the above "or unluckily delayed too long; or the patient injudiciously treated with sweating medicines, and bleeding, where the proof of infection is evident," recourse to blisters should have been speedily accomplished. If the head and limbs were affected, the blister should be applied to the back; if pain involved the breast, the blister should be placed in that area. Within 24–36 hours this treatment should cure the infection, after which the internal canal should be cleansed a second time by giving rhubarb with a small quantity of vitriolated tartar.

At autopsy, patients who died of yellow fever displayed nearly a quart of yellowish water in the left cavity of the thorax in which were many flakes of yellowish gluten. Other cakes of the same nature adhered to the pleura and lungs. In one who died on the tenth day of the fever without turning yellow, a quantity of pus and purulent crusts were found in the pericardium and the heart in different places excoriated. In another who died on the 13th day of the fever, more than two quarts of pus and purulent jelly were found in the cavity of the abdomen.[39]

The same year Dr. Lind presented his treatment for yellow fever, Dr. Peter Canvane, a physician at Bath, published "An Account of the *Oleum Palmae Christi,* or Castor Oil, a Safe and Efficacious Cathartic in Bilious Cases, Hitherto Almost Wholly Unknown." The opening paragraph in a review of the paper began, "It is universally allowed that nothing is more wanted in the art of healing, particularly in bilious cases, than a vegetable purgative that will act gently on the bowels in a small quantity, with little or no irritation."

(The oil was extracted from the *Ricinus Americanus major,* so called because the plant bore a seed like a *tyke,* for which *ricinus* is the Latin name, and *palmae Christi* because the leaves resemble the palm of the hand; it was also called *angus caslus,* from its cooling property and by a corruption of this name the oil has been called castor.) Canvane, like most other physicians of the 18th and 19th centuries, believed open bowels were the key to good health and ordered cathartics as a first line of treatment for nearly every disease. Stating that he used the oil for seven years in America and seven years in Europe, he argued for its use in fevers, stating, "Fevers being nothing else than a struggle of nature to throw off the morbific matter they sometimes indicate one evacuation, sometimes another." Finding the oil ineffective in treating low fevers, he had greater success in ardent and inflammatory fevers where "it has succeeded when nitrous medicines and *James's* powders have failed, giving every other day two spoonfulls of the oil."

Canvane claimed castor oil cured "the bilious yellow fever of the *West Indies;* first exhibiting an emetic, then the oil and the emulsion occasionally, at the same time giving diluting acids, which, especially in the beginning, are of great service." He added that for "bilious disorders in general, or disorders that arise from a vitiated bile, are more effectively relieved by this oil than any other medicine, as no medicine does in the same degree cool, purge, and correct the acrimony of that humour."[40]

If castor oil was almost wholly unknown, persons wishing to cure themselves of "consumptions, asthmas, all disorders of the lungs, and for the yellow fever of the East and West Indies" could purchase "Montpelier Royal Cordial Drops" in bottles for 6s and 3s each. Advice was offered gratis every day from nine till twelve o'clock.[41]

The Plague at Moscow, 1771

During the summer of 1771 an unspecified plague occurred at Moscow. In addition to fever, symptoms included itching or pain on those parts of the body where buboes and carbuncles were about to appear. The accession of glandular swellings or eruptions seemed to be the pathognomonic symptom of the disease. Its extreme violence "and the almost invariable affection of the lymphatic symptoms" appeared chiefly to distinguish it from typhus. The pulse was irregular from the onset of the disease, which was also characterized by headache, high delirium and a pulse that was "full, hard, strong, and quick." When those symptoms ceased, the pulse became "soft, feeble, intermitting, and not to be felt."

Treatments consisted of bleeding in the first, or "nervous stage," followed by the "putrid stage," where emetics, Peruvian bark and mineral acids were "administered in the most powerful doses." These methods were successful only in milder cases, however; doctors found no plan successful in violent attacks. Methods for arresting the progress of infection included removing contaminated persons into separate buildings, regardless of individual desires. "This," it was written, "is a fact which deserves great attention; as it proves that the progress of the plague may be impeded as effectually, and by the same means, as that of the common typhus."

As "the higher class of people were, as usual, less liable to infection than the poor," it was noted that the epidemic was greatly increased "by the warm attachments and superstitious prejudices of the lower ranks of Russians. They even broke into the plague-hospital, to carry images, to pray by the bed sides of their sick relations, and to embrace the bodies of the dead." In the month of September the number of dead was reported as high as 22,000, with a total mortality of upwards of 70,000.

In his 1799 work, *An Account of the Plague Which Raged at Moscow, in 1771*, Charles de Mertens asserted the claim "that *almost all physicians* now agree that the yellow fever is actually the plague," an idea that confounded reviewers. One in particular pointed out that "*we* cannot recollect *one* author of credit who has made the assertion," expressing his surprise that Mertens "confounded the yellow fever with the plague" and adding that "many respectable writers have of late denied that the yellow fever is communicable by infection."[42]

While it appears that the Moscow plague was not yellow fever, it is certainly indicative that a distinction of diagnosis persisted throughout the 18th century.

CHAPTER 3

A Question of Quarantine

> *Quarantine has always been incoherent; it arose when the idea of contagion first became rooted in the popular mind, and has never been saner than might consist with popular ignorance concerning the cause of disease. Its excesses have been the logical penalty of that ignorance, and to foster that ignorance was the grievous sin of medical men for centuries.*[1]

One of the most urgent considerations faced by politicians in the 1700s was the question of how to protect citizens from the importation of pestilential diseases. Selecting those distempers that spread rapidly, contaminated large segments of the population and left high mortality in their wake proved easier than identifying the direct cause of those maladies. Greatly compounding the issue was the fact that the medical community was divided over the spread of deadly killers such as smallpox, cholera and yellow fever. If a specific disease were transmitted by person-to-person contact or by touching a contaminated article, then it was classified as contagious. In that case, the argument could be made for quarantining infected people or goods. If, on the other hand, it was contracted by ingestion of food, miasmic effects, atmospheric or weather conditions or contaminated water, the subject became murkier.

In the 18th century there were few definitive means of establishing beyond a reasonable doubt how a disease was transmitted. Determining when and how to quarantine became a devisive issue between politicians, physicians, businessmen and lay people, all of whom had a vested interest in the outcome. While everyone wanted to feel safe and protected, quarantine was an expensive and onerous process, aspects of which disrupted the economy of individual cities and countries, seriously complicated travel and trade and often evoked international ire. The subject being of paramount importance, however, did not mean people would come together to make the best, most informed judgment and stand by it until more conclusive evidence was presented. On the contrary, just as the merits of quarantine for smallpox and cholera became vitriolic, there was no simple answer for how to handle outbreaks of yellow fever.

In 1754, the Reverend Dr. Hales, Clerk of the Closet to her Royal Highness the Princess of Wales, published "A Proposal for the More Speedily and Effectually Curing Men, Ships, and Goods, of Pestilential Infection." As yellow fever was considered a "pestilential infection" and the methods described were common ones, it provides a good understanding of the complex nature of the procedures required when maritime vessels and crew fell under quarantine regulations.

The method of fumigating a ship began by cutting one or more eight-inch diameter

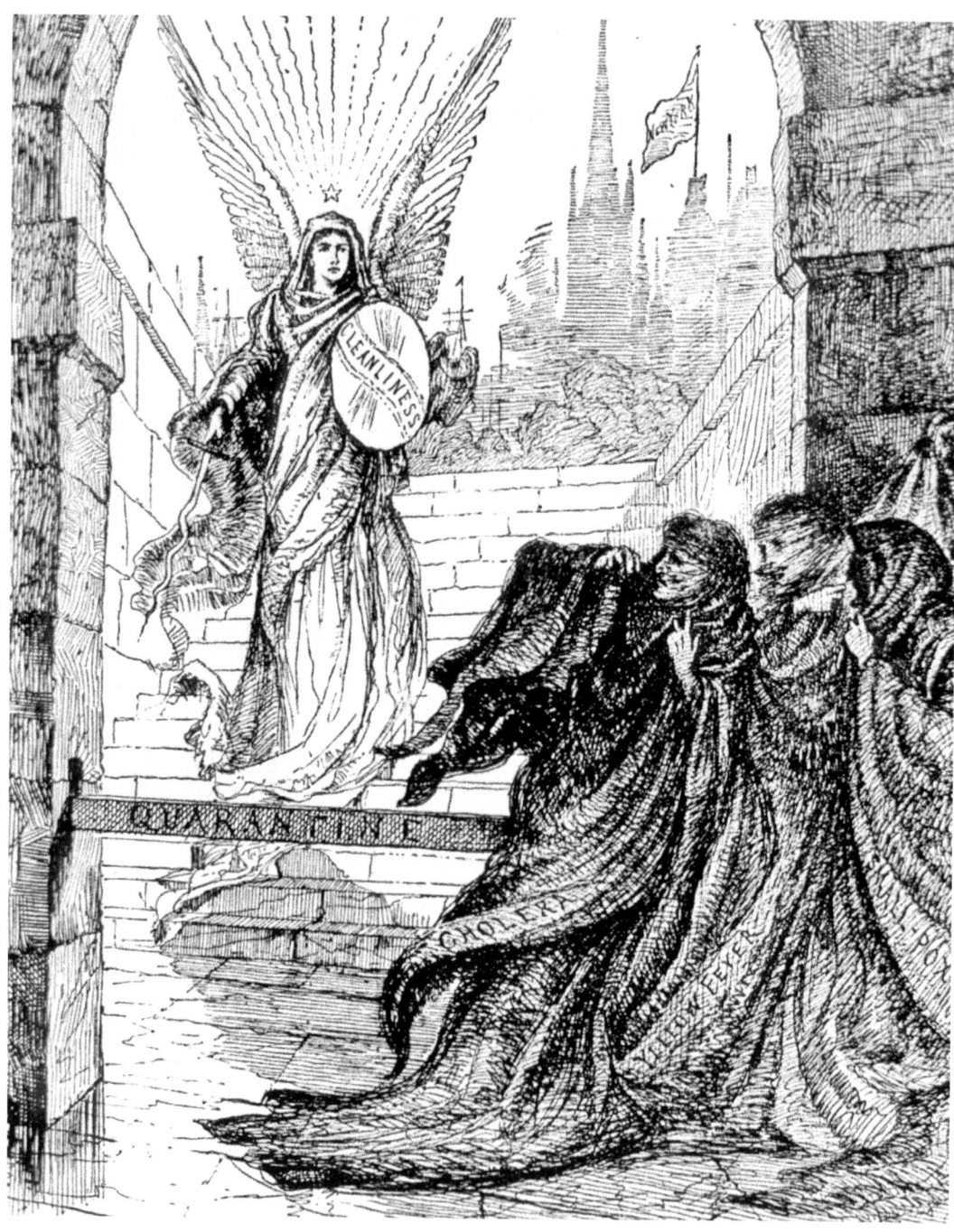

One of the most graphic illustrations of the times, the specters of cholera, yellow fever and smallpox tremble in fear at the angel blocking their entrance into the Port of New York. Her armament consists of a banner on which is written, "Quarantine," while her sword and shield represent cleanliness (from *Harper's Weekly,* Vol. 29, p. 592, published September 5, 1885) (courtesy National Library of Medicine).

holes through the windward side, below the lower deck. A bent iron tube of the same diameter was inserted into the hole(s), while the wider lower end was set over a stove in which about 50 pounds of brimstone with charcoal was to be burned. Significantly, the brimstone and charcoal were not to be burned in an iron pot unless there was a proper depth of earth at the bottom to prevent the pot from becoming red hot, as brimstone would instantly melt. Immediately before the mixture was lit, extreme care was to be taken to ensure all personnel were above deck in the open air to prevent their being suffocated. (Failure to take proper care not infrequently had dire consequences well into the 20th century. In the 1950s, five diseases were subject to international quarantine: cholera, plague, typhus, smallpox and yellow fever. Contaminated ships wishing to enter American ports were subject to fumigation. This was accomplished by placing canned cyanide-impregnated discs throughout the vessel. Combined with tear gas designed to drive people away, the discs, once exposed to air, released gas very slowly. The danger of this technique was demonstrated in New York when 13 stowaways failed either to heed or hear warnings and were later found dead.)[2] Once the fire started, acid fumes were distributed throughout the vessel. Hatches of the lower deck were opened to allow the fumes to ascend but gratings and other openings were closed with double tarpaulins. "This method," Hales added, "may also be used in slave ships, where a malignant and infectious fever is not only fatal to the people on board, but to the countries where they land the Negroes."

Lest some infection remain between the bales of goods in an infected ship (where the acid fumes could not penetrate due to close storage), it was recommended that as much brimstone as the crew could tolerate be continually burned as they were unloading. The merchandise was then to be brought to a lazaretto warehouse and more strongly fumed with burning brimstone, but not to such a degree as to discolor or spoil it. In plague countries, it was also stressed that before goods were boarded they be fumigated in as strong acid fumes as the packers could bear. This would not only prevent infection from being brought on ships, but would also prevent their being moth-eaten. Additionally, strips of cloth soaked in vinegar and spread throughout the ship during the voyage would likely abate the infection, especially if there were ventilators to circulate the foul air in the ship. For greater security, the ship was to be fumigated a second time after the goods were removed.

The clothes of the crew were fumed, washed in salt and then fresh water. Under the belief that "the evil is observed to manifest itself more in persons than things," the men also were ordered to bathe in saltwater and take antipestilential medicines. More extreme measures were taken in Turkey and on the Mediterranean coasts, where crews were placed in a closed room and fumigated by exposing them to a small quantity of burning brimstone to which had been added aromatic mixtures, supposedly to abate the noxious air. To avoid suffocation they were ordered to lie on their faces. This method, originally developed to kill insects, presented two problems when applied to humans: the fumes did not penetrate the lower half of the prostrate bodies and the poisoned air quickly ascended to the ceiling. It was observed, however (presumably in the case of insects), that continued fumigation eventually killed every living creature within the room and it was therefore suggested that lazaretto fuming rooms ought not to be too high-roofed.

The process of fumigating people, who required a much stronger degree of fumigation, was facilitated by first shaving their heads, then washing them in vinegar and covering their eyes, nostrils and ears with several folds of linen cloth. One of the layers was dipped in melted beeswax, which the acid spirits could not penetrate. For greater security, all the folds of linen could be covered in flannel dipped in strong lye, made with potash dissolved in water and wrung dry: "The obnoxious acid fumes of the burning brimstone will be turned, by the alkaline salt in the flannel, into a neutral, innocent, hard crusted salt." To facilitate breathing in people, a short faucet or pipe three or four inches long was fitted into their mouths and placed in holes drilled through the shutters or the boarded sides of the room used for fumigation, with a rail behind the men to rest against.

When the fumigation was thought to be sufficient, the doors and windows were opened, giving some time for the fumes to dissipate before the men were allowed to take their mouths from the breathing apparatus.[3] Considering the complexity of the technique, one wonders how many lives were sacrificed before it was "perfected."

Military ships returning to England during and after the French and Indian War inadvertently brought yellow fever with them, requiring fumigation to prevent the spread of what they believed to be a communicable disease. Referred to as "smoking," the process was accomplished by the vapor of burning tar. In the case of the *Edgar*, she was considered cleared of her infection by a large quantity of gunpowder fired onboard during an engagement. Dr. Lind believed "the only effectual means of destroying the noxious *miasmata* is by fumigation with tobacco, sulphur, arsenic, or gun-powder. I never heard of any ship, which after having been carefully and properly smoked, did not immediately become healthy." More specifically, he stated, in several ships the contagion of smallpox had been entirely stopped by means of wood fires, sprinkled with brimstone and kept burning and closely confined in the infected place.

From the good effects of fumigation in ships, the doctor advised like practice in the chambers where a person had died of any contagious distemper. He recommended immediate removal of the corpse and that the "doors close shut for at least eight or ten hours." Likewise, he believed burning Cascarilla bark or the diffusion of the steam of camphorated vinegar in sick chambers was likely to have a good effect. In order to purify household goods and apparel that were supposed to harbor infection, he prescribed long fumigation in a close place, while linen was to be steeped for some time in cold soap lees before being washed in hot water.

Peculiarly, Lind wrote, "The modern practice of burning large fires in the open air in the streets of places infected with the plague, or other contagion, is founded on principles groundless and erroneous; and hath therefore been experienced not only unsuccessful but hurtful." Countering that argument was the contemporary belief that smoke possessed a powerful antiseptic quality, "probably owing to the *ammoniac* it contains." Thus, in cases of contagious distempers, fires were "of singular benefit." As for Lind's proposed use of sulphur and arsenic, one authority noted, "[W]e cannot suppose any thing specific in them, unless we imagine the noxious *miasmata* to consist of certain *animalcula* floating in the air, and adhering to the inside of the ship; which possibly may be the case."[4]

Diseases Incident to Strangers in North America

With the termination of the French and Indian War in 1763, France ceded French Louisiana west of the Mississippi River to her ally Spain as compensation for Spain's loss of Florida to England. Britain in turn returned Cuba to Spain. With possession of these

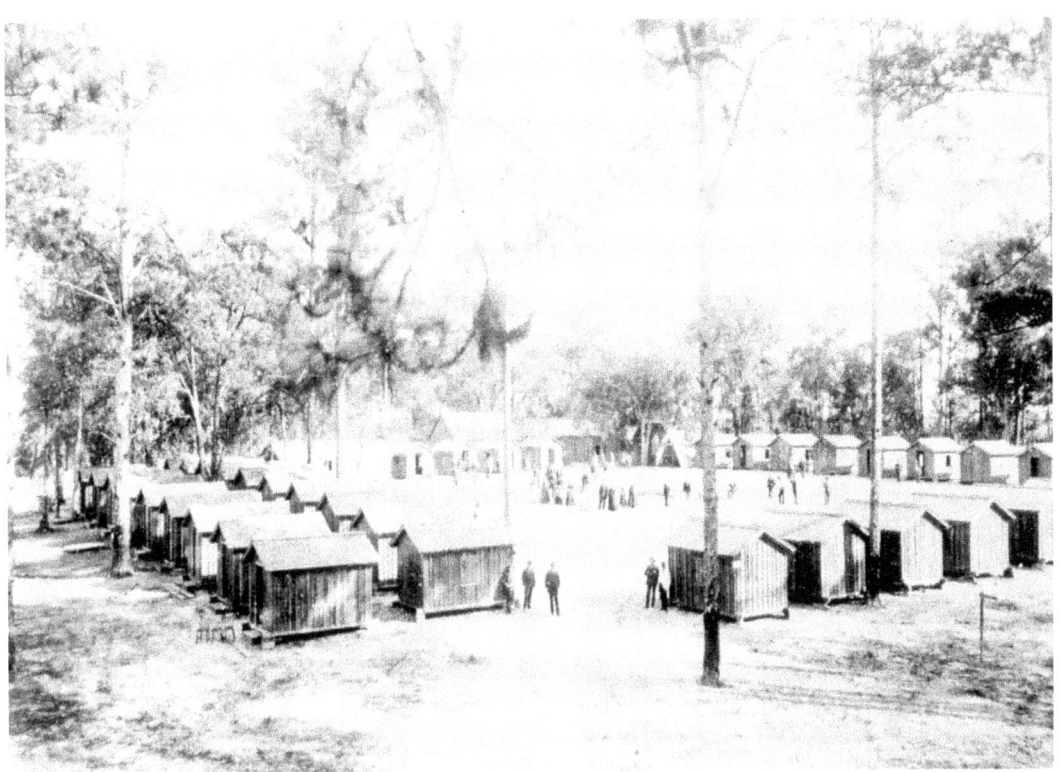

Dread of yellow fever spreading from areas of contamination gripped the United States throughout the 1800s. This illustration from 1888 depicts Camp E.A. Perry, situated on the border between Georgia and Florida. The sick were treated in makeshift tents such as this, while those capable of leaving the area often fled for their lives (courtesy National Library of Medicine).

territories temporarily settled, the idea of immigrating to America became more palatable to the British. There was, therefore, a need for more information on the weather and health of the colonies. The climate of New England, readers were informed, was similar to that of Great Britain, but southward into Maryland or Virginia the temperature was greater and the soils more moist. There were, however, fevers and fluxes very distressing to strangers, although natives in general were healthy and long lived.

In the latitude of South Carolina, diseases were "much more obstinate, acute and violent. In that colony, especially during the growth of the rice, in the months of July and August, the fevers which attack strangers are very anomalous, not remitting or intermitting soon, but partaking much of the nature of those distempers which are so fatal to the newly arrived Europeans in West Indian climates." The same was true of Georgia and east Florida during those months, but in west Florida diseases to newcomers more closely approximated that of the West Indian islands: "The excessive heat of the weather has sometimes produced in this place a mortal sickness similar to that which in the West Indies goes under the name of the yellow fever."

Pensacola, site of the 1765 fever outbreak, was believed to be healthier than Mobile, where intermitting fevers prevailed during July, August and September. Bark (quinine) was considered the best remedy for all fevers found in the American colonies. Treatments notwithstanding, in 1766 yellow fever broke out in New Orleans, "raging with great violence among the Spaniards," daily carrying off a great number of people and stagnating what little trade had been commenced between Pensacola and the New Orleans settlements. On the other hand, British troops and settlers in Canada faced a different set of disorders. One surgeon practicing in Quebec found that "true pleurisies, and other inflammatory disorders, were the genuine produce of the cold air of that climate; but that low, bilious and intermitting fevers were scarcely ever known there."[5]

The State of Medicine in the Mid–1700s

While a detailed account of battles and leaders is essential for the understanding of any war, there remain innumerable intangibles that play their roles behind the scenes. Perhaps the easiest example to offer regarding the Revolutionary War is George Washington's experience with smallpox. As a 17-year-old he accompanied his brother Lawrence to Barbados in the hope that a change of climate would cure the latter's tuberculosis. During their stay George contracted smallpox and was ill for nearly a month. Survival conferred on the future general a lifelong immunity and also impressed on him a respect for the disease and the ravages it could bring to a standing army. He supported inoculation, and when the Continental Army went into winter quarters in 1776 he decided to begin a massive inoculation program for all units joining the ranks.[6]

Washington's youthful experience influenced his later actions, and his insistence on inoculation earned him credit for achieving the single greatest contribution to preventive medicine during the war. Other soldiers' lives played similar roles in how they perceived and responded to the threat of disease. The prevalence of yellow fever during the summer or "sickly season" in the southern colonies was well known to officers on both sides of the conflict. Some chose to take their chances; others attempted to avoid major confrontations until the heat of summer and its harbinger of disease presented less of a threat. How they fared became part of the large jigsaw puzzle that fit together to make a whole.

The state of medical knowledge and the experience of the physicians also constituted many varied and disparate pieces of this puzzle. At the time of the Revolution, a medical license was not required for a man to call himself a doctor and only two institutions in the colonies, King's College in New York and the College of Philadelphia, conferred medical degrees. The College of Philadelphia granted its first bachelor of medicine diploma in 1768 and King's College did so in 1769. By 1775 fifty-one degrees had been conferred. By 1760 New York had enacted a medical licensing law and in 1772 the Medical Society of New Jersey petitioned the assembly to require subsequent practitioners to undergo qualifying examinations.[7]

The vast majority of those hanging out a shingle, however, learned their art through apprenticeships that often constituted little more than following the local doctor for a specified period of time. Studying the human body through dissection was rare and few surgeries other than trepanning and amputations were performed. Even these life-saving efforts were often in vain as there existed no anesthesia, no antibiotics as we know them today, no thorough understanding of what caused infection and little to administer if there had been. The judge of a surgeon's skill was often in how quickly he severed a limb rather than in patient mortality.

The knowledge of contagious disease was even more limited. Lacking any knowledge of germ theory, foundations were based on observation and as was clearly the case with many "maladies" there was seldom any consensus of how to interpret them. Authorities, influenced by personal bias, political pressure, economic forces and morality, often spent more time arguing with one another than in attempting to find common ground. Nor could the persuasive influences of superstition and religion be ignored. Arguments ranging from "God created disease, so man should accept and submit to its deadly power" to fear of being turned into a beast from vaccinations derived from "cow pus" slowed scientific advancements and often precipitated deadly consequences.

In 1785 Gilbert Blane, MD, physician extraordinary to the Prince of Wales, physician to St. Thomas's Hospital and physician to the "Fleet in the Late War" (having served as Admiral Sir George Rodney's chief medical officer in the West Indies during the American Revolution), set out several theories in his *Observations on the Diseases Incident to Seamen*. Included was his interpretation of the *vis medicatrix* (*vis mediacatrix naturae* the "healing power of nature," a guiding principle dating back to Hippocrates) that provides an insight into medical philosophy of the era:

> There is a tendency in acute diseases to wear themselves out, both in individuals that labor under them, and when the infection is introduced into a community. Unless there was such a *vis medicatrix*, there would be no end to the fatality of these distempers; for the infectious matter would go on multiplying itself without end, and would necessarily destroy every person who might be exposed to it. But nature has so ordered it, that this poison, after exciting a certain set of motions in an animal body, loses its effect, and recovery takes place; and those who happen not to be infected at first, become in some measure callous to its impression, by being habitually exposed to it. There is, therefore, a natural proneness to recovery, both with regard to that indisposition which takes place among a set of men living together, and with regard to a single individual who actually labours under the disease. Thus the most prevailing period of sickness is when men are new to their situation and to each other, and time of itself may prove the means of prevention as well as cure.

The idea that if left alone the body would cure itself ("nature is the best physician") became a tenet of physic. The philosophy was augmented by the early Renaissance physician Paracelsus, who advocated the idea of the "inherent balsam" within the body. Thomas Sydenham, who greatly influenced 18th century medical philosophy, considered fevers as a healing force of nature. In trying to explain contagion, Blane wrote, "There are some contagious diseases which cannot be propagated but by their own peculiar infection ... just as the seeds of vegetables are necessary to continue their several species; so that if the infectious poison were lost, so would the disease. Of this kind are the small-pox, and the other diseases to which man is subject but once during life. There are other diseases which produce infection without having themselves proceed from it. Of this kind are fevers and fluxes." Within the framework of animal economy laid down by Hunter—"at least a certain length in explaining this variable state of the body with respect to its susceptibility to infectious diseases"—Blane explained:

> This principle is, that the body cannot be affected by more than one morbid action at the same time. If a person is exposed to the small-pox, for instance, a fever, or while he is under the influence of the measles, he will not catch the first till the other has run its course. It may happen, therefore, that people escape the effect of contagion in consequence of being at the time under the influence of some other indisposition, either evident or latent.... It would appear from these considerations, that there are certain circumstances, or temporary situations on constitution, which invite infection, and render its effect more certain and violent in one case than another.

In summary, Blane perfectly described the state of the medical arts in the mid–1700s: "But there, as well as many other facts in animal nature, do not admit of a satisfactory explanation upon any principle as yet known. Even the most common operations of the body, such as digestion and generation, when considered in their causes and modes of action, are so obscure and mysterious as to be almost beyond the reach of rational conjecture."[8] This conclusion was easily translated into the extensively used expression "there are some things God never meant us to know," ironically used to excess in 1930–1940s horror films.

In the Revolutionary War era, the most recognized medical schools were at Paris, Rheims, Leyden and most notably Edinburgh, which approximately 200 physicians practicing in America had attended by 1800. At the beginning of the conflict, 400 out of 3,500 North American practitioners held medical degrees. From these learned individuals sprang the foundation of the healing arts, but they were limited by an art and a science in its infancy. The Hippocratic process of blood-letting was still a common practice to remove an excess of "humor" and thus restore the body's equilibrium, while depletion and stimulation were the most often prescribed treatments.

British medical practitioners labored under a highly defined caste that differentiated three distinct categories: surgeons, physicians and apothecaries. American doctors typically served the function of all three, handling primary care, performing operations and dispensing medicines.

With few exceptions, surgeries were limited to suturing cuts, open reduction of splintered bones and treating gunshot wounds. More extensive procedures such as repairing a hairlip, tonsillectomies, paracentesis and surgical removal of urinary stones were limited to the most skilled doctors. Postintervention infection rates were staggering, with a subsequent mortality rate in the 18th century estimated at over 50 percent.

The American War for Independence, 1775–1783

After yellow fever appeared in Philadelphia in 1762, British colonial North America remained free from major outbreaks for nearly 30 years. This was primarily due to enforcement of the "Commercial Monopoly" navigational act created by Parliament. Mirroring that of other colonial powers, it broadly prohibited trade between possessions of other nations.

British law became a moot point when leaders of the thirteen colonies declared their independence. While the war was fought with conventional weapons, it would not be an understatement to say that both sides in the conflict confronted a common enemy: disease. How their military strategy took the southern sickly seasons into consideration and how unforeseen circumstances dictated when and where battles were fought left troops more or less vulnerable to disease and significantly influenced the outcome of the war.

As an indication of how the factor of disease weighed on the minds of civilians as well as soldiers, an early notice from the *London Morning Chronicle* (April 18, 1775) touched on a double entendre for yellow fever:

> A correspondent, on reading an account in the papers of several subaltern officers being ill of Yellow Fever at Boston, says, the Public ought not to be alarmed, if in the next account they are informed, that not only several members of the General Congress, but some of the firmest among the American patriots, are likewise ill of the *Yellow Fever;* but from a different cause of a different aspect and symptom; and which, unless they should possess more that Spartan virtue, must operate very prejudiciously to their own characters in the first instance, and to the interest of their constituents in the second.

One of the earliest campaigns to be affected by fevers occurred in the spring of 1776 when the British sent troops and a fleet to capture Charles-Town (also spelled without the hyphen; the current spelling of "Charleston" and subsequent pronunciation of the word were changed in 1783). By late May after the attack had been delayed, a local man named Richard Hutson wrote that if the British did not move soon the city would be safe at least until November, "for it would be the height of madness and folly for them to come here during the sickly season." His view was shared by Sir Henry Clinton, commander of his majesty's troops, who lamented that as June approached and no action had been taken, "I have the mortification to see the sultry, unhealthy season approaching us with hasty strides, when all thoughts of military operations in the Carolinas must be given up." Under the command of Sir Peter Parker, the British fleet finally attacked on June 28 but their efforts were unsuccessful. Rather than lay siege to the harbor or attempt a land assault and face the dual threats of patriot counterattack and the dreaded summer fevers, Clinton removed his troops north. It was as well for him that he did, as Hutson later wrote to a friend that Charles-Town had been "very sickly, and the mortality unusually great so early in the season."

Americans proved less sanguine of their own country during the campaigns of 1776 and 1778 when soldiers from the Carolinas and Georgia attempted to dislodge the British from its Florida strongholds. Similar to what Dr. Lind had described when discussing yellow fever among British seamen at Pensacola in 1765, the patriots "suffered heavy casualties from fevers virtually without firing a shot at the British."

Although yellow fever was primarily a disease of the lower colonies it was by no means limited to the south. A letter dated July 30, 1775, written by a British officer and submitted to the *London Evening-Post* by a regular contributor who signed himself "Amicus," was published September 16 and offered some details of the Battle of Bunker Hill (June 17). After protesting British war policies in the colonies that had inspired the Americans to "court death to avoid [their own] slavery," he added that they all expected to fight to the death and, "to a man, to lay their execrated bones in this country." The unnamed soldier continued: "But should the scurvy, the bloody flux, and the yellow fever, continue to rage in our camp, as it has done for some time past, there will be no occasion for fighting to destroy us; death will make a sufficient and terrible carnage without it." Interestingly, a year later a similar letter was published in the London newspaper *Lloyd's Evening Post*. In a later edition (August 28–30, 1776) the editor drew a conclusion on the validity of the contents in part from its mention of yellow fever:

> We are sorry our Norwich Correspondent should attempt to impose on us, by sending a cooked-up Letter as from an Officer at Staten Island. What it says of the fatal effects of salt provisions, intense heat, hard duty, the bloody flux, the yellow fever, and the scurvy, manifesting themselves daily among the Troops, cannot be true, as salt provisions on Staten Island are as uncommon as salt provisions on the Isle of Wight; the intense heat at New York, a place in the same latitude with part of Great Britain, is ridiculous; the yellow fever is only known to the Southward of Maryland; and to talk of the sea scurvy, when they have made land, is absolute nonsense.

It is almost tempting to think the "Norwich correspondent" merely substituted "Staten Island" for "Boston" and submitted the letter to *Lloyd's* as original, but that does not obfuscate the fact that yellow fever had made a previous appearance in New York as early as 1702. And if the letter was actually an original, the two documents place yellow fever (or what was perceived to be yellow fever) in Massachusetts in 1775 and New York in 1776.

General Augustine Prevost captured Savannah in December 1778 and the following spring made an attempt to capture Charles-Town, but in the face of superior numbers under General Benjamin Lincoln and the coming sickly season he pulled back to Georgia. Lincoln followed Prevost only as far as the Savannah River. The British commander later excused his failure to capture Charles-Town by citing his poor health, "weakened by seven years in hot climates."

Worse news awaited Prevost on his return to Savannah. The troops he left behind to guard the city were suffering from widespread hot-weather sicknesses. However, those able to fight put up stiff resistance when attacked by American and French forces and maintained control of the city, albeit with heavy losses. In a more serious development, one of the Britain's most capable officers, Colonel John Maitland, died from a "bilious fever." Clinton and Prevost joined forces to surround Charles-Town and on May 11, 1780, General Lincoln surrendered in what was the greatest American defeat of the war. Not only did the patriots lose virtually the entire Continental Army in the south, it also lost the majority of the southern medical staff, most notably David Olyphant, Peter Fayssoux and David Ramsay, who worked independently of their northern brethren. With most physicians imprisoned on British vessels in Charles-Town Harbor, the remaining army re-forming in Virginia was forced to hastily reassemble a new medical staff.

Clinton returned to New York in June, leaving Lord Cornwallis to handle affairs in the Carolinas. The strategic city he had captured, however, was in poor shape as the sickly season approached. Devastated by protracted siege, a filthy and crumbling infrastructure, unsanitary prison ships, financial ruin of the upper classes and a black population reduced to utter desperation, health conditions were ripe for epidemic. By mid–July, smallpox and fevers—likely yellow fever, malaria, typhus and typhoid—had killed many ship-bound American prisoners, while thousands of slaves, fleeing bondage by escaping into British hands, were consumed by the same malignant disorders.

British troops fared little better, with Hessians suffering especially heavily. Although reports indicated that the health of the army was reasonably good in mid–July, the contingent in Charles-Town became increasingly ill during the late summer and fall. Surgeon Robert Jackson reported that the most common sickness were "intermittents." Other terms used were "agues and fevers," "malignant fevers," "putrid fevers" and "bilious fevers," any or all of which could indicate yellow fever, malaria and typhus. British reports from Savannah were no better. By early July the commander, Lt. Colonel Alured Clarke, reported that heat and sickness was "beyond anything you can conceive." By late August he pleaded for reinforcements and two months later wrote to Cornwallis that "our suffering from sickness in this vile climate is terrible and continues in a very great degree."

The local terrain continued to hinder British efforts to subdue the colonists. By August 1780 Cornwallis wrote Clinton, attempting to explain his failure to make inroads in the Carolina low country. His problems stemmed from the "the terrible climate, which except in Charles-Town, is so bad that within an hundred miles of the coast, from the end of June to the middle of October" troops could not be stationed there "without a certainty of their being rendered useless for some time for military service, if not entirely lost."

On July 29, Major Wemyss wrote from Georgetown, indicating his troops were "falling down very fast" with intermitting fevers; his next health report stated that six men had died of putrid fevers within the past three days and thirty others were ill. Accepting the inevitable, on July 30 Cornwallis ordered Wemyss to leave Georgetown and move inland along the Black River, warning him not to tarry long in any one place along the river, "which is a very sick place." He recommended "short and easy marches" and relocating in the High Hills of Santee, which he believed to be healthier. In that, Cornwallis's information proved faulty. Throughout the summer and fall he received news from his commanders detailing the deadly diseases that were seriously weakening their fighting forces. Particularly significant were the fevers that struck the 71st Highland Regiment at Cheraw Hill, east of Camden. By July two-thirds of the men had been seized with "fevers and agues and rendered unfit for service." By July 24, 1780, the commander, Major Archibald McArthur. was forced to abandon Cheraw, a move rebel forces took as a retreat. Nearly one hundred Highlanders sent to Georgetown for medical treatment were captured; this patriot success was followed by General Thomas Sumter's capture of 70 more sick men. Cornwallis regarded these losses as a "disaster."

In spite of the condition of his troops, Cornwallis defeated General Horatio Gate at Camden, but the victory also burdened the British general with numerous wounded and sick enemy soldiers. Fearing that staying in Camden would further exacerbate the situation, by September he moved his army to Waxhaws, hoping to leave the fevers and smallpox behind. The weather remained hot, however, and fevers among the troops increased rather than decreased. By late September he informed General Clinton that the 63rd was "so totally demolished by sickness that it will not be fit for actual service for some months."

Cornwallis hoped that by fall when "Good Doctor Frost" had done its work and removed the threat of fevers he could establish a base of supplies at Charlotte and then move into North Carolina. The sicknesses did not abate, however, and Lt. Col. Banastre Tarleton, cavalry commander of the British Legion, was ill from what was diagnosed as yellow fever. It was not until September 22 that Tarleton was well enough to be moved to safety and Cornwallis advanced on Charlotte, capturing the city on the 24th after a fierce battle. Victory carried consequences, as six other cavalry officers were overcome by yellow fever. (By this time of year, Peter McCandless argues in *Revolutionary Fever: Disease and War in the Lower South, 1776–1783* that the diagnosis is questionable given the army's distance from the coast. The *Aedes aegypti* mosquitos were poor fliers, but as the British were supplied via river transport from Charles-Town and Georgetown, it is entirely possible they were moved inland with the supplies.)

Five of the six cavalry officers died within a week, leaving only Major George Hanger. His health was so compromised, however, he was moved first to Charles-Town and then to Bermuda before he finally arrived in Britain, where he bitterly complained of the "baleful influence" of disease "in those intensely hot and sickly climates."

Although the weather finally cooled, Cornwallis himself fell to a fever that incapacitated him for weeks. Summing up the 1780 campaign, Patrick Tonyn, Royal Governor of British East Florida, wrote "sickness and disease have made more havoc in the neighboring colonies than the sword."

In the spring of 1871 Cornwallis faced a serious choice: return to South Carolina and hold the colony or march into Virginia and help secure it under British control. Justifying his northward move, he wrote that by doing so he hoped "to preserve the troops, from the fatal sickness, which so nearly ruined the army last autumn," and not inconsequentially to personally avoid a repeat of the dire fever. Cornwallis did march into Virginia, but even then he did not escape the dreaded specter of disease. A report from the *New York Gazette* of August 12, 1782, noted, "The French have brought the Yellow Fever into Virginia, and to prevent the Spread of this Pestilence, the Detachment moving Northwardly, are conducted by the back Road through Sussex." Nevertheless, the British appearance eventually set the stage for General George Washington's brilliant maneuvers at Yorktown in October. When Washington departed for the Hudson that November, however, he left behind 1,500 troops to recover from disease as well as wounds. James Thacher, a surgeon at Yorktown wrote, "Our New England troops have been very sickly, the prevailing diseases are remitting fevers, which are very prevalent in this climate during the autumnal months."[9]

The war was far from over but when the British evacuated Charles-Town in December 1782 principal fighting ended. However, General Nathanael Greene was ordered to maintain his army until formal declarations were issued. The peace treaty was not signed until April 1783 but by that time Greene's army was near mutiny, as the northern soldiers refused to participate in another sickly summer campaign.[10]

In summary, approximately 25,000 patriots died in the War for Independence: 6,800 in battle, 8,500 in British prisons, and 10,000 in camps or hospitals. Including seamen, the mortality rate was 0.9 percent of the population, "second only in the major wars of the United States to the mortality rate of 1.6 percent during the Civil War." Two-hundred thousand soldiers were under arms during the conflict, making the mortality for those who fought on the American side 12 percent, slightly under that sustained by Union forces against the Confederacy. The highest rate of illness in Washington's army (excluding the southern campaigns that would put the number significantly higher) reached 35 percent in December 1776 and 35.5 percent in February 1777.

Lowest Level of Sickness in Washington's Army for One Month (Excluding Southern Troops)

Year	Percent
1775	10.5
1776	9.6
1777	17.7
1778	16.0
1779	8.7
1780	8.2
1781	5.4

The average rate of sickness for the 8-year war was 18 percent.

Medical treatment during the war roughly equated to European techniques and standards of the 18th century. More medical supplies, medicines and physicians were available to those who fought in the northern colonies than in the southern, but both the Americans and the British suffered from poorly developed methods of retrieving the wounded. It was not until 1793 during the French Revolution that better organized, humane and efficient methods of battlefield removal were tried by Dominique-Jean Larrey.[11]

In 1775 only one permanent North American hospital, located at Philadelphia, existed. The war focused attention on the need for more formal medical establishments to be created but progress was slow. In 1798 the federal government established the Marine Hospital System, which provided medical assistance for seamen. The act was expanded in 1802 to cover those working on rafts and barges on the Mississippi, but it was not until 1830 that the hospital system was extended to steamboat crews working the western waters.[12]

The most significant medical contribution to the war was the success of the mass smallpox inoculations that prevented that dread disease from spreading throughout the army and contaminating cities near major conflicts. Some successful attempts at sanitation were achieved but no new standards were reached or established. The Revolution did create a need for the domestic manufacture of drugs and some (possibly niter, cream of tartar, castor oil and oil of turpentine) were made at army laboratories in Pennsylvania in 1778. It was not until 1786 that the first large-scale production of compounds such as Glauber's salts and muriate of ammonia began in Philadelphia, packaged by the firm of Charles and Christopher Marshall, who had supplied the Pennsylvania and New Jersey line in 1776.

One distinction that developed in the postwar era was that between physician and apothecary. The written prescription, used at the Pennsylvania Hospital since the 1760s, became more common and expanded the role of those who specialized in dispensing medicines at pharmacies and private shops.[13]

One factor that did hold powerful importance in the development of the new country was the experience garnered by those physicians who participated in the conflict. For good or ill, it was these men who would soon be called upon to face another great horror of civilization: epidemic.

Chapter 4

The American Plague

The medical art is the offspring of experience: yet life is too short, occasion too sudden, experiment too dangerous, and judgement too insufficient for any one person to acquire a competent knowledge of diseases, and their remedies, by his own experience.[1]

For thirty years significant outbreaks of yellow fever were absent from the Lesser Antilles. The British West Indies were likely saved from outbreaks by the enforcement of British trade laws beginning in the 1760s that prohibited foreign countries from commerce with their possessions. Yellow fever was not endemic to the islands and these regulations incidentally protected the inhabitants; the disease was introduced only when vessels from the Spanish colonies or Africa illegally managed to touch their shores.

During the American Revolution, British operations in the Caribbean against the Spanish Main were limited to two small expeditions against Central America launched from Jamaica. In both instances, troops were heavily afflicted by disease, possibly spread by newly arrived regiments to Jamaica in the fall of 1780. However, the disease did not spread to other British or French colonies.

After attaining independence in 1783, the newly formed United States lost the privilege of free commercial intercourse with British territories. That did not prevent illegal trade, and West Indian planters welcomed the Americans with open arms. The next decade provided relative calm from epidemics of yellow fever but it was not destined to last.

As though in anticipation of what was to come, in 1788 Dr. John Hunter, superintendent of military hospitals in Jamaica from early 1781 to May 1783, published *Observations on the Diseases of the Army in Jamaica; and On the Best Means of Preserving the Health of Europeans in That Climate.* He deduced that fevers and fluxes proceeded "from noxious exhalations from wet, low, and marshy grounds," adding that other circumstances coordinate with this miasma in either producing or aggravating these diseases, such as "the excessive use of rum, fatigue, hard labour, bad or scanty diet, long fasting, distress of mind, and exposure to rain." Dividing West Indian fevers into two categories, "remittent" and "intermittent," he considered remittent to be the most frequent and the most fatal. Discussing the work of several writers who minutely detailed the symptomology of warm climate diseases, Hunter concluded they actually described yellow fever, pronouncing it to be of the remittent type, accompanied with "the peculiar symptom of a yellowness of the eyes and skin." Furthermore, Hunter refuted "with strong arguments" the opinion "that bile is the cause of the remittent fever—that the remittent fever is putrid—that the yellow fever is putrid and infectious."[2] As the term "remittent

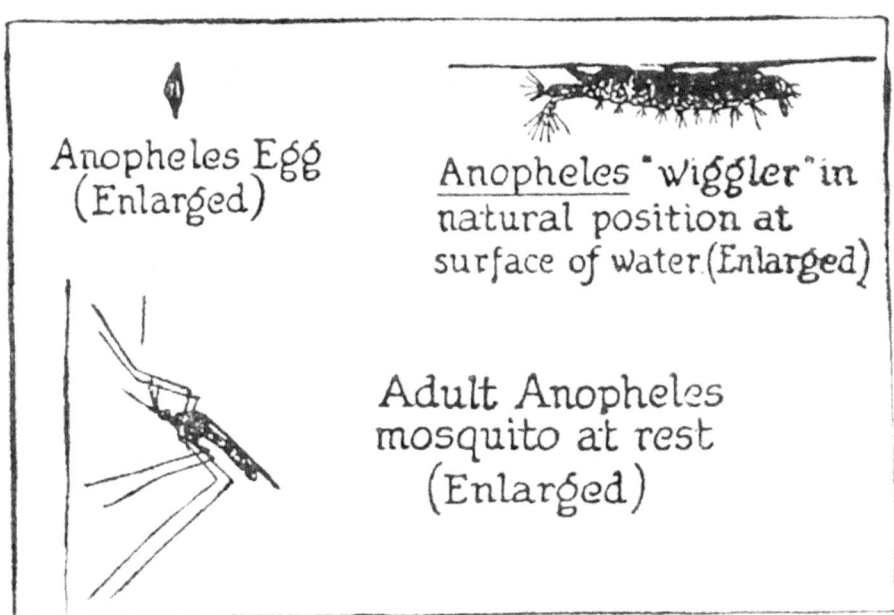

The idea that mosquitoes were the vector involved in the transmission of yellow fever was proposed as early as the 1700s but without proof no one believed it. It wasn't until the 1800s that the idea gained credence, but it took the American occupation of Cuba after the Spanish-American War to provide the research grounds for the brilliant collaboration that finally proved the theory (author's collection, from *Health Heroes*, 1926).

fever" generally referred to malaria, however, it is not clear which disease he was describing.

Hunter erred when linking yellow fever to the theory of poisoned air but he was far from alone. One reviewer of Hunter's book added his own comment to the miasmic theory: "By experience it is found, that fevers and fluxes are more prevalent in places abounding with these exhalations, than in those situations which are free from them; on which account, the exhalations are said to be the causes of the disease; and the fact must be admitted, although we cannot explain it."[3]

The evils of rum, dietary considerations, anxiety and exposure were common "throw-ins" for medical papers and lectures. They gave a bit of moral causality to the diagnosis, a theme expected and well received by their 18th and early 19th century audiences. During the sanitation movement to come, personal hygiene would also be included with those evils linked to a predisposition to disease. In the pre-microscopic era when doctors relied on observation and made grandiose assumptions based on extremely small case samples, miasma, atmospheric and cosmic influences and "filth," all linked to the lower classes, were often credited with the origin and continuation of outbreaks.

Scientific presentations aside, the idea that yellow fever was a bilious disease had taken hold of the public mind and "anti-bilious elixirs" such as Frith's were advertised in mainstream newspapers. This particular medicine promised to cure gouty and bilious complaints in the stomach and bowels, the jaundice and the yellow fever of the West Indies, indigestion, worms and "the effects of hard drinking or irregularity."[4]

In 1791 a joint stock company was created in England to colonize Bolama, one of the Bissagos Islands off the coast of Portuguese Guinea in West Africa. Organized by Henry Hew Dalrymple, he brought the former British soldier Philip Beaver in on the project. By April 1792 two vessels, one of which (the *Hankey*) Beaver captained, carrying a total of 275 colonists—153 men, 57 women and 65 children—set off to establish their settlement. From the outset, nothing went right. Nine days after the first ship set anchor, a Canhabaque war party from the mainland struck the colonists, killing or wounding ten men and carrying off six women and children.

After the directors of the project lost heart and returned to England, Beaver remained, although he later bitterly criticized the remaining colonists (48 men, 13 women and 25 children) for their want of discipline and dedication. Severely complicating matters was the outbreak of the War of the First Coalition (1792–1797) and the slave rebellion in St. Domingue, making it difficult for the settlers to receive supplies and protection from English ships. More directly, yellow fever or malaria or both were introduced from the African coast. Death from these diseases took a high toll on the colonists, finally compelling them to abandon their settlement and sail on the *Hankey* for Grenada, reaching that destination February 19, 1793.[5]

Unfortunately, Beaver's contingent brought yellow fever with them. Coming into immediate contact with the inhabitants of Grenada they passed the disease to them, and they in turn became carriers as their vessels traveled to other British islands. By July 1793 yellow fever had reached St. Vincent, Barbados, Tobago, Dominica, Antigua and St. Kitts as well as the Spanish possession of Trinidad, not only infecting those who lived on the islands but also French refugees from St. Domingue and European troops moving through the West Indies. As an indication that yellow fever had long been absent from the West Indies, many inhabitants were unfamiliar with the symptoms and took it for a new disease. One physician who had practiced in Dominica for 24 years declared he had never seen a similar outbreak, leading to the conclusion that increased travel to and between the islands and the influx of susceptible newcomers due to the various wars, as well as the unsettled social conditions and unregulated commerce, "provided an ideal setting" for the disease.[6]

This "ideal setting" was to play a significant role in bringing yellow fever to the United States. In 1791 St. Domingue (Santo Domingo; Haiti) was the most important of France's colonies, furnishing two-thirds of France's overseas trade and employing 1,000 ships and 15,000 French sailors. Not inconsequentially, the island was also the largest market for the African slave trade. Violent conflicts between the white colonists and the black slaves were common but the flash point may have stemmed from the French Revolution and the Declaration of the Rights of Man that stated, "In the eyes of the law all citizens are equal." In August 1791 an organized slave rebellion broke out; as matters worsened over the ensuing years, many individuals were forced to flee for their lives.[7]

A dispatch dated June 13, 1793, from St. Kitts complicated matters for those seeking asylum elsewhere in the West Indies by stating, "Admiral Gardner's squadron, with 3,000 troops, left Barbadoes on Tuesday morning for Martinique, where we are informed the aristocrats have been worsted, and that from Fort Royal to Trinity Bay every estate and house is laid to ashes. Upwards of a thousand more have been obliged to seek refuge in Dominica.... We are sorry to learn, that the fever which has lately made so much havoc at Grenada, is now equally bad at Tobago."[8] The next choice for a safe haven was the United States' temporary capital and her greatest port of trade: Philadelphia.

The "Philadelphia Fever," 1793

The Philadelphia winter of 1792–1793 was particularly mild, with no snow and only moderate frosts. January was so pleasant that the French balloonist M. Blanchard was able to ascend from the Prison Yard while Philadelphians sitting on the warm ground cheered. Fruit trees were in blossom by April and cold, dreary rains soaked the ground throughout May, swelling streams and creating pools of standing water in depressed areas and throughout city thoroughfares. Conditions underwent a dramatic change in June when the rains stopped and early summer heat dried the landscape. New pools that a month earlier had been maintained by surging creeks dried up, leaving stagnant marshes. The same held true for the city, which had no water system; wells were shallow and in the best of times people described them as polluted.

The sole sewer under the serpentine of Dock Street overflowed, creating small pockets of slimy, offensive puddles. The principal method of removing waste was "sinks" dug along streets to collect water from gutters. Without flowing water, human offal and animal waste collected in these sinks putrefied in the rising temperatures, while rotting city refuse piled along the banks of the Delaware created a stench powerful enough to taint the atmosphere. The city being unable to control the deteriorating sanitary conditions, insects found the perfect haven for reproduction.

When the rains did not come, drought appeared: wells dried, crops wilted and died, and people became ill with the annual "summer complaint" or the early appearance of "autumnal fever." The appearance of large flocks of pigeons was held to be a harbinger of "unhealthy air," and the overwhelming influx of mosquitoes were pronounced "a certain sign" of poisoned air.[9] And miasma meant the threat of death from those invisible particles, either animal or chemical, in the atmosphere.

Philadelphia was a low, level city, considered the hottest and dampest on the Atlantic seaboard, with temperatures greater than Charleston, Savannah and the islands of the West Indies. In 1793 it served as the temporary capital of the new country and was decreed by the Residence Act to remain so until 1800. President George Washington and his cabinet lived in this city that housed major seats of learning and medicine and supported the nation's most active seaport. With a population of 55,000, Philadelphians welcomed 2,500 births every year and mourned 1,400 deaths, ensuring a healthy increase of native-born citizens. In this mix were British-born adults whose families had colonized the land and fought in the Revolution, which had concluded a mere ten years earlier. There were also numerous German and French-speaking people and 2,500 Negroes.[10]

By July 1793 ships carrying refugees from St. Domingue began arriving at Philadelphia. Many were sick with fever; most had fled the slave revolt with little or no belongings, forcing them on the charity of the city. Citizens gathered together to raise money, among them John Bill Ricketts, the famous equestrian. Recently arrived from London, Ricketts had established a riding academy in Philadelphia while putting together a new form of entertainment called the "circus." The premiere performance was offered on April 2, 1793, and included such previously unknown feats as riding on his knees on the saddle, juggling on horseback, comic exploits, tightrope walking and the "Flying Mercury," whereby a boy posed on one foot stood on Ricketts' shoulder while Ricketts stood in the same manner with one foot on the saddle, the horse being at full speed. The entertainment was so unique even George Washington attended a performance, on April 22. Before the Philadelphia season ended on July 22 Ricketts' company held a benefit performance for

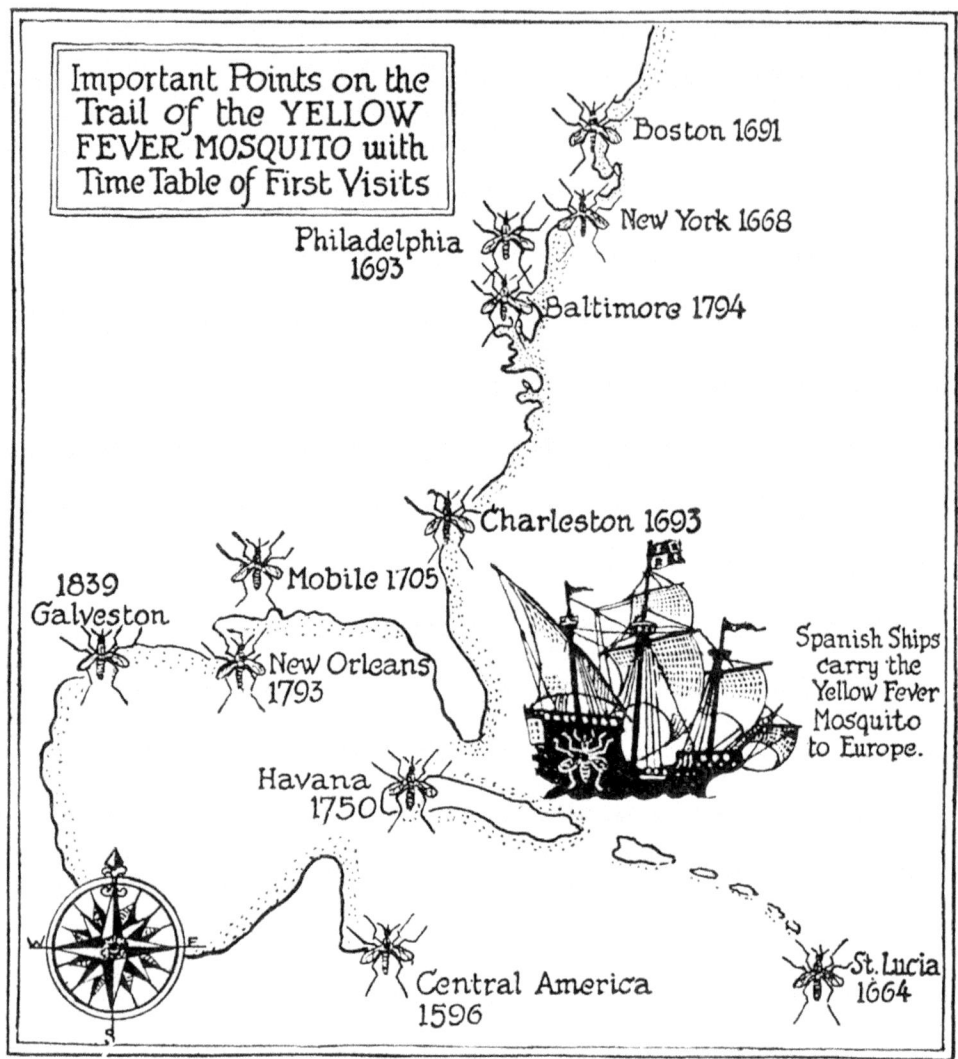

This map illustrates the major cities in the United States stricken with yellow fever during the 1500s through the 1700s. Many scientists believed the disease was brought to the United States on sailing vessels from tropical countries rather than being indigenous to the country. Intense debates over how yellow fever was transmitted often pointed the finger at fomites, or infected clothing and baggage, while others believed it was passed by contact with an infected person, contracted by inhaling miasma, or poisoned air, or through the soil, particularly that from swamps and cemeteries (author's collection, from *Health Heroes*, 1926).

needy immigrants.[11] In the coming yellow fever epidemic, several "Theatrical Adventurers" who also came to Philadelphia from London would perish, including Marshall, Miss Webb, Miss Brett, Hodgninson and the whole family of Mr. Milburne.[12] By the end of July more than 1,000 refugees had arrived. That number doubled in August. It was also the month when the dying began.

On August 3, Dr. Isaac Cathrall was called to treat a sick woman named Mrs. Parkinson, who lived with her husband, Richard, and two daughters at the lodging house of

Richard Dennie (also spelled "Denny") on Water Street. The couple and their two daughters had arrived in the brig *Ann and Mary* from Dublin at the end of June. Also residing at the house was an Englishman and two young Frenchmen. Mrs. Parkinson suffered from a violent pain in the head and back, fever and great thirst. On August 4 Dr. Physick treated the Englishman, who died the same night. By the 6th, Mrs. Parkinson had become delirious and crimson-colored spots appeared on her neck, breast and arms. She died on August 7 and was soon followed by one of the French seamen and Mr. and Mrs. Dennie, neither of whom survived more than seven days. The other Frenchman took new lodgings but died a few days later. Mr. Parkinson and his daughters escaped the infection.[13]

At the time, there was little apprehension of greater danger. In a letter written October 16 the writer offered details of what happened next: "Mrs. Parkinson, who appears to have been the first patient in this disorder, was seized on the 3rd of August, and died on the 7th.... From the first appearance, till towards the close of August, the dangerous enemy we had in the city was hardly known; the deaths of several persons were successively announced in the Papers, and read with the unconcern usual on such occasions."[14] Unconcern quickly turned to apprehension as the death toll steadily climbed, forcing locals to wonder whether the "Barbados distemper" from 1762 had reappeared. But just as the origin of that deadly fever had never been settled, the old question resurfaced. Had this malignant fever been introduced into Philadelphia by newly arrived refugees from the West Indies or was there a local source of contagion? One answer seemed to present itself, adequately summed up in a letter from a young gentleman in New York to his father in Bath, England: "A ship arrived at Philadelphia with a cargo of hides and coffee: the hides in the course of the voyage became putrid, and of course infected the coffee; the result of which was, those who were unfortunate enough to drink of it were seized with a mortal disorder called the Yellow Fever; its infections and direful effects have already been related."[15]

The ship referenced was the sloop *Amelia* from St. Domingue, which had arrived carrying cargo and refugees. The contaminated coffee was dumped on July 24 on Ball's Wharf, where it continued to putrefy, creating noxious effluvia. On August 19, Dr. Benjamin Rush assembled the known facts, identifying several other victims who had passed near the contaminated area and thus had become exposed to the miasma before contracting the fever. From these he deducted the illness sweeping the city to be "bilious remitting yellow fever," emanating from the fouled air of putrid coffee. The news was not well received, particularly among Dr. Rush's peers, who scoffed at his idea of local contamination, pointing instead to the immigrants they believed imported the disease from the West Indies.

Regardless of origin, the mysterious disease, under Rush's designation "yellow fever," spread like wildfire. On any average day in Philadelphia there were two or three deaths; but by August 21 twelve deaths occurred in the city and by August 24 the number had risen sharply to seventeen. The following day Rush wrote to his wife that the disease "not only mocks in most instances the power of medicine, but it has spread thro' several parts of the city remote from the spot where it originated."[16]

Rush applied to Mayor Matthew Clarkson, describing his case and warning that unless the putrid material accumulated in the streets and along the waterfront were cleaned, matters would quickly deteriorate. The mayor promptly issued an order for the "scavengers" (street cleaners) to clean the streets, alleys and gutters, beginning at Water Street. On August 24 newspapers also carried warnings that the law required residents to keep their property clean and to set out trash every Monday and Thursday for collection.

Clarkson also called on the College of Physicians to meet on Sunday, August 25, and render a judgment on the nature of the disease, its cause, effect and possible remedies. In so doing, he became the first American official to apply to an organized medical society for help on a public health emergency. Governor Thomas Mifflin also became involved, asking Dr. Nathaniel Falconer, health officer of the port, and Dr. James Hutchinson, port physician, to ascertain the existence of an infectious disease and explain its origin and advice on methods to cure or at least mitigate its deadly effects. On August 24, Rush wrote to Hutchinson, making his case for a malignant fever. Omitting his diagnosis of yellow fever he described symptoms that he considered of "a mild remittent, and a typhus gravior," the deadliness of which he had not seen since 1762. Stressing his belief that the putrid coffee was the origin of the disease, he mitigated his conviction by adding, "whether propagated by contagion, or by the original exhalation, I cannot tell."[17]

Falconer and Hutchinson were quickly overwhelmed by petitions demanding they visit every newly arrived vessel to determine whether there were sick aboard. On August 23 Falconer drafted a notice to the newspapers, providing details of the Act of 1774 under which the port officer and physician's duties were described. Added to the text was his blunt wish that the people of Philadelphia may see "that there is no such power vested in the officer."[18]

While doctors were arguing their various opinions, Philadelphians were desperate to try to protect themselves. Camphor and vinegar, old English standbys, were the main items used to ward off personal contagion. For wider areas, many suggested another ancient remedy: burning large fires in the streets to stop the progress of infections disorders. In a published letter dated August 24, one writer argued against such measures, citing Dr. Hodges' account of the 1665 pestilence in London. Desperate to stop the plague, the governors ordered fires to burn in the streets for three days, despite objections from physicians who "were different of the success, *as the air itself was uninfected,* and therefore rendered such a showy and expensive project superfluous, and these conjectures were supported by the authority of antiquity and Hippocrates himself." Before the three days had expired the rains poured down and immediately afterward "the most fatal night ensued, wherein more than *four thousand* expired."[19] Five days later Mayor Clarkson, after hearing from the College of Physicians, issued an order prohibiting such fires and warning that offenders would be prosecuted. Unconvinced, a writer signing himself "B" wrote to the newspaper, advising that the late Dr. Chevot, who had lived for a number of years in the West Indies, "found nothing so good to stop the progress of the yellow fever as firing of cannon." "B" repeated the story that a ship of war with putrid fever aboard often found the pestilence gone after an obstinate engagement and added that Philadelphians would "cheerfully pay the expense of the powder." Perhaps as a means of augmenting his argument, he added that despite the mayor's proclamation of August 24 the city was not cleaner than usual, at least where he lived between Sixth and Seventh, in Market Street.[20]

What was more important, one writer penned a letter to *Dunlap's American Daily Advertiser* August 29, making an astute observation:

> As the late rain will produce a great increase of mosquitoes in the city, distressing to the sick, and troublesome to these who are well, I imagine it would be agreeable to the citizens to know, that the increase of those poisonous insects may be much diminished, by a very simple and cheap mode,

which accident discovered.—Whoever will take the trouble to examine their rain water tubs, will find millions of the mosquitoes fishing about the water with great agility, in a state not quite prepared to emerge and fly off:—Take up a wine-glass full of the waters, and it will exhibit them very distinctly. into this glass pour half a tea-spoon-full, or less, of any common oil, which will quickly diffuse over the surface, and by excluding the air, will destroy the whole brood. Some will survive two or three days—but most of them sink to the bottom, or adhere to the oil on the surface within twenty-four hours. A gill of oil poured into a common rain-water cask, will be sufficient:—large cisterns may require more; and where the water is drawn out by a pump or by a cock, the oil will remain undisturbed, and last for a considerable time. Hickory ashes have been tried without effect. A. B.

The College of Physicians

Sixteen out of twenty-six members of the College of Physicians met on Sunday, August 25, 1793, to discuss the fever raging through Philadelphia and offer the government a plan that would it was hoped would mitigate and eventually stop its progress. The president of the College, Dr. John Redman, was absent, but three other officers attended: Vice President William Shippen; Secretary Samuel Powel Griffitts; and Benjamin Say, treasurer. Other members present included Adam Kuhn, Drs. Thomas Parke, Caspar Wistar, Jun., Benjamin and Samuel Duffield, John Gibbons, Andrew Ross, John Carson, William McIlvaine, Nathan Dorsey, James Hutchinson, William Currie and Benjamin Rush. Similar to the London Board of Physicians, these were a select association of famous men, those dedicated to the advancement of the art and science of physic. For the most part, they were separate in training and philosophy from the eighty physicians in the city and those in the outlying districts who fought disease through observation and experience.

Within this august college there existed a wide range of opinion. Because of the fact all people breathed the same air, Rush translated that into a belief that all fevers were caused by miasma, or putrid air. Calling malignant yellow fever *synochus icteroides,* Currie believed it to be a contagious disease of foreign origin, transmitted only from one sick person to another, although he acknowledged that infections were "strengthened by a particular construction of the atmosphere."

Once they had finished discussing their opinions, Rush, Hutchinson, Say and Wistar were asked to create a formal report; Rush agreed to write it and have it ready for review the following morning. On Monday, August 26, eleven of the Fellows met and unanimously passed the eleven-point document.[21] From there it went to Major Clarkson, who approved it and forwarded it to the newspapers. On Wednesday, August 28, Philadelphians got the chance to read it. The opening paragraph stated, "The College of Physicians having taken into consideration the malignant and contagious fever, which now prevails in this city, have agreed to recommend to their fellow citizens, the following means of preventing its progress."

(1) All unnecessary contact with infected persons should be avoided

(2) A mark must be placed upon the door or window of houses where infected persons reside

(3) Infected persons should be placed in large, airy rooms. Strict attention should be placed on cleanliness by frequent change of bed linen and by removing as speedily as possible all offensive matter

(4) A hospital should be set up in the neighborhood of the city for those poor individuals who did not have the above advantages in a private house

(5) The tolling of the bells at funerals should be stopped

(6) Persons who died of the fever should be buried in carriages [coffins] in as private a manner as possible

(7) Streets and wharves should be kept as clean as possible. "As the contagion of the disease may be taken into the body, and pass out of it without producing the fever, unless it be rendered active by some occasional cause. The following means should be attended to, to prevent the contagion being excited into action in the body."

(8) Avoid all fatigue of body and mind

(9) Avoid standing or sitting in the sun, in air currents or in the evening air

(10) Accommodate dress to the weather and to exceed rather in warm than in cool clothing

(11) Avoid intemperance, but use fermented Liquors, such as wine, beer and cider with moderation

The document concluded with the warning that the College conceived fires to be a very ineffectual and dangerous means of checking the progress of the fever, but they had "reason to place more dependence upon the burning of *Gun Powder*. The benefits of *Vinegar* and *Camphor* are confined chiefly to infected rooms, and they cannot be used too frequently upon handkerchiefs, or in smelling bottles, by persons whose duty calls them to attend or visit the sick. *Signed by Order of the College.* WILLIAM SHIPPEN, Jun. *Vice President.* SAMUEL POWELL GRIFFITTS, *Secretary.*"[22]

Without touching on treatments or cures or offering any "nosology" for the "malignant and contagious fever" (the words "yellow fever" were conspicuously absent), the proclamation offered little of value beyond outlining common-sense measures practiced during the outbreak of any epidemic during the mid-1700 and 1800s. The medical authorities made no allusions to what they believed caused the fever, nor was any reference made to putrid coffee or poisoned air, much less whether the fever might have stemmed from local contamination or imported disease. In actuality, it belied the danger by tacitly promising the "means of preventing its progress."

In fairness, although all the Fellows signed the recommendations, there was hardly any unanimity between them. Rush and his followers believed in the theory of local contagion but spoiled coffee was not the only possible culprit; others supported the idea that noxious fumes arising from graveyards poisoned the air. (This belief would also be extensively used to explain outbreaks of cholera.) One physician who had not attended the August 25 meeting quickly voiced his own ideas in a letter to the newspaper. Dated the day after the report was issued, "Quaestor Veritatis," who described himself as "a Physician whose reading has been extensive, and whose experience has not been more limited, than that of several of the members of that very respectable body," argued that what Philadelphians were experiencing "is only a modification of the influenza, or epidemic catarrh, which has prevailed more or less in this city, for the last four weeks."

Observing that the long, continued heat and drought had "relaxed, debilitated and disposed the bodies of the inhabitants to fevers, attended with symptoms of putrefaction, or a gangrenous tendency of the solids," he deduced "it is under such circumstances, that the small pox, and meazles, become highly putrid and malignant." In denouncing the idea that more people died in the vicinity of Water Street (thus indicating a specific local contagion), he offered the opinion that a more rational explanation would be that the air was less pure there, "owing to the situation of the houses half buried under ground;

and the quantity of filth and stagnant water, excrementuous substances in a state of putrefaction, whereby the air is not only more confined, but is robbed of its vivifying principle, for want of which, fire cannot be kindled, nor animals breathe."

Worse, in his opinion, was Article 2, which was, as he described it, "highly reprobated by many of the citizens, as setting a mark on the houses containing sick persons would give sanction to an opinion of the plague being among us, and be the means not only of effectually excluding all friendly offices, but would be the occasion of leaving the unhappy sufferers to perish without assistance, as wretches devoted by Heaven, to inevitable destruction." Not yet finished, the author added, "The publication of the Directions alluded to, appears to be unadvised and cruel, as they tend to give unnecessary terror," and would prevent "all commercial intercourse along the wharfs."[23]

Lacking specifics, both lay and professional healers were left to their own devices. None of them possessed the magic it would have taken to halt the fevers, and the number of deaths increased by staggering leaps and bounds. Details in a letter dated November 18, 1793, written by an accountant or business associate ("whose authenticity may be depended upon") to "a respectable House in Liverpool," attempted to explain the lack of correspondence by describing some of the miseries encountered. After noting the published opinion issued by the College of Physicians, which were "generally understood to be the same used in the East (and which we know from history was used in London), in times when the plague rages," he added that the marking of homes "was sufficient to alarm the inhabitants, and excite terror." The disorder spread quickly from the northeast parts of the city and threatened to become general: "It was so mortal in the beginning, that few survived the third and fifth [day], and it could not be ascertained for some time, whether any person had survived the eighth day; to be taken [ill], was considered nearly the same as to be dead: hence, there was a general abandoning of the sick to the care of the Blacks, who were supposed not liable to the infection. The nearest connections, with some exceptions, would not visit the chambers of their sick friends."[24]

Complicating matters, there were no pesthouses or lazarettos for the sick and destitute to go for medical treatment or shelter, and little money for the city government to provide for such services, transportation, treatment or medicines."

Budget for Philadelphia

Revenue		Expenses	
Personal taxes collected	£ 8,600	Watching & lighting the city	£4,000
Rent from public markets	£ 1,200	Paving & street cleaning	£4,000
Public wharves	£ 500	Salaries, maintenance and government expenses	£7,000
High Street ferry	£ 840		
Miscellaneous	£ 3,860		
Total	£15,000		£15,000[25]

Governor Thomas Mifflin wrote to Mayor Clarkson acknowledging that "a considerable alarm had taken place, in consequence of the appearance of an infectious disorder in the city." Clarkson forwarded the letter to James Hutchinson. On Tuesday, August 27, Hutchinson replied in a letter cosigned by Nathaniel Falconer. They stated that after consulting with their medical brethren and by observation they became convinced "a malignant fever has lately made its appearance in Water-street and in Kensington; principally in Water-street between Arch and Race-streets." A personal inspection made by Hutchinson the previous Thursday and Friday, August 22 and 23, revealed that east of Front

Street and between Arch and Race streets 67 persons were diseased, many with malignant fever. Thirteen, he noted, had since died. The disorder, he continued, "is spreading, and now appears in other places ... but in most cases, the contagion can be traced to Water-street."

In attempting to determine the cause, Hutchinson interviewed Dr. Say, "who has attended more in this disease than any other physician." Say stated that he first encountered the fever at Kensington on the 5th or 6th of August and that he did not perceive it in Water Street until the 12th or 15th, after which it spread rapidly. Noting that the "general opinion, both of the medical gentlemen, and of the inhabitants of Water-street, is, that the contagion originated from some damaged coffee," Hutchinson added that if Dr. Say's opinion was well-founded that he "observed the disease in Kensington previously to its appearance in Water-street, this cannot be the original cause of the contagion." The controversy would continue into September with some virulence.

Significantly, the port officers concluded that the malady "does not appear to be an imported disease; for I have heard of no foreigners or sailors, that have hitherto been infected; nor has it been found in any lodging houses; but it is, on the contrary, principally confined to the inhabitants of Water-street, and such as have done business, or had considerable intercourse, with that part of the city." He concluded, "The disease appears differently in different persons; its [sic] puts on all the intermediate Forms between a mild Remittent and the worst species of typhus Gravior."[26]

Reacting out of desperation to the expanding crisis, on August 26 the Guardians of the Poor took possession of John Bill Ricketts' amphitheatre, which had been left unoccupied since the troupe's departure for New York the previous July. Seven stricken paupers were brought there, but their presence was greatly unappreciated by those living near the enclosure, making the situation untenable. Three days later, Governor Mifflin again wrote to Mayor Clarkson. In a politely sarcastic letter he called his attention to the "infectious disorder" in the city, which had increased to "so great a degree" that it called for the "most vigorous and decisive exertions of the police ... to prevent the extension and to destroy, the evil." He added, with what must have been welcome relief to the mayor, "Whatever expense may be incurred upon the occasion if the Corporation [local government; no opening parenthesis to this sentence] should decline) I am confident the Legislature will defray."

Clarkson responded the same day, tersely informing the governor "every precaution which hath depended on the police of the city, has been attended to, in order to prevent the spreading of the calamitous disorder which now prevails. The streets have been cleaned, the wharves inspected for any prejudicial material and the market houses had been cleaned by means of a fire-engine." He added that the corporation had been convened and "entered upon such measures as appeared to them to be more likely to conduce to the relief of those, whose situations will require assistance. A Committee of their body have had an interview with the guardians of the poor, whose co-operation for the relief of the distressed, will, it is hoped, tend greatly to their comfort. An Hospital in an airy and healthy place is to be provided with all expedition: Indeed there is the most promising prospect that the benevolent disposition, for which the citizens have always been conspicuous, be exerted, in an extensive degree, and tend to the relief of suffering individuals, as well as to the safety of the community." He promised nitre would be burned on Water Street and another cleaning would commence the next day.[27]

Clarkson's committee, appointed on the 29th, resolved the same day to procure a suitable home for the sick at some distance from town. They also resolved that the Guardians of the Poor should appoint persons to seek out infectious diseases among the impoverished, and finally, they gave themselves permission to call upon the mayor "from time to time" for funds to enable them to carry out their duties. Moving quickly, by the 31st the committee had settled upon a house at Bush-Hill owned by the absent William Hamilton. As the owner had no local agent, Clarkson and Mifflin gave permission for the group to take possession of the mansion and the buildings adjoining the east wing without the consent of the tenant. That same day the four indigents still living at Ricketts' amphitheatre were removed and transported to the grand old mansion once so admired by Abigail Adams.[28]

Ricketts and his circus people may have fled, but as testimony to the fact the city of Philadelphia had not entirely lost their desire, if not their outright need, for relief from the grim news of disease, Jean-Pierre Francois Blanchard arrived. The famous aeronaut, having fled France to avoid the conflict of the Napoleonic wars,[29] began taking out advertising for his "46th aerial flight to the celebrated regions." Described as the "adopted citizen of the principal cities in Europe, pensioner of the French nation, member of several academies, &c.," he also brought his own invention, "a CARRIAGE, which runs without the assistance of horses, and goes as fast as the best post-chaise. *An Automation in the Shape of an Eagle*, chained to the tongue of the carriage, and guided by the traveller, who holds the reins in his hands, directs it in every respect. This extraordinary Carriage cannot only travel on all roads, but likewise ascend any mountain which is accessible to any common carriage. The distance it may proceed is unlimited, as there are no springs in the case, that require winding up."

On Monday, August 26, at his Rotunda in Chestnut Street, between 7th and 8th streets, Blanchard proposed to make two experiments, one of natural philosophy and the other of mechanism: "An Air Balloon of 11,498 2.3ds cubic feet, will be filled with atmospherical air in the space of six minutes (instead of ten hours, which were required formerly) by the help of a machine which he has invented and but lately brought to perfection. The Eagle fixed to the Carriage beginning its flight, the Carriage will come out from it, stand, and run round the place, carrying two persons." The entrance fee was half a dollar; gentlemen with dogs accustomed to the chase were requested not to bring them, "as experience has shown that they may prove very dangerous to the Eagle, which imitates nature to perfection." Blanchard promised to make experiments with his balloon and his carriage every day but Sunday. The expense and the plague notwithstanding, the entertainment must have proven successful, as advertisements ran in the newspapers until October 9.[30]

As the month drew to a close, Mayor Clarkson estimated 140 people had died of the plague; Dr. Rush believed the number to be as high as 325.[31] They hoped September would bring relief. They were wrong. Matters were about to take a turn for the worse.

Chapter 5

"Particulars of the Plague in Philadelphia"

The Physicians differed about the mode of treating the disorder, and published opposite systems; many of them were taken sick, and it became difficult to procure a visit; many were left to their own opinions, and adopted the mode published by the Physician that stood highest in their esteem, and many perished without any aid at all.[1]

The title of this chapter appeared over the contents of a letter written November 18, 1793, part of which was quoted in Chapter 4; a second segment appears above. Written by a businessman a month after one of the deadliest episodes in American history, the writer may well have added, "The physicians differed about the cause of the disorder, and published opposite opinions." The main bone of contention continued to center around Dr. Rush's and others' belief that "damaged coffee" was the source of the malignant fever.

On September 2 a letter penned by "Medicus" ran in *Dunlap's American Daily Advertiser* and began with the acerbic comment that "as this coffee has made as much noise, and with equal cause, as the scratchings of the *Cock Lane Ghost*, did in the city of London, it may not be amiss to enquire, how far the opinion is founded on truth." (The story of the Cock Lane Ghost began in January 1762, when William Kent married Elizabeth Lynes. She died in childbirth and several months later Kent married her sister Fanny and lodged in a house on Cock Lane owned by William Parsons. Kent loaned Parsons money that Parsons refused to repay, leading to a lawsuit. While Kent was away on business, Fanny claimed she heard mysterious scratchings in the bedroom she shared with Parsons' daughter, Elizabeth. Fanny attributed the sounds to her dead sister warning her of impending death. The Kents subsequently moved to new lodgings, where Fanny died of smallpox. The scratchings in Elizabeth "Liz" Parsons' bedroom increased after Fanny's death and her father began communicating with the ghost, using yes/no questions and a system of knocking to communicate with the supposed ghost of Fanny Kent, which revealed that Fanny had actually died of arsenic administered by her husband. The situation fascinated the public and the house became a popular attraction, with Parsons charging a fee for any who wished to communicate with the spirit. With the suspicion of murder thrown on him, Kent eventually succeeded in interesting a number of important people, including Samuel Johnson, to help him. There were suspicions that the Parsons were in collusion, and the fraud was uncovered when Liz was caught hiding a wooden clapper under her clothes. William Parsons was convicted of conspiracy, sent to the pillory and imprisoned for two years.² The Cock Lane Ghost became an international sensation, with Charles Dickens, Herman Melville and other Victorian authors touching on the story in their writing. The story was also included in a fascinating segment in the 1945 film *Dead of Night*.)

Medicus singled out a paper published by "R" (Rush) stating, "From what facts R has formed his opinion, I know not." He then proceeded to quote both ancient and modern authorities on the subject of "putrid matter" before pointing out that some inhabitants from Passyunk Road had taken the coffee from Ball's Wharf, brewed and drank it, yet remained in perfect health. The writer then added that recent investigation of the fever proved it had broken out at Kensington "long before it did on Water-street."

In what was to fester into professional antagonism and public feuding, Philadelphia physicians began questioning one another and the methods they used to treat the fever. Rush blamed Dr. Benjamin Duffield for penning the above article under the pen name "Medicus." Wounded by the charge, which he denied, Duffield wrote to his friend: "If to differ from you in medical Opinions is a Crime, it is one that every man must at one Time or other in his Life, be guilty of with some of his Fellow Travellers in the Difficult Road of Science."³ This fateful September there would be many difficult roads to follow and many disagreements. But through it all Dr. Rush would remain a constant. In a letter written to him on September 1 by Samuel Powel, Speaker of the Senate, he was asked for any positive word to allay the fears of the public and keep members of the government in town. Rush's answer was succinctly penned: "I know of but one certain preventative of the disorder, & that is to keep at a distance from infected persons and places."⁴

The unnamed writer of the November 18 letter cited at the beginning of the chapter observed how this advice was taken:

> In this situation, a great part of the inhabitants fled to the country in every direction: of these, some were taken with the disorder, and died; but we have heard no instance of any person, who had previously resided in the country taking the infection from them. Some few, from an apprehension of duty, more for the security of their property, and yet, more, because they had not the means of removal, or a place to remove to, staid in the city; and it is computed that above one-third of the whole number of inhabitants went away. Those who staid were cautious how they went about the streets, so that the city appeared in a degree to be depopulated: business of almost every kind was suspended; inward bound ships came to the villages down the river; and for nearly two months our streets were deserted by all, but a few sorrowful persons, walking, "as with their hands on their loins," about the necessary concerns of the sick, and hearses conducted by negroes, mostly without followers, to and from the different grave-yards.⁵

Death Toll for the First Two Weeks of September

Sunday, 1st	17
Monday, 2nd	18
Tuesday, 3rd	11
Wednesday, 4th	23
Thursday–Saturday	20 average
Sunday, 8th	42
Monday, 9th	30
Tuesday, 10th	30
Friday, 13th	37
Saturday, 14th	48⁶

Out of desperation and in keeping with traditional beliefs, on September 5 Governor Mifflin ordered quarantine for any vessel arriving from the West Indies. No ships were allowed to come farther up the river than Mud Island until it had been examined, and captains were instructed to hold any sick passengers or crew until they were seen by Nathaniel Falconer, health officer of the port. Six days later, Mifflin wrote to Falconer, confirming that an act of the general assembly had been passed sanctioning him to reiterate his instructions: "In doing so you will understand that I mean, particularly, to direct your vigilance to the patients in the hospital [at Bush Hill]." In addition he enclosed a warrant for $1,000 to be used in hiring two assistants at $3 per diem and to hire a boat with sufficient hands for the purpose of visiting all vessels "that are subject to examination, in pursuance of the laws, or my instructions for regulating the health office."

In the same letter the governor informed Falconer that he had appointed Drs. Samuel Duffield and James Mease as joint physicians of the port,[7] replacing James Hutchinson, who had died of yellow fever September 6. The same day they received a similar letter from Governor Mifflin, Duffield and William Allen cosigned under the title of Deputy Health Officer a letter to Mifflin informing him that the ship *Hope,* commanded by Captain Lowell out of Londonderry, had been inspected. After "strictest enquiry" they concluded there was no "contagious disease" among the 350 passengers. The fact that they found "only Seven persons died, belonging to this Ship, since she came to the Fort, which is now Eleven Days," apparently did not appear significant to them.[8] On September 7 Mifflin departed the city for his country estate at Falls of Schuylkill. That left only the steadfast Mayor Clarkson, John Barclay (his predecessor as mayor) and three Guardians of the Poor—James Wilson, Jacob Tomkins, Jr., and William Sansom—to govern the city.

As if Philadelphia needed any more controversy, Dr. Hutchinson's death sent shock waves through the city, not least because of the circumstances surrounding his demise. In late August Dr. Rush had re-read the folio of Dr. John Mitchell, originally given to him by Benjamin Franklin years earlier. Mitchell's descriptions of yellow fever epidemics in Virginia stood in stark contrast to conventional medical wisdom, the aim of which had always been to strengthen the body so that it might be enabled to fight off disease. Mitchell's primary tenet held that in malignant fevers the best cure was to purge poisons from the body to such an extent that the patient became weak almost to the point of death. Only through the "art" of extreme mechanical or chemical purges (as opposed to the natural course of evacuation) could the victim hope to recover.

Rush assimilated Mitchell's doctrine as inspirational. The most powerful purgative he knew was that prescribed by Dr. Thomas Young to soldiers in the Revolutionary army: 10 grains of calomel and ten of jalap, called "ten-and-ten." At the time, this was considered an exorbitant dose, far beyond the limits of conventional practice. (Thomas Young [1731–1777] was a New York physician in the 1760s. He later moved to Massachusetts and as a member of the Sons of Liberty participated in the Boston Tea Party. To avoid arrest by the British authorities he moved his medical practice to Philadelphia in 1775 and on December 14, 1776, he was appointed senior surgeon at the Continental Hospital in that city. He contracted yellow fever while working in the hospital and died June 24, 1777.)[9]

Rush first tried his remedy on August 29 by forcing his concoction down the throat of a dying man. When the man providentially recovered Rush guardedly believed he had finally found a cure. After several more successful attempts Rush increased the dose to 15 grains of calomel and administered a bolus every six hours until achieving four or five large evacuations. To further the treatment he added an antiphlogiston regimen consisting of cold drinks, cold baths, cool air and soft diet. These he used in combination with extreme bloodletting with the intention of removing all inflammatory stimulus that might operate on the "inquiline humours" of the body.

By September 2, Rush began spreading news of his unorthodox cure to his fellow physicians but many of them were skeptical. Nevertheless, when Dr. Hutchinson, the port physician and Rush's personal antagonist, fell ill from the fever, Rush offered his cure. It was summarily rejected on the argument that a purge was not required. The following day, Rush presented his cure to the Fellows of the college under the belief that he had successfully recovered 8 out of 12 patients with one day's treatment. By August 5, in a letter to his wife, Julia, he wrote that although the fever was still spreading it was no more fatal than a common bilious fever when treated with his mercury compound: "I now save 29 out of 30 of all to whom I am called on the first day and many to whom I am called after it." He added, "Never before did I experience such sublime joy as I now felt in contemplating the success of my remedies. It repaid me for all the toils and studies of my life. The conquest of this formidable disease was not the effect of accident, nor of the application of a single remedy; but it was the triumph of a principle in medicine."[10]

Dr. Samuel Powel Griffitts became an adherent, as did Dr. Charles Caldwell, among others. Along with Hutchinson, Dr. William Currie became the principal objector to Rush's extreme measures. In his pamphlet, *A Description of the Malignant Infectious Fever Prevailing at Present in Philadelphia; with an Account of the Means to Prevent Infection, and the Remedies and Method of Treatment, Which Have Been Found Most Successful* (1793), Currie, identified as a "Fellow of the College of Physicians, and Member of the American Philosophical Society," stated that the present disease, "like all other varieties of putrid fever, arises from, and is produced by specific contagion, and may be communicated from those labouring under the disease, to persons in the most perfect state of health." Bypassing the argument of whether it was of local or foreign origin, he added that the disease under consideration "though certainly infectious is nevertheless only communicable under particular circumstances. Those circumstances removed, no infection can possibly take place."

Dismissing the idea of a general contamination of the atmosphere as being contrary to, and contradicted by, observation and experience by reassured citizens that walking the streets placed them in no danger, "as the miasmata, or contagious exhalations from the bodies of the diseased have never been known to be conveyed by the air many feet beyond the chamber of the sick, except by means of clothes or other porous substances which have been in contact with, or very near to, the body of one labouring under the disease." The only way the fever was communicable was for a healthy person to spend extended periods in a small, closed sick chamber or to come in contact with the body or bedclothes. Exposing contaminated material to open air for several days and afterwards baking them in an oven effectively removed any risk of disease. He stressed that by "constant ventilation of their own as well as the apartments of the sick; tak[ing] moderate and frequent exercise in the open air when dry and serene; mak[ing] moderate use of relishing aliment copiously seasoned with salt and culinary spices, and drink[ing] wine or other strong liquors more liberally than customary; avoid[ing] intemperance of every description; but above all, the monstrous and abominable vice of getting drunk—I venture to pronounce with the most positive confidence, that the disease will not, cannot spread."

The various expedients made use of by all classes to preserve themselves—"camphor bags, amulets of dried frogs, tarred ropes, sponge dipped in vinegar of the four thieves, the salt of spices (as it is vulgarly called), the smoking of segars" were "productive of more evil than good," as they tended to depress the spirits. ("Vinegar of the four thieves" was a common expression reputedly dating back to the time of the Black Plague; similar recipes had been used since the time of Hippocrates. Herbs such as wormwood, marjoram, sage, cloves, rosemary, horehound, lavender flowers, fresh rue and large measures of camphor were added to vinegar, either red or white. The mixture was used by rubbing it on the hands, temples and behind the ears when approaching a plague victim. The story behind the name originated anywhere from the 14th to the 18th century and was said to have come about when thieves were caught robbing graves and in exchange for leniency promised to share the secret potion they used to ward off the disease.)[11]

Currie further avowed, "The best, and I believe I may say the only neutralizer or corrector of contagion yet discovered, is the pure vital air of the atmosphere." (The issue of "vital air" would reappear in 1799 at Albany, New York, when legislatures were attempting to determine whether contagious diseases such as yellow fever and cholera were of domestic or foreign origin. The lawyer defending manufacturers producing soap (believed to poison the atmosphere), introduced the work of Citizen Guyton, stating that "the chief difference between common air and pestilential are consisted merely in this; that in the former, the septon with caloric formed azotic air, and the oxygene constituted vital air, each distinct from the other; whereas in the latter case the septon and oxygene are chemically blended with each other, base with base."[12] Simply stated, vital air meant pure air or air rich in oxygen. Currie continued: "This salubrious aeriform fluid may therefore be most usefully employed for restoring to health the unfortunate sufferers under the present malignant disorder." The means of adding vital air consisted of "frequently deflagrating [burning with great heat] nitre on burning charcoal in different parts of the apartment: this is known to evolve considerable quantities of this vivifying air." Pouring vinegar on a hot iron, whitewashing the walls and growing pepper grass (known to have detoxifying properties) in vessels containing fresh water and cotton were also thought to purify the air.

Currie's cure consisted of tartar emetic in barley water or "camomile" tea until the stomach operated either upwards or downwards, followed by a mild purgative and a sudorific anodyne at night to promote free perspiration. A spoonful of camphorated vinegar or a solution of salt of tartar in lime juice given in barley water or gruel every two hours and the free use of lime juice or tamarind beverage also encouraged perspiration. Bed linen was to be soaked in vinegar and dried before use and windows and doors were to be left open. Once the pulse abated, the physician suggested half a grain of tartar emetic mixed in a peppermint or cinnamon draft with 25 drops of laudanum and 2–3 drachms of acetated ammonia.

Contrary to Rush's new belief that debility of the body was to be sought through purges and bleeding, Currie argued the opposite, stating bleeding led to a "state of debility" from "an increased action and apparent power in the arterial system." Likewise, he dismissed the use of mercury as being too strong, advocating blisters between the shoulders and on the legs. Indirectly refuting Rush's theory, he noted, "For nothing is more pernicious, or even fatal, than that any part or function should be forced to make exertions incompatible with its strength; and there is the more danger of ill-timed remedies in the present fever, as with the state of weakness there is conjoined a state of excessive irritability for the first two or three days." In any case, "where the skin becomes yellow, and the countenance appeared cadaverous, has hitherto proved mortal."

Instead of working together to restore Hutchinson to health, the divide between

Philadelphia physicians became even greater. Drs. Currie and Benjamin Smith Barton were called to treat the physician of the port. Ignoring Dr. Rush's loudly proclaimed successes with his new system of weakening the body to promote healing, the pair applied Currie's treatments. Hutchinson's death on September 6 only increased the animosity.

In an attempt to restore order, the College of Physicians met on Saturday, September 7. Presiding over the meeting was the president of the College, John Redman, who spoke at length about the fever of 1762 and compared it to the current epidemic, which had already proven far more deadly. Without offering any specific remedy of his own he called for cooperation. In support of Rush, his former pupil, Redman attempted to walk a middle road by noting that Rush's harsh evacuation treatment of mercury and jalap used at the beginning of the fever might very well succeed by immediately clearing the stomach and intestines, thus permitting the application of the more gentle curative remedies supported by Currie and his followers to ultimately heal the patient.[13]

"The poor negroes"

A letter written September 16, 1793, provides a firsthand account of how the situation in Philadelphia had deteriorated:

> The ravages committed by the Yellow Fever, or, as it is commonly called here, the Plague, are most alarming. It is supposed that it was brought from St. Domingo by the French who were obliged to quit that Island.
> Three of the Physicians in this city are dead, the rest have fled, except Dr. Rush, who still administers physical advice with the most humane attention. Philadelphia, so lately resounding with the "busy hum of men," is now desolate and dreary. You may pass in the middle of the day through the streets and meet no persons, save the poor negroes bearing the corpses in great numbers to the burying ground.[14]

There were more than 25,000 African Americans in Philadelphia in 1793, of which 2,000 were freedmen. There was little chance for economic improvement among them but they had the support of two leading Quakers: the Reverend James Sproat and Dr. Benjamin Rush. The city's Abolition Society was also a model for all other such groups in the newly formed United States.

"Early in September," as inscribed in Absalom Jones and Richard Allen's pamphlet, *A Narrative of the Proceedings of the Black People during the Late Awful Calamity in Philadelphia in the Year 1793*, a solicitation appeared in the public papers "to the people of colour to come forward and assist the distressed, perishing, and neglected sick; with a kind of assurance, that people of our colour were not liable to take the infection." This assurance, believed by most, if not all, physicians of the time, including Rush, stemmed from the early African slave trade. Lacking knowledge that the natives had likely been exposed to yellow fever as children and were therefore not susceptible to a second attack, it was deduced that the black population possessed a natural immunity. That this was not the case would prove tragic for those working amidst the dying in Philadelphia.

Leaders of the African American community met to discuss Mayor Clarkson's request: "After some conversation, we found a freedom to go forth ... sensible that it was our duty to do all the good we could to our suffering fellow mortals." After investigating the scenes of woe, representatives met with Clarkson on September 6 to consult with him on how best to proceed. Clarkson recommended strict attention to the sick and the procurement of nurses, which was attended to by Absalom Jones and William Gray. "Soon after, the mortality increased, the difficulty of getting a corpse taken away, was such, that few were willing to do it, when offered great rewards. The black people were looked to. We then offered our services in the public papers, by advertising that we would remove the dead and procure nurses."

The lack of help of any sort became so great that convicts in the jail were offered partial or complete remittance of their sentences if they would work as nurses at the Bush Hill facility. Matthew Carey later wrote they "conducted themselves with great fidelity," unfortunately failing to mention that two-thirds of the volunteers were persons of color prompted to service by the elders of the African church.

In the midst to misery where there were few physicians left to tend the sick, Benjamin Rush called on Jones and Allen "to attend upon the sick, knowing we could both bleed [cup]; he told us we could increase our utility, by attending to his instructions, and accordingly directed us where to procure medicine duly prepared, with proper directions how to administer them, and at what stages of the disorder to bleed." If they were unable to judge the case, either Rush came in person or sent his pupil, Dr. Edward Fisher, to assist. "This has been no small satisfaction to us; for, we think, that when a physician was not attainable, we have been the instruments, in the hand of God, for saving the lives of some hundreds of our suffering fellow mortals."

Tragically, this did not endear the African Americans to their fellow citizens, for although the whites desperately needed their services many treated them as diseased outcasts or hurled aspersions on the prices alleged to have been charged by those who removed and buried the dead. In response, the black community attempted to explain: "At first we made no charge, but left it to those we served in removing their dead, to give what they saw fit—we set no price, until the reward was fixed by those we served." When that failed to carry the point, they published a statement of cash flow:

Cash received for burying the dead	£233.10.4
Cash paid for coffins	£ 33.0.0
For the hire of 5 men for 70 days	£378.0.0
Total	£411.0.0
Debts due (uncollectable)	£110.0.0
Operating loss	£177.9.8

In addition, they said, they had the cost of hearses, maintenance of their families for 70 days, sundry gifts made to poor families and the burial of several hundred poor persons for which service no fee was asked or received: "How much then may we not say we have suffered! We leave the public to judge."

One of those who judged was Matthew Carey, who charged that "blacks alone" took advantage of the situation by charging extravagant prices. Black leaders defended themselves: "It was natural for people in low circumstances to accept a voluntary, bounteous reward, especially under the loathsomeness of many of the sick, when nature shuddered at the thought of the infection." They reminded the public that as soon as Carey had been appointed for the relief of the sick at Bush Hill Hospital, he fled the city. They concluded, "We believe he has made more money by the sale of his 'scraps' [tracts] than a dozen of the greatest extortioners among the black nurses."

Tragically, Bush Hill Hospital was a pesthole where the dead and dying were "indiscriminately mingled together," the ordure and other evacuations remained "in the most offensive state imaginable," and the attendants "rioted on the provisions and comforts, prepared for the sick." Ultimately, the staff was reduced to two black women and the hospital was finally "reduced to order and good government." Perhaps the entire contribution of the heroic African Americans is best described by those of that community who witnessed untold misery: "It is unpleasant to point out the bad and unfeeling conduct of any colour [yet] [w]e can certainly assure the public that we have seen more humanity, more real sensibility from the poor blacks, than from the poor whites."

One eyewitness described the scenes of Philadelphia with which both colored and white had to contend:

> Friday morning [September 13] the fever continued with great violence; about 100 were buried on Thursday. I rode from one end of the town to the other on Thursday afternoon, in order to view the situation of the place; pausing by four or five burying-grounds, I saw, as well as I could count them, fifty graves open to receive the dead that evening. I suppose Potter's Field and the other burying-grounds, would receive as many more. While riding a square and a half I saw about ten or twelve corpses carried by negroes, some few people walking after two of them. They bury them all in the evening, or early in the morning, and then by negroes.
>
> I advise no person to go to Philadelphia at present; for if they do, and are taken sick, they will be turned or carried out of their lodgings—no money would save them, or procure a nurse, except it was a negro.[15]

Around the middle of the month it became apparent that the African Americans were sickening and dying from yellow fever. At first the white community denied this, falling back on what had, until this point, been accepted as medical fact, that those of dark skin were immune from the disease. "When the people of color had the sickness and died, we were imposed upon and told it was not with the prevailing sickness, until it became too notorious to be denied, and then we were told some few died but not many. Thus were our services extorted *at the peril of our lives,* yet you accuse us of extorting *a little money from you.*"

Reference to the Bill of Mortality revealed that in 1792 there were 67 people of color buried, but in the following year of the plague there were 305 deaths, a fourfold increase.

The authors of the *Narrative* pamphlet paid homage to Dr. Rush for allowing them to serve the sick, particularly in the operation of bleeding. During a 70-day period they bled upward of 800 people. Confirming, at least by observation, the physician's theory of violent treatment, Jones and Allen wrote that before the bleeding had finished many "felt a change for the better, and expressed a relief in their chief complaints; and we made it a practice to take more blood from them, than is usual in other cases; these in a general way recovered; those who did omit bleeding any considerable time, after being taken by the sickness, rarely expressed any change they felt in the operation."

Concluding their stirring work, Jones and Allen offered an old proverb they justly thought applicable "to those of colour who exposed their lives in the late afflicting dispensation":

> God and a soldier, all men do adore,
> In time of war, and not before;
> When the war is over, and all things righted,
> God is forgotten, and the soldier slighted.[16]

On January 23, 1794, Mayor Clarkson published an open letter cheerfully giving testimony to the character of Misters Jones and Allen, stating, "Their diligence, attention and decency of deportment, afforded me, at the time, much satisfaction."[17]

"A most calamitous proof"

Conditions in Philadelphia continued to deteriorate. A letter written September 16 offered a view of the self-imposed quarantine faced by those who had not already left:

> The stage boats are forbidden to carry any person from Philadelphia; the officers of the Customhouse will not admit any person into the office, and receive all papers through the windows; the vessels are not allowed to go above Market-street to unload; the stores are nearly one half shut up, and a great number of those open are left without a single person to take care of the property; the Bank is expected to be closed this day, as little or no business is done in it at present.[18]

News of the disease drove those in other states to a frightful pitch of fear. Mayor Richard Varick (who served from 1789 to 1801)—reacting to the panic stirring New Yorkers to demand drastic action—reminded citizens that intercourse between Philadelphia and New York City could not "lawfully be interrupted by any power in this state." To ease fears and minimize the threat of infection, he notified his constituents that the "Corporation" (the governing authorities of the city) had opened a hospital for those who unhappily became subject to the prevailing disease. Notwithstanding, on September 13 a meeting was held at the Tontine Coffee-House "to consider the best means of preventing the introduction of the alarming disease, that now ravages Philadelphia." Among demands from many was the severing of all communication between the two cities by "*every rout, and by every kind of conveyance,* except by post." Varick quickly decided quarantine was within his legal rights and two days later issued a protective warning[19]:

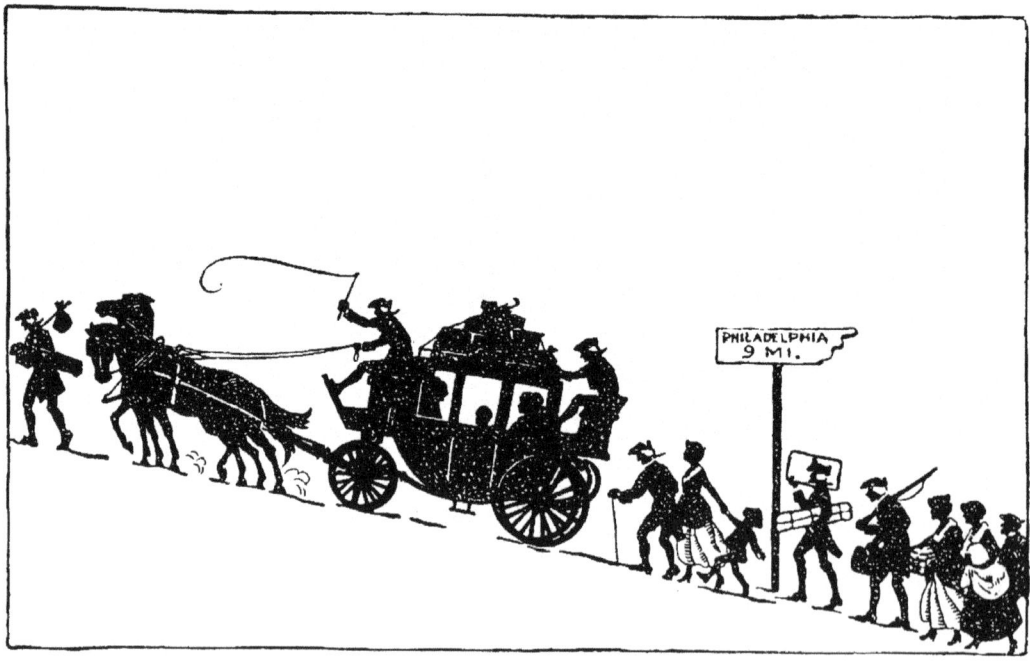

In the summer of 1793 Philadelphia was stricken with a horrific outbreak of yellow fever. Those who were able to fled the city, many heading toward New York. Unfortunately for them, "shotgun quarantines" were often established to keep them out for fear they would contaminate those in unaffected areas. The necessity for quarantine would linger into the 1900s, seriously crippling commerce both in and outside the United States (author's collection, from *Health Heroes*, 1926).

BY THE GOVERNOR

To prevent market-boats and others going on board or approaching too near vessels which may be performing quarantine, below the point of Governor's Island: Notice is hereby given, that the Health Officer will cause a Black Flag to be constantly displayed at the mast head of such vessels, respectively.

> Given at the city of New York, this 15th
> day of September 1793
> George Clinton.[20]

A letter written from New York City September 19 alerted friends in England not only of the tragedy but also the quarantine measures taken to keep the fever out of New York:

> We are much alarmed at the situation in which the city of Philadelphia has been for the last three weeks, in consequence of a malignant fever that has, and yet does, prevail there.
> The fever is called the yellow fever, and persons afflicted are usually taken with cold fits; and violent pains in the head and back; they then turn yellow, and become delirious and die in less than three days. The progress of this fever at Philadelphia is regular and rapid: through the streets great numbers have died, but such is the confusion every where occasioned, that no certain accounts can be procured, as to who is dead, or the precise number. Private letters say, that on Saturday last [September 14] 90 died; on Sunday 150; and on Monday 200. Considering that the average number of deaths, in healthy times, is not more than one a day, this will appear a large and alarming addition. The city itself exhibits a dismal spectacle; the shops all shut up, no business whatever is transacted, all the printers are either dead or sick, so that not even a newspaper is published, and more than 5000 of the most wealthy inhabitants have left it.
> Every precaution is taken here to prevent its entrance into this city; there have indeed been two persons from Philadelphia afflicted here, but they were instantly removed to an island, about two miles off, where they died. The Corporation and the inhabitants at large have come to a determination to have no intercourse with Philadelphia, and no person is suffered to enter this city from thence; for this purpose, the wharfs and every avenue are guarded, and the inhabitants patrole the different wards at night. These will, we trust, preserve us from this fatal calamity; a calamity regarded with more concern than that produced by the late war.[21]

One day later, on September 20, another New Yorker wrote, "All intercourse is prohibited between this place and Philadelphia; some folk, who had attempted a few days ago to come hither, were threatened to be sunk with the vessel, and they are now encamped on a small Island in the Bay.... Just now I have learnt that a person has been sent out of this town to the same island in the Bay, supposed to be ill of the Philadelphia fever."[22]

A Citizen's Committee was formed to assist the New York City Common Council, which in turn appointed a special committee comprising seven members to aid in the establishment of precautionary measures. Additionally, two physicians employed by the Citizen's Committee and three paid by the city joined the health officer in examining suspected cases of yellow fever. Not unaware that the health of Philadelphia affected those in the Empire State, the Bank of New York issued a loan of $5,000 to aid the needy there, charging only 5 percent interest, "in consequence of the benevolent use intended to be made of the money." Ultimately, only a limited number of fatalities from the disease occurred in New York, for which limiting intercourse with Philadelphia, cleaning the streets and ridding the city of nuisances (sanitation measures) were credited.[23]

New York's quarantine had unanticipated consequences. Alexander Hamilton and his wife, lately recovered from yellow fever, had departed Philadelphia for the safer confines of New York State. Unfortunately for them, a committee had been formed at Albany "and fixed a Gun-Boat at some distance from the city, where all vessels are stopt till the doctors examine the passengers." When Hamilton and his wife arrived they were denied admittance to the capital and sent to Mr. M'Gown's at Green Bush[24] (Greenbush, Rensselaer County, a suburb of Albany). The Hamiltons were not the only notable political figures to abandon Philadelphia. Although he was following his usual custom of spending the fall in Virginia, President George Washington's departure from the seat of national government on September 10 held the appearance of flight from the deadly yellow fever.

The secretary of the treasury had himself started a controversy in Philadelphia. Stricken with "the reigning putrid fever, and with much violence" on September 5 and his wife stricken soon after, Hamilton summoned Dr. Edward Stevens to his bedside. Stevens had lately arrived from St. Croix and carried with him a resume of having studied in Edinburgh. His mode of treatment, Hamilton wrote in an open letter to the public, "varies essentially from that which has been generally practiced—and I am persuaded, where pursued, reduces it to one of little more than ordinary hazard."[25]

Well aware of Hamilton's praise, Stevens wrote an open letter to Dr. John Redman, offering his cure to the physicians of the city. Describing the disease, he begins, "This disorder arises from contagion. Its approaches are slow and insidious at the commencement." Stevens recommended—at the first appearance of languor and lassitude—"a few extraordinary glasses of old Madeira," cold baths every morning and a gentle opiate combined with a few grains of the volatile salts and some grateful aromatic at night. If the condition "gained ground," he suggested relieving nausea with chamomile flowers or small doses of a cordial composed of peppermint and compound spirits of lavender, with cold baths every two to three hours. After each immersion a glass of old Madeira or a little brandy burnt with cinnamon was to be given.

Next followed an injection containing an ounce of powdered bark mixed with thin salep or sago to which a teaspoonful of laudanum had been added. Directly contradicting the regimen of Rush, Stevens stressed that "all emetics and violent cathartics should be avoided" and added, "all drastic cathartics do injury when the disease is in its advanced stage." If the pulse sank, he prescribed "small doses of the liquor mineralis hoffmanni" [hossmanni] or even vitriolic aether diluted with water. Musk and camphor in this stage also proved effectual. He concluded by reiterating the warning "against the ill consequences of debilitating applications of profuse evacuations in every period of this disease.... Should not violent evacuations which evidentially weaken and relax be avoided? These are hints which it would be presumptuous and assuming in me to extend or dwell upon; to gentlemen of such eminence as your colleagues it is sufficient to point out what reason and experience conjointly suggest to me."[26]

Add to this a letter signed "A.K." (Adam Kuhn), who quoted Dr. Stevens as saying "laxatives are never employed but when clysters are not attended with the desired effect of moving the bowels; that in violent attacks of the disease the bark clysters are repeated every two hours, and the water is applied to the body every 6 or 8 hours and even more frequently," adding "that the disease he has seen in this country is of the same nature with the malignant fever of the West Indies."[27]

For his part, Dr. Rush attempted to defend his use of the "short and simple mode" he adopted for treating the disorder. On September 11 he penned an open letter, allying himself with his first preceptor, Dr. Redman, then informing the public he had "waited upon Dr. Stevens" to obtain an account of his treatment for yellow fever while at St. Croix. Bluntly stating that he, in conjunction with Dr. Wistar, tried the method "and it failed in three cases out of four," Rush continued: "I had seen large doses of mercury given with safety in a bilious fever, in the year 1777, in the army of the United States, and I had read an account of its having been given with success in a disease in the East Indies, nearly related to our yellow fever; I therefore ventured to prescribe it." Rush said "the necessity and advantages of blood-letting after purging, are established," and he thought it prudent to defer bleeding until the morbid bile was discharged. Revealing how hurtful attacks on him had become, he added with bite, "The yellow fever now prevailing in our city, differs very materially from that which prevails in the West Indies, and in several particulars, from that of the year 1762. ... Prescribing for the name of a disease, without a due regard to the above circumstances, has slain more than the sword" (see Chapter 7 heading for the full quote Rush cited). He added that the success achieved by Dr. Kuhn's method were all on patients lightly affected and "they would probably have recovered much sooner, without the use of any of them."[28]

A day later, September 12, a more controlled but equally defensive Benjamin Rush wrote to the College of Physicians, again defending his regimen of bleeding:

> I have found bleeding to be useful, not only in cases where the pulse was full and quick, but where it was *slow* and *tense*. I have bled in one case, where the pulse beat only 48 strokes in a minute, and recovered my patient by it. The pulse became more full and more frequent after it. The state of the pulse seems to arise from an inflamed state of the brain, which shews itself in a preternatural dilatation of the pupils of the eyes. It is always unsafe to trust to the most perfect remissions of fever and pain in this state of the pulse. It indicates the necessity of more bleeding or purging. I have found it to occur most frequently in children.

Rush added that he lamented the contrariety of opinion among members of the College, which "seems to arise from the yellow fever being confounded with the jail or hospital fever." That thinly veiled insult was followed by a damning accusation: "The fevers of Breslau, Vienna, and Edinburgh, mentioned in some late publications, in which the cold bath was used with so much success, were of the latter kind. The two diseases are totally different from each other in their cause—seasons of prevailing—symptoms—danger, and method of cure." He signed the document, "Your Friend and Brother, Benjamin Rush."[29] It is doubtful those who opposed his system considered themselves either a friend or a brother after reading the tactless letter.

If Rush was tactless, Thomas Ruston was outright vicious. In a letter dated September 21, after giving his credentials as having practiced in Europe for several years where he treated putrid, malignant, jail, hospital and camp fevers, he offered his own cure from which he attained success both in Europe and America. In the early stages of fever he prescribed Ipecacuanha or tartar emetic, followed the next day by a purge of tamarinds, manna, rhubarb and water. He forbade his patients to eat animal food, allowing them to consume only ripe fruits and vegetables, especially potatoes and baked apples. The remaining part of the cure consisted in drinking plentifully of *cold* water or barley water with nitre.

In response to the idea that this cure might seem too simple to be true, he explained, "But let it be remembered, that nature is simple in all her operations, and this is the true and genuine method of nature." Regarding the use of bark, he found a fruit and vegetable diet and acidulous drinks served better to "resist debility and animal putrefaction." With respect to bleeding he firmly stated that in remittent fevers it tended to prolong the disease, but "in fevers that are purely putrid and malignant, you may almost as well, clap a knife at once, to the throat, as present a lancet to the arm of your patient."[30] Needless to say, Ruston did not precede his signature with "friendship" or "brotherhood."

Chapter 6

Most Unhappy Consequences

> *And there are not wanting cases of persons so deserted, as to be without a human being to hand them a drink of water. Parents have deserted their children—children their parents—husbands their wives—and wives their husbands. It is probably not exaggeration to suppose that a fourth or a fifth of the whole of the persons who have died, have been sacrificed through the consternation of those who ought to have taken care of them.*[1]

The above quotation, written by a Philadelphian on October 16, described the terrible summer of 1793. People abandoned their loved ones in a vain attempt to save themselves, and physicians, once the guardians of public health and security, fought one another, at times with vitriolic and sarcastic language, over proper methods of treatment. Businesses and banks were shuttered (the post office, the last public office to remain open, closed September 27), the highest ranking officials in the United States had fled, and many others were prevented from seeking asylum elsewhere "by the cruel, but indispensable regulations of other cities and places, to prevent infection."[2]

Even the indefatigable Benjamin Rush became ill with the fever on September 14. The next day he was bled of 10 ounces of blood before going out to treat his patients. That afternoon he took his prescribed mercury purge and went to bed. In the evening he took a second dose and was bled a second time, losing ten more ounces. For nourishment he drank weak tea and current-jelly water. On the 16th he bathed in cold water and slept better that night. The following day he felt well enough to write prescriptions and by the 19th he had resumed his rounds. Without mentioning yellow fever, a note in the *Federal Gazette* of the 17th reported, "Doctor Rush, we are happy to hear, is recovering fast from his late indisposition."

Unfortunately, Rush's miraculous recovery only strengthened his belief in his drastic system of bleeding and violent purging. Based on no scientific principles but that of observation (and those questionable), one of the greatest medical minds of the 1700s fell victim to one of the oldest and most dangerous of medical mistakes: that of forcing facts to fit a theory rather than allowing facts to confirm a theory. While he could not be condemned for his staunch support of bleeding, which had long been a foundation of medical practice, Rush, like many of his colleagues, acted on the false premise that the human body contained nearly twenty-five pounds of blood (in actual fact, it holds less than half that amount). Syphoning off a quart or more of blood at one time and then repeating the process over and over again until "four-fifths of the blood contained in the body are drawn away" actually induces cardiogenic shock, causing heart failure due to an inadequate supply of blood and oxygen to body tissues, in the same way as an acute myocardial infarction destroys the heart muscle.[3]

Equally dangerous, particularly in the long term or in excessive doses, was the use of mercury, now understood to be a deadly poison. In the definition taken from the *Lexicon Medicum* (1842), the author states, "Mercury is a very useful article both in the cure of diseases and the arts. There is scarcely a disease against which some of its preparations are not exhibited; and over the venereal disease it possesses a specific power. It is considered to have first gained repute in curing this disease, from the good effects it produced in eruptive diseases." That said, it soon became apparent that large doses were "attended with dangerous consequences." It was also observed that "mercury occasionally attacks the bowels, and causes violent purging, even of blood." The cure for mercury poisoning was "discontinuance for a time." Other remedies included purgatives, nitre, sulphur, gum-arabic, lime-water, camphor, Peruvian bark, sulphuret of potassa and blisters. *The Dispensatory of the United States* (1845), pages 377–381, stated the following:

> Mercury may also be resorted to in certain states of febrile disease. In some forms of the remittent fever of our own country, a particular stage of its course is marked by a dry tongue, torpor of the bowels, scanty urine, and an arid state of the surface. Here depletion by the lancet or leeches is often inadmissible, and the remedial measure most to be relied on is the judicious employment of mercury. It acts in such cases by increasing the secretions, and promoting the action of the exhalent capillaries, and, perhaps, by producing a new impression, incompatible with the action of the disease.

It was also noted that in Pearson's work on venereal disease he reported the occasional "disturbance of the vital functions," characterized by "small, frequent pulse, anxiety about the praecordia, pale and contracted countenance, great nervous agitation, and alarming general debility." In these cases, this indicated "a signal for discontinuing the mercury; as a further perseverance with it might be attended with fatal consequences." The potentially debilitating and deadly consequences of mercury poisoning were clearly established by 1793. Dr. Rush certainly would have been aware of that. Any layman knew the general principal that any living body would die from severe blood loss. Although both mercury and bloodletting were still recognized regimens half a century after the Philadelphia yellow fever epidemic, the difference lay in proportions. Rush's use of both was extreme and excessive. He dared break from established medical cannon and claimed wondrous cures. As J.M. Powell wrote in his exquisite work, *Bring Out Your Dead* (125), Rush "ignored the facts and kept his theory. He recognized no error, except in others."

Benjamin Rush recovered from his own bout of yellow fever because the men treating him (John Stall and John Redman Coxe, two of his five pupils who were living with him at the time) administered only two doses of mercury/jalap powders and bled only 20 ounces of blood from his body, a far less drastic regimen than the physician prescribed for his own patients. Regardless of this, Rush had no better proof than the success "upon his own body" and persisted in his methods.[4]

Such was Dr. Rush's reputation that his formula of 15 grains of jalap and 10 grains of calomel, given three times a day, lived long after the Philadelphia fever. Rush never patented a mercury pill or formula (although an individual—or individuals—with the surname "Lee" did receive U.S. patents for a bilious pill between 1796 and 1800, and 50 dozen pills of "Rush's Thrunderbolts"—aka "Rush's Thunderclappers"—were taken on the Lewis and Clark expedition).[5]

"...as for the federal government, it is neither here nor there."

So wrote a Philadelphian, the missive dated September 21 and published in the *Carlisle Gazette* on the 25th. "Half the citizens of Philadelphia (nearly 30,000) have become inhabitants of the country," he added. Huts in the environs of the city commanded as high a rent as the best houses, while a small tenement two or three miles away went for upwards of 300l. per annum.

By the second week of September, with the federal officers and the governor gone, responsibility for the deepening crisis fell on Mayor Clarkson. On the 10th he issued a call "to the benevolent citizens" pleading for help. The following day a letter appeared in the paper urging the mayor to inform the public of the true state of affairs at Bush Hill, "for many persons refuse to suffer their friends to be carried thither, because it is at present conducted mysteriously."[6]

Responding to the mayor's call, on September 12, a small group comprising Samuel Wetherill, Israel Israel, Thomas Wistar, Andrew Adgate, Caleb Lownes, Henry Deforest, Thomas Peters, Joseph Inskeep, Stephen Gerard (spelled "Girard") and John Mason came forward to assist Clarkson "to meet and consider a plan for the relief of the afflicted." (Others later included were Mathew Carey, Samuel Benge, Thomas Harrison, Thomas Savery, John Letchworth, James Swaine [also spelled "Swain"], John Connelly, Jacob Weaver, James Sharswood [or Sharfwood], John M'Culloch, Jas. Kerr, and Peter Helm.) James Wilson, a Guardian of the Poor, reported that Drs. Physick (also spelled Physic), Cathavel (also spelled Cathrall and Catharal), Annan and Leib (then indisposed) were in charge at the hospital. It was agreed that an investigation of conditions would immediately take place. At this meeting Wetherill was appointed as chairman and Lownes as secretary. Israel Israel later became chairman pro tem. With Matthew Clarkson serving as president, this group became his unofficial government. Wetherill accepted the position as vice president and Thomas Wistar became the treasurer; Lownes remained as secretary. They resolved to:

(1) Procure a sum of money
(2) Appoint a large committee from various parts of the city
(3) Have full power to act as circumstances required
(4) Keep a just account of their proceedings and expenditures

On September 13, Girard and Peter Helm, a cooper by trade, reported Drs. Cathrall and Physic's statement that "the hospital is without order or arrangements—far from being clean, and stands in immediate need of several qualified persons to begin and establish the necessary arrangements." On September 15 Girard and Helm agreed to superintend the hospital. Calls went out for an assistant apothecary, a steward, a "bleeder," and a barber. "Generous wages" were offered for nurses. Advertisements under Matthew Clarkson's name pleaded for a supply of old shirts and linen of any kind for use at the hospital. Work was done quickly. By the 16th, the committee reported "the Hospital is now fully furnished with officers and attendants except a few nurses ... [and] the sick are amply supplied with the necessary supplies and accommodations."[7] Their work did not go unnoticed:

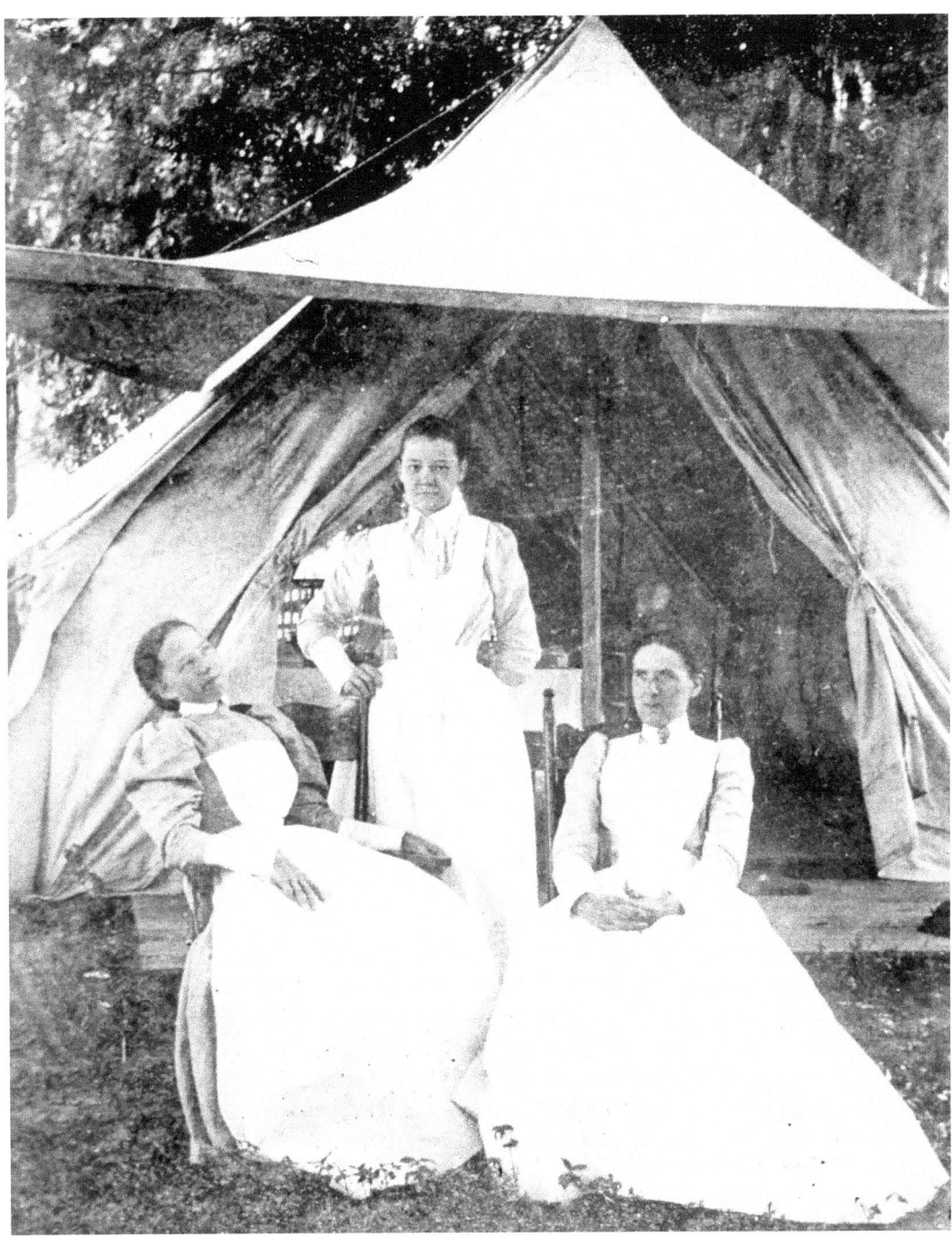

Nurses were the unsung heroes in the fight against yellow fever. Caregivers Ballard, Ferguson and Norsdoff pose outside a temporary yellow fever hospital in Franklin, Louisiana, 1898. Drawn from all walks of life, many such individuals left the comfort and safety of their homes to travel to a faraway state and volunteer to help the sick and dying (courtesy National Library of Medicine).

A number of citizens, however, with a courage that will always do them honour, formed themselves into a Committee, headed by the Mayor, borrowed money upon the credit of future subscriptions; established a hospital about a mile from town, for the poor; procured carriages to convey the sick to it; sat daily at the City-hall, to receive applications and administer relief; and two of them, Steven Girard, a French merchant here, and Peter Helm, born here, of German parents (men whose names and services should never be forgot) had the humanity and courage constantly to attend the hospital; and not only saw that the nurses did their duties, but they actually performed many of the most dangerous, and at the same time most humiliating services for the sick with their own hands. These gentlemen are mercifully preserved alive and well, though four of the committee who sat at the City-hall, took the disorder and died. Their names were Daniel Offley, Joseph Inskeep, Jonathan D'Sergeant, and Andrew Adgate.[8]

The money mentioned came from a $1,500 loan from John Nixon, president of the Bank of North America, supported by bonds from Thomas Harrison, Thomas Wistar and Caleb Lownes.

By September 25 the committee advised the city that those who had taken their loved ones away from the hospital only to find help "fruitless" should return them. On the 28th, the committee had the satisfaction of assuring their fellow citizens that Bush Hill was "in all respects in good order" and that children at the Orphan House were well taken care of. (John Swanwick donated the Loganian library to the committee, which converted it into the Orphan House. Approximately 100 children ranging in age from one week to 14 years were admitted.)[9] They added that Joseph Ogden, in charge of Potter's Field, had taken "every precaution" to maintain it in proper order.[10]

Interestingly, for those who believed in fumigation, a recipe invented by the Commission of Moscow (1771) was reprinted. "Powder of the First Strength" included leaves of juniper, juniper berries, ears of wheat, guaiacum wood, common salt petre, sulphur, and Smyrna tar or myrrh mixed together. "Odoriferous Powder" included a root called kalmus, frankincense, storax, rose flowers, yellow amber, Smyrna tar or myrrh, common salt petre, and sulphur mixed together.[11]

The Weather Changes

"Unfortunately we have had, for a continuance of time, a series of weather uncommonly favourable to this disorder. For above two months we have hardly had any rain; and during that time, there have not been above ten or twelve cool days. It is worthy of particular attention, that the degree of mortality has depended greatly on the degree of heat. On very sultry days, the number of deaths has been much greater than on cool days." So wrote a businessman from Philadelphia on October 16, describing the late summer of 1793. Putting their situation in context, citizens looked to history for an appropriate comparison. "This calamity, we conceive," wrote a second businessman, "has been nearly, if not quite as fatal, in proportion to the numbers, as the plague in London, in 1665; for, if we compare that thirty thousand persons remained in town, and that of these about four thousand died, which, when the accounts are all collected, we believe will be near the matter, it will approach to one seventh of the whole in about three months, which is nearly equal to the proportion who died in London in a whole year."

The cause remained obscure. "We leave it to the learned," one writer observed. Some insisted it was imported, others that it was generated locally by a long, hot, dry summer. Others believed it came from the West Indies, "but was much more general and spread more rapidly, owing to the season, which had disposed our bodies to receive infections of any kind." Elderly Philadelphians remembered two previous epidemics, once under the name yellow fever and another during the late war when it went by the name camp fever.

By October, people were weary of disease and infighting. "The discordant opinions and practices of the gentlemen of the faculty have been a great means of destroying the confidence of the public in their prescriptions." Another added, "a great variety of quack preventatives were offered to the public, and some placed confidence in them." No one knew what to do, whose direction to follow. "Dr. Rush and some other Physicians, have strongly advised bleeding, and purges of calomel and jalap. They have been very successful. Others have rested their hopes principally on the cold bath, bark, generous living, and a few occasional glasses of old Madeira."[12]

Conflicting opinions were not limited to private individuals. Clarkson's committee had assumed control over Bush Hill. Much had been done but a physician in residence was required. On September 16 citizen Girard recommended Dr. Jean Deveze's services as physician to the hospital. His appointment was accepted the following day with some trepidation. Like Girard, Deveze did not believe the fever to be contagious and his medical practice was founded on the use of stimulants and quinine, in direct opposition to the four American doctors presently serving the facility who followed Dr. Rush's methods. Rather than accede to the Santo Domingan refugee's request that he be placed in charge, the committee resolved that he "give his attendance." This did not suit Girard and the following day (September 18), Clarkson called in the four local physicians—Cathrall, Physick, Annan and Lieb. Well aware of what was at stake, they made their own demands: entire direction of the hospital, for which they pledged to attend the hospital every morning at 11 o'clock; they also requested they be paid 2 guineas for every visit and that James Graham serve as "prescribing Apothecary."

A compromise was struck. Dr. Deveze would be given a room at the hospital for those desirous of his services, meaning, in plain terms, those who did not wish to be subjected to Rush's system. The agreement, such as it was, was untenable and would clearly place two opposing systems in one very crowded hospital. After six days of back and forth argument, on September 22 Cathrell, Leib and Physick resigned, leaving Girard's choice of Deveze the only viable option. Graham was discharged and Dr. Benjamin Duffeld, another anti–Rush practitioner, agreed to serve under Deveze.[13] By September 27 "Doctor Graham, who has attended at Bush-Hill Hospital, for two week, both day and night, by appointment from the committee," quickly advertised that he was "at leisure now to attend such sick families in town as may need his assistance," having during that period "administered medicine to nearly one hundred sick persons," and having observed the different methods of treating the disease, was ready to practice "that which appeared to him most successful."[14]

Quiet, tactful Deveze and his associate Duffeld treated 807 cases of yellow fever, kept meticulous notes and performed autopsies. In a comparison of treatments performed for David Nassy, postmortem results of a victim treated with Rush's system were contrasted with that of a victim who had undergone the gentler French method. For Dr. Nassy this small study to be proved conclusive: the harsh mercurials were proven to have "caused great havoc in the stomach and intestines, increasing the corrosive damage of the disease." Benjamin Rush had been wrong all along but he never acknowledged his mistakes. By 1854 Jean Deveze was considered the highest authority on yellow fever.[15]

The cold weather and rain that Philadelphians anticipated to put an end to the outbreak were "six weeks after their usual time in coming," wrote one man on November 18, 1793:

> [A]nd we were left under the affliction till about the 24th of last month [October], when it pleased Divine Providence, who permitted the affliction, to give it a check, without much apparent change in our atmosphere; from that time the number of deaths rapidly decreased, and of convalescents increased; and some rains and cool weather, which have succeeded, seem to have nearly, if not altogether eradicated it, as we have heard of no new cases for many days past; and most of those who had it before, are recovered and recovering, though from the violence of the remedies recommended by several physicians, and most generally adopted, many are left in a very weak state, which will require time to restore them to their former strength.... The physicians are all agreed, that the infectious disorder is no more in the city, and the citizens are rapidly returning.[16]

"The white Flag was hoisted on Bush-Hill[,] Philadelphia, the 1st of November," another wrote. "It was the Signal of Health; and, in two days, more than 7000 of the absentees had returned to the city.—The number which fled was calculated at 20,000." On November 3 two churches were opened for divine services, several stores opened the following day and after a suspension of several weeks one of the newspapers resumed its office on November 5. The good news traveled fast: "Certificates of a general convalescency have been transmitted by Dr. RUSH and other physicians to New-York; and it appears by the New-York prints of the 7th, that a communication between these places would immediately be opened. The frost has been very inveterate since the 23rd of October at Philadelphia."[17]

The epidemic had ended in Philadelphia but it was far from conquered, either in outbreaks (as it was said to be "raging in a most cruel manner" in St. Croix in December 1793) or in the preferred method of treatment. While history ultimately condemned Rush, that remained for future generations to prove. In the same article that mentioned the disease raging in the West Indies, it was also noted, "It is now generally agreed by the Citizens and Physicians of Philadelphia, that the great mortality of the yellow fever has principally arisen from the use of the Bark, Wine, Hot Baths, and the various preparations of Opium."[18] If that quote was not written by Rush, it certainly originated with one of his followers. Rush was not through defending himself. In 1794 he wrote *An Account of the Bilious Remitting Yellow Fever, as It Appeared in the City of Philadelphia in the Year 1793*. Still promoting the idea that the epidemic was generated in Philadelphia "from the putrid effluvia of damaged coffee, thrown upon one of the wharfs of the town; when the state of the atmosphere, from an uncommonly hot, and dry summer, was fully adequate to produce the effect," he suggested the 4,044 deaths, like those from the West Indian yellow fever, were "of a truly inflammatory origin; —and after a great deal of unsuccessful and fatal practice from bark, opiates, and cordials," through his influence he was able to stop its ravages. A reviewer in London sadly concluded, "We cannot but entertain an apprehension, that the mortality among our seamen and soldiers in the West Indies, at present, must arise, from the nature and treatment of this disease not being thoroughly understood."[19]

Unfortunately, by 1850 medical science had not advanced as much as might have been supposed. In that year, when an ancient building in Philadelphia was torn down, a mahogany coffin containing the remains of a body that had been nearly destroyed by quick lime was discovered embedded in the masonry of an arch under one of the chimneys. On the coffin was an ornamental breast plate, formed of copper silvered over. The metal was too corroded to decipher any wording and the general belief prevailed that the individual had died of yellow fever either in 1793 or 1798 and was secretly interred for some urgent reason. A panic nearly arose from fear of contagion and the body was quickly disposed of.[20]

Chapter 7

The Controversies of Yellow Fever Continue to Rage

"The names of diseases kill more patients than the diseases themselves" (Frederick Hoffman). The present yellow fever of the West Indies was at first called contagious; it is now known not to be so. The mistake has hitherto, perhaps, prevented the invention of an adequate remedy to its ravages.[1]

Yellow fever was gone from Philadelphia but that did not mean it had disappeared from the scene. Reports from Kingston, Jamaica, dated July 20, 1794, stated that yellow fever was raging dreadfully, especially among those in the shipping trades, and had made its way to the windward parishes, "where its ravages are truly shocking." The mortality at Port-au-Prince was so great that no one dared venture there; upwards of 24 officers and 700 soldiers had already fallen victim to the malady. Questions, however, lingered as to the true origin of these deaths. Some supposed that deserters from the brigands had impregnated the water with some poisonous substance. There was "scarcely any person left" who could remove the "poisonous stuff," as those who remained were starving from their inability to purchase food. The same report lamented the death of Dr. Ford, one of the most eminent physicians on the island."[2]

The mention of troops concerned the War of the First Coalition, which had started in 1792 when France declared war on Austria. After two years of fighting, the revolutionary government of France executed Louis XVI on January 21, 1793. This act united Europe against France, causing that nation to declare war against Great Britain, The Netherlands and Spain. When Portugal, Naples and Tuscany declared war against France, these six principals became the first coalition. The following year the conflict extended into the West Indies, where a British fleet captured Martinique, St. Lucia and Guadeloupe. Later that year a French fleet reclaimed Guadeloupe.

War had its casualties, but disease proved an even greater threat. In May 1794 General White arrived with troops from England; Port-au-Prince was carried. Colonel Lenox arrived with flank companies from the Leeward Islands, but in consequence of this reduction in force Guadeloupe was lost: "As soon as they arrived the troops seemed death-struck; 40 officers and 600 men died in the space of two months." By September 1794 yellow fever had become "more destructive in the *West Indies,* within the last eighteen months, to the young men from Britain and Ireland in the Mercantile and Planting line, to the Seamen in the Navy, and Merchant Service, and to the Military, than in any period ever remembered."

The outbreaks prompted the Faculty of Physicians in Jamaica to pool their ideas for ways of preventing the fever and the means of assisting people to recover from it. The belief that yellow fever was of a putrid nature prompted the suggestion that yeast was a remedy. Unfortunately, due to heat and high humidity, yeast could not be preserved in the West Indies. This prompted the London Society for the Encouragement of Arts, Manufactures, and Commerce to offer the premium of a "Gold Medal or Thirty Pounds, for discovering a substitute for, or preparation of Yeast, that may be preserved six months." Submissions were due on the last Tuesday of November 1794.

A letter to the editor signed "Benevolus" suggested that as the prize for so useful an invention was so low the government add something considerable to it so as to encourage competition. The preservation of yeast, he argued, would allow ale or beer from malt to be produced at sea or locally manufactured in those climates "where the health of seamen and soldiers are impaired from the use of new rum, or other spirituous liquors, either by the scurvy or yellow fever."[3] The same month, under the assumption that yellow fever was contagious, the British Admiralty ordered chests and bedding imported to Shields by transports lately at the West Indies to be taken out to sea and sunk in deep water.[4]

The year 1795 brought little relief. Yellow fever was reported at Grenada and prevailed in some of the other islands. Jamaican papers of May 23 warned that "without great precaution the yellow fever is nearly as fatal as ever to new comers; and as the season advances, may prove equally destructive as that of last year." The same report advised that a body of troops was forming at Martinique for the purpose of taking possession of Demerara in the name of the stadtholder, or provincial executive officer of Holland. A later report stated that yellow fever raged in Jamaica before the British ship *Carteret* sailed for home, with two passengers dying of the disorder on the voyage. In consequence, the inbound mail was delayed because of the requirement for fumigation. News from passengers indicated that Jamaicans feared the French meditated a design against the island, while a "plot for seducing the negroes was frustrated" several months before "by a timely discovery."[5]

While war dominated news from the West Indies, reports of deaths from yellow fever continued. On July 12, the British at St. Domingo indicated that during the previous four to five weeks its troops continued to suffer very severely from the disease, while at Havannah (the 18th century spelling) the approaching war with Great Britain was the prevailing topic. A second report lamented the fact that at St. Domingo "our officers and troops, employed upon that ill-fated expedition, have mostly fallen a sacrifice to the yellow fever; and most of the principal posts on the Island, which we had taken, have been since relinquished, on account of the pestilential air of the climate." Remaining forces were confined to keeping possession of Cape St. Nicholas and Port-au-Prince, which, however, were thought to be abandoned and with them "all further intention of possessing ourselves of St. Domingo."

Among those who fell victim to yellow fever were Daniel Clarke Dornford, assistant commissary of accounts to the expedition to St. Domingo, and Captain Lewis of the *Hannibal* man of war. News from the *Grantham* was worse. At the time of her sailing from Jamaica, seven of the crew and Captain Bull were sick from yellow fever; ten more died by August 28. In the same report bleak news from the Court of Portugal indicated authorities had agreed to pay twenty-five million crusades demanded by the French government and a further demand that they exclude all English vessels from the Tagus was likely to be granted.[6]

As French troops were winning victories on the continent, the *Fair American,* arrived at Dublin from Cape Nichola (also spelled "Nicolas") Mole (Island of Hispaniola; Haiti), dated August 5, 1796, and reported that yellow fever had made "unparalleled ravages amongst the French troops, particularly at Aux Cayes," where one regiment of 1,000 men had lost all but a corporal by July 23. Further news stated that the "famous Mulatto General Regow, to whom the French were indebted for the continuance of their power in St. Domingo," had been superseded. Conscious of the indignity, he had gathered 25,000 men "of different colours" in St. Domingo and outlying islands, but "7000 of the troops, most of whom were Europeans, had been carried off by the fever."[7]

As the war wore down, a 10-month drought on Jamaica in 1797 threatened to ruin most of the sugar and coffee crops: "The same drought has also favoured, unhappily, the progress of an epidemical disease, somewhat similar to the yellow fever, to which not only the new comers, but several old and native inhabitants of the Island have already fallen victim."[8]

In a 1797 excerpt from the House of Commons concerning the war in the West Indies, members concluded, "The ravages of the yellow fever were so fatal that our forces were obliged to confine themselves to acting on the defensive.... After four years of war, in short, it appeared that no acquisitions of any importance, except Port-au-Prince, had been obtained, more than had been acquired within the first ten days." Notwithstanding that the harbor of Cape Nicolas Mole remained under British authority, privateers from Aux Cayes committed great depredation on English shipping. In four years, bills on the treasury from every part of the world amounted to 16 million, while those from St. Domingo alone were between four and five million, more than a quarter of the whole.

"But the mortality, which attended our continuing to occupy these positions, were still more serious...." Up to September 3, 1796, there were 7,500 deaths, few of them by the sword; through October 1795 not more than 100 had died in the field. "In March 1796, there had died 129 officers, and 5,840 men. So the number of those who had fallen victims to the pestilence of the climate might easily be gathered. Nor were the men seasoned by time to the climate. The attack of the yellow fever was almost always mortal, and it was even apt to recur."[9] Those arguments aside, Great Britain and France remained at war as other members of the First Coalition conceded the contest in 1797.

The news was not all grim if you happened to believe a report stemming from an American merchant ship that stopped at one of the West Indian islands where the crew contracted yellow fever. After the ship's surgeon died of the disease, the captain dosed the remaining men with half water and half "Spirit of Spruce." Most taking the turpentine concoction recovered, "and it is supposed all would if some of them had not been in a bad State of Blood. This Remedy was applied with equal Success by the Captain of another Ship (the *Sampson*), where the Men were infected by the Yellow Fever." A new book on the same subject, *An Account of the Yellow Fever, with a Successful Method of Cure,* was by James Bryce, and *Surgeon, Late of the Busbridge East Indiaman* was published by William Creech the same year. According to Dr. Bryce, yellow fever occurred aboard the *Busbridge* during the summer of 1792, after the ship had been 40 days out to sea. The disease infected the seamen around the time of the initiation ceremony of "ducking" (dunking) novice crew members who had never before "crossed the line" (equator). Without access to recent medical publications on the subject, he liberally dosed the crew with a mixture of calomel and gamboge, jalap, "and other drastic measures." Out of 250 cases (300, counting relapses), only three terminated fatally. Bryce was unable to determine whether the disease was carried aboard at some point prior to departure or was generated within the ship; the identity of the disease, however, was considered sufficiently strong to be associated with that which "depopulated America and the West Indies." A reviewer of Bryce's text noted that from 1793 to 1797 there had been numerous works professing to reveal "successful methods of treatment," yet yellow fever continued unabated. He questioned whether these books ever reached the army surgeons and, if so, whether they read them. Or, perhaps more likely, the reviewer wondered if the treatments advocated were "less successful in the hands of others than in those of the first proposers?" Ironically, the same year, "an infallible method of cure for the yellow fever" was announced by a young graduate from Scotland, wanting "only a trial beyond the Atlantic to demonstrate its efficacy."

As if to prove the point of "numerous works" professing cures, *A Treatise on the Yellow Fever as It Appeared in the Island of Dominica, in the Years 1793, 4, 5, 6, to Which Are Added, Observations on the Bilious Remittent Fever, on Intermittents, Dysentery, and Some Other West India Diseases*, by James Clarke, MD, was released. He recommended the free use of mercury, as both a remedy and a preventative, suggesting that upon arrival in the West Indies soldiers undergo two courses of mercury and "a few laxative medicines" with "a moderate use of wine." Used in conjunction with a diet of fruits and vegetables for the first two months after arrival, they might "rely almost to a certainty, on escaping the fever."

Doctors were not alone with their claims. A seaman named Edward Rock wrote to the Lords Commissioners of the Board of Admiralty in 1798, claiming that he contracted yellow fever in the service while stationed in the West Indies. Declared incurable by navy physicians and London specialists, he wished it known that a wine prepared by a Mr. M'Bride of Fenchurch Street called *Tue-kay de Espagna* cured his fever and heart palpitations in less than a quarter of an hour. "I have been a witness," he wrote, "to scenes of mortality in the West Indies too shocking to relate; I have seen the Doctor of the ship harshly tell a man that nothing ailed him, who the next day, was a corpse. I have seen men in the yellow fever walk out at the port-holes into the sea." Rather than have the government pay "some hundred thousand pounds for medicines, which are proved by the publications of Physicians themselves to be of no use in those dreadful disorders," he suggested the purchase of this cordial for fevers and fluxes.[10]

For those who did not have access to McBride's miracle cure, there was always "Dr. Norris's Fever Drops." In 1795 the success of this medicine was based on the namesake's 40-year medical practice. Advertisements claimed that aside from their renovating powers, the drops were invaluable in preventing and curing yellow fever, asthma, gout, piles "and many other fatal and obstinate Complaints." A year later the claims leapt a decade as it was declared, "Dr. Norris's Drops for half a century past have been esteemed the safest and most efficacious Medicine ever discovered, for the cure of the YELLOW FEVER, and every other species of Fever." In 1797 the proprietor of Dr. Norris's Drops opted to use a testimonial from James Frazer, master of the good ship *Hector*. Noting he had "seldom lost a Slave to whom the Drops were administered," Frazer avowed "there is nothing so efficacious in the Yellow Fever, as well as in those fatal disorders arising from contaminated Air in Ships, Camps, or Prisons." By 1798 the advertising emphasis changed to preserving health and curing colds and stomach and bowel complaints. While continuing to promote the drops for yellow fever, added to the list of accomplishments were putrid fever, consumption and "the decays of advanced Life".[11]

Under the heading "Yellow fever in England"—a paragraph that as easily could have substituted "smallpox" or "cholera" as the disease of choice—it was reported that clothes belonging to a young man who had died of that dreadful malady in the West Indies were received by his relatives at Lancaster. Upon the family opening the package, the infection was communicated to five persons present; within a few days two of the five had died. Some neighboring families also caught the contagion but "providentially it has been arrested in its progress."[12]

On an equally "contagious" note, the *London Herald* ran an article mentioning that a "beautiful and amiable young Lady" from the region of Bath had recently died from symptoms resembling, "in a great degree," those of yellow fever. She was supposed to have caught the infection from having worn "a fashionable wig, *a-la-Brutus*, made of hair imported from America, which, it is thought, was cut from the head of some person who died of the fever." The *Evening Mail* promptly responded, "We are no advocates for the wigs; but the story may certainly be considered as 'a weak invention of the enemy.'"[13]

A Review of Medical Publications

In the final year of the 1700s the causes and cure of yellow fever had not advanced to any significant degree and the medical publications of 1799 were stale and repetitious. Perhaps the most egregious was *A Voyage to the South Seas*, written by Captain Colnett of the Royal Navy, who "served under the celebrated navigator Captain Cook." In treating seamen who suffered from yellow fever he "recovered them," he wrote on page 80, "by adopting the method that I saw practiced by the Natives of Spanish America when I was a prisoner among them." When the first symptoms appeared, the fore part of the head was immediately shaved and the temples washed with vinegar and water. The whole body was then immersed in warm water to give a free course to perspiration; "some opening medicine was afterwards administered, and every four hours a dose of *ten grains* of *James's Powders*." By this mode of treatment, "the whole crew improved in their health." Run as an advertisement in *Lloyd's Evening-Post* (London, February 15–18. 1799), the text added, "A more judicious treatment of this disorder could not have been derived" (see Chapter 2 for a discussion of James's Powders). The same text ran in the *Scots Magazine* of April 1, 1799, without being labeled as a promotion. No explanation was given on how the "Natives of Spanish America" received their ample supply of James's cure.

An interesting explanation of how yellow fever was introduced into the Royal Navy was given by Mr. Elliot, a surgeon in the African and West-India Merchants' service, in his book, *The Seaman's Medical Advocate*. His theory on how 500 seamen were lost annually through yellow fever was simple: these were impressed men "who have been wandering on shore, and who by intemperance and exposure to the night air have contracted the disease before they are taken." The obvious remedy was "the abolition of that tyrannous and most cruel practice." As that suggestion was not likely to be heeded, Elliot recommended all impressed men and those who impressed them "be lodged in houses in the most dry and healthy part of the islands, and there be detained under the care of a surgeon until it can be ascertained that they have not caught the infection."[14]

William Lempriere, apothecary to his Majesty's Forces, wrote *Practical Observations on the Diseases of the Army in Jamaica* (1799). Referring to yellow fever as "the *tropical continued fever*," he considered it an endemic disease and not contagious, supposing it

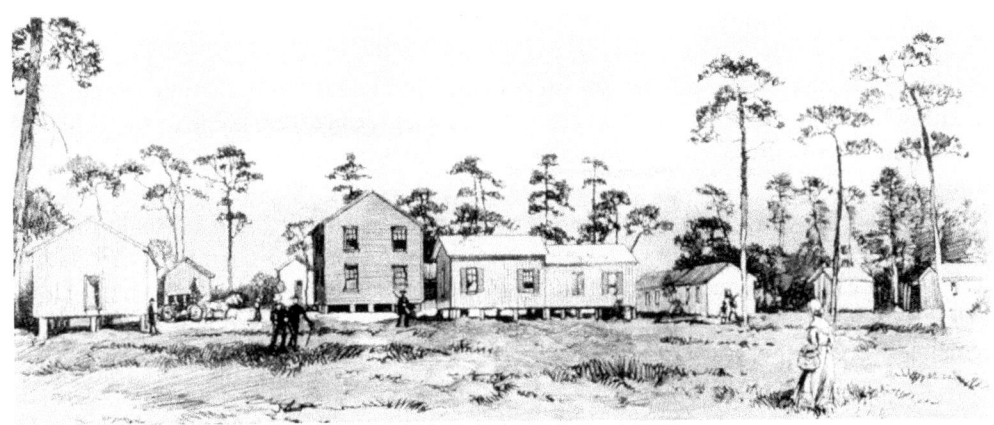

Above: The fear of yellow fever being transported into other states prompted authorities to do everything in their power to prevent its spread. Without a proven cure, however, control was based on quarantine and sanitation. This view of Sand Hill Hospital looks northeast (originally published in *Harper's Weekly,* September 29, 1888). *Below:* In the 18th and 19th centuries it was commonly believed that African Americans were innately immune from contracting yellow fever. This was based on the assumption that slaves imported from Africa seldom displayed symptoms. Their immunity actually came from early exposure to the disease in their native land. Subsequent generations who did not have this immunity fell victim to the disease in large numbers and, like their white counterparts, those who were able often fled the seats of contagion. This illustration, from *Harper's Weekly* (Vol. 23, p. 652), published August 16, 1879, is titled, "En route for Kansas, poor Negroes fleeing yellow fever in Memphis" (both photographs courtesy National Library of Medicine).

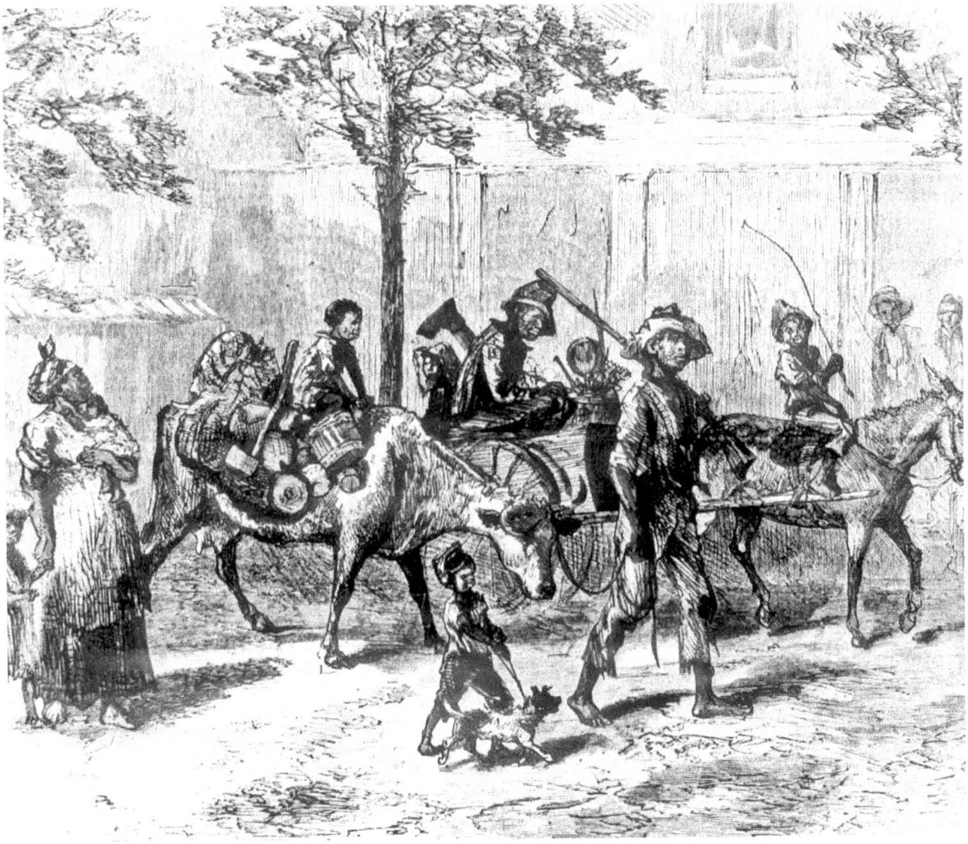

to have originated "in the effluvia of animal matter, in a state of putrefaction." Apparently learning the wrong lessons, he observed that "the Negroes are less liable to the action of contagion than whites, from the history of the Philadelphia fever." He attributed the unusual prevalence of yellow fever in 1793 and succeeding years to "to the action of a very hot season, after uncommonly heavy rains" and the constitutions of the Europeans newly landed on the island in consequence of the war. Correctly surmising that subsequent cooler months checked the disease, his description of a victim stands out: "[T]he whole surface of the body exhibits an appearance as if recovering from Mosquito bites, which however is soon succeeded by a general yellow suffusion." The author's preventive plan harkened back to Benjamin Rush and chiefly consisted of bleeding and repeated purging before men arrived in the West Indies. He added that "the debility produced by a course of mercury, during the voyage, has been found a protection against the epidemic."[15]

Robert Jackson's *An Outline of the History and Cure of Fever* stressed the fact that endemic fevers, which incidentally proved more fatal to tall men, arose from marsh-miasmata and the prevalence of these miasmata in the atmosphere, while contagious fevers arose from human effluvia, making them an "accidental" and "artificial" disease occasioned by an improper mode of living. Numerous dissections of patients who died from yellow fever revealed "congestion in the head, and of inflammation, or effusion of blood, in the villous coat of the intestines." To cure yellow fever Jackson recommended "bleeding at the arm, to the amount of twenty ounces," followed by purgatives; calomel and James's powder were particularly stressed. Similar to Dr. Rush's practice even when the patient was evidently sinking, Jackson advocated brisk purging, friction of the abdomen, ablution with cold water, moving the patient into direct sunlight and repeated bleeding.[16]

Perhaps the best way to end the century is with a letter written after authorities at Glasgow announced plans to clean the streets. In objecting to the scheme, the writer observed the adage "Dirt bodes luck," referencing New York City. He stated that as long as it "continued distinguished for its dirt" it remained free from yellow fever, but "cleanliness contributed materially to the nurture and encrease of that destructive malady." His point was that a dirty street fermented by the "scorching noon-tide sun" created nitre, the all-powerful "antiputrescent" that provided wholesome acid to inhale.[17]

Forty Days and Forty Nights: Prodigious Ravages Throughout the Former Colonies

Yellow fever disappeared from Philadelphia when the weather turned cold in 1793 but it was far from gone. The disease appeared the following year in that city, where it was attributed to the "appearance of some few cases of the bilious remitting-fall fever." While in some instances fatal, it was "if taken in time" perfectly "under the control of medicine." Unlike the previous year where outbreaks were substantially confined to that one city, by 1794 yellow fever was found in Baltimore and at various points across the Eastern seaboard.[18]

A letter from Charleston, South Carolina, dated August 18, 1794, advised that yellow fever had been making "such prodigious ravages in that State, that all business is at a stand." Its effects, according to the writer, were confined to Europeans of the male sex; few women or children were seized. Of importance, he noted, "The cause of this destructive malady is attributed to the rains, which have been so incessant, for forty days and nights, as to have inundated the whole country and entirely destroyed the crops."[19] Rain, of course, led to stagnant water where mosquitoes bred, but no connection was made. Even without that connection, however, it was a point to be noted. The state of the atmosphere (rainfall, thunder and lightning, temperature and miasmic conditions) were becoming important considerations that astute men correlated when attempting to determine the dread cause of this devastating disease.

There was less cause for concern in New York City. During 1794 twenty to thirty cases of yellow fever were diagnosed. Fearful that worse epidemics lay on the horizon, the common council spent £2,000 for the lease on the Brockholst Livingston estate and its four acres of ground. Situated on the bank of the East River, opposite the Three Mile Stone, Belle Vue, as it was called, was converted into a hospital where patients could be isolated.

On May 29, 1795, two infected sailors were removed from the *Antoinette* docked at Whitehall and taken to Belle Vue. On July 19, the brig *Zepher,* Captain Frederick Bird, arrived at New York from Port-au-Prince with a cargo of sugar and coffee. The health officer, Dr. Malachi Treat, boarded the vessel and discovered that several men had died from yellow fever on the voyage, a boy had died that morning and other crewmembers were ill. Dr. Treat became sick on July 22 and died on July 30, suffering from the characteristic symptoms of yellow fever. As panic began to spread, suspicion was placed on all ships arriving from the West Indies. Disease was discovered on the *William,* arrived from Liverpool on July 25, and the rumor started that her crew had contracted it from the *Zepher.* Although it was later proven that the two vessels had not come within half a mile of one another, the fever spread ashore to those living on Water Street, close to where the *William* lay anchored.

With panic came suspicion, and attention was drawn to a bale of cotton delivered by the brig *Caroline* to the store of Lawrence and Mott on Dover Street. Reports stated that after a man thrust his arm into the cotton the arm turned a livid color from the contagion. When news of the outbreak reached Philadelphia, it was stated that New Yorkers were "popping off like rotten sheep" and that all the glass in the city had been broken by the preventive measure of firing cannon. On August 31, Pennsylvania's governor returned the "favor" of quarantine by forbidding all communication with New York.

Scenes similar to those played out in Philadelphia in 1793 were now witnessed firsthand in New York. On August 15, a group of medical men styled the "College of Physicians" held a meeting at city hall and reported "that no contagious fever, in any particular different from what this city has been accustomed to, for some years past, at this season, exists at present." Following their example, the Committee of Health noted on August 29 the fever was "a local malady" and the number of sick had considerably decreased. And just as typical, a letter mailed from New York to Philadelphia expressed the concern that the fever raged chiefly at Water Street, noting eight or ten people were buried every night. The letter concluded, "God only knows what will become of us."

Calling the College of Physicians "some characters who are out of the pale of the medical society," the New York Medical Society reported that the disease was not "specifically contagious," while the common council informed Governor Jay that the city had a greater degree of health than was usual at that time of the season. Unconvinced, the

New York Hospital refused to admit fever patients because officials there considered them contagious. That October the citizens of Philadelphia sent $7,000 to the mayor for the relief of the poor.

In the pamphlet *A Collection of Papers on the Subject of Bilious Fevers* (1796) compiled by Noah Webster, Dr. Valentine Seaman wrote "the musquetoes were never before known, by the oldest inhabitants, to have been so numerous as at this season, especially in the southeastern part of the city; they were particularly troublesome to foreigners, many of whom, had those parts of their bodies that were exposed to them, covered with blisters from their venomous operations."[20]

During the epidemics of 1795 and 1796, among the prominent New York physicians called upon to treat yellow fever were Drs. David Hosack, his associate Samuel Bard and Hosack's brother, Alexander, Jr. David Hosack divided fevers into two categories, one arising from "sensible changes of the atmosphere" (including pleurisy, acute rheumatism and inflammations of the brain, stomach and intestines), and the second caused by "matter of a peculiar quality, introduced into the system." This included smallpox, measles, chicken pox, influenza, "hooping-cough," scarlet fever, dysentery, yellow fever and plague.

Hosack's abiding principle in regard to the second category was "to attend to the different functions of the body, that the action of the poison may be rendered as moderate as possible, and that every other source of irritation be removed, until the cause producing the disease be entirely exhausted" in the least debilitating process possible. His first step consisted of removing from the bowels any matter that might aggravate the yellow fever, and then to restore perspiration, "which is for the most part obstructed." For this, he relied on sweating, the success of which, he believed, had been proven by Dr. John Bard of New York and Dr. Warren, from his studies of the yellow fever of Barbados. Equating the success of Peruvian bark in intermittent fever to sweating in yellow fever, he asserted that if induced within the first twelve hours from the commencement of the disease the practitioner would rarely be disappointed in its effects.[21]

The 1797 work of Alexander Hosack, Jr., *History of the Yellow Fever, as It Appeared in the City of New York in 1795*, stated very similar ideas while adding, without discussion, his opinion that the disease was contagious. After briefly discussing purgative medicines used by some physicians during yellow fever epidemics in Philadelphia (calomel and jalap; rhubarb and magnesia with cinnamon or mint-water), he recommended Glauber's salts dissolved in a pint of gruel made of Indian meal; if the stomach was irritated, recourse was made to glysters composed of vinegar and water, quickened by the addition of molasses. To promote sweating, sudorific medicines were employed, including James's powders and antimony. The best approach, however, was to wash the whole body with cold vinegar and water and then cover the patient with blankets. Thereafter spiritus mindereri and saline drafts of Riverius succeeded well, especially when given with warm drinks containing an infusion of snake-root, gruel, toast water, tamarind water or lemonade. Some physicians, he noted, including Professor Gregory of Edinburgh and Dr. Currie of Liverpool as well as Dr. Samuel Bard of New York Hospital, promoted cold bathing. Hosack himself considered this technique acceptable in the early stages of yellow fever but injurious in the last stages of the disease. He also added that in New York Hospital, where bleeding was frequently employed, the result was "very injurious and unsuccessful," often terminating fatally.[22]

Yellow fever broke out at Lynnhaven Bay, a "watering place for ships, a few miles from Norfolk," Virginia, in August 1795. The disease was believed to have been imported by a West India ship that had touched at St. Lucia before departing St. Domingo in July. Before departing for more northern ports, the vessel landed some infected passengers and seamen who had complained of the usual pain in the back, head and limbs, with shivering and external cold. The fever spread rapidly and by August 25, twenty-two inhabitants had died, most within the third or fourth day after exhibiting symptoms. It was felt that emetics, large drafts of diluting liquors and in some instances the consumption of pure water had proven efficacious.[23]

In a strange twist that may have been a consequence of the epidemic, the *American Eagle* departed Norfolk with a crew of ten on September 15, bound for Havre de Grace with a cargo of tobacco. On October 28, after being disabled by a storm, the vessel put in at Cowes, where the second mate reported that the master, William Little, had perished from yellow fever during the voyage. Another crewman told a different story, however. He testified that the second mate and three other conspirators had actually murdered their two superior officers at the mouth of the Channel. Their object was to run into some distant country and sell the ship and cargo for their own profit but stormy weather forced them into Cowes. Local magistrates committed the entire crew to Winchester jail before removing them "by Habeas Corpus" to Newgate for trial at the next Admiralty Session.

That trial was held January 22, 1796, where Francis Cole, George Colley, Michael Blanche and Emanuel Bether were charged with murder. (Only Cole and Colley were

---

YELLOW, TYPHUS, and other FEVERS.
Dr. Wm. Stevens, in his work, says, "Whenever the saline treatment is adopted the otherwise fatal yellow fever is deprived of its terrors." In one thousand cases treated on the saline plan in the Island of Trinidad, the astonishing number of 989 recovered. Dr. Stevens has certified, of which a notarial copy is to be obtained at 113, Holborn-hill, that Mr. LAMPLOUGH is the sole manufacturer of the EFFERVESCING PYRETIC SALINE, a term signifying in the words of Dr. Johnson, the lexicographer, a "remedy having the power of controlling fevers."

Messrs. Orr and Sons, of Madras, in a letter dated 23rd September, 1866, state Surgeon Major C. Murray Duff, M.D., &c., had called for a further supply of all that we could give him, and spoke of its remarkable effects in the jungle fever in quite enthusiastic terms, directing a further supply to be sent overland, besides what had already been forwarded by the Cape.

A case of jungle fever had been treated with the partial contents of one bottle with perfect success; the medical attendant, of considerable repute, likes the medicine much, and wants more.

In another case of severe vomiting the patient was relieved after the third dose, and fell into a refreshing sleep.

Sole Maker, H. LAMPLOUGH, Chemist, 113, Holborn-hill, London.

"Deprived of its terrors"; "astonishing number" recovered; "remedy"; "perfect success"; "refreshing sleep." Who wouldn't want to try the Effervescing Pyretic Saline to treat the "otherwise fatal yellow fever"? (*London Daily News*, November 29, 1866).

actually tried; the other two, being Spanish and not his majesty's subjects, were required to be tried by a jury consisting of one-half foreigners.) According to testimony of three crew members, shortly after the ship departed Norfolk the mate, Richard Little (the captain's brother), and two others died of yellow fever. Colley assumed the mate's position. On October 27 they encountered a squall about 50 leagues from the Isle of Wright. Captain Little remained on deck until midnight and then retired to his cabin. There he was repeatedly stabbed by Francis Cole "with malice aforethought." The body was dragged onto the deck, undressed and pitched overboard. Attempts were then made on the lives of those not involved in the murder but they managed to talk themselves out of a watery grave.

After removing and dividing $245 stolen from the captain's chest, Colley doctored the ship's log to read that Little died of yellow fever on October 13. They planned to make for France but when it was discovered none of the remaining men could navigate without reading the sun (that being obscured by the storm) they made for the nearest land. The jury deliberated for ten minutes and returned a verdict of guilty and the two prisoners were ordered to be executed Monday, January 25.[24]

Ironically, a ship called the *Norfolk Eagle,* departing that Virginia port sometime in October, apparently carried the remnants of the yellow fever epidemic with it. Reaching the Motherbank, Portsmouth, on November 2, the crew reported having buried the master and three seamen who reputedly died of the disease. The vessel was immediately put into quarantine.[25]

The first major yellow fever epidemic at New Orleans occurred in 1796. At that time the city had a population of fewer than 10,000, and the official mortality reached 300.[26] Officials in New York City had a greater task on their hands and passed an act in 1796 for the appointment of health commissioners who were to serve along with the health officer, the object being to prevent major outbreaks of contagious diseases by enforcing quarantine regulations. They were also to make recommendations to the common council concerning sanitation and supervise a lazaretto on Governor's or another island. The measures were so successful for the years 1796–1797 that Bellevue Hospital was leased as a place of entertainment, with the stipulation being that if it was needed as a medical facility it would be immediately surrendered.[27]

Yellow fever proved more troublesome in Providence, Rhode Island, Baltimore and Philadelphia in 1797. In the latter case, the College of Physicians traced its origin to two ships carrying the infection—one from Havana and the other from Port-au-Prince. The year 1798 would prove to be an even greater calamity, as the disease was more widespread and fatal.

Chapter 8

The "Great Epidemic" of 1798

> *The FEVER: The alarm of both citizens and country friends, on the subject of the fever, has exceeded all bounds—Divested of reason, philosophy, religion, what a poor creature is man!*[1]

Yellow fever was not the primary consideration on the minds of Americans at the beginning of 1798. The Treaty of Campo Formio in October 1797 had temporarily ended the War of the First Coalition, but tensions had remained high between France and Austria. Eventually, the Habsburg Monarchy, the Russian Empire, the Holy Roman Empire, Great Britain, Portugal, Naples, the Ottoman Empire and the French Royalists formed a new alliance to prevent Napoleon Bonaparte from taking Egypt and conquering Germany and Italy. The War of the Second Coalition (1798–1802) threatened to involve the United States and preparations for warfare against France soon dominated public consciousness in the U.S.

The state of public health was expressed on September 1, 1798: "The prevailing sickness has alarmed many of our inhabitants. It is called a *putrid malignant Fever,* and has been very fatal, particularly in some parts of Queen-street, on Goldenhill, and in Cliff-street. Many parts of the city are as healthy as usual—and as there seems to be no instance of its communicating, even to Nurses, we are in great hopes our city will soon regain its wonted state of health and vigor."[2] By September 4, the same newspaper (*Greenleaf's New York Journal*) observed that fear of the fever had driven off four of their apprentice boys but noted there was not a solitary case of the sickness on Wall Street; several died but "none of them took it here." The editors were happy to hear that authorities intended to publish the number of deaths to decrease the prevailing alarm. They believed if it were "*officially* ascertained, that not more than *ten* deaths per day occurred in all the month of August, including all disorders" and the "subjects at Bellevue" were "short of the usual dog-day mortality in this city" matters would return to normal. This did not prove to be the case.

Authorities had limited options to rein in panic and they used them all. The "few cases of disease" were attributed to effluvia from sewers or miasma coming from rotting provisions meant for the West Indies but unshipped for fear of French ships preying on American commerce. In the first week of September politicians at Albany proclaimed the outbreaks were "due to local causes and engendered among themselves." On September 10 the Common Council appointed a standing committee "for the duration of the crisis" to make provision for the sick and indigent and to facilitate admissions to Bellevue, which had been reopened June 12. The hospital was placed under the charge of Dr. Isaac

S. Douglass, while the health officer, Dr. Richard Bayley, sought other medical assistance. Douglass later contracted yellow fever although he denied having been contaminated at the hospital, noting that no other cases of infection were reported among the 16 nurses and attendants working there.

When reports of the malady indicated an epidemic of even greater proportions than had ever been seen in New York City, attention was drawn to the East River. Businesses including the custom house on Mill Street and the insurance office on Water Street were temporarily transplanted to the Tontine Tavern on Broadway, where conditions were considered healthier.

As boys dragged hand carts through the city crying, "Coffins! Coffins of all sizes!" for sale at $4 apiece, dead carts carted away innumerable corpses to the dreaded Potter's Field. In his *Account of the Malignant Fever Lately Prevalent in the City of New York* (1798), J. Hardie went into some detail about conditions at Bellevue. As it was considered to more closely resemble a house of death than a facility where people went to get well, charges were brought that the dying were kept in close confinement with those convalescing, while many of the staff earned reputations as "improper persons." In response, the Common Council ordered two new buildings, each 60 × 20 feet, to be constructed. Eventually, Hardie opined, such strenuous efforts succeeded and the hospital came to be looked upon "as a place where they stood a greater chance of recovery that anywhere else." Yet people still fled the city. To address fears of looting in these temporarily abandoned properties, on September 24 the city doubled the number of watchmen assigned to keep the peace. The surrounding population aware of the growing crisis, from the end of the month until the New Year charitable contributions of food, clothing and medicines were sent from the Hudson Valley, New Jersey and Connecticut, aiding more than 500 families.[3]

Complicating a situation that could not be resolved, medical authorities were divided between the idea of imported contagion versus that of local origin. On September 19 a writer signing himself "Theorist" argued that yellow fever "is known to be most contagious in close dirty streets and alleys which do not admit a free circulation of air ... [so] does this not shew that something exists in such contagious places, that is necessary to support contagion that does not exist elsewhere? I believe it to be that offensive effluvia or myasmata which assails our senses as we pass the streets." He deduced there was little danger of contagion during a high windy day; that stagnant water contributed toward producing miasma; the infection could exist in one part of the city and not another; all persons would not be infected at all times; and the infection could be imported where myasmata existed in sufficient quantity to support and nourish it. He concluded "that the noxious effluvia is heavier than the common air, and occupies the lower space—consequently the highest and most airy apartments of the house will be found to be the safest."[4]

Dr. Valentine Seaman believed yellow fever to be of foreign origin and urged quarantine of ships from the West Indies and southern ports. Noah Webster took the opposite argument, purporting that nearly all epidemics resulted from local circumstances in conjunction with meteoric influences and the appearance of comets.[5]

Proving that cures were equally controversial, Drs. Isaac Rand and John Warren offered the results of two dissections of yellow fever victims, "which evinced a deficiency of secretion in the biliary organs," indicating a cure that "might obviate the inflammation in general of the organs diseased, and open the excretory ducts of the liver, that the fluid might resume its course into the intestines." Toward this end they recommended the use of calomel, given in small doses every 1-2 hours. They mentioned with pleasure the "learned Dr. Rush of Philadelphia" and his use of mercury and then cited the mercurial system used by Dr. James Clarke in the island of Dominica (see Chapter 7) as the method most "explicitly and highly recommended."[6] Theories and cures to the contrary, 2,086 people died from yellow fever in New York City during the epidemic of 1798.[7]

The Manhattan Company

In light of the disagreements over the origin of yellow fever, a joint committee was formed on November 19, 1789, "to investigate the Causes, Progress and Probable Means of preventing a return of the fever." Comprising representatives of the common council, the Chamber of Congress, the medical society and the commissioners of the Health Office, the team issued its report February 4, 1799. The opening paragraph stated the sources producing pestilential diseases were "filthy sunken yards, where the offal of the house and wash of kitchens be until the earth absorbs or the sun exhales them—lengthy sewers without floors, and of little descent—foul ships exposed to the sun great part of the tides—decayed docks out of repair—vacant water lots—ground under stores and houses built on piles or timber, and running bare part of the tides; these are generally receptacles of every description of impurity and carrion."

Among their suggestions were the following:

(1) Enact strong, energetic laws and hire inspectors who are to receive reasonable pay

(2) Remove accumulations of winter filth after the last frost to prevent substances from penetrating the ground and allow spring winds to pass over a clean rather than a filthy surface. Have trash picked up every Tuesday and Friday mornings

(3) Raise or fill in all sunken cellars that were used as boarding houses for sailors, particularly along the East River; fill in all sunken yards

(4) Descents in streets ought to be made wherever possible, especially between the Coffee house and Fly market in Water street to drain off stagnant water

(5) Common sewers be projected on an incline plain

(6) All slips ought to be filled with wholesome dirt

(7) Heavy fines should be imposed on boatmen tossing refuse into slips or docks

(8) All water lots ought to be filled with wholesome earth

(9) All salted beef and pork in casks, all dried and pickled fish and all imported hides and skins removed to the northward of Corlaer's Hook to the North River; tainted or corrupted beef and pork should be destroyed

(10) From June 1—October 1, no fresh meats or dead fish ought to be offered for sale after 10:00 o'clock AM.

(11) Slaughterhouses should be prohibited south of the East River along Grand-street and Bayard's lane to the North River

(12) No glue manufactured, no blubber stored, no animal skins brought in or manufactured between May—October

(13) Pitching, levering and repairing of streets by order of the Common Council

(14) No cellars, sink holes or cisterns dug out between June—October 20

(15) All empty carts to be arranged one behind another to allow for street cleaning and to protect foot passengers from vicious horses

(16) Cartsmen shall carry shavings, litter and straw in tight boxes

(17) A fine of 20 shillings for feeding a cow, horse or hog on side walks and streets

(18) Goods brought into Wall-street shall be removed before 5 o'clock PM

(19) The interment of bodied between June 1—November 1 ought to be prohibited; all graves shall not be less than 6 feet deep

(20) Authorities shall correct the noxious fumes arising from sinks and privies

(21) Correct the evil of taverns, tippling and boarding houses on the low ground of the East River where sailors, the lower class of emigrants and other disorderly persons collect because they often produce fevers of the most serious nature

(22) No street shall be laid out without the approval of the City Council

(23) Provide a plentiful supply of fresh water to the city

(24) Provide tents for at least 5,000 sick persons as a means of sheltering them away from areas of contagion

Of all the provisions, number 23 drew the attention of the wealthy and powerful of New York. It read in full: "In suggesting the means of removing the causes of pestilential disease, we consider a plentiful supply of fresh water as one of the most powerful; and earnestly recommend that some plan for its introduction be carried into execution as soon as possible."[8]

Dr. Joseph Browne, a New York physician, believed that contaminated well water was the overriding cause of yellow fever. He also happened to be the brother-in-law of Aaron Burr. After a consultation, they concocted a plan to draw water from the Bronx River and distribute it throughout the city under the auspices of a private company. They presented the idea (which also included provisions for fighting fires and repairing streets damaged by the laying of pipe) to the Common Council. They liked the concept but preferred a public company be formed to operate the business. That proposal did not serve Burr's purpose, which, tragically for the people of New York, had nothing to do with pure water. Aaron Burr was actually interested only in obtaining a bank.

In 1799 New York had only two banks: Alexander Hamilton's Bank of New York and the New York branch of the First Bank of the United States. Burr wished to enter into the banking business and the easiest way to do so—with the aid of public money—was through a subterfuge. In order to make his proposal appear legitimate he assembled a bipartisan coalition of six partners that included three Federalists and three Anti-Federalists (soon to be known as Republicans). The prominent (albeit duped) supporter of Burr's plan was Alexander Hamilton, who had been the first secretary of the treasury in 1790.

On February 22, 1799, Burr and Hamilton gave their proposal to Mayor Richard Varick and the Common Council. Hamilton's presentation convinced the council and it was sent to Governor John Jay, who signed the act into law on April 2 without anyone's realizing that Burr had removed language from the original proposal concerning street repair and providing water for fire companies. In place, he substituted the proviso "that it shall and may be lawful for the said company to employ all such surplus capital as may belong or accrue to the said company in the purchase of public or other stock or in any other monied transactions of operations." This, in essence, allowed the newly formed Manhattan Company to become a financial institution.

When Burr's true intentions were made clear, Hamilton was quoted as saying, "He has lately by a trick established a bank, a perfect monster in its principals, but a very convenient instrument of profit and influence." Realizing the pretense, Dr. Browne wrote to Burr: "I expect and hope that enough will be done to satisfy the public and particularly the legislature that the institution is not a speculating job."

Dr. Browne hoped in vain. The company began doing business on September 1, 1799, at 40 Wall Street. After raising two million dollars, a scant one hundred thousand dollars was spent in failed efforts to lay pipe and dig wells; the remainder went into Burr's banking efforts. By 1808 the company sold its "waterworks," making a profit of 1.9 million dollars. Outliving its owners if not its purpose, the Manhattan Company became one of the original 52 members of the New York Clearing House Association. It merged with Chase National Bank in 1955, becoming Chase Manhattan. In December 2000 the bank acquired J.P. Morgan to become JP Morgan Chase & Company.[9] New York City did not get an adequate water system until October 1842, when the Croton Water System brought fresh water through 40 miles of aqueduct and pipes from the Croton Reservoir in Westchester County to Manhattan.[10]

The Tragedy in Philadelphia Returns, 1798

The reappearance of yellow fever at Philadelphia in 1798 was especially devastating to local authorities who had been persuaded that adopting strict measures of sanitation would ensure a summer with little, if any, infection. They admirably succeeded in cleaning the city and improving sewers and the water supply, but by failing to adopt any quarantine measures they unknowingly left themselves open to importation of the deadly source. Baltimore, on the other hand, enacted a strict quarantine against all ships arriving from the West Indies and also against any persons or baggage coming from Philadelphia and entirely escaped contamination.[11]

Extracts of letters from the summer of 1798 reveal a tragic picture of the city:

August 25: The Yellow Fever, in Philadelphia, continues to be very alarming to its citizens, and distressing to every friend of humanity. It has spread its deadly effluvia thro' almost every part of that unfortunate city. During the last week, the deaths averaged about 20 persons per day. The Inhabitants are quitting it in every direction.

By direction of the Board of Health, of Philadelphia, a Camp has been formed on the bank of the Schuylkill, near Walnut street, for the reception and relief of the Poor.

Forty-nine new cases of the prevailing fever of Philadelphia have been reported for the 14 hours ending Sunday morning, by 33 Physicians, and fresh cases make their appearance daily.

August 29: The deaths have now increased from 20 to 40 daily; and four-fifths of the Inhabitants have left the City.

August 30: One hundred and eleven new cases have been reported for the 48 hours ending on Tuesday at noon, in Philadelphia. The number of deaths for the last 48 hours is 82.

August 30: The pestilential Yellow Fever has broken out in this City, and threatens us with a renewal of the calamities of 1795…. Philadelphia is nearly deserted. The last day's report states 111 new cases! The confusion this curse occasions is not to be described.

Our Custom house and Coffeehouse are removed nearly out of town, to provide in some measure for the safety of their Clerks.[12]

As noted, the Custom House was moved to Chester, about 15 miles from the city, and the offices of government were transplanted to Trenton. Another missive noted that in Philadelphia "not more [than] *one house in fifteen open,* and yet the deaths were from 60 to 70 a day," while the newspaper editor of the *Aurora,* Mr. Balche, died of the disease. "At New York," a letter dated September 16 observed, "the mortality and desertion were similar; and Boston, which had hitherto escaped this destructive malady, is now involved in all its horrors. Such persons as had the means of flight, had retired to the country; most of the shops are shut up; all public places are closed; and large fires, composed of ropes, tar-barrels, &c. are constantly kept in the streets to carry off the infection." The only hope they had was that the coming winter would "happily repress its virulence." In a similar vein, the *London Observer* (November 4, 1798) wrote, "Trade, and even the printing of news-papers, is said to be suspended at Philadelphia and New-York, in consequence of the yellow fever. Humanity unites in the wishes of the inhabitants of those Cities, that the frost may destroy the infection."

Frost was as long away as any meeting of the minds concerning the origin of yellow fever. In discussing the 1798 outbreaks, after reporting that the summer had been exceedingly dry and sultry, the *London Monthly Magazine* (September 1, 1799) summarized what they had gleaned by stating, "A pretty general opinion seems to be prevailing, that in all these instances the disease was not imported by any contagion, but produced in each place by a variety of putrescent animal matter; in Boston especially, by a large quantity of raw hides and ill-cured fish and beef, which remained during the whole summer in warehouses, owing to a prohibition of all exportation to the French West India Islands." At the same time, in a public letter to the mayor and inhabitants of New York, Philadelphians proposed the states recommend to Congress a general prohibition of all communication with the West India Islands during the months of July, August and September. In their *Facts and Origins* published the following year, the College of Physicians stressed this point.

Nothing on that subject was done and mortality continued to climb during the summer of 1798. Yellow fever was said to have killed 1,500 in New York and 800 in Philadelphia during the month of September. In the latter city "the numbers had so greatly increased, that they had ceased to give [daily mortality numbers] publicity; and in order to conceal the dreadful effects of the pestilence, the unfortunate suffers were buried in the night. The distemper has made nearly as mortal a progress at New York, where about 20 persons died every day, and all the principal families had deserted the city. Not a single person was to be met in the streets without a handful of segars, and one smoking in the mouth as a precaution against the disease."

Nor were these cities alone. Reports also indicated that a disease of a similar species, "infinitely more malignant than the former diseases with which these places have been visited," had appeared in Vermont at New Milford, Royal Towns, Windsor and around the "Grand Isles of the Lake Champlain." By September 17 yellow fever was reported to be raging "in different degrees" at Newburyport, Portsmouth, Portland, Providence, Newport and New London, whereas at Albany and Boston the sickness was said to be on the decline.

Mortality from Wilmington, Delaware, during August 7–19 listed 97 dead; from

August 13 through September 19, at the Borough Hospital 46 patients were admitted: 18 died, 12 were dismissed cured and 16 remained. Private accounts indicated "nearly one half of the inhabitants have already left the place." Not surprisingly, authorities at New London, Connecticut, were unable to trace the source of the contagion either to the West Indies or any infected town in America. They ultimately determined that the malady spread from a quantity of putrid fish or meat and was "probably a domestic disease."

Mortality in Philadelphia, Late October, Early November 1798

October/November	Deaths
27	23
29	47
30	17
31	15
1	20

In good news for Philadelphia, if it could be called that, it was announced that as of October 29 seventy persons had died that day, "which had for some times carried off about 400 in a week." Cold weather did eventually arrive, and by October 17 "the fugitives were returning to New York ... where the disorder has considerably declined." At Boston, by October 23 "it had wholly disappeared," but "we fear no preventative has been discovered to guard against its reappearance next summer." By November 4 the Philadelphia Committee of Health invited the inhabitants to return to their homes "under the assurance of perfect safety, under proper precautions as to cleaning and airing their houses, bedding and clothing." One newspaper side note added that if New Yorkers had taken the precaution of having their city houses opened and fumigated before they returned from the country the contagion that "hung about the buildings" would have been dissipated much sooner.

Mortality for 1798 was depressingly high. Newspaper tallies from Philadelphia dated November 17 indicated 3,446 persons died in the city; when numbers from those who perished in the country were added, the number reached "not less than 5000 inhabitants." Bills of mortality for New York would eventually reveal that "no less than 3000 of the inhabitants died during the few months the disorder prevailed."

On December 30, news of the discontinuance of quarantine observed against all vessels coming from certain ports in America by order of the British Council (originating from their issuance on September 28 and October 24) was announced, officially ending international recognition of the yellow fever plague of 1798.[13]

No Relief from Yellow Fever in 1799

As testimony to how seriously matters were taken in Philadelphia, a letter dated June 28, 1799 indicated that when the ship *Thomas Wilson* out of Jamaica (where yellow fever had been raging for some time) arrived at a point below Chester, it was met by the surveyor and two inspectors from the custom-house barge. After the mate reported that four hands died on the voyage (a 12-day trip) and that the captain and one passenger remained ill from yellow fever, orders were issued to the pilot not to proceed further until the ship was inspected by the health physician. Early the next morning the same three authorities, accompanied by Drs. Allen and Duffield, were surprised to see the vessel in the offing (beyond the anchoring ground). Rowing to her, they discovered that during the night four English passengers forced the pilot to bring them ashore. Once the physicians confirmed the presence of yellow fever, warrants were issued to locate and return the escapees to the boat, where it was to serve quarantine down the river. An armed sloop was dispatched after her with orders to fire upon anyone attempting to leave.[14]

Interestingly, the incident with the *Thomas Wilson* turned into an imbroglio for everyone involved. The *Gazette* originally reported (March 23) that the ship, under Captain Jones, arrived from Kingston after a 31-day voyage. The question of the captain's illness, the presence or lack thereof, of yellow fever, and conflicting testimony of the principals would remain an issue for weeks. According to newspaper reports, James Hall, resident physician to the port, Samuel Duffield, consulting physician and William Allen, health officer of the port, affirmed that they went aboard on March 23 and found all the people in perfect health except Captain Jones, who claimed he had been "sick in the West Indies in October last, from which he recovered, and was again taken sick soon after he left Jamaica, on his passage home." He appeared not much indisposed but "his throat [was] bound up in consequence of the operation of mercury, which he had been using." They also reported that four of his crew had died at Petit Guave and Kingston in October, and that their bedding and clothes were thrown overboard.

The ship appeared to the inspectors to be "rather dirty" but did not exhibit "any such stench as would be likely in our opinion to produce a contagious disease." However, being unable to decide whether she was a sickly vessel or not, "from prudential motives and to prevent alarm" they directed her to be moved down opposite the marine hospital and there await directions from the board of health.[15] William Jackson, one of the inspectors, deposed that Doctor Hall reported to him that after visiting the ship he stated Captain Jones had the yellow fever.[16] Complicating matters, the owners of the *Thomas Wilson* denied any responsibility for what the captain or passengers reported.

These would be only the first salvos in the epidemic of 1799. As unrest grew, one editorialist who signed himself "Urbanity" drew the conclusion that should yellow fever become a threat "all agree that a dispersion of the inhabitants is all that is necessary to check its progress.... But this dispersion is at present attended with ruinous consequences," owing to a scarcity of affordable housing outside the danger zone. He suggested the authorities and "rich holders" erect convenient buildings on the commons, while "the humanity of Mr. Hamilton, Mrs. Powell, and all the other holders of property" on the other side of the Schuylkill join in a "general plan for construction of small back buildings for those whose occupations render it necessary to remain as near as safety would permit."[17]

By July, the authorities were forced to publish an uninformative statement of non-facts: "For two weeks past the most contradictory reports have been in circulation respecting the existence of the Yellow Fever. During this period much alarm and apprehension have been excited. The insidious nature of this disease forbids us to pronounce either upon its existence or its probable extension. It may however be satisfactory to observe, that if any cases of the fever are among us, they are on all hands allowed to be few, and to have produced no instances of contagion."[18]

In late July yellow fever, "or some malignant fever which resembles it," was reported at Newburyport, Massachusetts. Locals responded by appointing a board of health to investigate and take action. Neighboring Boston promptly issued orders for all vessels from Philadelphia to perform quarantine. This raised the ire of Edward Garrigues and in his position as president of the Philadelphia Board of Health he issued an official complaint to the Boston Board of Health. Arguing that the action was hastily entered into and would prove injurious to his city, he asked they rethink the action, promising that if it were discovered contagion existed he would duly inform them and any other place "which we may have connexion by commerce or otherwise, so they may rightfully adopt those measures deemed necessary for their safety."[19]

By August 22, the situation had altered significantly, requiring the Philadelphia Board of Health to issue a more precise proclamation. Admitting that within the past six days a number of persons had been taken ill by a disease they did not name, principally in the lower part of the city and suburbs, President Edward Garrigues and Secretary P. Hollingsworth held out hope that a change in the weather would check the progress of the disease. Based on the list of interments, they declared there was "not sufficient ground for the great alarm which pervades the City" but promised that if matters worsened they would further inform their fellow citizens.

The College of Physicians immediately issued a communication to the board of health offering their opinion that "a contagious and malignant Fever, similar to that which raged in the years 1793–97 and 98, at present exists in this City, and rages to an alarming degree." The list of interments indicated that within the 24 hours ending at noon on August 22, eleven grown persons and eight children "had been deposited in the several Burial Grounds of the City and Suburbs."

Under the same date, news from New York City indicated that since the 30th of May there had been frequent isolated cases of yellow fever, but at the present time it was thought to be more general, although the board of health had not published any notice on the subject. Country people were deterred from coming into the city and in consequence the markets were ill supplied.[20]

Bellevue Hospital remained closed during 1799, indicating early fatalities were not as severe as in the preceding year. Perhaps this was due to Dr. Angelis's "Four Herbs Pills," which contained "a certain and infallible cure of the Malignant or Putrid Fever," universally known and approved by eminent physicians and all ranks in Italy. Aside from the stupendous self-promotion in his June 15 advertisement, Angelis stated that febrile disorders generally originated from "an aflection in the blood," and that he felt it his duty to assure the public that "the Infection originates in this country, and that it will exist in this city by the last of July next." Rather than alarm people, he noted that it was in his power to remove this dreadful calamity "with trifling expense" if only citizens would buy his product.[21]

If they were not saved by "Four Herbs Pills," at least New Yorkers maintained their sense of humor concerning yellow fever. In a "marvelous" story that made the trades as far as Philadelphia, a farmer purportedly appeared in the city and saw a number of men digging in the middle of the street. Racing home he declared "that the town folks were dying so fast that they had to bury them in the middle of the streets!" On inquiry, it was found that he had mistaken the excavation of waterworks canals for graves.[22]

By September 10 letters indicated yellow fever was raging in New York and Philadelphia "with extreme violence ... and the number of deaths was as great as at any preceding period of this calamity." The fact that the disease had not appeared in any of the more southern states was "considered by many as a proof that it is an imported malady." (Later reports indicated yellow fever had "found its way to Carolina, where numbers of persons had been carried off by it.") As testimony to the fact the controversy concerning its origin raged as greatly as the fever, another newspaper reported that the disease at Philadelphia was attributed to the "numerous Docks, which being exhaled by the immense power of the sun, fills the air with putridity."[23]

On the Subject of Letters, Commerce and "Delusive Quackery"

Americans were great letter writers and many of these seemingly innocent missives eventually found their way into the newspapers. The information these notes contained often present an insight into the temper and the conditions of the times. That does not necessarily imply that what the authors conveyed was accurate or that people reading them appreciated their judgments. One such, dated July 8, 1799, prefaced, "Extract of a letter from a respectable merchant in Philadelphia to a mercantile house in this city" appeared in the *Philadelphia Gazette* of July 11. It read as follows:

> I assure you nothing is more untrue or unfounded than the prevalence of a contagious fever here. As many as three or four persons have died of a fever, which, it is said, appeared to have some affinity to the late yellow fever. These, it is said, derived the infection from a certain prize schooner from the West Indies; and we trust, that with the last of these unfortunate victims, (if any such there were as applicable to the disease in question) with them expired also the contagion.... From these and from no greater causes have the various and idle reports of the prevalence of the yellow fever here arisen. I flatter myself that you will cheerfully do a commercial sister city the justice to contradict reports so false and detrimental to our trade, which from various causes is already too much destroyed—but whatever may be our misfortunes in this respect, you may depend upon it the Philadelphians will never suppress the truth.

Interestingly, a letter with a slightly different slant, reprinted from the *Gazette of the United States,* appeared in the *New York Commercial Advertiser* of July 9, 1799:

> There is no set of men among us who make so much uproar about the restraints imposed to prevent the introduction of the fever as the merchants; and yet they are always the first people to sound unfounded terror, and extend unnecessary alarm. The first serious accounts we receive of this scourge being among us is generally from extracts of letters from our own merchants, returning upon us from all quarters. A merchant is informed by his clerks or runners perhaps, that the fever is very bad; this is enough for him: all his letters of the day are burthened with this precious authentic intelligence, and flies to every corner of the continent, and comes back to us in "extracts of letters from a respectable mercantile house in Philadelphia." The very obliging correspondents of these gentlemen never lose a moment to carry their letters to the press; and thus from our own counting houses an absurd terror is diffused over the whole country to be exceeded in its pernicious consequences only by the yellow fever itself.

The first letter decries the "various and idle" for spreading false rumors; the second blames gossip. In both cases, the concern is for commerce, or more specifically the potential damage to business in light of the threat of yellow fever. If, in fact, the threat from disease were slight or nonexistent, merchants could hardly be blamed. But if the danger were real, that cast such arguments in an entirely different light—one that had a tendency to cloud rather than illuminate the situation.

While those questions remained open to debate, others were equally significant. These could be summed up in two interrogatives: Real or imagined? Cure of quackery?

Perhaps nothing better illustrated the breadth of the spectrum than a man named Elisha Perkins.

On August 7, 1799, *Greenleaf's New York Journal* published a brief note: "We understand the celebrated Dr. Perkins, the inventor of the Metallic Points, has arrived in this city." It is likely this tidbit was slightly delayed, for the "celebrated" doctor had already began running ads for his services:

DOCTOR PERKINS
INVENTOR OF THE METALLIC POINTS CALLED TRACTORS,

> HAVING obtained from various experiments satisfactory evidence that the Yellow Fever is as much within the control of means safe, simple and easily obtained as any fever whatever, thinks it his duty therefore, in this explicit manner to make it known to the public in general, and to the inhabitants of this city in particular. He wishes to administer in the presence of the best judges that a just decision on the subject may be obtained by others. He flatters himself he shall, altho a stranger, meet with that candid and liberal treatment which ever characterize a learned and virtuous people.
>
> It [is] his intention to give advice in the various complaints that come under the care of Physicians, and if he finds suitable encouragement, to continue his residence in this city.
>
> His office is at no. 59 John-street, where he will be happy to see his friends.[24]

Born on January 16, 1741, at Norwich, Connecticut, Perkins practiced medicine in Plainfield and became a member of the Medical Society of the State of Connecticut. On February 19, 1796, he received a 14-year parent for his "Tractors." These consisted of two 3-inch metal rods with pointed ends that he claimed were constructed of "unusual metal alloys" but that were actually steel and brass.

The method he used consisted of stroking the affected parts of the human body with the pointed metallic instruments, "giving out that such stroking will radically cure the most obstinate pains." Naming his therapy, "Perkins Patent Tractors," he gained a considerable following in the United States and abroad, including surgeons at the Royal Frederick Hospital in Copenhagen, Denmark. Considered to be a technique in the category of animal magnetism, Perkins claimed his "points" were able to cure cases of rheumatic pains, agues, pains in the head, face and side, and distressing inflammations including those of the eyes. Even George Washington was said to have purchased a pair of the tractors, and being "convinced of the importance of the discovery from experiments in his own family, availed himself of its advantages."

Sadly for Perkins, the same year he received the patent, the Connecticut Medical Society cited the Tractors and the philosophy as "delusive quackery." They expelled Perkins from their group on the charge he used "certain pointed Perkins' Instruments, pretending they were an invention of his own; and also that they possess inherent powers of curing many diseases."[25]

Dr. Perkins was hardly defeated. In a preface to his book, *Certificates of the Efficacy of Doctor Perkins' Patent Medicine Instruments* (1796), he wrote the following:

> Sensible that every attempt at improvement in any of the useful arts, ever has, and probably ever will, meet with opposition, either from interested or *certain* other motives, which in a greater or less degree influences the generality of mankind,—the subscriber takes the liberty to cite a few among very many cases in which his method of removing pains, inflammations, and spasmodic affections from the human body, has been attended with success. The novelty and apparent simplicity of this practice, may possibly, influence some, before they have attended with candor to the subject, to treat it with ridicule. That the public may be more satisfactorily informed as to its utility and importance, he publishes the following certificates, as received from several respectable characters.
>
> Elisha Perkins, Plainfield, August 12, 1796

In his book he reprinted testimonials from "characters" residing in eight states: Massachusetts, New Hampshire, Rhode Island, Connecticut, Vermont, New York, Pennsylvania (Philadelphia) and Delaware.

Perkins also invented an antiseptic medicine that he was interested in trying on yellow fever victims. Drawn to New York City by the epidemic of 1799, he set up practice, undoubtedly encouraged by the flattering newspaper mention. Unfortunately, the following three instances his name found its way into the papers were not what he would have wished:

> September 4: Dr. Perkins, the celebrated inventor of the Metallic Points, is extremely ill of the fever.[26]
> September 5: Dr. Perkins, inventor of the Metallic Points, (we are informed) in a fair way of recovering from his late indisposition.[27]
> September 6: We mention with sincere regret, that Dr. PERKINS, inventor of the Metallic Tractors, fell a victim to the prevailing epidemic this morning, after an illness of 6 or 7 days.[28]

While it would appear this was the end of the metallic points, it was not. Dr. Perkins' son Benjamin Douglas Perkins went to England and settled in Leicester Square. As his father's therapy was already well known and required little introduction the younger Perkins obtained a patent on the tractors and sold them for 5 guineas a pair. This price was prohibitive to the poorer classes, prompting the Society of Friends, of which Perkins was a member, to construct a hospital for the poor that they called "Perkins Institution." Treatment was offered to all comers free of charge.

The phenomenal success of the therapy aroused interest in the medical community, prompting Drs. Haygarth and Falconer to put it to the test. Shaping and then painting two wooden sticks to precisely resemble Perkins' tractors, they selected five patients from a hospital in Bath and repeated the stroking technique. Patients reported immediate pain relief and great satisfaction. The experiment was repeated the following day but this time with the original equipment. The results were the same, indicating that the therapy worked as a placebo rather than an actual treatment employing magnetism or some electrical powers. After Haygarth published *Of the Imagination, as a Cause and Cure of Disorders, Exemplified by Fictitious Tractors,* the metallic points and Perkins Institution fell into disrepute and the hospital closed. Benjamin Perkins returned to Philadelphia with a £10,000 profit and presumably lived out his life as a wealthy gentleman.[29]

Yellow Fever: The View at the End of the 1700s

Toward the end of a century it is common practice for people to become retrospective, to cast one long, lingering look over their shoulders and summarize the major events of the past one hundred years before turning the page and moving forward. An extract from Dr. Hillary's *Treatise on the Yellow Fever* offered one definitive view:

> I know no disease, in which the recovery of the patient so much depends upon the *right* or *wrong* method of treating it, at the very first attack, or beginning of the disease, as this fever does:—For by thus discharging and carrying off the putrid, acrimonious, bilious matter, out of the body, before much of it is carried into the blood; not only most of the bad symptoms, which attend the second state of the fever are prevented from coming, but hamorrhages, and the yellowness of the skin also;

and the fever soon taken off; For I have never seen any hamorriage come on, and but little yellowness, or in some none, when they were thus treated.[30]

In 1799, *Lloyd's Evening-Post* (January 16–18) published, "A Short Essay on the Origin of the YELLOW FEVER, Which Has Appeared in the Towns of the UNITED STATES of NORTH AMERICA." In it, the unnamed author drew a number of conclusions.

(1) Yellow Fever, like the Plague, is certainly a disorder originating in the warm climates of Asia or Africa. It was introduced into the West Indies by African ships and is now general to the Islands

(2) In times of peace it is little regarded, but during war, when the inhabitants are confined in besieged towns and fleets and armies maintained in situations favourable to disease, yellow fever rages with uncontrollable violence

(3) Europe is preserved from it by the length of voyage from the West Indies, and, perhaps, by the fleets arriving generally in seasons sufficiently cold to check it. The United States, with the shortness of the voyage which is a little more than a fortnight, renders the West Indies the same source of contagion that the Levant is to Europe

(4) There is strong collateral evidence, arising from the identity of the disorder (differentiating it from diseases of an inferior tribe, such as intermittent, bilious, putrid and jail fevers) that yellow fever is imported rather than of local origin. The idea of its originating in the U.S. "was first mentioned by a Physician in Philadelphia [Benjamin Rush] in 1793, who is remarkable for the eccentricity and enthusiasm of his systems, which were prosecuted almost to a degree of insanity, contrary to the general opinion of the faculty, and the good sense of the citizens at large."

(5) No regulations in Europe proved effectual against the Plague until quarantine was generally adopted; the partial regulations of that kind in the U.S. proved useful, but have never been adopted with the rigour of Europe and evasions have been too little noticed or punished

(6) American cities are generally as healthy as those of Europe, but at no time in their history until a few years past have they been ravaged with yellow fever. Yellow fever has never appeared in any town which does not have some immediate connexion with the West Indies. Since these vessels have recently been prohibited from reaching Philadelphia, they have been forced to unload cargo in towns along the Delaware River; almost immediately outbreaks of the disease have been reported

(7) Yellow fever appears most in the Middle and Northern States where trade is carried on to a great degree; it is seen less often in Southern States, where the climate is more favourable, but where there is less commerce

(8) Rather than credit yellow fever as an imported disease, numerous stories have been propagated relative to the crowded construction of cities, want of common sewers and poor sanitation. Yet the disease does not remain in cities from one year to the next but each outbreak is produced by fresh contagion. Cold and rain have in all instances totally destroyed it.

In conclusion, the author noted that the differences among various individuals as to the origin, nature and treatment of yellow fever "have been prosecuted with an enthusiasm and rancour, which have proved one of the severest afflictions that has accompanied it, and has robbed the unhappy sufferers of all the comfort which confidence in a physician is capable of." This circumstance, he hoped, should teach the world to beware and trust only those opinions with good sense and an attention to facts.

That said, two "dueling" works of note were published in 1799. The first, "Facts and Observations Relative to the Nature and Origin of the Pestilential Fever, Which Prevailed in the City of Philadelphia, in 1793, 1797, and 1798," by the College of Physicians of Philadelphia, offered arguments for two basic tenets: the Philadelphia fever was imported from the West Indies, not generated in the city, and it was highly contagious. Yet there was more to explain: "A striking peculiarity, which does not occur in any other disease, attends the yellow fever in the West Indies. The natives and persons who have resided long in those islands, are very seldom seized with this fever." Indicating that few, if any, Creole French immigrants suffered from the disease during the epidemics, the Fellows observed that children born to them after their arrival in the United States were as likely to die from the fever as were those of European blood. They concluded:

> It is an observation founded in long and extensive experience, and which admits not of an exception, that strangers are the greatest sufferers from the diseases of the country into which they migrate; were the yellow fever a disease of our country, the Creoles would probably have been among the first to experience its fatal effects; but as it is of West Indian origin, and their constitutions are assimilated to it, they escaped it here as they do in their native country.

Attempting to put together a medical jigsaw puzzle, the authors were compelled to work in some pieces that did not quite fit, noting that their theory was not "quite so clear as might be wished," as army physicians asserted that "tropical continued (or proper yellow) fever" is not contagious, "but that it arises from a particular state of the atmosphere." The difference, therefore, lay in the precise type of fever, acknowledging some species to be contagious and others not. Their recommendations included:

(1) Create a Board of Health consisting of 5 persons, two of which should be practitioners of physick

(2) Set aside a sum of money for the use of the Board. The Board to meet daily during the months of July through October; during these months establish a quarantine for every vessel from the Mediterranean, Coast of Africa, West Indies, and that territory to the southward of Florida

(3) Assign a resident physician to the islands and a consulting physician in Philadelphia

(4) Punish masters of vessels and passengers who evade the law by a charge of murder in the second degree

(5) Let co-operative laws be procured from neighboring legislatures or Congress

(6) Give the Board of Health power, with the concurrence of the governor, to cut off intercourse with infected persons and places. Establish a fever hospital

(7) Clean and water the streets, gutters and wharfs[31]

The second article, written by Benjamin Rush, was entitled "Observations upon the Origin of the Malignant, Bilious, or Yellow Fever, in Philadelphia, and upon the Means of Preventing It, Addressed to the Citizens of Philadelphia" and served, in some measure, as a rebuttal of the above. Dr. Rush explained the remote cause of yellow fever by stating, "This disease is the offspring of putrid vegetable and animal exhalations in all countries.—It prevails only in hot climates and seasons." The sources in Philadelphia were, he enumerated:

(1) The docks, containing a large quantity of filthy matter in a highly concentrated state. In New York City, the disease goes by the name of *dock fever*

(2) The foul air of ships
(3) The common sewers
(4) The gutters
(5) Dirty cellars and yards
(6) Privies
(7) Masses of water that lie in the neighborhood of the city
(8) Impure pump-water

Rush noted that in *Facts and Observations* the College of Physicians stated common bilious fever and dysentery had very much diminished, but as the putrid exhalations remained the presumption must be that "they produce our highest grade of bilious, which is the yellow fever." He likewise stated, "The cold in these cases cannot act upon the disease in our houses, and of course it does not alter the quality of the matters discharged from the bodies of the sick. It acts only upon the putrid exhalations which float in the atmosphere." He was also of the belief that there was "a remarkable sympathy between the stomach and lungs" and ascribed the type of yellow fever in Philadelphia "to an unusual quantity of oxygen in the air." Rush's discussion on prevention centered entirely on sanitary measures.[32]

British surgeon James Anderson, late of the 60th Regiment of Foot, published his own book, *A Few Facts and Observations on the Yellow Fever of the West Indies*, asserting that there existed two "species of fever" that had been described under the same name but proceeded from very different causes. He claimed "proper yellow fever" was not contagious but that a highly infectious fever raged in the islands that "resembled the endemic in many of its symptoms." His practice consisted of giving large doses of calomel with James's powder in the first days of the disease, "so as to keep the bowels very open." In agreement with him was an unnamed correspondent to the *Philadelphia Gazette* (July 10, 1799). Under the heading "Medical Communication" he stated that there actually existed "two distempers which differ essentially in certain important particulars, viz, the yellow fever, and the malignant pestilential fever." Yellow fever, he believed, was marked with a horrid effusion of bile but was seldom or never contagious, while the malignant pestilential fever was hardly ever accompanied by "this shocking appearance, is highly contagious, terrible in its symptoms, and very fatal." Both diseases, he concluded, made their appearance at the same time in North America but were not distinguished with sufficient accuracy, causing numerous contradictions "which appear to disgrace a liberal profession."

Hector McLean, MD, the assistant inspector of hospitals for St. Domingo, added his own theories to the mix with his book, *An Enquiry into the Nature and Causes of the Great Mortality Among the Troops at St. Domingo*. He considered yellow fever to be an "endemic remittent of that island, not infectious," that acted on Europeans because of their "plethoric state, and from habits of free living." Candidly admitting he met with much disappointment in his treatments, he found that bleeding and cold bathing afforded more relief than other methods.[33]

"More irritating than profitable"

During the summer of 1799, in an effort to limit yellow fever, lawmakers in Albany, New York, passed a bill prohibiting certain trades and manufactures, including those involved in the production of soap and candles. Those directly involved in these businesses hired Dr. Mitchell, a physician from the New-York Hospital, to argue against the act. Mitchell presented his "Theory of Pestilential Fluids" (first published in 1795) to the legislature, arguing that substances composed of "carbone and hydrogene," such as fat, grease and oil," were incapable of yielding pestiential air but that substances containing septon (the skinny, lean, muscular and membranous parts of animals, together with the blood and alimentary faeces) were the substances whence unhealthy and noxious exhalations proceeded.

Further developing his theory on the origin of yellow fever, Mitchell believed the pestilence "to be occasioned by azote [septon] in its uncombined state, or only united with those qualities of oxygen necessary to constitute it respectively oxyd of azote, nitrous gas, and nitrous acid. The production of azote from putrescent animal matter, and the *septic properties* of this acid of pestilence, which would 'threaten ruin to the animal world,' he conceives are best kept under by alkalies and alkaline earths, and hence their use in cleaning and purifying from the contagion of putrescence." "Mitchell then expounded on the idea that privies and collections of human ordure (excrement) had long been observed to contain septic (nitric) acid, and the effluvia of privies had been known to excite dangerous sicknesses. Additionally, many articles of diet contained septon; and oxygen, in some form, always existed in the alimentary canal. It was therefore probable, he concluded, that septic acid might be formed in the cavities of these abdominal viscera, and that 'irritation and inversion of the motions of the stomach, in some forms of *yellow fever,* as well as spasms of the colon, griping pains and tenesmus in some of the cases of *dysentery,* PROCEEDED FROM THE SAME EXCITING CAUSE.'"

Drawing on his private practice, Mitchell found watery solutions of the carbonates of pot-ash and soda to be an excellent antidysenteric remedy, while the acid/base relationship was used to explain yellow fever and elucidate dysentery. Giving azote the name "septon" created other nomenclatural conjugations, including *septic acid* for nitric acid, as well as *septate of lime* and *septate of potash*, which became fashionable with medical men in the United States.

It was not surprising that after listening to Dr. Mitchell's learned discourses the Albany politicians abandoned any attempt to determine whether yellow fever was imported or of local origin by declaring the city had enough causes for the production of diseases without any need for external sources.[34]

Perhaps the best way to end a discussion of yellow fever in the 18th century is to quote a commentary taken from the *London Monthly Review* of September 1, 1799: "We cannot help noticing the acrimony with which this controversy concerning the origin of the [yellow] fever is carried on; even in the letter from the General Committee of Citizens in Philadelphia to those in New York, they begin by declining to enter upon this controversy, more irritating than profitable."

It would take more than a century for the acrimony to be resolved.

CHAPTER 9

Is Yellow Fever More Deadly Than the Plague?

> *THE YELLOW FEVER: This dreadful disease baffles all our skill and ingenuity; reason cannot discover its principles, nor account for its operations, no further proof of our ignorance is necessary than the many and various opinions we have about its origin and cure. And its great mortality under our most skillful Physicians.*[1]

The first decade of the 1800s carried on where the last century left off. With so many questions still unanswered, debates raged as violently as the yellow fever itself. Was it contagious? Did it originate locally or was it an imported disease? Did it arise spontaneously from putrid matter or was it generated from poisonous air? What part did weather play? How did atmospheric conditions, meteors, electricity and oxygen factor into the equation? Did quarantine help prevent its spread or merely hinder commerce? And which health care practitioners had the cure? Or was there a cure at all?

These were all weighty subjects and everyone, it seemed, wanted to express an opinion. Those who did so for obvious gain—to say nothing of notoriety—were the hucksters of nostrums and notions. It is difficult to determine whether these profiteers actually believed what they sold were authentic cures. Three things are certain, however: the concept of "truth in advertising" was nonexistent; the advertisements promoted concoctions as cures for a wide variety of diseases, never failing to mention the prevailing "disease of the month" (whether it be smallpox, cholera, typhus or yellow fever); and sellers proclaimed their products to be the one and only effective means of dispelling the horrors of the reigning malady—often equated with that most terrifying of mortal diseases—the plague.

One advertisement in 1800 promised to "supply the Wealth"—figuratively, of course (which would have made a nice rhyme with "to maintain our health" had the proprietor thought it through, but then again, this was a serious notice), by "a medical Gentleman of the first eminence." Stating his "preventative" was "the only substantial Cure for the Yellow Fever, and the train of bilious Diseases which it perpetuates," the inventor clarified the situation further by warning, "This Medicine has no Connection with the common System of Quackery, which promises unprecedented Effects from the feeblest Nostrums." A careful reader might have been impressed with the guarded claim of "substantial" and the implied separation from "feeblest Nostrums," but his patriotism—and common sense—might have been stretched by the further boast that his preventative would eradicate the "horrors of almost certain Infection" sailors contracted when supporting "the

> Did you ever;
> No I never,
> See'd a feller,
> Half so yeller,
> How's your liver?
>
> Why, all upset, of course. Then take the remedy, Dr. Pierce's Golden Medical Discovery, and you won't go around looking the color of a yellow fever victim. It means good bye biliousness, headachs, lost appetite and sour stomach, indigestion, impurities of the blood, and countless miseries of suffering humanity. It is guaranteed to benefit or cure in every case of disease for which it is recommended, or money paid for it will be refunded.

In the 1800s "cures" for yellow fever were as common as deaths caused by the disease. This advertisement attempts to interject a little humor with a short poem before making exaggerated and false promises of cures for all sorts of ailments (*Whitesboro News* [Texas], September 6, 1889).

glory of their Country." The medicine sold for one guinea per parcel or six for five guineas.[2]

If a bolder approach were possible, S. Solomon, MD, took it when promoting "Cordial Balm of Gilead." In a staggering eight-paragraph ad be promised to cure "all delicate, weakly, and relaxed constitutions, lowness of spirits, hypochondria, horrors, tremblings, weakness of sight, loss of memory, impaired vigour, tabes dorsalis, nervous consumption, those who have revelled in the midnight cup," while adding, "It has been the only means of restoring thousands afflicted with the YELLOW FEVER in America." Dr. Solomon missed the chance to make a play on his name with "wisdom," traditionally associated with another famous Soloman, but he likely compensated for that oversight by requiring the fee of one guinea in advance for consultations and the "saving of one pound-six shillings" when his balm was purchased in bulk.

The following year, in an even longer ad obviously geared for a higher clientele, Solomon lamented the fact that if Laurence Sterne (1713–1768, author of *The Life and Opinions of Tristram Shandy, Gentleman*) or Tobias Smollett (1721–1771, author of *The Adventures of Roderick Random*), who suffered from debilitation and hypochondria respectively, had access to the Balm of Gilead, they would have been restored to health. Even more audaciously, he associated his preparations with Cullen's nosology, while noting that in "the prints of the day, that inestimable 'Guide to Health' and other productions, continue to waft its praise to all civilized countries. In America it has stayed the ravages of the Yellow Fever; in Europe it hourly saves the Consumptive, Asthmatic, and debilitated victim from the jaws of death." Without mincing words, Solomon concluded, "The Balm is the Cape stone of medical research, and is resorted to with that confidence no other medication ever was in the memory of the oldest man living."[3]

In 1801 "the progress of Science and the triumph of Labour and perseverance, united with Art" combined to create an Important Discovery in the Materia Medica: A 'SPECIFIC'" for the prevention and cure of "this desolating distemper, to which the appellation of the Yellow Fever is now generally given…. The Nation at large, so justly interested in the fate of those who devote themselves to her welfare must highly rejoice at this discovery." This patent medicine was sold in boxes for one guinea each.[4]

Dr. Brodum had a more unique take on how to sell his "Nervous Cordial and Botanical Syrup" for the treatment of gout, rheumatism, evil, scurvy, nervous consumptive, yellow fever, jaundice, bilious complaints and debilities of both sexes arising from natural or acquired causes ("evil" and "debilities of both sexes" a polite way of expressing sexually transmitted diseases). His pitch was to encourage patients to apply to him by post, signing only their initials, where they could state their case without reservation rather than confess their "weakness to the physician he is intimate with, and in which case the female in particular often falls a sacrifice, rather than divulge the secret of their guilt." The cordial was sold in bottles for 22s, 11s and 6s, duty included.[5]

Rather than use his own name in promoting his "REMEDY," one unnamed promoter began his 1804 ad by announcing that Dr. Willich, late physician to the Saxon ambassador and author of the *Domestic Encyclopaedia,* approved and recommended his product as a means of curing and preventing the yellow fever. The promoter noting that it was an easy, safe and pleasant preserver of health, the product with the generic name "Remedy" came supplied with full directions, also sanctioned by Dr. Willich. For the price of one guinea, a box was sufficient for one person for twelve months.[6] Curiously, the following year, the proprietor, who had expanded the product name to "Yellow Fever Remedy," published a letter from Dr. Willich in which he stated he had the powder analyzed and concluded that the examination proved the ingredients "cannot fail to be of eminent service in malignant fevers, and especially such as prevail in tropical climates." A caveat warned, however, that he (Dr. Willich) had no actual experience with treating yellow fever.

If that were not peculiar enough, in the same newspaper a bold caption announced, "One Hundred Guineas Reward. Warehouse for the Yellow Fever Remedy, No. 40, Charing-cross, London." The text notified the public that the company had recently "billed upwards of Three Hundred Thousand Magazines, each with one sheet of paper, containing their Advertisement and several Cases" (testimonials), only to discover some "Person or Persons" removed a great number of said bills "and for malicious purposes sent them by the post, inclosed as double Letters to persons residing in the county," presumably charging the cost to the proprietors. Whoever helped bring the criminals to justice would receive the reward upon conviction of the perpetrators.[7] (See Chapter 12 for two court cases involving the sale of shares in this yellow fever remedy.)

By 1807 a new notice appeared wherein Dr. Willich "recommended, in the strongest manner possible," the YELLOW FEVER REMEDY. In order to convince surgeons of Garrisons and other eminent Medical Gentlemen of the worth of this remedy, a sufficient quantity was offered GRATIS to preserve health in foreign climates.[8] A bolder proclamation was made in 1807 when it was announced that yellow fever had disappeared in America: "This may be greatly accounted for by the large Exportation which had taken place a considerable time before of the REV. WM. BARCLAY's PATENT ANTIBILIOUS PILLS, which are known to be the most infallible Remedy for this and every Bilious Disorder."[9]

Occasionally a nostrums peddler was able to get his name in the paper without paying for it. A year after his advertisement for "Four Herbs Pills" ran in New York newspapers, Dr. Angelis's name appeared in London's *Lloyd's Evening-Post* (October 22–24, 1800), where he attributed yellow fever to eating immoderately of peaches and cucumbers. And then there were those good souls who offered free advice. One gentleman lately returned from Martinique (1803) recommended a small tumbler of water strongly impregnated with "camomile" and magnesia, with a tablespoon of citron narbonne honey to cure yellow fever. A letter writer from Nassau (1804) reported that a Spanish physician cured the disease by having victims drink an infusion of the rind of the common sour orange; and an American doctor (1806) discovered that the principal ingredient in Castile soap was sure to cure the malady. (See Chapter 10 for an additional discussion.)[10]

The "Barbary Triangle"—Cadiz, Gibraltar and Malaga

The first decade of the new century would not be good to Spain, especially regarding that territory encompassing the small inverted triangle that began along the Barbary Coast of northern Africa and extended to Cadiz on the southwestern tip of the country, crossing through the Rock of Gibraltar and concluding at Malaga on the southeastern side. Situated on the southwestern top of Spain at 36° 30' N. latitude in the temperate zone, Cadiz had a population of 64,838 in 1768; by 1801, the year after the Great Epidemic, it had been reduced to 57,837.

The heath of the people was generally good, although historically there had been a number of "plague years."

Health of Cadiz

Year	Disease
1466	An unnamed "infectious disorder" nearly depopulated the city.
1507	The same or a similar disease raged through Cadiz and Barcelona.
1649–51	A disease referred to as the plague lasted three years and carried off more than 14,000 souls. The disease was believed to have been introduced by a vessel that came from Malaga and Murcia and anchored at San Lucar.
1730	"El vomito negro," or black vomit, made its first appearance.
1731	A disease referred to by the vague name of "la peste," struck with equal fury. It had one distinguishing symptom: spots of a livid, yellow or dark color covered the body and were the certain forerunner of the black vomit. It was considered pestilential in nature and was believed to have been introduced by a ship newly arrived from Spanish America
1764	An epidemic raged between September and October and was thought to have originated from old and corrupted corn. Dr. Lind described it by writing that it "gave rise to epidemic bilious disorders, resembling those of the West Indies, of which a hundred persons often died in a day." The disease began with alternate chills and heat, pains in the head and back and pit of the stomach. Within 24 hours, the patient suffered violent retching and vomiting of green or yellow bile, and some threw up humour as black as ink. Lind speculated that this disease might be communicated by contagion but only a slight one unless commingled with bad air. For those affected aboard ships, the disease was greatly checked by putting out to sea

Thirty-six years elapsed between the epidemic of 1764 and the terrible ravages of 1800. In that year a ship named *Dolphin* arrived from Spanish America. It was thought its crew of smugglers broke quarantine and managed to reach land for the purpose of hiding their goods. At the time, quarantine measures were lax, particularly for smugglers working the coast of Africa; crews of Spanish privateers were also permitted to land without quarantine. In a further relaxing of regulations, on February 1, 1800, ships coming from the United States were also exempt.

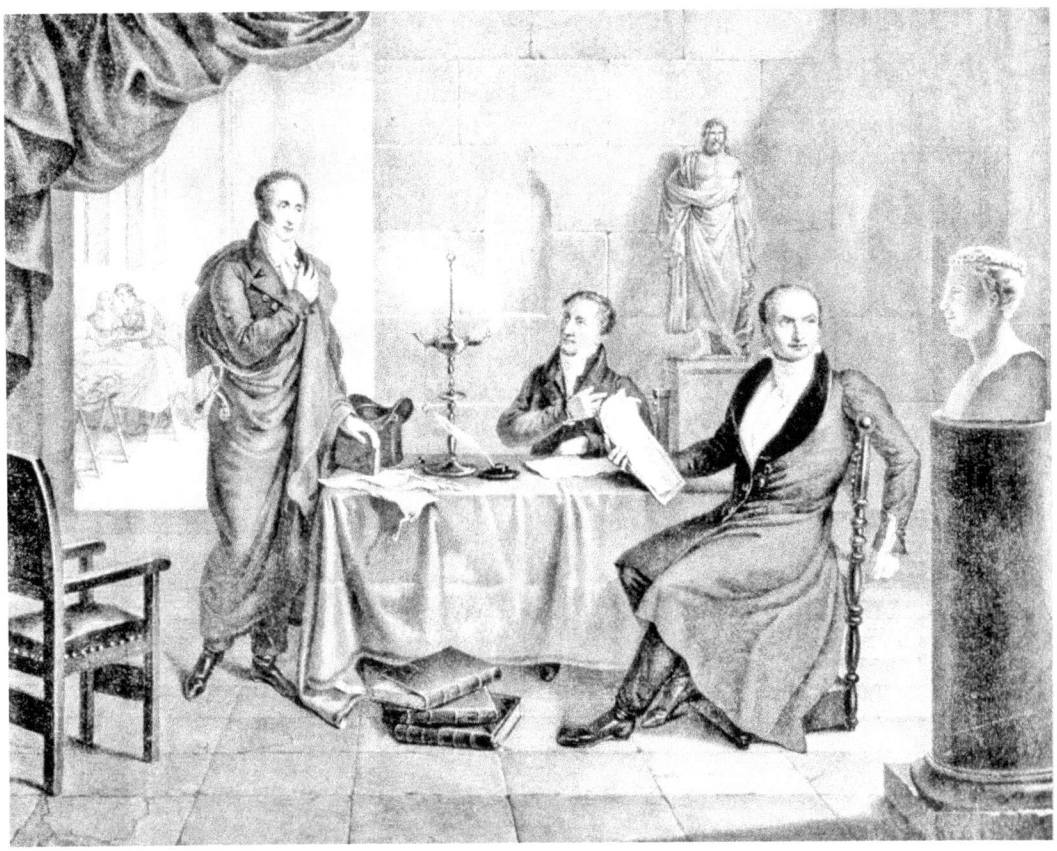

Yellow fever was not confined to the Caribbean and southern United States but presented a grave threat to many European nations where epidemics destroyed thousands of lives. Among the countries most affected was Spain. This painting, "Commission des Medecins," depicts three gentlemen gathered in "Barcelonne," 1821. Without knowing how the disease originated, their almost hopeless goal was to try and contain the spread of yellow fever while vainly seeking a cure for those suffering from the deadly symptoms (courtesy National Library of Medicine).

By the middle of August, 25–30 deaths from the fever were occurring daily at Barrio de Santa Maria. According to letters from Cadiz, during the period from August 18 to September 5, total mortality in that city reached 3,600, with 207 persons expiring on September 5 alone. Those contracting the disease usually died on the third or fourth day after the initial attack. The first symptoms were pain in the limbs and bones and violent vomiting.

It was not surprising that those who could flee did so, and by early September it was reported 30,000 had left the city, leaving behind 40,000 to try to survive as they might. To limit the spread of disease an order was issued warning that no further exodus would be permitted; to enforce this, Spanish troops were drawn along the peninsula to prevent any intercourse with the country. In another step, authorities broke with tradition and ordered bodies to be buried outside the city limits rather than in nearby churchyards. Furthermore, as had been done elsewhere, the tolling of death bells was prohibited. Traditional remedies such as covering the face with a handkerchief steeped in thieves vinegar, wearing aromatic amulets and dosing with cordials were resorted to, with little effect.

Deaths remained as high as 200 per day by mid–September. French papers, "without giving a name to this horrible malady, deny that it is either the yellow fever or the plague,"[11] and attention was directed toward the "stagnant, noxious air" as a contributing factor. (This idea was supported by English authority Dr. Edward Bancroft. In his essay on the prevailing disease at Cadiz and Gibraltar, he stated that the fever was brought on by the "morbid effect of marsh miasmata in both these places," and, therefore, "any precautions founded on a belief of the importation and contagion of the disorder was objectionable.") In a curious development it was also observed that animals were victims of the fever, especially dogs, cats, horses and poultry. Locals reported that "no sparrow ever appeared during the epidemic" (as opposed to other species of wild birds that fell victim to the disease), so that the continuance of sparrows in a dwelling was held as certain proof of its being free of contagion.[12] It was also noted that the pestilential fever of Spain was never known to attack persons a second time.

In response to military maneuvers during the War of the Second Coalition (1798–1802), the British fleet under Lord Keith appeared before Cadiz in early October. This threat broke the lethargy of disease and death, prompting the people of Cadiz to rise up and defend their city. Whether this sudden action or a change in the weather affected the course of the epidemic, mortality lowered so much that it was hoped the worst had passed. Those who had fled returned to Cadiz, but with their arrival it reappeared in some force. Authorities ordered the firing of cannon to disinfect the air, which continued until November 12, when the city was declared free of contagion.

From August 1 until the first week of November 1800 a total of 48,688 people were sickened: of these, 7,292 perished and 40,699 recovered. At Seville mortality exceeded 22,000 and at Xeres 10,000 succumbed. Symptoms preceding death were described as a yellowness of skin, discharges of black blood from the mouth, nostrils, anus and eyes, hiccoughs, coldness in the extremities, convulsions and black lips. Elderly people seemed less prone to the fever, while newborns and the very young were more likely to recover than individuals beyond the age of puberty and in middle age. Females had a better prognosis than males.

The Rock of Gibraltar is situated on a peninsula in the province of Andalucía, in latitude 36° 9' N. In 1804 there was a civilian population of approximately 6,000, with an additional 4,000 stationed in the British garrison. In healthy years the average number of deaths per year was 72. Because of its close proximity to the northern coast of Africa, trade between the two areas was of great commercial value. In the early 1800s this included irregular contact with privateers and smugglers. Well known along both coasts, these seafarers were either notoriously exempt from quarantine or were savvy enough to slip through the lax measures enacted by authorities.

In 1799 and 1800, a disease simply called the "plague" broke out with virulence along the Barbary states of northern Africa. At Fez in particular many thousands fell ill but Fez was far from alone. By the end of July 1800, upwards of 2,000 Moors living in Tangier had died, while the tragedy at Tetuan was little better. According to Mr. Matra, the British consul, the disease eventually extended as far south as Arzillo.

Aware of the dangers presented to Gibraltar, General O'Hara, governor of the Rock, cut off all intercourse with the coast of Barbary. Issuing such wide-ranging orders proved impossible to execute and the prevailing fever soon broke out on the island. According to a letter written August 10, 1800, by the secretary of state, the Duke of Portland, evidence suggested that Gibraltarian smugglers had landed a cargo of tobacco in Spain but had subsequently been pursued by the authorities in armed boats. They managed to escape to Barbary but there they came in contact with fever victims. On their return, several of the crew were landed at Santi Petri near Cadiz, while the remainder went on to Gibraltar, gaining free access to the garrison.

Soon afterward fever appeared among them. The smugglers and nineteen others with whom they had been in contact were seized and placed in a lazaretto under quarantine. To prevent their escape and further contamination, authorities also burned their vessel. These measures limited the outbreak at Gibraltar, but the disease at Cadiz gained a foothold through those smugglers who had been left at Santi Petri.

By 1802 the Spanish fever had subsided locally but was far from gone. Reports from the Caribbean in August of that year noted that yellow fever had "occasioned considerable mortality at the Canash, in Grenada. Many vessels lost the whole of their crews there."[13] The following year a May 10 article warned, "The disagreeable news has been received in Holland, that the Yellow Fever having broken out at Curacoa [northern South America], has there carried off the greater part of the troops, many persons in official employment and several Gentlemen, the loss of whose talent and personal worth is exceedingly regretted."[14]

By October 1803 rumors reached the garrison at Gibraltar that disease, thought to be the same species as that which prevailed at Cadiz in 1800, had been introduced at Malaga by French ships newly arrived in the Bay of Malaga. By October 22 Malaga was reported to be seriously infected, prompting the lieutenant governor of Gibraltar, Sir Thomas Trigge, to issue orders to cut off all communication with parts of the Spanish coast. By December 17 it was finally determined the malady had run its course and quarantine regulations at Gibraltar were relaxed. The disease was destined to reappear with horrific severity at Malaga in 1804, prompting Sir Thomas Trigge to issue a proclamation on August 27 prohibiting entrance into Gibraltar Harbor of all vessels arriving from east or west of Malaga. The following day a man named Santos, accompanied by his family, arrived at Gibraltar from Cadiz. Although he denied exposure to the disease at Cadiz, family members soon fell ill. Mr. Kenning, assistant surgeon of the Royal Artillery, was called to see them. He reported to Dr. Nooth, chief of the medical department, that the group labored under the "bilious remittent fever common to warm climates." By the time the authorities discovered the falsehood of Santos's assertion and he acknowledged having been sick before he left Cadiz, the fever he introduced had spread, creating a general alarm.

On September 12 a bombardier and his wife died, marking the first fatalities in the garrison. Kenning and a French practitioner named Monsieur Jay expressed the opinion that the disease resembled that which had swept through Cadiz in 1800. Three days later their diagnosis was seconded by a Spanish priest named Hoyera, who reported to Captain Dodd, secretary of the garrison, that what they had in their midst was "a very malignant and fatal disorder" that appeared to be the same as that which had been identified at Seville in 1800. Thomas Trigge ignored their warning and no precautions were taken. The number of sick increased rapidly, in some measure augmented by the Feast of the Tabernacle held on September 15 or 16. Prior to that celebration, Jewish residents had remained relatively isolated in small family units. Coming in contact with large numbers at their synagogues for the Day of Atonement on the 18th further exposed them to contagion and by the 19th four of their company had died of the fever.

In response to the growing threat that would ultimately kill 700–800, the officer commanding the artillery ordered the discharge of cannon on September 25, despite Nooth's protest that the action would not correct "the vitiated atmosphere," especially as the weather was calm. The doctor finally succeeded in having street bonfires prohibited and guards were appointed to assist the newly formed Committee of Health. Comprising five British merchants, the group established a lazaretto and saw to it the noncommissioned officers and men of the Royal Artillery were transferred to Windmill Hill in the healthier southern district. On September 30, the barracks were fumigated with alum and brimstone.

During the first three days of October deaths in the town of Gibraltar reached 167; one day later the death toll climbed to 175. With people in a panic and life in disarray, carts were ordered to pass through the community collecting dead bodies left unattended in the streets. The high rate of mortality among cart drivers, however, made it impossible to recruit replacements and ultimately soldiers were ordered to perform the deadly task.

Major-General Barnet, second in command, was applied to for help, but the highest medical authorities asserted the malady to be no more than a simple, noncontagious bilious fever caused by a contaminated atmosphere. The physicians argued against precautionary measures as being unnecessary, stating that "every inhabitant of the rock would be attacked sooner or later." They were correct on one count, as Barnet contracted the fever and died on October 7 or 8, 1804.

On January 6, 1805, a letter from the camp at St. Roch reported more grim news: "The winter has occasioned no check to the rages of the yellow fever among the garrison of Gibraltar; it has been observed, that many more English than natives in proportion, have died of it, which is ascribed to the former being less temperate in the use of strong liquors. We have now double reasons to hold Gibraltar strictly blockaded."[15]

The city of Malaga, situated at 36° 44' of latitude, had its own history of "plague."

Health of Malaga

Year	Disease
1600–1602	Great mortality was occasioned by a "Peste," a vague name for a malignant fever that reputedly carried off more than half the population.
1637	A similar calamity occurred with the loss of 40,000 in two months.
1648–1650	Another extremely fatal disorder lasted three years.
1678	A pestilence year.
1741	The first year symptoms of the "Vomito Prieto" or "Vomito Negro" appeared. The disease was believed to have been introduced by a vessel from Spanish America that landed infected goods and was augmented by the low, marshy situation of the town and by heavy rains immediately preceding the disorder. About 10,000 perished
1800	The disease did not return until the end of this year and only after it had prevailed at Cadiz. It was also believed to have been introduced by a ship from Spanish America.

A much more serious outbreak was recorded in 1803. The fever that prevailed this year was thought to have been introduced by one or more vessels. The first was the *Young Nicholas,* a Dutch ship that left Smyrna on March 14 and arrived at Malaga on May 22. The second and third were ships chartered by the French government to transport troops to St. Domingo. The *Dessaix* sailed from Marseilles on April 26 filled with 171 conscripts, deserters, prisoners and convicts. It entered Malaga on May 17. The *Union* left Marseilles on May 5 with 150 men of the same character. It lost at least 67 men on the voyage and arrived at Malaga on June 3. The last of the suspected vessels was the *Providence*, late of Montevideo laden with cocoa, hides and tallow. It arrived June 9, 1803.

On or about July 14, 1803, a local man came down with fever and died on the 5th or 6th day after his symptoms first showed themselves. Thirty-five days elapsed before a second person died of the same malady and medical authorities considered this the start of the epidemic at Malaga. The disease spread slowly through mid–September but from this point there was little agreement as to its true diagnosis. Local physicians believed it to be the true yellow fever of America, introduced by the two French brigs from Marseilles on their way to Sr. Domingo. This theory was supported by M. Delestra, the French practitioner in change of both vessels and argued against by the English doctor, Edward Bancroft. To defend his position, Delestra described how those crew infected by the fever had vomited dark fluid prior to their deaths. His treatment aboard ship consisted of cold effusion, immersions and fomentations.

However, there were apparently other ships blamed for the importation. A letter dated October 8 puts another light on the subject:

> A calamity has befallen us here, from which the most serious consequences are apprehended. Several vessels lately arrived in this port from New York, and other parts of America, have communicated [introduced] to us that fatal disorder, the yellow fever, so destructive to the Americans. Some of the inhabitants in the town and suburbs die daily; all the crews in the harbour are more or less afflicted with it.... All communication between the Town, the Harbour, and the Mole, is excluded, which prevents us from learning the true state of those on board of the different ships; but we fear the worst. At present the vessels are restricted from all intercourse with each other, notwithstanding sometimes the most urgent calls of business.[16]

Other locals believed that the epidemic was somehow related to atmospheric conditions or at least was exacerbated by them. Consequently, villagers resorted to burning aromatic plants such as thyme, rosemary, lavender and myrtle to permeate the area in a cloud.

Mortality at Malaga had reached 7,000 by mid–November. Hundreds of people were said to be dying daily and those who could fled the area. A letter dated November 30 offered a glimpse into the hopes and disappointments of the month:

> When I wrote to you a short time ago, we were all here in great spirits; it was not doubted that the malignant fever, which had proved so destructive to the inhabitants of this place, as well as the strangers trading here, was considerably abated; and that the cold weather, which was then setting in, would soon completely annihilate it. We were, however, unhappily mistaken; the cold days were of short duration, and were succeeded by close dull weather, and incessant rains. At this period (about the middle of the month), the pestilential fever began to rage with increased fury; the daily returns of deaths, by the Board of Health establisher here, were between 60 and 70.—Our calamity, as it appears, is unfortunately not at its height; for yesterday 90 persons were reported to have died in 24 hours. Where this fatal disorder will stop, God knows! It is, however, some consolation to find that the fever, owing to the great precaution of the Board of Health in cutting off all communication wherever it can be done, is contained within the limits of the town, with the exception of two or three small villages.[17]

Newspaper reports dated December 21 (typically a month behind the times), indicated "the yellow fever still raged at Malaga, and it was still reported that it had reached Barcelona, and Barceloneta, which is without the walls." A further notice, dated November 30, added, "The destructive ravages of the yellow fever seem to be little, if at all abated in Malaga.—All public meetings are prohibited; no person is allowed to quit his house except on public business; and to shake hands in the street is prohibited under pain of being sent to the gallies."[18]

A letter dated November 27, 1803, gives another firsthand account of the disaster:

> I can hardly give you an adequate idea of our melancholy situation here, which seems daily to get worse. Notwithstanding upward of forty thousand people have left the city, and mortality still increases and now amounts to one hundred and forty daily. About seven thousand have already died of the disorder, and about twelve hundred are now sick of it. A great majority of those who are seized die, and it generally proves fatal in three days.... Almost all the attendants and nurses of the sick have fallen victims to it, and many whole families have been carried off. It has now got into several of the nunneries and convents, where it makes great havoc. The faculty have as yet been very unsuccessful in their mode of treating the disease which appears more nearly to resemble the plague than yellow fever, and a great variety of opinion prevails with respect to its origin.

Among the symptoms were violent pains, an uncommon lowness of spirits and great debility accompanied by thirst and great heat, followed by the appearance of black, livid spots on the third day. The writer noted that many ships lying in harbor had lost entire crews. By December 10 the disease at Malaga had "so much diminished, that instead of 80 or 90, not more than 60 persons die daily."[19]

In what likely triggered numerous debates among scientists and those interested in correlations between weather, natural phenomenon and the occurrence of disease, on January 13, 1804, an earthquake struck at Malaga, with effects felt as far away as Gibraltar and along the Barbary coast from Oran to Tangiers. Aftershocks continued for over a week, with six striking on January 21. Summer heat proved intensely hot on August 16 and 17; on the 18th, fever broke out at Malaga, described as a "contagious disorder, on the nature of which, people did not seem to agree." A week later, Spanish physicians declared the prevailing malady to be nothing more than "a tertian [recurring] fever, which was not contagious." Further statements indicated that treatments were working. Private correspondence indicated otherwise, as letter writers indicated between 80–100 persons were dying daily. This apparently prompted reconsideration, and the disease was then diagnosed as "tabardillo" (spotted fever), but no precautions were adopted by the Spanish authorities until the end of August.

The pestilence spread quickly. From Malaga it traveled to Cordoba (75 miles inland); Granada (65 miles distant); Velez-Malaga, Cathagena and Alicant. News that yellow fever had appeared at Leghorn in November sent shock waves throughout Europe. The Italian Commission of Health reported 54 deaths in the third week of November and 74 in the final week of the month. Physicians there asserted it to be nothing more "than a common putrid fever, notwithstanding its being the received opinion, that it was the same disease as that which raged in the southern provinces of Spain, namely, the yellow fever." In order to seek help higher than that offered by physicians, on October 30 the vicar general ordered that the miraculous image of the Madonna del Montenero be conveyed to a meadow where the "incessant peals of bells, and the sacred benediction, accompanied by discharges of artillery from the fortress" were "pronounced over the city of Leghorn." Thirty thousand persons were said to have witnessed the spectacle and the disease was apparently contained.[20] However, the threat prompted a December 1804 notice: "The trade of Hamburgh is embarrassed anew by a cordon of numerous troops which the Danish Government intend to draw along its coast and along the Elbe, to preserve it from the contagion of the yellow fever." The Board of Health of Copenhagen also persuaded the authorities to prohibit, "in the most rigid manner," all importation of wool and cloth.[21]

Significantly, the fever also reached Penon de Velez on the coast of Africa, where the Spanish garrison there received supplies originating from Malaga. On a similar note, in November yellow fever was reported present at Sicily, where English agents were making considerable purchases of provisions for supplying the magazines of Malta, from which the whole of Admiral Nelson's fleet derived its subsistence. Proving a capacity for travel, the fever also reached the towns of Antequea, Cadiz and as far away as Ayamonte, severely attacking those who lived there. The fever eventually crossed the river Guadiana separating Spain and Portugal. The malignity of yellow fever was also present in the West Indies. One traveler there observed that the disease "had so much increased, as to baffle every established method of treatment." The disease was particularly prevalent among British ships; aboard the frigate *Diana,* every officer in the gun room except the purser succumbed to the fever.[22]

The fever of 1804 was described as attacking most commonly at night, sometimes in the evening and very frequently at daybreak. On hot days or during the Levant winds, a greater number were taken ill. During the course of this epidemic it was noted that no precautions taken by individuals, including those who had recourse to injections (enemas), purgatives, cordials, or "other supposed remedies," were effective in either preventing or curing the disorder. Symptoms included a yellowness of the skin (not as common as observed in the epidemic of 1800) and black vomit (more frequent than in 1800). Forerunners of the fever included a more or less intense sensation of cold, violent pains in the forehead, shoulders, loins and extremities. After a universal sweat accompanied by loose, bilious stool, the fever remitted for 24 or 48 hours. If the fever reappeared it usually resulted in death.

In reference to prevention, Sir James Fellowes, the English physician who wrote the above text from which this summary was taken, ultimately declared "there is scarcely a disease known, however infectious, which may not become milder, or lose its infecting power by early attention to *separation, cleanliness,* and *ventilation.*"[23]

The Diffusion of Yellow Fever, 1800–1810

Sporadic yellow fever outbreaks appeared in the United States with some regularity during the first ten years of the 19th century. One succinct newspaper report offered a view from 1800: "We are sorry to perceive that the Yellow-Fever still rages with great violence in Baltimore and Norfolk, and that Providence (in Rhode Island) has been added to the list of infected places. People were still flying from those places on the 15th of September. Philadelphia and New-York had prohibited all communication with them; and so great was the dread of infection at Philadelphia, that guards had been stationed to prevent persons arriving from Baltimore, from entering the former city."[24] On October 3, 1800, a lady at Baltimore wrote her friend: "Our situation here is very distressing at present, owing to the yellow fever having visited our city. Every person who could procure a [cart] of any kind to put their families into have left the city; the contagion increases daily; 853 have died between the 5th of August and the 25th of September, in this cruel disorder. The three banks, with all their officers, &c. have been removed to Valcks Place, about a mile and a half from town."[25]

By mid–November cold weather put an end to the disease in Baltimore. Newspaper exchanges carried similar grim tidings on a wider scale in 1801. On September 6 the Health Office of Philadelphia informed the public of six new cases of malignant fever, exclusive of one death and five recovering from their previous report. The Health Office of Baltimore, on September 2, stated an increase of ten cases of infectious fever since its last report, with nine deaths within the previous three days. The *Boston Gazette* denied the presence of any contagious disease in the city but added that the weather was "very unfavourable to the health of the inhabitants, particularly children."

Alarmed by news coming out of Philadelphia that the malignant fever there was assuming a more frightening aspect, and having "reason to believe" that the malignant disease in that city had been introduced into their own borough, the board of health resolved, on September 5, to rescind a previous proclamation permitting open communication between the two cities and to put back into force the order restricting all intercourse with Philadelphia. This restriction did not sit well with New Yorkers, who immediately demanded an exception. Authorities there contended "that any apparent increase in its obituary beyond the usual proportion, is to be imputed to the arrival of the French squadron, which landed 162 sick, chiefly of the dysentery, at the marine hospital, of whom 11 have died." In a bit of editorializing, the Wilmington papers noted, "The city of New York, it will be recalled, has long been accused of exaggerating its own happiness in this respect [the health of the city], and the calamities of its rivals, Philadelphia particularly, with a selfish view to the advancement of its own commerce."[26]

Scattered reports from 1802 during mid–August indicated nine patients remaining in City Hospital at Philadelphia; cool weather and several deaths at Portsmouth; only three active cases of malignant fever at Baltimore, with 12 deaths; New York healthy; and several cases of yellow fever at Elizabeth City, North Carolina, but none since August 15. By the following week, yellow fever at Philadelphia was "still rag[ing]," with 9 deaths registered at City Hospital and 16 patients admitted. The fever at Baltimore "appear[ed] to increase"; one victim at Peachbottom, on the Susquehanna, was stricken with black vomit during the first 24 hours. "It is advanced as a proof of the domestic origin of the disease."[27]

The year 1803 proved more devastating to New York City residents. The hospital at Bellevue, which had been closed since 1798, was opened to admit yellow fever victims. Between August 4 and August 10, seventy-nine deaths were registered and 188 new cases reported. At Catskill, New York, the *Hudson Bee* reported the existence of yellow fever at Catskill Landing and added this commentary: "But from the importance of establishing the doctrine of the *domestic origin* of this terrible disease, to which cause alone we understand it can be attributed in this instance, we think it our duty to publish the fact." Newspapers as late as October 20 stated that yellow fever at New York City and Philadelphia was "greater than at any former period."[28] While not precisely accurate, it expresses the extreme pressure experienced by those living through such frightful times.

Just as yellow fever was never far from the minds of those living under its terrifying umbrella, questions pertaining to its cause and cure remained in the forefront of peoples' minds. One author with an eye toward sanitation reminded New Yorkers of the dangers associated with night soil, or human feces. Adroitly observing on September 21, 1803, that such "nuisances have been collecting within our City ever since its first settlement," he warned that excrement had spoiled most wells and deteriorated the rest: "They are accumulating prodigiously on us; and, as yet, no general and permanent plan of removal has been adopted by our police. From this foul colluvies, increasing most rapidly from year to year, a world of febrile mischief may be expected to arise in our hot climate.... Thus exposed, we find the contents of unalkalized British ships turn to pestilential air in our harbour, and excite yellow fever in the British seamen on board, when there is no such disease, or any thing like it, in the City."[29]

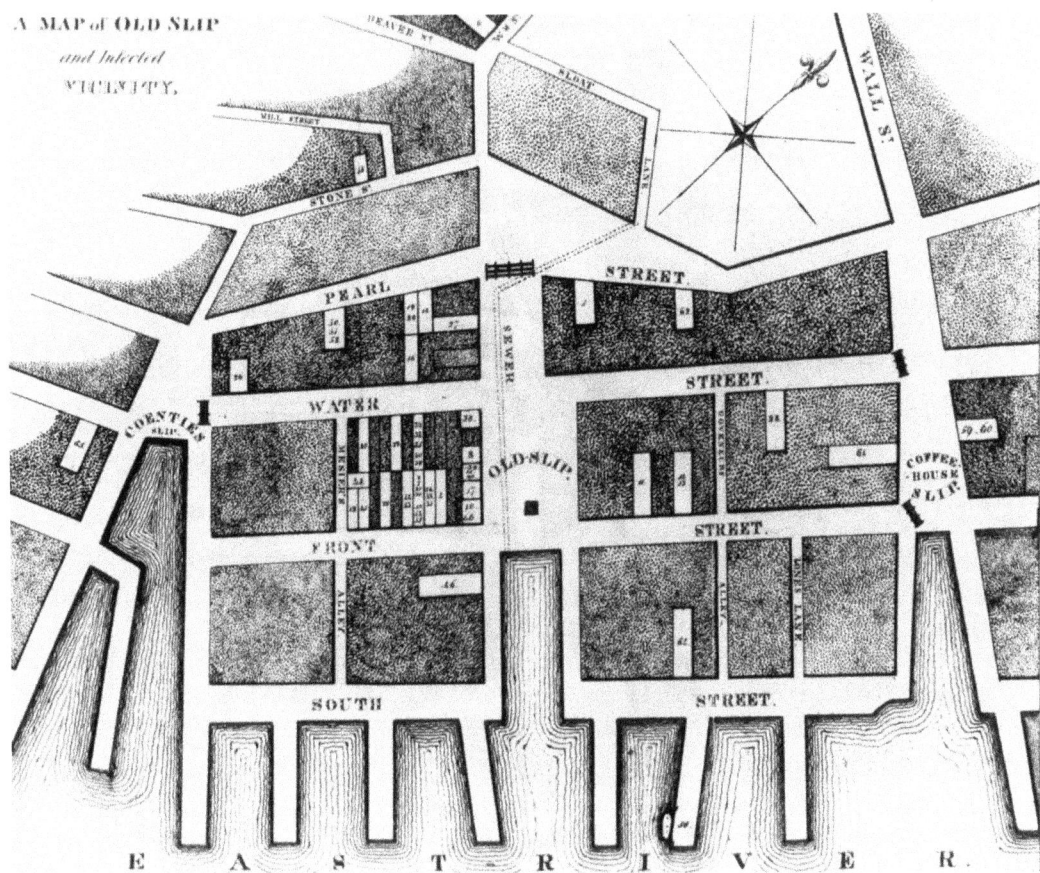

Yellow fever was a serious and deadly problem in the United States during the 1700–1800s. No one knew where it came from, how to control it, or even how to treat victims. Quarantines were often established between cities, causing disruption of travel and major economic loss. This map of the Old Slip (lower Manhattan and the East River), New York, identifies infected vicinities (courtesy National Library of Medicine).

Even in years when outbreaks were less serious, mild cases were considered noteworthy. On July 20, 1804, yellow fever made an appearance at "Waalebought [sic]," Long Island. In this case, it was thought to have originated from a brig that arrived from Port-au-Prince. Three persons died and five labored under the influence of the disease. Later in the year, the New York Board of Health confirmed the existence of yellow fever in the City of St. Domingo and Port de Paix on the same island. They also informed the public that the contagion had been found at "Guadaloupe (19th century spelling), New Providence, Charlestown, Darien, Georgia, Detnararn, and Tobago (though there is some doubt with respect to the last two places)."[30]

Yellow fever also made an appearance at New Orleans during 1803–1804, causing high mortality. Following the advice of those who advocated sanitation reform as a means of preventing the disease, on July 9, 1804, William Charles Cole Claiborne, the first American governor, commissioned the "Permanent Health Committee," which included two physicians. Members met weekly and issued ordinances to clean slaughterhouses and cemetery dumps. Furthermore, they took the laudable step of establishing examinations for physicians, surgeons and apothecaries who did not already hold diplomas. They also assumed responsibility for maintaining sanitary conditions at Charity Hospital.[31]

In the summer of 1805, outbreaks of yellow fever prompted the reopening of Bellevue and an asylum was built on public grounds adjoining the hospital gate for the sick and poor who had been removed from the seat of contagion by the board of health. The almshouse on Chambers Street was also opened and rations were eventually issued to 1,640 families. An earlier report by John Pintard, city inspector, provided an insight into conditions not much improved seven years later:

> The buildings called hospitals erected at Bellevue appear to have been set up on the spur of the occasion, and on the presumption that the fever would never recur again. Fatal experience has proved otherwise, and points to the conviction that we may expect repeated attacks from this insidious disease. The wards, the one appropriated for the men especially, are every way inadequate to the wants of the patients or the comfort of the nurses and physicians. The buildings are on too contracted a scale—of materials too slight to repel the summer heat or autumnal colds. The crowded state of the hospital, during the last season, must have had an unfavorable influence on the spirits of the patients. Those newly arrived were evidently depressed by the shrieks of convulsed and dying subjects.[32]

By August 20 1805, there was only one case of yellow fever in New York City, a circumstance attributed to the vigilance of the board of health, which removed "all who had the smallest symptom of being infected, either to the city hospital, or sent into the country."

However, success was not going to be so easily achieved. A letter written by Englishman John Davis remarks that yellow fever broke out about September 5 and although he begins hopefully enough it is not long before he gets to the crux of the situation:

> I am sojourning at New York. It possesses by nature a spot the most beautiful in the world, not excepting even the classically celebrated Bay of Naples; but it is subject every summer to a fever which makes terrible havoc among its inhabitants. We have just experienced a visitation of this yellow fever, or plague; and notwithstanding the flight of the citizens, 250 persons were arrested by death, of whom 166 were males and 84 females.
> Scarcely had the dreaded disease made its approach, when the inhabitants, taught by fatal experience of its nature, fled to the neighboring town of Greenwich. Soon the streets and roads were covered with the goods and furniture of the fleeing citizens, and, both in and out of the city, all was solicitude and bustle. Others again, who chose a more distant retreat, hurried away by water in every direction; so that in a day or two, thousands had disappeared, and the most populous part of the city was left uninhabited....
> [I]t was a painful lot to see the sable and solitary hearse "slow moving to the mansions of the dead"; while perhaps a single mourner, or two, followed at an awful distance.... It is a fact, that many who fled, and hugged themselves in their flight with the idea of safety, carried with them the seeds of the disease, and died in agonies, a few days after on the neighboring shores.... The prevailing talk now was, who were suffering from the fever, or numbered by it among the dead.

Davis added that with the return of cold weather the fever terminated and on October 25 the board of health expressed their opinion "that the citizens might return in perfect safety," enjoining them to throw open the windows of their houses.[33] Taking the position that yellow fever was not contagious, city physician Edward Miller, wrote that the nurses at Bellevue Hospital, "became entirely free from all apprehensions of the contagiousness of this disease, so that they often slept on the same bed, with the sick," without ever contracting the disease.[34]

Occasional outbreaks of yellow fever were reported over the next five years, including news that as of October 28, 1808, yellow fever raged with great violence at Barbados. No fewer than 20 surgeons or assistant surgeons in His Majesty's service fell victim to it, all dying in a short time. Also in 1808 the mortality lists of Philadelphia indicated that 70–80 persons were daily dying; that same year the major of New York prohibited all intercourse with Brooklyn in consequence of its having been visited by the calamity. The fever was also reported to have broken out in North Carolina in 1810. Similarly, an outbreak at Santa Cruz in the Canary Islands occurred in October 1810. Three hundred persons died within the course of one month and by November 16 five thousand remained afflicted, with 25–30 dying every 24 hours. "In general," it was stated, "the poor people died from want of assistance, and there was a great scarcity of medicines of every description in the island." All communication with the town was severed, effectively stemming the spread of disease.

One of the more interesting incidents of this decade was a report in a Charleston paper of 1806 that yellow fever had broken out in New York City. The New York papers "satisfactorily contradicted" the charge "and a reward has been offered for the discovery of the malicious author of the above fabrication."[35] In a bit of Americana, in 1851 when Grant Thorburn (widely known as the hero of John Galt's *Lawrie Todd; or, The Settlers in the Woods* (1830) and a man who considered himself under the care of a special Providence), was rewriting his autobiography for the *Home Journal* he mentioned the yellow fever epidemic of New York in 1807. Upon observing a driver pass by with a cartload of corpses, he said, "O for the chisel of Powers, or the pencil of West, for now would I sketch a second edition of Death on the Pale Horse!" The statement was remarkable for the fact that Hiram Powers (American sculptor, 1805–1873) was a child at the time, far removed from fame and fortune.[36]

Chapter 10

The Repository of Knowledge

Nothing is more idle than to suffer alarms from the repetition of old proverbs. That a "green Christmas should make a fat church yard["] is not to be admitted, without caution, as a general truth. We should at least be able to prove that the fact is common, and that a "frosty Christmas makes a lean church yard." How stands the facts for the last ten years?[1]

Put simply, yellow fever was a terror, a poorly understood enemy of life. By 1800 it had raged at times with unmitigated violence. People feared it as a visitation of the Grim Reaper. The very words "yellow fever" or "the plague" meant the possibility of outbreak. Outbreaks led to epidemics and epidemics brought on mortality lists that numbered in the thousands. Those who could flee did. Those who could not remained behind to face the invisible enemy. Within a day or a week, a man, woman or child who had been healthy and strong became wracked with pain, burned by fever and dehydrated by loose stools and black vomit. Newspapers were filled with advertisements for cordials and tonics supplemented with the most glowing testimonials. Purchased with hard-earned coin and greater hope, these sure-cure remedies failed. People continued to die. Elected officials, who knew no more than their lay constituency, turned to the medical men as authorities and received conflicting opinions. Some advocated quarantine; others dismissed it as a waste of effort that affected commerce more than the progress of contagion. Doctors on the front lines attempted their own remedies. If one patient out of ten or twenty recovered they touted their "cure" to the profession. When others in the profession attempted to duplicate this guarded result they were unsuccessful. In times of desperation, everyone had an idea and no one had an answer. Did yellow fever originate locally or was it imported? What role, if any, did weather—temperature, rainfall, atmospheric conditions—have? How was miasma or poisoned air involved? Would improved sanitation or fumigation with acids delay or prevent the disease? Did copious bleeding or violent cathartics help or hinder the symptoms?

In the first ten years of the 19th century numerous essays and learned texts were devoted to answering these questions. In a brief overview on the subject of the "Phlegmatia Dolens," or cause of the disease, in 1800, little substantial or insightful breakthroughs had occurred. Noah Webster's *Brief History of Epidemic and Pestilential Diseases* argued that all epidemics were, to a degree, periodical, resulting from "comets, or the natural convulsions of the globe, volcanos, and earthquakes." He believed the disease had depopulated the Indian tribes of America before the West Indies were settled by Europeans and argued that it usually originated in America. He further contended that the plague and yellow fever could not be spread by contagion or infection, except at certain seasons of the year, and that this period never commenced before the end of July or August.

Dr. Trotter, in his *Medicina Nautica*, believed the cause might "be fixed in the extremities," forming a "malignant ulcer." Dr. Chisholm, in his short treatise, "On the Malignant Yellow Fever Imported from Bulam," considered at least one form of the disease to be imported. In his essay, "An Enquiry into the Causes of the Insalubrity of Flat and Marshy Situations; and Directions for Preventing or Correcting the Effects Thereof," William Currie concluded that yellow fever and summer and autumnal febrile diseases were "not owing to any invisible miasmata or noxious effluvia, which issue from the soil, and lurk in the air, but to a very different cause, *viz.* to a deficiency of the oxygenous portion of the atmosphere in such situations, in consequence of vegetable and animal putrefaction, in conjunction with the exhausting and debilitating heat of the days, and the sedative power of the cold and damp air of the nights...." "It was a concurrence of these circumstances," he added, "which gave origin to the yellow fever which appeared in Grenada in the beginning of the year 1793, and which was afterwards imported into Philadelphia, as appears from the account published by Dr. Chisholm" (Vide Chisholm's "Essay on the Fever of Grenada in 1793").

Dr. George Fordyce, who had never seen yellow fever, wrote in "A Fourth Dissertation on Fever" (1802) that he believed it to be a "femitertian, the product of animal and vegetable putrefaction, exalted, or rendered virulent by heat, by which it is supported and propagated; consequently, that the opinion of its having been imported into those countries, and propagated by contagion, is not well founded."

In an interesting study on the subject of how weather affected the frequency and severity of disease, the *Adams* (PA) *Centinel* of January 21, 1801, from which this chapter heading was taken, offered a comparison between winter temperatures and summer

In cities threatened by yellow fever, authorities were desperate to determine the origin and explain the erratic spread of the disease. Was it imported or did it spring from local conditions? Was it contracted by eating fruit, breathing bad air or spread by personal contact? Local, state and national boards of health were assembled to try to answer these questions and whenever those bodies made a determination, "cures" were sure to follow (*Galveston News*, July 4, 1880).

health. The disease referred to as "scarlatina" is better known as scarlet fever; "angina" or "angina scarlatina/Scarlatina angino" refers to scarlet fever with ulceration of the throat (see the glossary for more symptoms).

Judgment of Weather

Year	Weather
Winter of 1771–72	Latter part of winter as mild as ever known; peaches bloomed in February; summer uncommonly healthy.
Winter of 1774–75	A green Christmas and a very mild winter; during the summer, malignant dysentery was very prevalent.
Winter of 1775–76	Remarkably mild; vessels sailed from New York to Albany in January; no general sickness but some dysentery and angina affected several towns.
Winter of 1776–77	Unusually severe winter; dysentery more prevalent in summer than in 1775.
Winter of 1777–78	Winter of usual severity; disease caused more deaths than in 1775.
Winter of 1788–89	More severe than usual; the summer following brought measles and influenza but no mortal diseases.
Winter of 1789–90	Remarkably mild. Snow, sleet and rain fell in abundance but no frost until February. No unusual mortality that summer.
Winters of 1791–92 and 1792–93	Both winters unusually severe. In 1791 malignant fever in New York and mortal angina scarlatina. Yellow fever appeared in 1793 and angina raged.
Winter of 1793–94	Less severe than the two previous winters but not mild. Same malignant complaints and dysentery prevailed.
Winter of 1794–95	A green Christmas and a mild winter. A sickly summer but not universally.
Winter of 1795–96	Normal winter. The summer was more healthy, but yellow fever and angina affected many towns.
Winter of 1796–97	Winter more than usually severe. The summer was generally healthy in the northern states but several towns there and in the southern states were afflicted with yellow fever.
Winter of 1797–98	Winter more severe, followed by the most general prevalence of malignant fevers and dysenteries.
Winter of 1798–99	Occasionally severe and more lengthy; the summer less sickly but not free from malignant fevers.
Winter of 1799–1800	Much milder winter and the summer remarkably healthy.

The newspaper concluded "that heat and cold are not the most influential agents directly in generating epidemic diseases."

If there was little agreement on causation, treatment remained an even greater mystery. In a second essay for the American Philosophical Society, "A Sketch of the Rise and Progress of the Yellow Fever" of 1799, Currie offered a threefold discussion: that yellow fever was imported from two infected ships from Havana and St. Domingo; that yellow fever was not, as he formerly believed, the same disease as the Typhus Gravior; and to provide a means of treating it. After objecting to the mode of practice proposed by Drs. Warren, Wright, Jackson, MacLean and Chisholm, he proposed a system employing the free use of cathartics and up to four treatments of moderate bleeding. If, however, symptoms were severe, he argued bleeding "did manifest irreparable injury." He added that the "liberal use of sulphuric acid, sufficiently diluted with water, was occasionally useful. Wine, bark, and opium, so frequently beneficial in bilious and typhus-fevers, were decidedly injurious in every case of yellow fever."

Dr. Chisholm relied on calomel. Dr. Fowler, in his "Practical Treatise on the Different Fevers of the West Indies," advised bleeding only at the onset of symptoms. (Fowler also conjectured that the yellowness seen in fever victims was merely a concomitant symptom "and by no means such as could be sufficiently characteristic of any one fever.") Dr. Lempriere's "Practical Observations on the Diseases of the Army in Jamaica" stated he was "cautious in his bleedings," except in the early stages and afterward trusted more to mercurials. Dr. Benjamin Rush continued to support "his favourite remedy, the lancet," while Dr. Jackson, in his "Outline of the History and Cure of Fever," defended both these practices.[2]

Volume five of Rush's *Medical Inquiries and Observations* went into details of the yellow fever epidemic of 1797. Countenancing the ideas of Webster that pestilential fevers were preceded by some disturbance in the weather, Rush noted that in July 1796 "a beautiful corona, or halo appeared, and in the spring and summer of the following years, unequal quantities of mosquitoes, ants, and cockroaches, were observed, and the martins and swallows were said to have disappeared for a time from the city and its neighborhood; a disease also prevailed among the cats, which was generally fatal." Far from moderating his views, Rush alleged that during the months of August and September, when between a thousand and eleven hundred persons died, this mortality resulted from "the neglect of bleeding and other evacuants, in the commencement of the fever." Arguing that 150–176 ounces of blood could be drawn from a patient, Rush then devoted a considerable part of his argument speaking against those physicians who refused to adopt his practice. In the same light, Dr. Rush considered bleeding (with a loss of blood usually between 100–200 ounces), purging and "a salivation" as a cure for gout and hydrophobia, which he attributed to yellow fever. The reviewer for the *London British Critic* (July–December 1801) concluded, "It is melancholy after all to consider, that, notwithstanding the sublime discoveries of the new philosophy, and the confidence with which this author, and other of its proselites [proselyte: convert], speak of the application of its tenets to the practice of medicine, that the yellow fever, gout, hydrophobia, and all the other diseases that have been acknowledged to be difficult to manage, or totally intractable, continue the same ravages they were accustomed to make, before these discoveries were divulged."

Thus the search continued, but nearly always along the same lines. In 1803 Chief

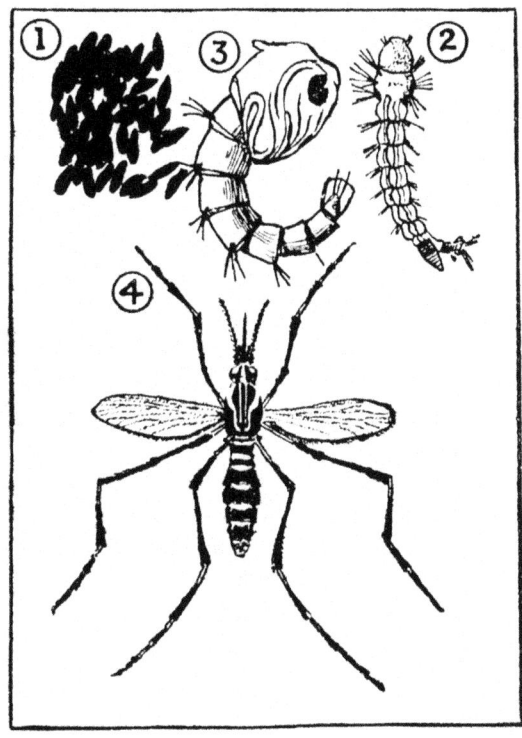

These enlarged illustrations depict the stages in the life of the yellow fever mosquito: (1) A view of mosquito eggs deposited in a close-lying mass; (2) a view of a full-grown "wiggler"; (3) mosquito pupa; (4) female adult mosquito, the carrier of yellow fever (author's collection, from *Health Heroes*, 1926).

Physician Gilbert published *Histoire Medicale de l' Armee Francaise* (*A Medical History of the French Army at St. Domingo, during the Tenth Year*). After denominating the medical topography of the island (seasons, temperatures, soil, botanical products), he offered the opinion that yellow fever would "cease to be dreaded the moment that proper regulations are adopted." Unfortunately, disease among the troops reached "such a dreadful degree of violence" that M. Gilbert called for a medical conference with all the army physicians serving on the island. After Gilbert posed eleven questions, the only conclusion reached was that the approach of the rainy season was the only positive "treatment" they had.[3]

Another study on weather-related illnesses came from *A Short Essay on the Nature and Cause of Influenza ... Together with a Hint for Stopping the Ravages of the Yellow Fever in the West Indies* (1803). The "hint" consisted of a notation that, as warmth was known to foster yellow fever, temperatures could be reduced by watering the streets during the heat of the day, at public expense.[4] The same year, an American author noted "the very striking analogy which subsists between the effects of the venom of the rattlesnake and those of the poison inducing malignant yellow fever." That led him to the conclusion that emetics might be useful in both cases.[5]

Scientific works published in 1804 argued that yellow fever was not contagious. Metzger's *Gerichtlichmedecinische* (*Dissertations on Medical Jurisprudence*) and Dr. Ruston's *A Collection of Facts; Interspersed with Observations on the Nature, Causes, and Cure of*

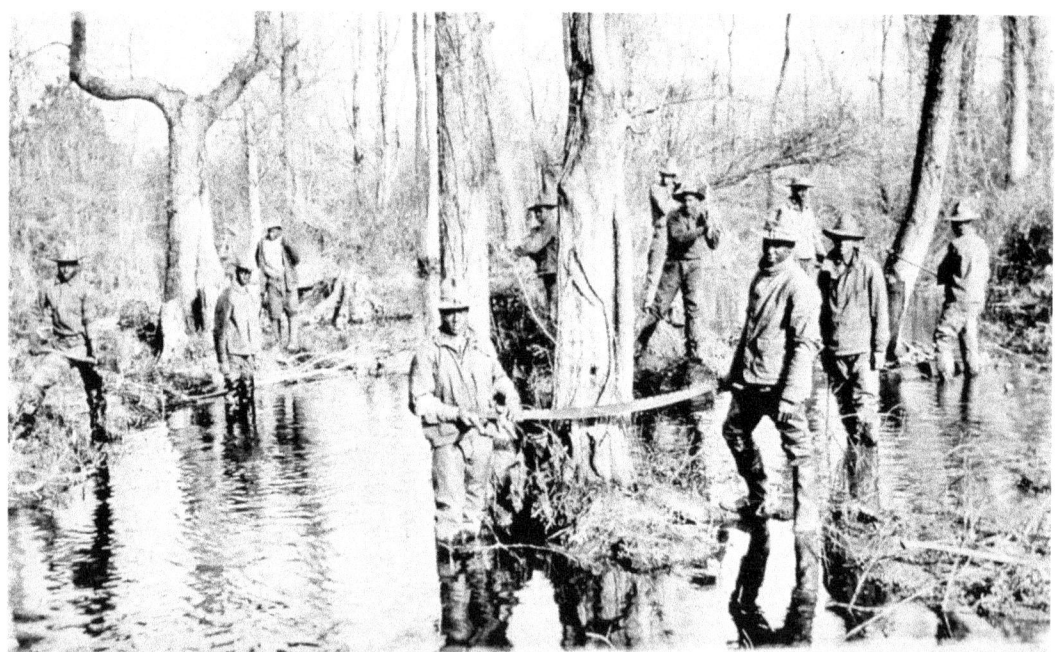

Mosquito extermination was of paramount importance in the control of yellow fever and malaria and the idea was suggested (although for the wrong reasons) one hundred years earlier. Felling trees and draining swamps was backbreaking work but strenuous efforts paid off as the number of laborers suffering from disease fell off drastically after the United States took control of the project. This photograph was taken at New Market Creek Swamp in 1910 (courtesy National Library of Medicine).

the Yellow Fever, published in the form of letters to the people of the United States, confirmed the same opinion. W. Blackburne's *Facts and Observations Concerning the Prevention and Cure of Scarlet Fever* lectured on febrile infections generally, including plague, smallpox, measles, scarlet fever and yellow fever or those of the jail, hospital, putrid, low, nervous, malignant or typhus fever. Their joint origin (considered to be "single and identical"), he believed, stemmed from "certain exhalations or marsh miasmata" (generating "paludous" or "limose gas") and the effluvia from febrile animal bodies, generating contagious gas.

In summary, Blackburne considered hydrogen ("or the principle of humidity") to form an essential confluent part of both types of pyrexial gas, and that "by depriving these gasses of their aqueous or hydrogenous principle, they are for a time annihilated." This argument, he explained, confirmed the well-known fact that extreme heat or cold arrested the progress or destroyed the existence of all epidemic and contagious diseases. Oddly confounding "hydrogen, or the principle of humidity, with humidity or water, itself," the author went to great lengths to suggest preventive measures on a grand scale. These included clearing away or "ventilating" jungles, woods and forests and cultivating the grounds they covered. He also wished to drain swamps, remove mud and mire and eliminate humidity (or "moist unwholesome exhalations") by the proper construction of housing. All this, he suggested, could be done by employing "unfortunate criminals of all countries ... where their labours can contribute to the beneficent end here proposed."

In arguing the theory of "pneumatic medicine," Dr. Robert John Thornton stated "pure air is the antidote against infection," noting "the admission of the purest air is of infinite service in fevers." The basis of his argument was the work of Dr. Lind, whom he quoted as observing the "benefits resulting to the sick in fevers, when removed from the cabin of ships to the better air of Haslar hospital," adding that he had seen seamen recover from yellow fever "solely by having the benefit of a free and constant admission of the pure sea air into a ship anchored at a distance from shore ... while gentlemen, on the contrary, shut up in small, close, and unventilated chambers, at Kingston, or Portroyal, expire with their whole mass of blood dissolved, flowing from every pore; the bad vitiated air of their room having produced a state of universal putrefaction in the body even before death."[6] Perhaps the best review on the state of medical writing in 1804 came from the *Monthly Magazine* (London, March 1, 1804): "'A physical Inquiry into the origin and causes of the Pestilential Fever,' is full of the wildest and most unintelligible notions. The anonymous author takes it for granted that the ancient doctrine of the four elements is right, as far as it goes; but he thinks two others ought to be added, viz. the *electric fluid,* and another universal agent, to which he ascribes very whimsical properties."

The year 1805 started out promisingly enough with the introduction of several new American publications: *The Medical Repository, and Review of American Publications on Medicine, Surgery and the auxiliary Branches of Science,* by Drs. Mitchell and Edward Miller of New York; *The Philadelphia Medical Museum,* by Dr. Coxe; and, *The Philadelphia Medical and Physical Journal,* by Professor Barton. However, with all these new works, one British reviewer noted, "Upon the cause and *modus medendi* of the yellow fever we perceive the American practitioners are much divided as ever; but we have no desire to enter into the contest." With that said, published medical thought was depressingly stagnant. In opposition to Dr. Blackburne's 1804 theory, Dr. Richard Dinmore, of Cleveland, Ohio, argued that defoliating large areas of the United States (as was currently being done as the population expanded into new territories) would lead to an immense quantity of vegetable matter decomposing into carbonic gas. He explained that this gas was "irrespirable" and, being heavier than atmospheric air, rolled from the higher to the lower country. When combined with hydrogen (also an irrespirable air emitted by the marches and elevated by the heat of the burning sun) and absorbed by the lungs, he suspected this caused bilious intermittent and remittent fevers. The similarity between these and yellow fever suggested to Dinmore that the latter was produced by similar vapors, "heightened by azote emitted in the decomposition of animal matter." He did not, however, hold that yellow fever was contagious. From his own experience at Alexandria, Ohio, in 1803, when the "cruel disease" burst out in the lower parts of town, he observed that only those who lived there or visited that section were affected.

In August 1805 Dr. A. Fothergill of the American Philosophical Society published "Friendly Cautions of the Prevention of Pestilential Contagion, and of Premature Interment." He belonged to the ranks of those physicians who believed plague, smallpox, measles, yellow fever and other malignant diseases were not only related but "communicated by contact, or effluvia alone emanating from the sick." Noting surprise that so little had been accomplished toward arresting the career of these diseases, considering they existed only within a few paces from its source, he determined the poisons were actually spread through inattention. By this he meant improper cleaning of sick rooms and ships, furniture, vestments or other bodies, where the malignancy lay dormant "till a warm atmosphere renews its activity, and calls it into action."

The remedy he suggested, taken from methods used at Smyrna by Leopold Count Berchtold, consisted simply in powerfully rubbing the whole body with tepid olive oil. If performed properly, Berchtold believed the copious sweat that resulted would wash contagion away. This association was confirmed by the British Consul, Mr. Baldwin, who informed Berchtold that "among the numerous tribe of oil porters, not a single individual was known to die of that disease [plague]." As further proof, Fothergill quoted passages from the Sacred Writ — "Let the sick be anointed with oil, and be healed" — adding that the Catholic ceremony of extreme unction served as a preventative to priests, while the Jewish priesthood was saved by performing frequent sacrifices and burnt offerings with the fattest (and consequently most oily) animals. Fothergill concluded, "If olive oil can then resist the Plague ... why may it not be reasonably presumed sufficiently powerful to counteract the Yellow Fever, which, from its entire history, evidently appears to differ from the real Plague only in degree, not in essence?"[7]

Two interesting points of interest originated from Prussia in 1805. The king issued orders that as the mineral fumigations of Guyton Morveau were considered to be the safest preventative against yellow fever, they were to be adopted in all Prussian harbors and in all vessels under quarantine or coming from an infected place. The second had to do with a prize of "100 milled ducats" to be awarded to any person providing answers to the following questions concerning yellow fever:

(1) Is there proof to induce the belief that yellow fever attaches itself to inanimate bodies without losing its contagious properties?

(2) If such is true, or the contrary is asserted, provide experiments and facts

(3) Is it true that the miasma that occasions yellow fever is produced by the fever itself? Is the virus inherent in animal excretions?

(4) Have they any notions of the chemical properties of the contagious virus and is there a chemical agent capable of destroying it?

(5) Is there a space of time after which the contagious virus loses its efficacy?

(6) What are the differences between those who become infected and those who do not?

(7) Is the disease that rages in North America, southern Spain and Leghorn the same malady?

(8) Does yellow fever rage only along the coasts or can it rage at distances from the sea?

Submissions were to be sent to the Supreme College of Medicine and Health at Berlin, no later than January 1, 1807. This type of contest was not uncommon in the 19th century when heads of state offered substantial awards for medical innovations or proofs, but more often than not (especially in the case of cholera) entries were often useless or repetitive reworkings of known theories. Often, entry dates were extended or prizes never awarded.[8] Dr. James Currie, of Liverpool, in his new edition of *Medical Reports on the Effects of Water, Cold or Warm, as a Remedy in Fever and Febrile Diseases* (1806), offered communications from various practitioners in the West Indies and East Indies, Egypt and the United States, demonstrating the efficacy of cold and tepid "affusions" in the raging fevers of hot countries. Currie considered cutaneous perspiration as the principal agent in regulating the temperature of the body and the increase of temperature the most essential and important of the symptoms of fever: "Hence the diminution of temperature is the principal indication in the cure of this [yellow fever] disease." The application of external cold was, therefore, the best remedy, while emetics, sudorifices (diaphoretics) and blood-letting had an indirect, less safe and less efficacious result. Nor did Mr. McGregor's account of the plague and yellow fever offer any hopeful solution. His system purported to cure yellow fever and opthalmia by the use of mercury and nitric acid taken internally and by the use of the nitric bath.

In direct contrast, in 1806 a Baltimore paper published a lengthy self-promotion under the heading, "Highly Interesting to the Public in General: On the Yellow Malignant Fever." The author, Dr. John J. Girand, began his editorial with this weighty sentence: "Humanity being the first virtue of a physician worthy of a profession so distinguished, and the desire of preserving the existence of his fellow citizens the principal inducement to all his researches; it is with the most heartfelt satisfaction I announce to the public the discovery of a specific remedy for the Yellow Fever, that terrible scourge, which for several years past (beginning in 1793) has rendered the most flourishing cities of this fortunate position of the globe the seat of desolation." After turning his attention to the "alkalescent and turgid bile which always exists in the commencement of the yellow fever," Girand discovered that Castile soap was the ultimate remedy: "Its properties which are opening, dissolvent, alkaline and sudorific, always causes it to neutralize the poisonous quality of the bile, and never fails to bring on a salutary crisis." Although the simplicity of the remedy might cause doubt to some, it appeared "to have been, by Providence, scattered with profusion" and was "in all families ... in daily use" and could be used "not only as a cure for the yellow fever, but also as the means of preservation from it. Opportunely administered, it decreased muscular agitation, promoted the flow of urine, abated fever, calmed irritation of the stomach and dryness of the throat, and from the 6th to the 7th day affects a favorable crisis by means of a sweat or stool, and a bilious vomit, destroys the fever." At the end of his essay, the doctor swore by Almighty God that he had used Castile soap in his practice since 1800 and effected cures in the course of eight days.[9]

Castile soap did not revolutionize the treatment of yellow fever. In 1807 *Dr. Pinckard's Notes on the West Indies* stated that the disease continued to attack Europeans, particularly in the month of August. The author himself was assailed by the malady and if there were any doubt about the horrors suffered by victims, his description bears repeating:

> I knew not from which I suffered most, the excruciating pain, the insatiable thirst, or the unappeasable restlessness; for all were equally insupportable, and either of them might have sufficed to exhaust the strongest frame. Combining their tortures, they created a degree of irritation amounting almost to phrenzy; and which, but for the means used to alleviate it, must have destroyed me in a few hours. No place nor position afforded a moment's rest. I rolled about the bed—turned every instant from side to side—laid it low—threw my limbs from under the sheet, hung them over the side of the bed—tumbled off the clothes, and moved about incessantly to find a resting place; but all in vain—no case was to be found, not even a momentary respite was granted from this excessive torment.

Acting as his own physician, Dr. Pinckard treated himself with bark, opium and the cold bath, effecting his recovery. The remainder of his text found less favor, as one reviewer concluded "that it is likely to fill a chasm in useful knowledge, we very much doubt." Two years later the doctor apparently rose in at least one man's estimation. In critiquing the 1808 book *Suggestions for the Prevention of That Insidious and Destructive Foe to the British Troops, in the West Indies, Commonly Termed the Yellow Fever*, by Dr. Stewart Henderson, a reviewer noted, "The author is indebted to Dr. Pinckard, for these Suggestions on the Yellow Fever; we do not even find a single remark upon the subject, which has not been made by that intelligent physician." Henderson's original ideas were to design a hospital in which every patient had a separate room and to create a corps of regularly appointed hospital attendants. His last suggestion put him in serious conflict with the Royal College of Physicians when he deprecated young licentiates being appointed as army physicians because they were "young, inexperienced, and unacquainted with the diseases of tropical climate." Most, he added, "either died or were rendered totally useless in the course of a few weeks."[10] Although unappreciated, Henderson's point was well taken.

One writer for *Bell's Weekly Messenger* (London, July 19, 1807) opted for sarcasm when attacking the "Directors of the Institution to secure Health in hot and unwholesome Climates." Noting they claimed to be "actuated by motives of humanity," he informed the public they had taken a House near the West India Docks for the benefit of mariners and "as a Warehouse for the Sale of the Yellow Fever Remedy.... The business of this House, it is understood, will be conducted upon the same liberal plan as the Warehouses appointed for the sale of this invaluable Remedy at Charing-cross, and in Castle-street, Liverpool."

The issue of yellow fever in 1808 remained muddied. In describing the disease at Andalusia, Don Juan Manuel de Arejula wrote, in his *Description of the Yellow Fever*, that the disease was highly contagious, while a contrary opinion was expressed by Don Francisco Salva, who studied the disease at Barcelona. Considering it noncontagious, Salva attributed the cause to exhalations from the port of that city, which was daily becoming shallower "and [was] likely to be in time completely filled up by the accumulations of filth thrown into it."[11] The following year a more interesting conclusion that might have appealed to the Gothic imagination came from the unidentified author of *An Account of Jamaica, and Its Inhabitants, by a Gentleman Long Resident in the West Indies*. After concluding yellow fever to be nothing more than "a malignant bilious fever, the extravasated [escaped] fluid, diffused through the system, producing the deep yellow tinge on the skin which gives name to the disease," he stated that much of its fatal effects actually arose from "the horror and despair" the prevalence of the disease produced: "On many estates, every white person on them was swept in succession off within the space of a week or two. But why, it may be asked, if this disease was thus infectious in its nature, and rapid and certain in its effects, were not the medical attendants infected and carried off by it? They were generally exempt from its rage, while their patients were thus in such numbers dying around them. In short, there can hardly be a doubt of many of these unhappy men having become martyrs to self-created terrors."[12]

By 1809 the situation concerning yellow fever had regressed to a point of making those interested in the subject shake their heads in despair. "A Gentleman Long Resident in the West Indies" critiqued Dr. W. White's *A Treatise on Inflammation, and Other Diseases of the Liver, Commonly Called Bilious,* noting it was little more than a republication of his former work under a new title. Finding the section on *Synochus biliosa* particularly unhelpful, the reviewer wrote, "[W]e are told, in one place, that it is 'a distinct genus of fever'; we are afterward informed that it differs only in degree from cholera; and a third opinion given respecting it is that it 'is only a diminutive species of the bilious, or yellow fever, which occurs in hot climates.' The reader, we trust, will excuse us if we do not consume his time in examining what the author says respecting the treatment of so indefinite and incomprehensible a disease." Even better was a review of William Saunders and A.S. Fellow's text, *A Treatise on the Structure, Economy, and Disease of the Liver* (4th edition): "From a note in p. 103 we expected a new remedy for the yellow fever, which would have been, we believe, the *eleventh cure* on sale for this *incurable disease;* but in p. 186, with more candor and truth than some other pretenders, he announces calomel, jalap, and neutral salts, as the best medicines."[13]

The last major epidemic to strike the eastern seaboard of the United States occurred in 1805; thereafter, although minor outbreaks visited the new nation nearly every year, the country remained free of devastating mortality until 1819. Being directly proportional to death lists, public interest in the malady waned, although fear lurked behind the scenes. John Lambert, a traveler visiting the United States during the years 1806–1808, penned his observations on the health of Americans. Echoing an oft-opined European sentiment, he wrote, "The constant use of segars by the young men, even from an early age, may also tend to impair the constitution, and create a stimulus beyond that which nature requires, or is capable of supporting. Their dread of the yellow fever has induced a more frequent use of tobacco of late years; but it is now grown into a habit that will not be easily abandoned."[14]

Arguments between contagionists and noncontagionists, between those who believed in a local origin and those who supported the idea of importation, and the vital issue of quarantine continued unabated within the scientific community during the next decade, achieving little consensus.

Chapter 11

Daily Mortality Is Now More Considerable

Perhaps there is no disease more alarming in its approach, more fatal in its consequences, nor one that has excited deeper interest and speculation among medical men than the yellow fever. Whether this fever, or epidemia of Andalusia, is imported from the coasts of Africa, or brought from the far distant sickly shores of America, or generated at home through the agency of known or unknown causes acting upon peculiar locality, it is now the subject of gloomy speculation among the French troops of this garrison [at Cadiz, letter dated July 20, 1824].[1]

After the Berlin contest that ended in 1807 failed to elicit the requisite information on yellow fever, in 1811 the Medical Society of Brussels offered what might be considered hopeful on one hand and desperate on the other: a gold medal (worth 200 francs) to the author of the best dissertation on yellow fever. Topics were required to cover:

(1) What is the nature and cause of the disease?
(2) What are the symptoms that essentially characterize this fever?
(3) Are the yellowness and black vomit to be regarded as essential or characteristic symptoms of the disease or merely as accidental symptoms?
(4) Is the fever contagious?
(5) What are the means of protection against it?
(6) What are the most effectual means of cure?

Submissions were open to the world at large although they had to be written in either Latin or French. The prize was to be awarded in 1812.[2]

That the world needed answers to these questions was undisputed, but it would not get much help from the hucksters. There was, of course, "Dr. James's Powder for Fevers, and all Inflammatory Disorders" (now sold by Dr. James' grandson, Mr. James) and still advertised as being "attended with the most perfect success in the Yellow Fever." If that proved less than promised, American sufferers could try "Dr. Crary's Anti-Septic Family Physic, IN PILLS, justly celebrated for preventing and curing Bilious complaints, viz. Yellow Fever, Remittent Fever, Intermittent or Fever and Ague, Jaundice, Dysentary, and the Bilious Cholic." This remedy was promoted by this claim: "They differ from all other physic—for during their operation they stimulate or strengthen as ... durable as spirituous liquor: common diet may be taken." The pills sold for 50 cents (small box) and $1.00 (large).[3]

One desperate letter writer who noted that, "when that dreadful distemper is so very prevalent," the cure for yellow fever might be found in a book published in 1746 by Thomas Prior entitled *An Authentic Narrative of the Success of Tar-water*. Prior described a passage aboard a ship bound from Portabello to Jamaica. The men were suffering from a want of water, "which threw many of them into the yellow fever," when a heavy rain finally fell. All hands set to work collecting all the rain they could, "and the deck of the ship, and cordage, having been newly daubed with [vegetable] tar, all the water they could get was impregnated with tar; notwithstanding which, they drank plentifully of it; and it had this good effect,—that *all* those who were ill of the fever, and drank of it, recovered in a short time, to the great surprise of them all, as it was reckoned the most fatal distemper in that part of the world." For those interested, a recipe for tar-water followed:

Dr. Munroe's Method of Making Tar-Water

Take the best Norway tar (or any vegetable tar) one quart, add one gallon of boiling water and stir for several minutes and let it remain, covered, for 24 hours. Then skim it and remove one quart, replaced with one quart of water. Let stand another 24 hours then take off another quart and add another quart of water. Repeat the process until there is 12 quarts in the whole. Mineral tar will not do to make tar-water and may be distinguished from the vegetable as it makes the water black; whereas the vegetable makes it a yellow colour.[4]

Aside from protecting the wood and ropes of ships at sea, vegetable tar was used in the 17th and 18th centuries as a medicine both in its original state and infused in water. It was used in the "cold and phlegmatic habits of mankind" by raising the pulse, accelerating the circulation and at the same time raising the animal spirits. By the early 19th century it was used primarily as an external application for stings.[5]

Remarkable Occurrences

So severe was the yellow fever outbreak of 1811 that at least one publication listed it as number 29 in its New Year summary of significant events for the past year: "The yellow fever broke out at Carthagena, and several other places on the coast of Spain, and continued to rage through the rest of the season." Reports of the epidemic began around the middle of August 1811 with notices that yellow fever was "fatally prevalent" at Carthage. By the 26th, letters from Gibraltar "gave very afflicting accounts of the progress and ravages of the malady at Carthagena." The newspaper continued: "The deaths, according to the latest intelligence received at that fortress, amounted to about thirty per day; and to such an extent had the apprehension of the possible introduction of the dreadful disease into Gibraltar being felt, that the most timely and effectual precautions had been resorted to. Soon afterward the gates of the garrison were closed by order of the Governor until the return of a physician who had been dispatched to Carthagena to ascertain the precise state and condition of yellow fever, with which many were afflicted."[6]

On September 1, R.Y. Vance, surgeon to the forces, presented his findings on Carthagena and Alicant. He began by stating that after an investigation in the Lazaretto, City and Royal hospitals he "had no hesitation in declaring, that the same disease exists there at present which prevailed in the years 1804 and 1810, and which, with some variations, I have witnessed so many Europeans fall victim to in the West Indies." He continued:

On the first attack, the patient is generally costive; but, previous to death, diarrhea often takes place, and what is voided has always a black, putrid appearance, and excessively fetid small. All these symptoms have not made their appearance in the same patients, but I have observed the whole in the numerous cases which presented themselves in the Lazaretto, and other hospitals in Carthagena. The disease has not been contained to any particular part of the town, nor is any person exempt from it who has not had it in the years 1804 and 1810....

The number of deaths may appear trifling for a town the population of which is generally calculated at 36,000 souls (the estimate in 1806); but, when you consider, that the fever last year reduced this number considerably, and that every person who had the means of escape has left it this year, leaving little more than a population of 9,000 in the city, most of whom had the disease upon former occasions, you will be able to form a more just idea of the mortality.

Of more significance, Vance added the following:

The physicians cannot account for the disease making its appearance this year at Carthagena; but I have good reason to suppose it might have remained dormant during the winter, till roused into action again by the summer's heat; and I am more disposed to favour this opinion, from the circumstances of their using so little precaution last year; neither destroying the bedding, clothes, or other furniture, liable to preserve contagion, of any of the people who died of the disease, as they had done in the year 1804; and I am sorry to observe, that they have gained little by experience, as they pursue the same system to the present moment.

The report continued by stating there was not the slightest degree of disease at Alicant but at Elche, about four leagues distant, yellow fever was present, believed to have been brought there by a soldier and five or six people who aided him from Carthagena, all of whom died after a few days of sickness. Immediately thereafter a cordon was placed between the two towns and a rigid quarantine established, limiting the spread of contagion. At Murcia, the capital of the province (distant 13 leagues from Alicant) the disease was carried there by refugees from Carthagena. The town was placed in a state of quarantine but with so many fleeing there after the French made their appearance he feared a greater spread of the disease.

Deaths from Yellow Fever at Murcia, Summer 1811

July 29: 12	Aug 6: 4	Aug 14: 24	Aug 22: 17
30: 4	7: 11	15: 16	23: 19
31: 5	8: 7	16: 12	24: 24
Aug 1: 7	9: 7	17: 6	25: 29
2: 8	10: 16	18: 20	26: 34
3: 9	11: 7	19: 23	27: 20
4: 4	12: 20	20: 22	28: 20
5: 3	13: 21	21: 21	29: 26

On September 4 the lieutenant general in charge of the Gibraltar garrison issued a proclamation. It began with the warning that as an alarming fever had broken out at Carthagena and other places on the coast of Spain he found it necessary to cut off all communications with Spain by sea and land. He called for volunteers to keep improper persons out of the garrison. He also called for a 14-day quarantine from all ports of Spain and the Mediterranean.[7] Amid reports that the enemy was gathering in great numbers at Marbella, gates of the garrison at Gibraltar remained closed until the return of Dr. Vance.[8] By the end of the epidemic it was stated that 45,000 persons living in and around Elche, Orihuela and Murcia had perished from yellow fever.[9]

Health matters would not get appreciably better in the ensuing years. The situation being complicated by war maneuvers, the spread of disease along the southern coast of

Spain continued to be a matter of pressing urgency. In August 1812 the British troops of General Ross were to be united with those of General Maitland. Ross, having an official communication to the governor of Carthagena, made inquiry into the true state of affairs there. In a report of August 23 the board of health reported that yellow fever had lately broken out within the walls but that "the most active measures" were being taken. This included preventing all communication with affected individuals. Physicians, however, warned that such measures were ineffectual and that it was impossible to completely check the contagion.

The sick troops encamped at Carthagena were permitted to be attended in their own houses but without free access to the rest of the inhabitants, while the poor of the city were taken to King's Hospital. Since August 11, the day on which the Lazaret had been formed, 10 persons had died of yellow fever and by the 23rd of the month 231 were reported sick. Reports dated October 8, 1812, indicated that sickness was abating at Carthagena and that "our medical men deny the existence of the yellow fever." The claim may have been more political than factual, as it was further stated "there has certainly been a fever of some sort, which affected our troops in the Goleras. Nearly 200 of the 67th regiment were in hospitals and several of the townspeople had died."

The situation appeared to be better at Alicant. On October 9 a report by E. Brown, deputy inspector of hospitals to Major General McKenzie, stated there existed no malignant or contagious fevers in the city. The same state of health apparently did not apply to the French. Three days later a directive from Alicant reported that the infection had "certainly broken out" among the enemy, with 7,000 of their troops being placed under "observation." This outbreak was attributed to the incursion of a party to plunder Zugar, where yellow fever was known to be present.[10] Reports of yellow fever arrived early in 1813 and persisted throughout the season.

Deaths from Yellow Fever at Malta, 1813

Month	Mortality
April	1
May	110
June	800
July	1,594
August	1,042
September (to the 25th)	603

Of these 4,150 fatalities, 1,634 were at Valetta.[11]

Yellow fever ("i.e. the Plague") was acknowledged at Gibraltar on September 5, 1813. Not atypically, official reports from Cadiz dated September 6 denied reports that the disease had also broken out in that city, but by September 26 newspapers in Lisbon "distinctly [mention] the existence of putrid fevers of the nature of the yellow fever, with the melancholy addition of that dreadful disorder being present at Gibraltar, where it is stated 25 persons died between the 8th and 13th ult." Subsequent reports mitigated the severity of the outbreaks, noting that several persons had been "carried off" but their malady was not believed to have been of a contagious nature. Lieutenant General Colin Campbell, the lieutenant governor of Gibraltar, issued a statement dated September 13 avowing that the alarm was "no more than the disease peculiar to the station." In what might be considered a touch of sarcasm, after commenting on the "agreeable and positive accounts" that the plague and yellow fever were incorrect, one Lisbon reporter added, "So decided and so generally credited was the report, that our Government had taken the most decided measures to prevent its introduction here." In any case, by December 4 a notice from Lisbon assured its readers "the yellow fever at Gibraltar, the plague at Malta, and the black vomit at Cadiz, have all ceased, or so nearly ceased, as to cause no further alarm even to the inhabitants of those places: this may be confidently relied on."[12]

Between 1814 and 1818, reports of yellow fever were scarce. On September 2, 1814, a notice from the junta of health at Madrid was charged by his majesty to "prevent his States from the contagion of the yellow fever" at Gibraltar by ordering all vessels from that port to perform a rigorous quarantine. The same year, in a discussion on international travel, it was stated that the extreme slowness in which temperatures increased during the passage from Spain to the "New Continent" was "highly advantageous to the health of Europeans, who go to settle in her colonies. At Vera Cruz and at Carthagena, the creoles who descend from the high savannas of Bogota, and the central elevated plain of New Spain, are more exposed on the coasts to the attack of the yellow fever, or *vomito*, than the inhabitants of the north, who arrive by sea."[13]

"Memoir on the Fumigation of Letters"

While it is tempting to look back on historical events and wonder at the measures taken to avert the spread of contagion, it is difficult for anyone to put themselves in the place of an individual faced with almost certain death from a disease little understood. Without any positive explanation, cause, preventative or cure, the mere mention of yellow fever must have caused a shudder of fear, while the actual presence of this plague meant a horrific, life-altering tragedy, if not actual loss of life. In that light, the effort Bernandino Antonio de Gomez went to in determining the effects of fumigation on letters suspected of being contaminated is not to be wondered at but applauded.

In 1816, Senor Gomez, of Lisbon, posed a question to the junta of health. He asked whether, in order to preserve Portugal from the introduction of the plague or yellow fever, it was sufficient to make incisions in letters received from countries suspected of being infected and to fumigate them without fully opening or soaking them in vinegar. The junta recommended opening letters so they could be well penetrated by vinegar, the most powerful of all anti-epidemics. If, however, the letters contained articles susceptible to infection they should undergo chlorine fumigation according to the anti-contagious process of Guyton Morveau, who had earned success from his successful treatment of miasma of different contagious maladies. Authorities in the junta disagreed as to which measures were sufficient, however, and with the assistance of Gomez they conducted a number of experiments that he minutely described in his study, "Memoir on the Fumigation of Letters."

Experiments on Decontaminating Letters Received from Countries Contaminated by Yellow Fever, 1816

First Experiment: Some opened letters were placed perpendicularly in a stove of Baume and exposed for 5 minutes to the action of chlorine as developed by Morveau. Upon their removal, some characters had a yellowish hue and the letters had a strong scent of chlorine or muriatic acid.

Second Experiment: One letter was treated as above after 3 parallel incisions were made, each 1" long. Upon removal the letter retained the chlorine odor but not as strongly as in the first experiment.

From this Gomez determined the first experiment to be more efficacious because of the more powerful odor, but he argued that not all letters were composed on a half sheet of paper such as that used in the study. He argued more voluminous letters might not be fully penetrated.

> Third Experiment: Encasing two sheets of paper covered by a third and sealed with wafers, he made four slits, each 1" long and placed them in the stove. Using chlorine, he added 1 ounce of common salt, $2/8$'s of manganese, $1/8$'s of water and $6/8$'s of sulphuric acid. After 15 minutes he discovered the sheets smelt inwardly of chlorine.
>
> Fourth Experiment: Three sheets of paper were put in an envelope and folded in two; three 1" incisions were made in the envelope and processed in the same manner as in Experiment 3. The paper smelled strongly of chlorine.

The letters thus fumigated retained their odor of chlorine for many days, prompting Gomez to deduce that the gas did not introduce itself into the letters only through the incisions. To confirm this theory, he conducted further tests.

> Fifth Experiment: The 4th experiment was repeated without making incisions in the letter. Afterward the letter smelled strongly of chlorine but he wondered if the gas might have insinuated itself into the letter through the openings of the envelope.
>
> Sixth Experiment: The 5th experiment was repeated, closing all openings of the envelope with sealing wax. He observed the odor of chlorine was perceptible in the paper but to a lesser degree than when incisions had been made.
>
> Seventh Experiment: The 6th experiment was repeated but the letter was placed inside two envelopes, both hermetically sealed. The result was the same and after two days still retained the odor of chlorine.

Gomez concluded that if chlorine actually did extend "its power to the plague," then Morveau's process of fumigation was successful, even without making slits in the letters. The questions thus became how long fumigation should continue and how to prove the process actually disinfected the letters.

> Eighth Experiment: Six ounces of meat were set out to putrefy in a saucer; above the meat was suspended cotton, silk, hemp, wool, feathers and fur. The whole was placed in glass and corked shut. When it was determined the meat had putrefied all the items smelled bad but the odor was strongest in the feathers and the skin (fur). Twelve letters were then enclosed with the six substances infected with cadaverous odor. Two incisions were made in each letter. Fumigation was performed as in the 3rd experiment. After half an hour the letters were examined. Only the hemp preserved the odor of the chlorine; the cotton was free of it; the feathers and skin still smelt of the putrefied flesh; the odor was weaker in the silk and still weaker in the wool.

Gomez concluded that animal substances (feathers and skin) impregnate themselves more with the cadaverous odor than do vegetable substances; that the latter lost it altogether or were easily purified; that the effect of the fumigation was less at the close of the operation than on preserving the letter sealed until the following day, and that animal substances required a greater duration and intensity than fumigation.

> Ninth Experiment: On a paper pricked with a pin the animal substances infected with cadaverous gas were placed. Fumigation was performed on the outside of the stove by suspending the paper 2" above the fumigating cup. In 5 minutes the bad smell was not perceptible.
>
> Tenth Experiment: The same substances and the paper were infected as in the 9th experiment without the half ounce of water which in the 9th test moistened considerably the substances susceptible of infection. The bad odor was not so strong, supposing that it was either exhaled, its communication with the exterior air not having been intercepted by the water, or arising from some other cause.

Eleventh Experiment: Fumigation was performed on letters containing paper, silk, wool, cotton and hemp and infected by the same process. They remained in the stove for one night. The following day all the substances smelt of chlorine and had lost the cadaverous smell.

This confirmed the 8th experiment.

Gomez ultimately concluded that on account of the exhalations of the chlorine not being uniform or the letters not being equally exposed to its action the results of Morveau's process were not always the same. He was satisfied it worked sufficiently well but ultimately warned that a better process for the fumigation of letters was necessary.[14]

The mistake Gomez made is readily apparent: he based his experiments on the idea that miasma or bad smells were the same as, or similar to, the process that caused yellow fever. Clearly they were not but his efforts demonstrate the advances in scientific technique and the grave error involved when the original premise was incorrect.

"Important accounts were received....": 1819

The above quote, interchangeable with "according to the latest advices" or "letters from," typically began 19th century newspaper articles designed to alert readers of significant foreign news. In October 1818 one brief paragraph, similar to so many others, began somewhat deceptively: "Letters from Madrid state, that the yellow fever has not only reached Cadiz, but also Seville, Cordova, Grenada, and other cities." What followed would portend a calamity of international consequences.

"Famine, as well as pestilence" raged in Cadiz, the Isle of Leon and Seville, the account continued. "The fever is advancing upon Madrid. Seville is infested. The gates of Madrid are closed." The number of sick in the Isle of Leon (a mile distant from Cadiz) attained its height with 1,086; by September 24 it had been reduced to 495. At Cadiz, however, numbers registered on September 29 indicated the number of sick there was 4,075. Death from a more insidious enemy was also to be reckoned with: "This is not all of evil which the Almighty permits in that afflicted kingdom. Murcia rings with the groans of wretches on the rack. Two persons of distinction, of whom one was a colonel of artillery, perished under the torture in that city. No confession could be torn from them; and the executioners, who are stated to be attendant devils of the inquisition, screwed the instruments to a tension beyond the life of a man to endure. The crime with which they are charged is freemasonry."[15]

The presence of yellow fever began in late July and early August 1819. Letters from Gibraltar on August 2 warned that the disease raged at Cadiz with great malignity, not only on the inhabitants of the town but the military personnel in the neighborhood. It was believed the fever had been introduced by the *Asia*, from Havana, where the fever had made considerable ravages during the prior months. Half the crew of the *Asia* were said to be infected or dead of the dreadful malady. At the British fortress precautions were taken by the governor to prevent all communications with Spain, and a cordon was to be established without delay. All intercourse, it was added, would thus be interrupted unless the regulations of quarantine were observed.

Measures adopted August 20 failed to protect Madrid from the contagion raging on the Isle of Leon and in consequence the authorities and troops of the expedition (Spanish armament) prepared to leave town and orders were issued for the establishment of a cordon of health 10 leagues in circumference. On August 29 General Don, the governor of the garrison and territory of Gibraltar, announced his own four-point plan to prevent the "yellow fever, or epidemia" from spreading.

(1) All communication with the Isle of Leon, whether by sea or land is prohibited

(2) No person coming from the territory of Spain shall be permitted into the garrison except as reside in the neighborhood

(3) Persons coming by sea shall be quarantined; vessels coming from the Isle will not be admitted without passing through the Lazaretto

(4) A register of persons passing in and out of the garrison will be kept by the Inspector of Strangers. Persons with urgent business in Spain may apply for a pass. A cordon of troops is established across the Isthmus of the territory; sentries are ordered to fire on anyone attempting to pass without permission

On September 7 the Spanish government officially acknowledged the existence of yellow fever on the Isle of Leon and expressed apprehension of its spreading. That concern proved correct; by September 15, yellow fever had "shown itself with symptoms of progressive aggravation, in the town of St. Ferdinand and the Isle of Leon."

Partial Record of Deaths on the Isle of Leon, 1819

Date	Deaths	Recoveries	New Cases
August 1–20	105	392	723
August 20–31	345	663	1,313
September 4	57		
September 5	10		
September 6	10		
September 7	35		

The rapid and fatal progress of yellow fever was attributed to "the indigent class, which is very numerous, being destitute of all resources and means of cure for any kind of malady, particularly the yellow fever."

At Cadiz it was believed measures adopted by the board of health would contain the fever and no great fears [were] entertained of the fever spreading."[16] As often happened, such optimism was doomed to disappointment. Authorities first acknowledged the presence of yellow fever at Cadiz on September 13 but a letter dated September 14 from that city contained information that in consequence of excessive heat for the past week the fever had increased to an alarming extent and it was "calculated that upwards of 3000 persons are laid up with it; the number of deaths is from 30 to 40 daily, out of a population of 70,000 souls. The Governor, and all the troops intended for the expedition, left this last week; since [then] we have been completely shut in. The communication with the vessels in the bay is also closed." It was observed that those who had previously suffered from the disease were not attacked a second time.

At Cadiz it was "remarkable that the daily mortality is more considerable now than at other periods, when the town was afflicted by the same disease, although the population was then more numerous." From September 13 to the 29th, there were 939 deaths; on the 30th alone 74 deaths were reported, with letters indicating 83 died on November 1 "and the number of the sick had then augmented extremely." Notices from Madrid on September 19 added that, because the fever was spreading, many inhabitants from Seville, Cordova and Grenada had fled to Murcia or La Mancha. Contradictory news indicated that "under these circumstances it is impossible for the grand expedition to sail, since it would be imprudent to risk a great fleet and army which may be infected by the miasma of this cruel disease."

Death tolls continued to mount. Between September 14 and September 21 inclusive, 333 persons died at Cadiz and 337 from the Isle of Leon. Since all communications were cut off from Seville beginning September 26 it was further supposed the pestilence also raged there. This proved to be accurate: between September 24 and September 30, twenty deaths from yellow fever were reported. Between the 24th and the 28th the number of dead at Puerto Santa Maria was given as 23, with 343 still affected. By October 2 seven more had died and 396 remained ill.

Mortality at San Fernando (Isle of Leon) September/October 1819

Month	Date	Number of Deaths
September	28	56
	29	17
	30	20
October	1	16
	2	16

Between August 28 and November 7 a total of 5,306 persons died on the Isle of Leon.

At the end of September mortality in Cadiz had reached 1,212, of whom 684 were men, 186 women and 342 children. By October 1 an estimated 9,230 remained ill of the fever. By the 2nd intelligence indicated that at Cadiz the yellow fever had grown more malignant, business was suspended, counting houses closed and shops shuttered, reducing the inhabitants to want for the necessities of life. Average mortality per day rose from 69 to 89, a staggering increase.

Mortality in Cadiz, October 1819

October	Number of deaths
1	89
2	91
3	79
4	82

Aboard the Spanish ships meant for a war "expedition" to South America pestilence also raged, taking the lives of seven captains, while thirty seamen were listed as dead. The great disproportion between captains and common sailors was explained by the fact the men were not allowed ashore, where it was supposed they became infected, and the officers were. In light of the mortality among officers, orders arrived from the government at Madrid ordering all ships into dock for the winter. Preparations were also made to prevent the spread of yellow fever, "or as some will have it, the plague," from Cadiz to Madrid. All travelers arriving from the southwest were subjected to a temporary quarantine, but by October 9 it was rumored that the disease had made an appearance in the suburbs.

By October 7 reports indicated that the disease had run its course on the Isle of Leon, as no person had died of yellow fever during the last week of September or the first of October. News was little improved at Cadiz. On October 11 the cases of fever were 105 and at Seville not much less. "The only prospect the inhabitants had of being relieved from the distemper," noted one newspaper, "was the approach of the winter season."

Between October 19 and 23, there were 73 deaths reported at Cadiz. The change in weather did not occur until October 24 when rain set in, announcing the arrival of lower temperatures. At the time, 7,680 remained sick with fever and the number of daily fatal cases (reaching 82 on October 25) was expected to significantly decrease. In light of those numbers, one newspaper account that deaths were "few in number" at Seville, "not exceeding 20 to 25 daily," was at least somewhat justified. Reports from Port St. Mary's on October 20 indicated 434 were sick and the town was averaging 9 deaths per day. Official mortality returns from yellow fever to the end of November listed 4,537 deaths at Cadiz within three months; of these, 2,849 were men, 694 women, 602 boys and 392 girls.[17]

CHAPTER 12

The Baneful Effects of Yellow Fever

The New York papers of the above date [September 28, 1819] are filled with the most melancholy accounts respecting the progress of the fever. The Health Office at New York publish Bulletins every day. The Banks and shops have all been shut up, business suspended, and the number of people who have fled from New York within three days was estimated above 30,000; the fever is one of the most malignant description; as there appears no instance where a person infected ever recovered.[1]

Reports from Teneriffe (19th century spelling) in the Canary Islands indicated that yellow fever at Santa Cruz "continued to be prevalent there" through the middle of December 1810. Mortality was high, "and what added to the distress of the inhabitants, no medical aid could be obtained, nor had they any medicines adapted to their unfortunate cases."

The disease carried over into 1811 as reports continued to warn that yellow fever was raging violently at Santa Cruz and that mortality was excessive, with the inhabitants "carried off in great numbers daily." Vessels leaving the islands for Madeira were immediately put under strictest quarantine. After tapering off during the mid-part of 1811, yellow fever again appeared in the Grand Canary during the month of September. It raged throughout the rest of the year, and more than 3,000 perished.

By October 4 the disease had appeared at Port Orotava. Merchants and principal residents fled to the country "in the greatest consternation, abandoning everything." Ultimately, more than 500 out of a population of 3,000 fell victim to the malady. At Santa Cruz it was noted that the disease had been less destructive "owing to the greatest part of the inhabitants having previously been affected by it." For those who attributed yellow fever to the weather, reports indicated that there had been no rain since the fever commenced and the temperature was "hot almost to suffocation." Adding to the misfortune, the island had twice been visited by scorching winds from the desert of Barbary, bringing with it clouds of locusts which devoured "every atom of vegetation."

Business came to a standstill and several American and English ships were unable to land their cargoes owing to the lack of people to unload or receive them on shore. Reports indicated that the sickness prevailed mostly among the laboring classes.[2] For British troops serving in and around the Leeward Islands, exposure to yellow fever was always a hazard although the caprices of the disease were inexplicable to ship surgeons. The homeward-bound *Nyaden* left St. Thomas on May 5, 1811, and lost 100 men, including its captain, Frederick Cottrell, who died April 28 at Barbados. The *Thetis* lost the same number of seamen, while the *Castor*, which lay at harbor beside it, had not a sick man aboard. The following year yellow fever was prevalent at Antigua and St. Kitts but not at Nevis, although "three shocks of earthquakes ha[d] been felt here,"[3] a fact that would have fit into Webster's theory that yellow fever was predicated by natural disasters.

Information on yellow fever in 1816 was accompanied by political news. Writing from the British standpoint, one newspaper remarked that the disease had broken out at Point-a-Petre, Martinique, "as soon as we had given up the Island to the French." Another noted that at the time of its surrender to the French troops, yellow fever had broken out. "Happily, the Commander-in-Chief of the Britannic forces (Sir James Leith) taking all the measures that humanity commanded, offered to Lieutenant-General Count de'Lardenoy, to leave provisionally some black troops at Point-a-Petre, and all the French garrison was accordingly cantoned in the field of Beau Soleil, till the malady should cease. All necessary precautions were also observed to preserve the rest of the island from the contagion." The same year, yellow fever was prevalent at Antigua. On September 19, 1816, one resident wrote that there were great expectations that recent storms would have abated the violence of the fever "now too long prevailed here," but they were "painfully disappointed, as each succeeding day has added one or more names to the [mortality] list. With some few exceptions, the fever has been confined to persons resident here but a short time." The contagion was thought to have been brought to Antigua in a vessel from Guadaloupe.[4]

By the 5th of October British ports in the Bay of Honduras were opened to American vessels laden with provisions, but on November 6, after several cases of yellow fever were discovered, the governor of St. Bartholomew's issued a proclamation rigidly prohibiting all vessels from Guadaloupe and Antigua from entering that port. Through mid–November, hurricanes considerably damaged cane and coffee crops of the Antilles, while yellow fever continued to desolate those colonies, especially Martinique.

With the Napoleonic Wars finally over, England's presence in the West Indies was solidified. That meant, however, troops were subject to attacks of yellow fever and notices typical of that published by the *Military Register* (London, February 19, 1817) were common: "We have to regret the loss of many officers of both Navy and Army, by the Yellow Fever, in the West Indies. Active exertions are, however, making to stop its progress. To prevent unnecessary pain, Lists of the Army may be seen at the War Office by relatives." Sporadic news in 1817 and 1818 from the West Indies revealed that outbreaks of yellow fever persisted, particularly on Martinique, where the minister of the interior at the Havre "commanded the adoption of sanitary measures," subjecting vessels from that island to undergo a 30-day quarantine, while during the latter half of the year 300 victims of the disease were reported dead at Port-au-Prince. Yellow fever was also said to be making extensive ravages at Havana. Interestingly, while writing of La Guayra (La Guaira), Venezuela, one resident noted that "the scourge of yellow fever, or *calentura amarilla*," had been known for only two years and mortality was not considerable "because the confluence of strangers on the Coast of Caraccas was less than at the Havannah and Vera Cruz."[5]

Yellow fever persisted in Bermuda throughout 1818 and the island was placed under quarantine. Attrition among British servicemen from the disease continued to reach distraught families back home. Among those listed as having perished from the fever were Mr. Llewellyn, surgeon, Mr. Bartie, master, and Mr. Young, assistant commissary general. Closer to home, the same article reported that yellow fever had broken out in Ireland during September: "A great number of the artificers who had recently arrived at the Naval

Dock-yard were attacked by it, and twenty are dead. Five soldiers, also, belonging to a detachment of the 62d regiment, died in the Hospital." The remainder were placed in strict quarantine. Many other residents of Ireland fell victim and the disease was said to have spread to the neighboring islands.

At the Newry Fever Hospital, Ireland, a two-week report from September indicated 1,308 admissions with 34 deaths. In describing symptoms of several cases where a disordered state of the liver caused the patients to turn yellow, one in particular was diagnosed as "typhus thus modified, and which, by the nurses, was called 'yellow fever,' was brought to the hospital at an advanced period of the disease, and the patient died."[6]

The year 1819 was a particularly fatal year not only in Spain but also in Jamaica, where yellow fever raged during the summer. Particularly affected were troops of the 50th and 92nd regiments, which arrived there from Ireland in June. By the end of the month fever appeared among the 50th, "in the most aggravated and appalling form"; nine officers, about 190 men, 23 women and 15 children fell victim. In the 92nd, three officers and 150 men and children were lost. By September 3 the ravages had not ceased, prompting Sir Home Popham to offer the *Seraphis* as a convalescence ship. Among those who died was Colonel Hill, who had served in the 50th regiment for 47 years. When he heard his men refused to act as nurses for the sick he performed the work himself and died within a few days from the same dreadful malady.[7]

Letters dated early November continued to mention the "awful malady" that had extended, "in a particular degree, throughout the troops garrisoned here." The Highlanders of the 92nd were so affected that upwards of 200 men were swept away in five weeks. By the end of the year official totals from the various regiments were as follows:

Mortality from Yellow Fever Among British Troops in Jamaica, 1819

Regiment	Men Landed/Died	Women Landed/Died	Children Landed/Died	Officers Landed/Died
92nd	661/290	77/36	65/27	27/10
61st	–/40	–/–	–/–	–/1 major, 1 captain
50th	–/230	–/–	–/–	–/12
58th	–/–	–/–	–/–	–/1 paymaster
Royal Artillery	–/40	–/–	–/–	–/1 captain[8]

Nor were Martinique and St. Domingo exempt. When the disease became epidemic during the summer, orders were sent to French ports to quarantine all vessels from the West Indies for at least 28 days. Similar conditions prevailed at Havana, where 3,000 newly arrived troops were made to march in the hot sun. Of these, nearly 400 were later sent to the hospital and died from yellow fever.[9]

"The die is cast": Yellow Fever in the United States, 1810–1819

Scattered outbreaks of yellow fever in the United States between 1810 and 1815 garnered little attention from local newspapers but were significant enough that a later newspaper account quoted General Andrew Jackson as declaring, after his victory in the Battle of New Orleans in January 1815, "Long may the city stand, uncursed by war or Yellow Fever." By 1816, however, notices from New Orleans dated October 18 were giving warnings:

> The sickness has been more fatal than was ever known before at this place, affecting alike natives as well as strangers. Nearly all the physicians of any note have either died, or been rendered by the epidemic incapable of duty. From 20 to 30 die daily, and the alarm and consternation is such as to render it difficult for the sick to procure assistance of any kind. Advices have been received from many districts in the Southern States, Georgia, and South Carolina, which state, that the great numbers had fallen there also victims of the yellow fever.

News of yellow fever outbreaks persisted into the following year. During one week in the summer of 1817, out of 48 deaths at Charleston 16 were attributed to that malady: "Great numbers of the inhabitants had removed to, and lived in, tents on Sullivan's Island." From November 2 to the 9th, only 3 of 27 deaths were recorded by the board of health as having resulted from yellow fever.

In order to ward off a repetition of the yellow fever epidemic of 1817, the Charleston Board of Health published regulations meant to prevent or limit the severity of new outbreaks. Among the new rules was a fine in the staggering amount of $2,000 issued to anyone who neglected to open his cellar doors for a few hours every day. The situation in New Orleans remained hopeful for the writer of a letter dated September 5, 1818, indicating that while yellow fever had made its appearance it was "by no means malignant in its character, or alarming to the citizens."[10]

In Europe the subject of yellow fever in North America was occasionally discussed with a disparaging connotation. In 1817 Dr. Butte of Frankfort wrote an article stating "Europe alone can be the abode, at present, of civilized people." In order to discourage emigration he supported the popular notion that the ravages of yellow fever were spread "in proportion to the opening of the grounds by cutting down woods." In reviewing his work, one author "disbelieved" his assertion: "A disorder that is contagious may go any where without doubt, but the originating cause of the yellow fever assuredly sprung up in places and under circumstances very different from letting in the light of the sun and the sweeping action of the winds upon tracts which, confined by their primeveal forests, have never before seen the one or felt the other."

A retrospective study covering over two decades offered a more scientific conclusion. When records and tables from Philadelphia between 1793 and 1817 were reviewed, findings revealed that when the temperature in June and July did not exceed 70 degrees, yellow fever did not prevail; but when the average heat of those months exceeded 79 degrees, the fever raged and was most mortal in those summers when the thermometer indicated the greatest temperature.[11] As proof that not even the correlation between temperature and yellow fever was established, a report from Baltimore in 1819 stated, "It seems that during the hot weather the seeds of the yellow fever are planted and lying dormant until a cooler air brings them forth—this supposition is corroborated by the fact, that in 1793, when it prevailed in Philadelphia, the number of deaths encreased as the weather became moderately cooler, until the 11th of October, on this day 119, the highest number of deaths occurred."[12]

In June 1819 the governor of Louisiana issued a proclamation stating that he had received news yellow fever existed in the ports of Havana and Vera Cruz. He therefore ordered all vessels arriving from said ports to perform quarantine. Officials in New Orleans had reason to fear the disease. Yellow fever was a frequent and dreaded visitor to the city. It had appeared in 1817, killing 80 persons. The following year that number increased to 115. As early as 1804 New Orleans had established a Permanent Health Committee. By 1817 the city's sanitary code included 24 ordinances that included street, sidewalk and gutter cleaning and a mandate that privies be at least three feet from a dwelling and dug to a minimum depth of seven feet. A moratorium had been placed on hog raising, slaughterhouses and tanneries; requirements were stipulated on how to bury the dead in cemeteries; and a prohibition was placed on selling oysters during the summer, particularly between the months of June through November when yellow fever was most dangerous.

Following yellow fever epidemics in the late 1810s, the "Act to establish a Board of Health and Health Office to Prevent the Introduction of Malignant Pestilential and Infectious Diseases in the City of New Orleans" was passed. Its function was to administer new quarantine laws. Not surprisingly, businessmen and political leaders found the quarantine laws counterproductive to commerce. These individuals "ignored, or purposefully covered up the problem of disease and death," going so far as to make a concerted effort to convince newspapers not to publish news or mortality lists resulting from yellow fever. This second board of health did not survive long, but a new board was created by the "Act Against the Introduction of Infectious Diseases." Within its scope was a provision for quarantine against any ships carrying yellow fever victims: 15 days for those sickened and 10 days for those without symptoms. At this time (1817) the epidemiology society began tracking daily accounts of death in New Orleans.[13]

In 1810 Henry Sellon Boneval Latrobe, son of the famous architect Benjamin Henry Latrobe, presented a plan for a waterworks system to the New Orleans City Council. The concept was based on the Center Square Water Works project that Henry Latrobe had designed and created in Philadelphia as an attempt to improve sanitary conditions to ward off future yellow fever epidemics. The New Orleans project was also to include desalting water using steam-powered engines. The council agreed to commission the work in 1811 but the project was delayed by financial problems and the War of 1812. Henry Sellont remained in New Orleans and fought during the war. Afterward, he continued to work on the project but, tragically, died of yellow fever in 1817. Benjamin Latrobe arrived in New Orleans on January 10, 1819, and resumed work on the waterworks project. He finally succeeded in getting an engine built to run the massive machinery required and the work progressed. His timing was critically unprovidential: the year 1819 proved to be a devastating one for the city. A massive yellow fever epidemic swept through the environs, claiming 2,190 people, most of whom were immigrants, children, laborers and the poor. The following year, on September 30, 1820, Benjamin Latrobe himself perished from yellow fever.[14]

Charleston newspapers of August 11, 1819, exercised their painful duty to state yellow fever had made its appearance in the city. One paper actually apologized, writing that it had "been guarded in not exciting unnecessary alarm, and have therefore made this statement on the authority of the Board of Health," as well as with the approbation of respected medical gentlemen who had attended a stranger who died that day and who were also in attendance on two others afflicted. The notice went on: "The general health of the city is good. We forebear to say more at present." That guarded statement foreshadowed the tragedy to come. On August 22, the board of health reported four new cases; by noon on the 23rd, the number had doubled. Five additional people were stricken August 30. Subsequent reports through September added more to the mortality lists although it was noted that several cases of recovery had occurred after an illness of three to four days.

On August 28 dire news arrived from Baltimore that at the remote part of Fell's Point 50 cases of yellow fever had broken out. Although still confined to narrow limits, the disease had been traced to the same spot but exhibited indications of slowly spreading. The board of health was not a moment too soon to add that they "earnestly advise the citizens of that district to move away as speedily as possible." Unfortunately, a terse report from the *York Gazette* of August 29 informed readers of worse news: "Pitt street at Fell's Point, all sick but a few—George street the same—Wolf street ditto. Dr. _____ says the sickness will run through the place. The sickness first came among the apprentice boys, because they had to work in the sun, when the journeymen would not work.—We bury night and day—Fell's Point is all in an uproar, and people are moving away." This uproar was heard as far away as Philadelphia, where that city's board of health issued a proclamation on August 30 declaring that "all vessels from the city or port of Baltimore shall stop at the Lazaretto, and be proceeded within the same manner, and under the same penalties and forfeitures as are provided in cases of vessels coming from foreign ports." The order further stated "no person's goods, wares, merchandise, bedding, or clothing, coming from the city of Baltimore, shall enter or be brought into the city or country of Philadelphia before the 1st day of October next, by land or water, without the permission of the Board of Health, under the penalty of 500 dollars, and the forfeiture of the goods."

By August 31 the Baltimore Board of Heath advised that the situation of the 28th had "not marginally varied.... New cases still occur in full proportion to the number of inhabitants remaining in the diseased districts; they are, however, of a milder character, and evidently more yielding to medical treatment." Warning that it was the duty of every citizen to assist in counteracting the progress of the disease, the board expressed hope the disease would speedily terminate, "but on this subject the Board are not authorized to speak with confidence."

It was as well the Baltimore authorities mitigated their expectations, for the disease prevailed throughout the month of September. On the 9th, nineteen deaths occurred within a 24-hour period; by the middle of the month the mayor, at the request of the clergy, ordered September 23rd set aside "as a day of humiliation, fasting and prayer, for the purpose of imploring Almighty God, that he would be pleased to arrest the progress of the malady prevailing in that city, and restore it to its wonted health." Between September 25 and 26 sixty-eight new cases were reported. By early October mortality had finally begun to decrease: on the 3rd, two died of malignant fever and seven died on the 4th.[15]

When rumors began circulating that yellow fever had again reared its ugly head in New York City in the summer of 1819, representatives of the "whole commercial interest, and that of all moneyed men" gathered at the Tontine Coffee House to determine how best to prevent news of the disease (as opposed to the disease itself) from spreading and thus destroying commerce. The resident physician of the city was declared "incompetent" for his public statement that the disease existed at No. 13 Williams Street; efforts were begun for his removal and his person was threatened with violence.[16] Urging the dismissal of one man was not enough to calm the city. Rumors turned to facts, as a letter dated September 18, 1819 proved:

> The die is cast; the yellow fever is proclaimed, and New York is declared a fellow sufferer with her sister cities, Baltimore and Boston. Philadelphia is, as yet, stated to be free from the devouring

pestilence. The alarm which lately existed here is now becoming a woful reality: thousands have already left the city; and in a day or two hence, the probability is, that the lower part of the city will be completely deserted, which, in fact, is in great measure already the case. In Pearl, South, Front, Water, Hall, and Pine streets, with all the intermediate parts, forming the principal section of the town for business, not one store in fifty remains open. For the present, many have located themselves in the highest part of the town, particularly in Broadway; but of those the greater number will follow the current, and remove out of town, entirely. At Greenwich, a village about 3 miles distant, an attempt will be made to rally and concentrate business. The Banks, Post-office, and auctioneers, will fix at it; and there we must look for business, if any is to be done.

Sept. 20

It is almost impossible to describe the uproar of the town to-day; all is bustle and confusion; cartloads of furniture and goods moving in every direction. After all, perhaps, the danger is deemed greater than it really is. But Mr. G. Aspinwall and one of his clerks having been carried off, and the former being a man so generally known, and of such high standing, has tended not only to increase the alarm, but to cause a general panic.[17]

Interestingly, Greenwich would become known as "the Village" because it was a safe haven outside the city during yellow fever epidemics.[18]

Baltimore packets were blamed for importing the disease (in 1798 and 1805 as well as 1819), as yellow fever was especially prevalent in a small district near a low, shallow, land-locked piece of water, in a part of the harbor called the "Old Slip," where they generally anchored.[19] As news of the spreading plague reached Nova Scotia, Earl Dalhousie issued orders that every vessel arriving in the harbor of Halifax from any port or place of the United States where yellow fever had made an appearance was to undergo strict quarantine. Similar action was taken in Liverpool when the collector of the port placed all vessels from the United States under quarantine. Those ships coming from New York, such as the *Ann* under the command of Captain Crocker, often carried "upwards of 100 returned emigrants" who found returning home safer than remaining in a city infested with plague. The letters they carried told a harrowing tale. One such indicated "the principal streets of that city are deserted by the inhabitants, who have fled to the country to avoid the contagion. Business was suspended, and there were not any hopes of the fever abating until the end of October." Contrary to foreign port authorities, "Washington and other places, have continued an uninterrupted intercourse with New York and Baltimore, notwithstanding the disease prevalent in those cities."[20] Another letter, dated September 28, paints the melancholy picture in vivid detail:

The number of deaths have been few, but almost every person who has caught the infection has fallen a victim to the malady. The consequence is, that there is as great an alarm in this city as in former years, when the number of cases, as it is termed, or number of persons who became daily infected with the disease, was ten times as great as it is at present. The disease is, however, of a much more malignant nature than has heretofore prevailed in this city. It is very different in many of its symptoms from the Yellow Fever in the West Indies, and much more fatal. It is an undoubted fact, that every one who has caught the infection has received it in a particular part of the city, not more than the eighth of a mile square. This part of the city has been completely encircled, and therefore I am in hopes the fever will soon terminate. It is a fact in which most of the medical men are agreed, that persons moving from an afflicted to a healthy part of the city, with the disease upon them, will not communicate it to their nurses or attendants; or in other words, the fever is not contagions. Nothing confirms the fact more strongly than this, that there is not a single person who has been afflicted with the fever, who has not recently visited the infected part of the town. This part of the town is now shut up, and therefore there must now soon cease to be any new cases. Mr. _____, who laughed at the idea of a fever, has fallen a sacrifice to his temerity; both he and the young men in his store, which is in the affected part of the town, died last week. He was in such a state of putrefaction immediately after his death, that they were not able to move him from the bed in which he died.[21]

A letter from New York, dated September 25, 1819, had a slightly different take on the situation:

> I fear, however, that we shall have but a poor fall trade, in part owing to the inability of the country merchants to make payments, and in part owing to the alarm (for a fortnight past) of the yellow fever making its appearance in one part of our city.... I have removed my family to Newark, but have my store continued open in town, as usual. We have had an unusual warm and dry summer, and most of our sea-port towns have suffered most.... Boston and Philadelphia have not escaped; thus, you see, that in addition to the general depression of the times, we are scourged with pestilence. I am much concerned and grieved to see the accounts of the Reform Meetings in England, which I consider as pestilential, and as much to be dreaded as the yellow fever.[22]

By the second week of October no new cases of yellow fever had been reported and the epidemic came to an end. Notwithstanding, on November 6, 1819, the Lords of the Privy Council, Whitehall, having approved the quarantine restrictions against vessels from New York issued by the collector at Liverpool, approved and had "transmitted orders in conformity to Collectors and Comptrollers of the Out-ports, generally."[23]

"An action to recover..."

In 1819 two actions to recover investments in yellow fever remedies came before the Court of the King's Bench. The lead paragraph in the second case more than adequately summed up the circumstances: "This was a case of peculiar interest to the incautious, who are apt to be caught by the *gull-traps* daily set for them in newspaper advertisements, by artful imposters, promising enormous advantages to all who will suffer themselves to be lured to advance their capital upon plausible speculations, which ultimately turn out to be mere swindling stratagems to cheat the credulous and unwary."

The first case, brought July 10, 1819, pitted Admiral Charles Powel Hamilton against George Frederick Stratton, Esquire, in an action to recover £2,310. As presented by Mr. Caselee, the plaintiff, an admiral in the navy, gave money in 1807 to a Mr. Hardacre. Hamilton had patronized Hardacre, "who, through his interest, from a midshipman became a lieutenant in the navy." Hardacre believed he had discovered a medicine which would prove a specific for curing yellow fever and had succeeded in establishing an arrangement for disposing (selling) his medicine in the West Indies. The concern was divided up into 80 shares and Hardacre was to hold 30; the admiral purchased one share at £2,100, for which he held the option of retaining his share or selling it back for the original purchase price plus interest (£2,310) after two years had elapsed. The defendant had become joint surety with Hardacre in this deed.

Hamilton did not make his option until 1817, at which time Hardacre had become bankrupt. Hamilton thus proposed to sue Stratton. Mr. Scarlett, for the defendant, stated, "It was by the plaintiff's recommendation that the defendant had first become acquainted with Mr. Hardacre, who had set up the preposterous pretension that he had discovered a specific for the yellow fever, by means as absurd as had ever entered a visionary's head. Admiral Hamilton had only affected to give £2,100 for a share in this concern; he had never given the money. It was, therefore, a fraud upon the defendant." The chief justice ruled this plea was inadmissible. Scarlett then argued that as Hamilton had not made his

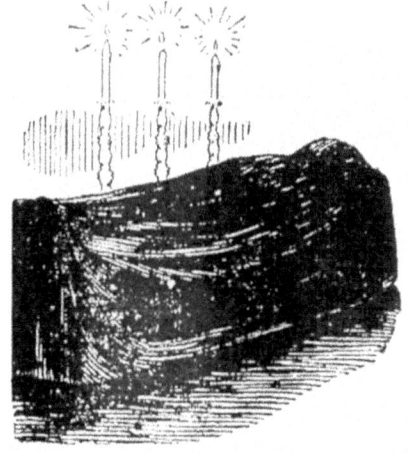
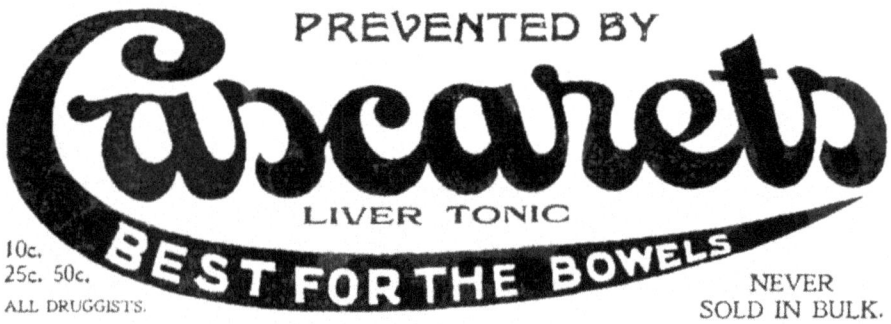

DEATH

begins in the bowels. It's the unclean places that breed infectious epidemics, and it's the unclean body—unclean inside—that "catches" the disease. A person whose stomach and bowels are kept clean and whose liver is lively, and blood pure, is safe against yellow fever, or any other of the dreadful diseases that desolate our beautiful land. Some of the cleanest people outside are filthiest inside, and they are the ones who not only "catch" the infections, but endanger the lives of all their friends and relatives. There's only one certain way of keeping clean inside so as to prevent disease and that is to take CASCARETS. Perfect disinfectant and bowel strengtheners. All diseases are

PREVENTED BY

Cascarets

LIVER TONIC

10c. 25c. 50c.
ALL DRUGGISTS.

BEST FOR THE BOWELS

NEVER SOLD IN BULK.

If shock had any value in selling products, then Cascarets Liver Tonic must have been a best seller. The idea that death began in the bowels was a nearly universal theme and tonics that cleaned the body from the inside were thought to cure everything from female complaints to yellow fever (*Mitchell* [Indiana] *Commercial*, March 7, 1901).

option after two years, it was presumed he had received payment and asked for the case to be discharged. This motion was also denied. Defense then claimed that in 1812 the plaintiff had written to Hardacre claiming only £1,360, indicating he had already received £1,040, "in bad bills, of course, but in such a way as to preclude him at least from claiming more than £1,360 from the defendant. He had, besides, proved only £1,450 under Mr. Hardacre's commission of bankruptcy." The chief justice remarked "that each party was now naturally anxious to disclaim a foolish project," and the defendant's offer of £1,450, including interest, was accepted.

On December 8, 1819, before the Court of the King's Bench, the case of the *King v. Hardcastle, Sir Fred. Stratton, John Stratton and Higgon* was held. This criminal indictment stated that Hardcastle had been a lieutenant in the Royal Navy and about the year 1804 "promulged [promoted] a specific medicine for the effectual cure of that dreaded disorder the yellow fever … and for the dispensation of it he opened a Depot at Charing-cross. He advertised for purchasers of shares in this speculation, and proposed most lucrative results to those who should choose to become adventurers." Hardcastle proposed to divide the property into 80 shares, which he valued at 2,000 guineas each. He retained 15 shares. Stratton, "a Gentleman of high character and great landed property," was induced to take 10 shares, his elder brother took 5 shares and Mr. Higgon took 5 shares. Several others took fewer shares, "all encouraged by the most confident hopes to make above 100 per cent. upon their respective adventures."

According to testimony, Hardcastle then advertised his 14 shares to "some person willing to take a share in a lucrative concern, by which a rapid fortune might be acquired in a very few years." A Mr. Bird wrote to No. 40 Charing-cross and met with Hardcastle, who at first informed him the speculation would yield 20 percent; he later stated it would produce 100 percent yield. He offered to sell "one eightieth share" at 2,000 guineas and invited Bird to dine at his house in Gloucester Place, where Bird met, among others, Mr. Stratton and Mr. Higgon. "There was an elegant dinner, consisting of turbot, venison, and other luxuries, various wines, and all the appointments in a style of fashionable elegance."

Duly impressed, Bird was invited to review the company books but was presented only with the petty cash accounts. When he requested to have his friend inspect all the records, Hardcastle diverted him by offering him a position as manager. His duty would be to inspect the other two offices that offered the medicine for sale, one at the West India Docks and the other at Liverpool. For this service he was to receive a salary of one guinea per day and travel expenses. Induced by these additional advantages, Bird agreed to purchase one share. The signatures of both the Strattons and Mr. Higgon were affixed to the contract in early 1811.

Bird received no more than £480 and subsequently Hardcastle became bankrupt. Bird appealed to Stratton and Higgon, telling them he was advised to indict them on criminal conspiracy unless his money was repaid. Solicitors for the men responded that they too were innocent victims and had "lost their money in the concern." At trial a Mr. Copeland deposed that, like Bird, he had purchased one share for £2,000 guineas and never received one farthing profit.

The prosecution argued that the Strattons and Higgon "must have known by experience that the concern was wholly unproductive; and they must also know that such a sum was utterly beyond the real value." The judge advised the jury that if they found this to be so they must find the defendants guilty, but if they believed only Hardcastle acted fraudulently they must find a general verdict of acquittal. "The Jury, without hesitation, returned their general verdict—*Not Guilty.*"[24]

Although the record does not reflect this, the defendant, Mr. Stratton—named "George Frederick Stratton" in the first case and "Sir Fred. Stratton" in the second—is clearly the same individual. His residence in the first case was "New-park, Oxfordshire," and in the second he is described as "a Gentleman of high character, and great landed property in Oxfordshire, and not many years since High Sheriff of his county." Presumably, the names "Hardacre" and "Hardcastle" were either purposely corrupted to complicate and separate the frauds or one was misspelled in the court report.

Proceedings of Public Societies and Monthly Reviews

David Hosack, MD, opened his essay, "Observations on the Laws Governing the Communication of Contagious Diseases, and the Means of Arresting their Progress" (1816) with this statement: "That the plague, when once generated, whatever may be the sources whence it derives its origin, is communicated by a peculiar virus secreted by the diseased body, will not, I trust, be questioned at this day." Dr. Hosack, professor of Theory and Practice of Physic and Clinical Medicine at the University of New York, linked the plague, dysentery, typhus and yellow fever together, remarking that they were not generally contagious, "depending on the qualities of the air to which it may be communicated." The history of every visitation of yellow fever in the United States, he added, "establishes this truth." By way of proof he cited the appearance of the disease in seaport towns where the air was most impure and during those seasons "when such impurities acquire their greatest virulence."

Supporting the work of Drs. Chisholm and Stewart that decomposed animal or vegetable matter could not of themselves produce the pestilence, Hosack agreed that the disease was generated in the human system and communicated from one person to another by a peculiar secretion from the morbid body. His object in the essay was to "show that when such virus is introduced into a certain state of atmosphere, the disease is readily contracted but that beyond that atmosphere it is rarely infectious." Contrary to what Dr. Adams of London and other authorities believed, that a *tertium quid*, or a new kind of air, was generated when the atmosphere was deprived of its due proportion of oxygen and loaded with "mephitic materials, especially the confined excretions of the human body," causing an extraordinary degree of malignancy, Hosack believed that the combination of the peculiar virus of those diseases "is in no way changed, but multiplied," and that the multiplying power resembled the fermentation process, called the "assimilating fermentation" by Drs. Walker, Cullen and Mr. Cruikshank.[25]

On the subject of dissention, Edward Doughty, in his text, *Observations and Inquiries into the Nature and Treatment of the Yellow or Bulam Fever, in Jamaica, and at Cadiz*, took exception to the work of Mr. Pym and Sir J. Fellowes respecting the nature or origin of fatal fevers. These two authorities particularly stressed the point that yellow fever "was always propagated by a specific contagion; and that this alone was adequate to its production, although the symptoms might be rendered more violent by other concomitant circumstances, such as peculiar states of the constitution, or certain conditions of the atmosphere." Doughty, on the other hand, viewed the subject much like Dr. Edward Nathaniel Bancroft (who published "An Essay on the Yellow Fever; with Observations Concerning Febrile Contagion, Typhus Fever, Dysentery, and the Plague" in 1811), in that yellow fever was not generated from animal effluvia and did not propagate itself by emanations from bodies laboring under its influence.

In "proving" the domestic origin and noncontagious nature of yellow fever, Doughty offered the test of taking patients suffering with yellow fever into the mountains, believing the disease would not be spread to those caring for them. On the other hand, if healthy individuals from the mountains were exposed to the disease in Kingston or some similar place and returned home, one or more would become affected, because their residence in the mountains "would not destroy the susceptibility to the influence of the morbid cause." This led to the conclusion yellow fever "cannot be propagated in a soil which does not itself impart the seeds of the disease." He furthermore denied Pym's doctrine that the fever "attacks the human frame but once," although he allowed that after one attack the body became "less susceptible than before, though the susceptibility gradually returns."[26]

Edward Bancroft himself offered a "Sequel to an Essay on the Yellow Fever" (1818), in which he discussed the diagnostic symptoms of the Bulam, or pestilential, fever, indicating that the most important was the absence of remissions, "in opposition to the paroxyms [paroxysms] of the disease which has, from this very circumstance, obtained the specific name of remittent fever." Bancroft emphasized that "although the ordinary form of *miasmatic* fever derives its popular name and most obvious character from the remissions which accompany it, "abundant facts" proved that when it existed "in an exasperated degree, the remissions are no longer perceptible." Second, he argued that the Andalusian fever was remittent. The remainder of chapters 1–3 lay in discrediting the theories of Dr. Pym.

Perhaps the most interesting argument was that of contagionists. Stressing the moral or political effect of the doctrine, they acknowledged that while their opinion might possibly be false, "it is more useful than the contrary idea, prevents much mischief, and can do no harm." Bancroft "warmly" opposed this position.[27]

Dr. John Mitchell, in a lecture before a select committee of the House of Commons (1819), argued that "the diseases of a place are in their nature, even though they go under the same name as subject to variations, as are the manners, customs, and circumstances of its inhabitants." Arguing against Drs. Pym, Russell, Fellowes and Warren (strenuous supporters of the contagion theory), Mitchell accused "the prejudice of system and the dogma of the schools which have upheld this phantom of contagion" to have caused unnecessary loss of life. Instead of permitting inhabitants to flee when the scourge visited, contagionists, Mitchell accused, prohibited them from quitting their abodes for fear of spreading the disease, condemning them "to breathe a pestilential atmosphere" and remain in their own abodes where "death and horror raged." Mitchell also advocated a clearer definition of terms, using "contagion" to refer to that disease "capable of separate self-existence, and of propagating its species *ad infinitum*, through its operation on the human body; while 'infection' should rather denote a quality or affection of a substance or body."[28]

A further study conducted in Spain in 1820 by Dr. Jackson, a venerable Englishman "on the verge of 70" years, asserted that yellow fever was never imported nor was it contagious. "The poison," he stated, "or malaria, which produces the disease, is the product of the soil itself, elicited by particular seasons, and the fever so generated, if directly exported to other countries, could not there be propagated, for want of its primary pabulum."[29]

CHAPTER 13

Corpses Still Animated: Yellow Fever, 1820–1829

A French physician has discovered that scrofula may be cured by a preparation of gold, which same disease another of the same faculty, with wonderful simplicity, denominates a species of yellow fever. Such, indeed, are all diseases that gold will cure.[1]

Remembrances of the staggering mortality from the yellow fever epidemic of 1819 had hardly faded from consciousness when its reappearance in early August 1821 at Barceloneta (a suburb of Barcelona) elicited great fear it would spread throughout the south of Spain. The distemper was believed to have been imported by a Spanish brig directly from Havana; three carpenters who worked on board and four seamen who belonged to other ships who communicated with the brig became early victims. The fever was thought to be contained and on August 29 the Superior Council of Health at Catalonia declared it to be noncontagious. Notwithstanding that assurance, the fever spread to Barcelona. Within days, the state of health in the city was described as "most alarming." Shops were shut and people huddled indoors for fear of contracting the disease. The fever being a particularly malignant type, patients were "generally carried off within three hours from the commencement of the disease."

On September 3 authorities at Catalonia published a notice warning that the number of sick at Barceloneta had increased to the point where it was judged necessary to sever communications with that town and others in the province. The constitutional municipality also declared measures would be undertaken to prevent the spread of disease. By September 11 the chief authorities and the garrison were removed and a precautionary cordon was formed a league from the city; three days later Spanish troops were also prepared to create a cordon around the Isle of Leon to protect the city of Cadiz, but this precautionary measure was not adopted as it was determined "the greater proportion of the inhabitants have suffered under it, and would probably escape its ravages."

By September 13 the situation had seriously deteriorated. Bulletins from Barceloneta stated there were between 20–30 deaths per day and all persons not infected were compelled to leave. These, estimated at 2,000, were lodged in a convent at government expense.

The *Journal de Leon* of September 20 indicated that yellow fever had manifested itself in the Lazaretto of Marseilles, brought there by a Danish vessel from Barcelona. Another Danish ship arrived on September 7, also carrying yellow fever victims. In consequence, the prefect of the Department of the Pyrenees issued an order on the 15th cutting off all communication with Spain, except by Porthus, where a Lazaretto had been established. French troops were ordered to reinforce the cordon and if necessary the national guards would be summoned to establish a second cordon.

Simultaneously at Gibraltar, the governor issued restrictions and although "they proved injurious to the trade of the place, he was unwilling to run the risk of repealing them." It was as well that care was taken, as reports of September 6 stated that the *Superb* and the *Auspicious,* recently arrived from Malaga, carried yellow fever. Both were ordered away and were thought to be proceeding to England.[2]

Reports of September 22 indicated that Barcelona was in the greatest misery and desolation. Returns of this period, including the Hospital of the Vice Queen of Poru (outside the walls of Barcelona), indicated that not a single patient had recovered. The number of deaths was given as 42, none cured, 66 remained ill and 67 new cases were reported. The clergy no longer attended victims to the grave and death carts passed through the streets twice a day. Upwards of 60,000 people were said to have abandoned the city but their condition was described as "most deplorable; to prevent the propagation of contagion they are repelled from every place where they claim hospitality, and have only the dreadful choice of perishing by hunger or pestilence."

A physician of Madrid argued against quarantine, writing, "The fears which these measures excite, the want of care experienced by the sick who are abandoned, and the famine which follows the suspension of all communication with a town, are all circumstances which extend the ravages of the fever to those who would otherwise have resisted the contagion." He suggested sanitary measures and allowing persons not affected to remove to healthy districts. Unfortunately, the latter idea was a double-edged sword. After studying the Spanish epidemic of 1820, Dr. Jackson confirmed the above observation by noting that those who fled "were treated like contaminated deserters from a pest-hospital, and either left to starve, or put to death by their barbarous countrymen."

Fatalities continued to mount. A letter dated September 29 and published in the *Gazette de France,* described conditions at Barcelona: "Our situation becomes daily more cruel; in vain did we hope that the last days of September would bring with it a cooler temperature, and consequently put an end to the fatal scourge which devours us, or at least lessen its progress. The season continues the same, and the victims to the yellow fever increase in number. Ninety died yesterday, and 600 new cases were declared. Death closes rapidly upon us; perhaps my turn is at hand."

At Tortosa 600 died within a five-day span and the garrison at Mont Jouy was infected by a soldier exposed to the disease in town. The commission of health, comprising four merchants, three physicians and two counselors, conjectured that the yellow fever circulating along the coast of the Mediterranean never extended from the coast beyond a certain distance inland or to places situated at more than 350 or 400 toises above sea level. Letters from Catalonia also painted a picture of despair. From September 23 to September 24 they indicated that 260 died at Sarragossa; outbreaks were also reported at Lerida, Barbastro and several other towns of Catalonia and Arragon. Advices from Madrid attributed the fever at Catalonia, "in great measure to the miserable deficiency of the system of Police and Municipal regulation."

From September 23 to September 25, recorded deaths at Barcelona reached 199, Barceloneta 146 and 44 at the seminary where people had congregated for safety, three-fourths attributed to yellow fever. The number of patients in these three places and the house of the vice queen were placed at 431, an increase of 31 since the day before. On the 26th, 76 died, 13 recovered and 120 new cases were added.

News up to September 29 indicated Barcelona to be an ill-fated town prey to the most appalling scourges of contagion and famine: "The children, whose mothers have fallen victims to the deadly contagion, are suckled by goats.... It was contemplated to evacuate the town, and encamp in the vicinity; but this last resource was found impracticable. Despair and stupefaction increase the evil. The physicians do not agree in opinion respecting the nature of the pestilence; some think it is the yellow fever, whilst others affirm that it is the Guinea negro malady, or black vomit. Some regard it as a stationary malignant fever." As accounts of mortality filled foreign newspapers, the Sisters of Charity of San Vincent Paul at Tortosa offered their services. They were aided by the Committee of the Junta which supplied some vinegar, chocolate and rice. If those foolish enough to pass the cordon around the city were caught, they were "given up to the rigour of the laws."

More promising accounts did not reach the public until October 27 when one letter from Barcelona stated:

> I have been 6 days in this city. I have witnessed the most distressing scenes. I arrived at the moment when the dawn of more auspicious days appeared. Up to that period death carried off, upon an average, 300 persons per day, and on some days, the deaths amounted to 400 or 500; but since the 22d. the date of my arrival, the number is under 170; yesterday it was reduced to 140.
>
> Yesterday the guns were fired at Barceloneta because no deaths, no new cases had occurred. There remains 60 sick out of a population reduced to about 4,000. It was in that suburb that the fever first broke out and infected the rest of the town. The citadel and Mont Joui, which shut their gates in time, have not been affected by the contagion.
>
> Some houses have lost the whole of their inhabitants, while in others no case of fever had occurred. The city is composed; tranquility prevails, the markets are tolerably well supplied, and the poor are supported by the Government.
>
> There still remains in Barcelona, 40,000 souls; the emigrants amounted to about double that number; and about 14,000 have fallen victims to the pestilence. It is remarked that this large portion that emigrate and spread throughout the different towns and villages of Catalonia did not transport the disease to any part, and the opinion most to be relied on is, that the fever is not contagious without the walls of the town. It is the yellow fever. The French physicians, except Bailly [Bally], have been invulnerable to the contagion.[3]

Dr. Bally, mentioned above, was a member of the French commission sent to Spain to study the progress of the disease. Fears had been entertained that he had died of yellow fever, but he survived his illness. A report by these physicians (Bally, Pariset, Francois and Andouard) was summed up in a letter written October 30, 1821. Supporting the idea that yellow fever was contagious, Francois wrote that the disease "appears to show itself visually. Its point of departure is marked; its progress followed; it may be said that it is seen passing from one individual to another. Those who devote their cares to friendship rarely fail to pay dear for their humanity." Describing symptoms, he continued: "The body of the patient then exhales miasmata, not perceptible to the senses, which attaches it to the bedding, clothes, furniture, and even the walls of the apartments (as, from numerous facts, there is reason to believe), which then becomes capable of infecting individuals, more or less promptly, according to their disposition. The disease appears to have its seat in the nervous system. It successively paralyzes the different viscera. The kidneys cease their functions first. The body, which may be called a corpse still animated, exhibits all the symptoms of decomposition.... It requires courage, I assure you, and the most perfect self-resignation, to approach and touch certain patients."[4]

13. Corpses Still Animated: Yellow Fever, 1820–1829

Dr. Pariset added his voice to the others. In an interview dated October 31 he avowed, "Yes, I repeat it a thousand times, it is contagious." Furthermore, he believed the disease to be imported and identical to the yellow fever of America. He added, "With only five good police and firmness, both Barcelona and its commerce, might, humanly speaking, have been preserved, even on the avowal of the anti-contagionists of this country. But what has been the fact? They wrangled, they disputed; the scourge entered, raged, proved fatal, and nobody knew how to remedy it. Hence all labour, all industry, all prosperity is here extinct for a long time. The heart itself has partaken of this depravity. The father shuns the presence of his children, and there is an adieu to every feeling of humanity!"[5]

Death Tolls Come Marching In

The number of dead continued to add to already depressing death tolls.

State of Yellow Fever in Spain, October 1821

Locale	Date	Dead	Cured	Remaining Sick
Port St. Mary's	13–23	89	190	235
Xeres de la Frontera	14–23	20	10	221
Lebrija	13–20	19	31	46
San Lucar	14–22	8	4	13
Barcelona	24	58	24	664
Barcelona	25	43	21	629
Barcelona	26	45	17	625
Barcelona	27	–	–	629

If one story could encapsulate the horror of yellow fever in Barcelona, a letter dated October 31 would suffice: "The other day the Municipal Junta was informed that a noxious odour issued from a house in Nomada-street, and that a child was heard crying within the house. Upon the house being visited there were found the body of a man greatly disfigured by the ravages of the yellow fever, and who had been dead four or five days. Beside this corpse was a woman expiring, and, lying upon her, a suckling infant, which, in the torment of hunger, was crying and gnawing the breast of its mother."

Reports of October 28 indicate that yellow fever had broken out at Malaga "with increased vigour, and there appears no hope of its being got under at present. Trade continues, of course, completely at a stand." On the Isle of Majorca (Mallorca) off the eastern coast of Spain, one bulletin announced more than 1,200 deaths from "plague" had occurred. The city of Palma was said to be deserted and barracks established in the neighborhood contained 6,000 persons. Effective quarantine measures added famine to the misery, leaving the island "absolutely without resources."[6]

Indicating how serious yellow fever was considered to be, a public notice dated October 26, 1821, from the Portuguese consulate general warned that all vessels, persons and effects from the ports of Marseilles, Catalonia, Malaga, Majorca, the Bay of Cadiz, and the American ports of Baltimore, Virginia, North Carolina and Long Island "shall not be admitted into any port of this kingdom." Vessels from these areas arriving at Lisbon were to undergo a rigorous quarantine of at least 30 days and in all cases vessels were required to supply documents from the authorities of public health at the port of departure stating that no disease existed aboard before departure.[7]

"*Much alarm was spread....*"

"[T]his morning among the merchants reading [about] Gibraltar, [there was] an account of the intelligence by the Steam-boat, that a disorder, supposed to be the yellow fever had broken out at that place." Almost generic in form and content, this one single sentence had the power to alter human life and well-being. Written September 19, 1828, it foreshadowed another epidemic of that dreaded malady. Typically, private letters were the first to announce news of yellow fever. When those receiving such communication forwarded them to newspapers, word was spread throughout the community, province, country and internationally, although not always in that order, for it was more likely foreign citizens were alerted before those more closely affected ever received official confirmation. In this instance, letters from Gibraltar dated as early as September 4 announced the presence of an "infectious fever," producing excessive consternation. As the rumor spread, an immediate cessation of business occurred and most of the Spanish families fled without waiting for confirmation. The number of fugitives increased so rapidly the governor of Gibraltar issued an order that no one was permitted to leave without permission. "All the remaining residents," it was dolefully stated, "had therefore no alternative but to stay and face the evil."

Increasing the terror, two sentinels were placed outside dwellings where persons were sick with the disorder, but authorities refused to confirm the nature of their disease, stating only that the infection was not contagious. Physicians from the board of health in San Roque and Algesiras were called in, but they differed on their conclusions. Nevertheless, a cordon was placed on September 5 and "fever of a *suspicious nature* was declared" to exist; "foul bills of health were issued" and precautions taken. No official returns were published, but a letter of the 8th noted that there were rumored to be 40 cases and 12 deaths.

Shortly thereafter, George Don, the lieutenant governor, issued orders calling on the inhabitants to cooperate with the government by following newly issued health regulations. He also ordered places of worship and the courts of justice to be closed. Three days later, another letter from Gibraltar bemoaned the fact that "from some unaccountable cause there has been no report of the public health published here, when, in fact, it is notorious that the yellow fever has prevailed for several days, which omission gives rise to vague and exaggerated rumours, and may be the means of attaching unnecessary suspicion to us on future occasions in other ports." The writer added that by close inquiry he determined the actual number of cases to be 104 (including the military), of which 31 were dangerous, 51 slight and 22 convalescent.

Proving how contrary opinion could be when the true state of affairs was unknown, a different writer informed his correspondents on September 8 that he believed "very energetic measures" would stop the progress of the disease, adding, "Nevertheless, the evil has been done by a complete stoppage to our trade, and all the concomitant mischief. For the 24 hours previous to 9 o'clock this morning, one patient only was admitted in the Hospital. Numerous of our friends and neighbors have gone off (not dead, but run away), and in short the panic is perfect. We of course remain: if it is the fever, we hold ourselves to be indigenous to it: if it is not, we console ourselves with not having abandoned the interests of our friends." There was, apparently, little for which that writer had to console himself. Up to October 11, new cases amounted to 100–110 daily with an average of 20–25 deaths. There remained on that date 344 serious cases, 217 slight and 210 convalescent. Deaths from September 10 to October 11 totaled 2,377, of which 454 were directly attributed to yellow fever. The governor ordered two carts to proceed through the streets to take up dead bodies at the doors of their houses; the military was forbidden to enter town and smuggling vessels were prohibited from entering the harbor.[8]

In an interesting commercial side note, in an article titled "Spanish Cigar Factory" (*Logansport* [IN] *Journal*, October 8, 1853) the writer offered a history of tobacco, noting that, as in most places of continental Europe, tobacco was a government monopoly. In Spain, where cigars were considered a necessity of life, the tobacco monopoly for 1852 amounted to 190,000,000 reals, minus 46,000,000 reals expense, leaving 144,000,000 reals ($7,200,000) clear profit. These figures were exclusive of the tobacco brought in by smugglers, which was especially lucrative considering the inferior quality of government tobacco. At the height of the yellow fever epidemic when smugglers had a difficult time bringing their contraband into Gibraltar, the authorities were forced to employ several thousand extra hands to work in the tobacco factories.

By early December the disease had run its course.

End of an Epidemic Gibraltar, December 1828

Date	Dead	Remained Ill	Admitted	Under Observation	Officers Sick
2	1	178	12	25	13
3	4	181	4	25	13
4	2	178	5	25	13[9]

As an indication of the state of medicine, an "officer of high rank in the Royal Navy" suggested a remedy for "the dreadful disorder that now ravages Spain being a species of *Plague* formed by a mixture of the *Yellow Fever and the Negro Disease.*"

(1) When the disease first appears, large fires should be lit and fumigations of gunpowder made in streets and public places

(2) To preserve oneself, "an oil skin silk should be worn *next the skin,* with the head and ears covered, as well as the whole body, and a *mask* worn strongly impregnated with garlick: five or six wine glasses of *Madeira* and *bark* should be taken daily

(3) If attacked by the disease, immediately drink a large glassful of *pure lemon juice,* and then have *arms, legs and thighs* rubbed with cantharides until large blisters form. He must also drink 0 times a day a large glass of Bourdeaux (sic) wine mixed with an equal quantity of lemon juice, in order to excite and keep up a profuse perspiration; continue until convalescence[10]

The Mississippi River: The Nile of America

In a recurring series entitled "America," the *British Press* (May 19, 1820) ran a study of New Orleans that might have served as a travel brochure. After lauding the steam engine boat that went "up the Mississippi, the Ohio and the Missouri, against the current, and require[d] only thirty days to traverse a distance of 2,000 miles, which separates our city from Pennsylvania," the article bragged that "they thus establish an immense and rapid circulation until now without example in any country in the world."

As far as health was concerned, the writer noted that it was "unfortunate that our city should be the focus of the yellow fever. We remember the ravages which it spread among us in 1817. The Mississippi is the Nile of America; the town is built below the level of the river on a slimy soil, which suffers the water to escape only to the depth of a few feet; it is surrounded by cyprus trees and marshes. The river, on its retiring during the summer, leaves an extended slimy plain covered with the refuse of animals and vegetable matter, which owing to the heat of the sun is promptly decomposed; hence the cause of our yellow fever, which attacks new comers in particular." This scourge, however, did not "prevent our population from increasing more rapidly than in any other part of Louisiana. It consisted of 130,000 inhabitants in 1810; it is now 277,235.... Natchez, which was only a miserable assemblage of cabins on the banks of the Mississippi, near an old fort, is now a beautiful town, peopled by 4,000 souls, where there are tribunals, a sheriff, several public establishments, a press, and a journal."

News of a yellow fever outbreak in July 1822 reached Ohio by the steamboat *Robert Fulton*. Confirming previous accounts, eyewitnesses reported no less than twelve deaths occurring daily. The disease had become so alarming, they stated, the mayor recommended inhabitants leave the city. By September 5 eleven new cases and several deaths were reported daily, prompting the board of health to fit up a county hospital for the reception of victims, particularly those not residing in the city. During the month, 550 persons eventually perished, 250 in one three-day period. A letter written November 2, 1822 depicted the state of affairs:

> Since I wrote you last, the fever and black vomit have, if possible, raged with augmented violence, and have been more deadly in their effects, baffling the skill of the most eminent physicians. Whole families have been swept away in the course of a few days, and in several cases absolute visible mortification has taken place before life has been extinct. Such is the dreadful putrifying state of the air at this place. Still, notwithstanding this, you see no alarm, no apprehensions for the consequences. As soon as the breath is out of the body of a person, he or she is placed in a ready-made coffin, hurried off to the grave, and when covered, you hear nothing more. Death, in fact, has completely lost its terrors, and business is totally at a stand.[11]

News for the remainder of the decade was similar. On August 20, 1823, all was "bustle and confusion" at Natchez, with 75 cases of yellow fever reported that day. Accounts warned that some "who were well at breakfast, are in their coffins by nine o'clock at night." The frightened inhabitants were removed and "expected to out *en mass* to day." The following year, the New Orleans Board of Health reported that on August 27 no less than 34 yellow fever cases were reported, "most of which are now in the grave"; between August 28 and 29, nineteen more fatalities were recorded. Newspapers indicated that there was scarcely a native or an old inhabitant among the dead: "they are all strangers, who have unwisely braved the climate, which experience has proved to be almost inevitably fatal, in the hot and autumnal months, to those who are not habituated to it."

A report from 1824 stated that yellow fever was raging with increased malignancy at New Orleans and that from August 10 to August 21 there were 65 deaths. Following the pattern, in 1825 yellow fever turned Natchez into a gloomy affair, with no fewer than 8–10 dying daily. The place, it was said, was literally deserted "and the most of those who have had the rashness to stay, pay the forfeit of their lives for their temerity."

In 1827 the fever broke out at Opelousas and proved very fatal—"the great bulk of its worthy citizens having fallen victims"—and in 1829 one letter writer observed that yellow fever was "raging here with great violence. Yesterday [August 2], it is said, thirty persons fell victims to it."[12]

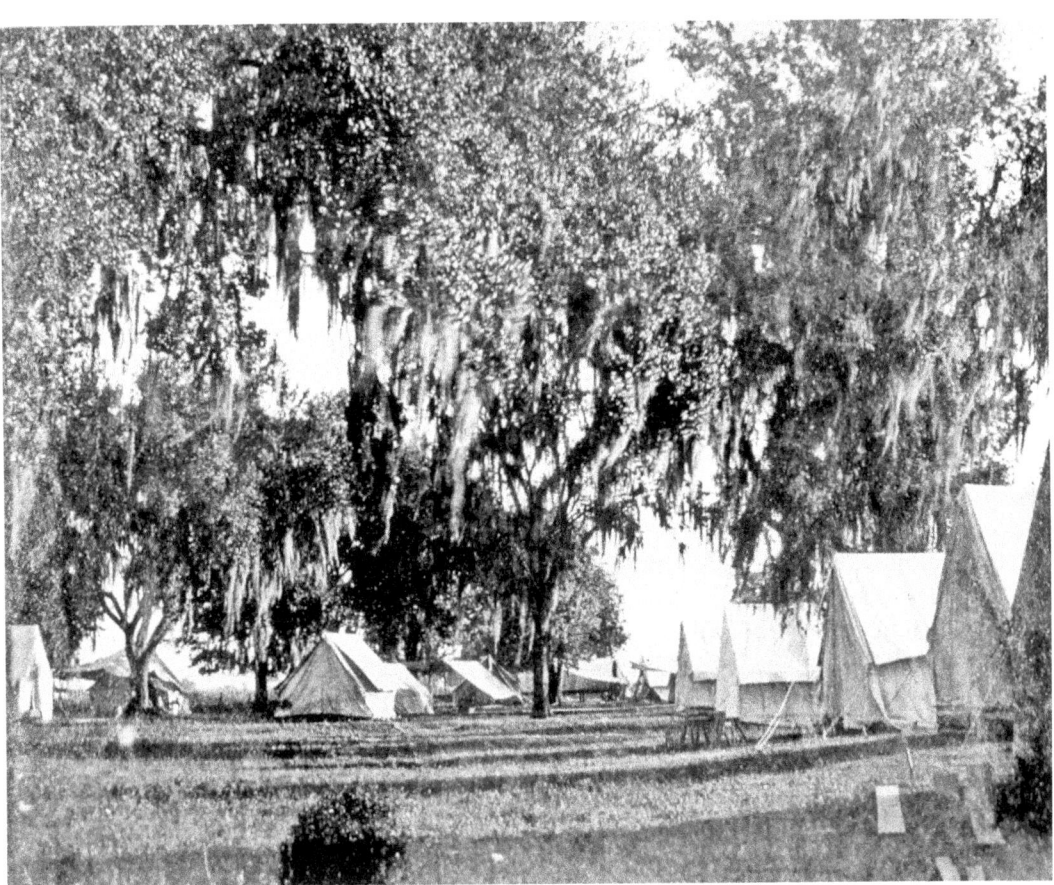

This detention camp, serving as a quarantine site during the yellow fever epidemic of 1888 at Franklin, Louisiana, was maintained by the United States Marine Hospital (courtesy National Library of Medicine).

Deaths from Yellow Fever in New Orleans, 1820–1829

Year	Mortality
1820	–
1821	–
1822	237
1823	239
1824	108
1825	49
1826	5
1827	109
1828	150
1829	215[13]

Fortunately, through the decade of the 1820s there were no great epidemics such as occurred in 1819, and after several years of low mortality the third New Orleans Board of Health was abolished and quarantine repealed in 1825. The fear of renewed attacks did, however, have an impact on health care in the city. After the scare of 1817 French-speaking physicians formed their first professional organization, *La Societe de la Nouvelle-*

Orleans, and in 1820 the English-speaking physicians created the Physico-Medical Society.[14]

The Bancker and Rector Street Outbreaks and the Infant Prophet

Isolated incidences of yellow fever appeared at Charleston and Poughkeepsie, New York, in 1820. An epidemic was also reported in Philadelphia during the summer and on August 18 the mayor of New York issued a proclamation interdicting all intercourse with Philadelphia by land or water for 30 days, asserting that city was "the seat of pestilential yellow fever." On September 13 the Grand Jury of the New York Court of the General Sessions of the Peace toured Bancker and Lombardy streets, finding a "variety of disease, filth, misery, and depravity, not only distressing to humanity, but disgraceful to our species." The following day the jury declared these areas to be "a nuisance," in consequence of the representations of resident physicians. It was later ascertained that a fever had prevailed at New York since August 21, at the time the mayor issued his interdiction against Philadelphia. This was excused because the New York fever was not considered contagious *"because it had not the yellow suffusion"* associated with yellow fever.

"Politically and commercially," noted a writer at the time, "the decision was of great importance to New York, which, by a different one, might have run the risk of being interdicted by all the other cities of the Union, entertaining apprehensions of yellow fever." The controversy did not end with the outbreaks. On November 9, 1820, Dr. Hosack, holding a system of trust under the Quarantine System, supported the idea of contagion and demanded new and more rigid measures enforced by pestilential police. To strengthen his argument he cited British contemporary authorities Sir Gilbert Blane, Dr. Chisholm, Dr. Wright, Sir James M'Grigor, Dr. Pyne, Sir Joseph Gilpin, Dr. Charles Maclean, Dr. Currie and Dr. P. Russell as agreeing with his views. In reply to Dr. Hosack, the Medical Society of New York issued a report on December 22 on the "causes and character of the Epidemic Fever which prevailed in Bancker-street and its vicinity in the summer and autumn of 1820." They concluded, with "authors, from Hippocrates to the present day," that the disease was "the yellow fever of tropical climates and our own harbors."[15]

In 1821 reports from Amelia Island (off the northeastern coast of Florida) were "extremely calamitous." The entire population was said to have come down with the fever and the island itself was "a perfect hospital." New York City, Long Island, Norfolk and Baltimore residents were also attacked by the fever, while at Baltimore the malignant fever was said to have made "serious ravages," although in neither year were death tolls high.[16]

In 1822, what became known as the "Rector Street Epidemic" (so named from the street on which yellow fever was first discovered that year) struck New York City. By early August new cases were reported almost daily and the disease was said to be spreading in all directions. On August 6 the board of health issued a statement with respect to the fever in Rector Street. Harking back to the days of Benjamin Rush and the supposed threat of contaminated coffee, the board attributed the illness to "a quantity of old boxes of Havanna segars, that had been landed in that vicinity, during the warm weather in July, from the Spanish Soldier and Eliza Jane."

By Monday, August 26, the post office, customs house, seven banks, ten insurance companies, three printing offices (the *Gazette*, the *Evening Post* and the *Mercantile Advertiser*) and 146 commercial firms had removed from areas of contagion. In reference to the panic in New York, the *Evening Post* of that date observed, "It is useless to attempt to disguise it from ourselves, that, owing to a fatal confidence in a single individual, (who it too certainly now appears erred in judgment) those early and efficient measures which alone can extinguish yellow fever in its early stages, were neglected by those in whom we were led to place our reliance, and *that the disease has, at last, gained such a head, as to threaten to become a sweeping epidemic.*"

The board of health met daily, including Sundays, during the epidemic. At one meeting considerable doubt was expressed that physicians "scrupulously fulfilled their duty in reporting all the cases of fever that came under their cognizance," prompted by "the anxiety of many families to prevent their situation being publically known." By September 5 the number of dead was calculated at 70, with a few cases occurring daily. Although this was hardly a devastating number, authorities in Philadelphia evoked the "Non-Intercourse Act," ordering that no persons, goods, wares, merchandise or clothing from New York be allowed to enter the city.

By the first week of November the New York Board of Health announced that there had been 401 cases of yellow fever in the city, 355 of which occurred in the lower district and 46 in the upper. Of these, 230 persons died. The board also acknowledged that in "several cases" physicians did not report finding yellow fever. A proclamation was issued, inviting those who had fled to return and open their houses for a day or two for cleaning; those from the infected districts were urged not to return until the weather turned cold, at which time they were to clean and fumigate their dwellings. As proof of the desolation during the growing season, "green beans grew in Liberty street and muskmelons grew upon the pavements of Greenish street."

Isolated cases of yellow fever were also reported in the upper counties of Virginia and along the James River. By October 24, however, the presence of frost "was expected to produce beneficial consequences." In Petersburg, bilious cases had been numerous and violent but not generally fatal. At Savannah, the number of deaths from yellow fever was placed at 175.[17]

Perhaps the most significant event to happen in New York during 1823 was the birth of an infant prophet.

The story, as related by the *Commercial Advertiser* (June 16, 1823), concerned a newborn baby inBrooklyn who, immediately after arriving into the world, proclaimed "*that the whole of New-York was to be desolated with the yellow fever the present season, beyond any former affliction of the kind that had ever befallen it, & that those who should escape the ravages of the pestilence* WOULD NOT BE SUFFICIENTLY NUMEROUS TO BURY THE DEAD." The words were uttered in "deep and solemn tones, & we learn, in verse, rivalling, probably, the loftiest efforts of the muse of David, Solomon, or Milton":

> Let us talk of the Ghost without head,
> That kiss'd Mother Mump in the cellar—
> That frightened the barber's boy dead,
> And let us all be unhappy together.

Having uttered this portentous warning, the messenger "immediately closed its eyes, and its spirit departed to the regions whence it came." The house where the baby prophet was born was "for several days as completely thronged as was ever the tomb of Thomas Becket." Ironically, during 1823 and for rest of the decade, New York was remarkably free from yellow fever.[18]

Putrid Potatoes and Cabbages

Proving that little advancement had been made in expanding established ideas, news out of Philadelphia in 1820 revealed that the origin of yellow fever in the vicinity of Race and Front streets was traced to a cellar filled with water and potatoes in a putrid state. That correlated with 1819 when the bilious fever in the neighborhood of New Market, Frederick County, was traced to a quantity of cabbages in a state of putrefaction; the person employed in removing this rotting mass from the cellar "did not live four days after he executed the office."

Sporadic outbreaks occurred at Baltimore and Norfolk in 1821 but news proved more deadly in 1823. A terrible epidemic of bilious fever struck Pensacola in August, killing 150 in twenty days. "Never," reports stated, "perhaps, was a fever more universally fatal, utterly defying the aid of medicine; no instance of a recovery after an attack, has occurred." The report continued: "Such was the alarm, that many of them [the dead] were conducted to the tomb without a single attendant but the man who conveyed them in his cart; and sunk, on the bed of pain and despair without a single friend to shed a tear, or soothe their last moments with offices of sympathy and kindness." Those who could fled the area, including the legislative council, but "in a country so thinly settled, it was not easy for fugitives to obtain shelter, the neighboring houses are consequently much crowded, and many of the poor are compelled to be exposed to the wide expanse of the heavens."

At Baltimore it was said there "never had been more sickness in that state."

Death Tolls Per Week at Baltimore from Bilious Fever, 1822

Month	Day	Mortality
September	17	35
September	24	36
September	30	46
October	7	40

It was also reported that yellow fever existed along the Ohio and Muskingum rivers "to an alarming degree," and more than 300 cases had occurred in the neighborhood of Marietta.[19]

Yellow fever struck again in 1824. From the 10th to the 21st at New Orleans 65 deaths occurred, primarily from this cause, while for the week ending August 5, sixteen deaths at Charleston resulted from the same cause. On September 6 the board of health reported six new cases one from the schooner *Fame*, sent to the hospital; one in Tradd Street; one in Broad Street; and one in Whim Court. The following day, Elliott, Tradd and Broad streets reported one new case each, while two cases from Gillon Street were sent to the poorhouse. Deaths in Charleston for the previous week were 40, sixteen from yellow fever. The disease had run its course by November 15, when only one death was reported. The total for the season amounted to 240.[20]

Ships returning from Vera Cruz, Mexico, in July 1826 delivered news that yellow fever was raging with great violence and "that the deaths had for some time averaged 100 a day. Those who were attacked generally survived only 12 or 14 hours." Three years later yellow fever again appeared at Charleston. On August 7, 1829, sixty-two persons were interred, and there were no fewer than 40 daily between that date and August 14. Not only did the fever attack natives, but many recently arrived Spaniards from Mexico also fell victim in great numbers. Deaths were said to occur within 60 hours of the first attack. By mid–November, the disease, then referred to as "the broken bone fever," had become less malignant, yielding to medical treatment. Other cities in the south were also affected: as late as October 23 Mobile still labored under its malignancy and strangers were warned to keep away. Interments for the week ending the 20th were 35. Accounts from St. Augustine to October 17 indicated there were still 185 persons down with the yellow fever, but at New Orleans, by October 22 the heath of the city was said to be restored and strangers might visit in safety.[21]

Contagious or Noncontagious? The Argument Continues, 1820–1829

In the October 30, 1821, edition of the British newspaper *Courier* William Fergusson noted, "Medical treatises are not often read by the community at large; and it is only through the public press, of the universally read Journals, that we can expect the information, which is interesting to all, to be universally diffused." In arguing against the contagiousness of yellow fever, he pointed out, "It is notorious, that during former epidemics of yellow fever in Spain, that no infection was conveyed to the people in the immediate neighborhood outside the walls of the pestilential town; and if it could not be carried so far as the ring of the fence (if I may use the expression) that enclosed the infected, how can it possibly be conveyed beyond the sea in ships?" He added his belief the fever had "never yet" been carried beyond a cordon, "and that its breaking out in other places can only therefore be considered as a simultaneous event, or an event close in the order of sequence, resulting from the same, or similar, causes of temperature, season, climate, and situation." He suggested that all those who could afford to leave the area do so, and those who could not, be removed to an encampment on well-ventilated ground, where they would be permitted to return to the town during the day but return at night, "the malarious poison which generates the fever, being presumed on good grounds to exert its baneful operations, principally upon those who pass the night and sleep within the theatre of its influence."

Two days later Fergusson wrote another letter to the *Courier* (November 1, 1821), clarifying medical definitions. He stated the term "contagious" was synonymous with "infectious" and that by "yellow fever" he meant "the malignant remittent fever, frequently styled the boulam, attended with black vomit and hoemorrages on its fatal termination, which, on account of the livid discolorations often seen on the skin ... has very improperly obtained the general denomination of yellow fever," while the milder remittent bilious fever, "accompanied with more or less of jaundice, which is by no means so fatal a form of the same disease, would more properly bear the name of yellow fever." He considered neither one contagious, "under any of their forms or stages, from one person to another."

In December 1823 the opposite point was argued by Gilbert Blane, who had spent 44 years in the medical service of the navy and army, or in contemplating yellow fever. In a letter to the British Admiralty, he took great pains to describe an incident concerning the sloop of war *Baun*. Immediately before its departure from Sierra Leone there had been an unprecedented loss of life among the white inhabitants of the settlement. Complicating matters, some of the men were sent over to the *Caroline* (where yellow fever had destroyed all 20 hands but the master and two others) to bring her to an anchor. When the *Baum* departed in late March the crew was in perfect health but within a few days, until her arrival at Ascension on April 15, thirteen men died of yellow fever. Although there was no disease on the island when they arrived, 20 more crew members perished between that time and June 2, or nearly one-third of the complement of 107, not counting the 29 African supernumeraries who were unaffected.

There had been no instances of yellow fever at the garrison on Ascension between September 1821 and May 1823 until shortly after the *Baun* arrived, when it was transmitted ashore, killing 16 men, 5 women and 4 children, or three-quarters of the population living there. The disease was described as having the true characteristics of the fever of the West Indies, North America and Spain, with "the skin tinged with yellow, assuming a deeper and deeper hue," and "before death, the vomiting of a dark-coloured fluid like coffee-grounds."

Greatly disturbed that most naval and army doctors persisted in the belief in the noncontagion of yellow fever, Blane begged the Admiralty to "enlighten and guide" these officers on the facts of Ascension, to prevent future disasters.[22] Although Sir Gilbert Blane was considered an authority and his arguments on the contagion of yellow fever coincided with the 1821 French Commission's report on the disease at Barcelona, disagreement was loud and persistent. In 1825, exception was taken to Dr. Pariset's view of contagion by offering eyewitness accounts and citing numerous instances where free communication with the sick in private homes and lazarettos failed to result in any transmission of yellow fever. The same year, M. Dupuytren argued before the Paris Academy of Sciences, demanding more scientific evidence. He wished to determine how "the influence which heat, humidity, and the greater or less elevation above the sea" affected the rise and progress of yellow fever, as well as the influence exerted by crowded housing: "For instance, to see if the emanations from the bodies of negroes are more hurtful than those from whites. Would not the exact proportion of men assembled in the same place be another condition of the problem?"

Answering the second part of his own question, he stated that at one hospital ward constructed to hold 200 patients there was little spread of contagion but when that same ward was overcrowded in 1815 to contain 300, "the air suffered an alteration, the nature of which could not be ascertained by a chymical analysis, but which was known by a nauseous odour, and by the appearance of rottenness in the hospital, and by fevers of a violent character." The Academy concluded that too much haste could not be made to determine the nature, mode of transport and cure of yellow fever.

Two years later the topic was presented to the French Royal Academy of Medicine in order to discuss documents collected by Dr. Chervin, "with the design of deciding the great problem as to the contagion or non-contagion of the yellow fever." Dr. Sedillot read a memoir of considerable length, concluding the issue was not definitively established, and moved that further discussion on Chervin's documents be indefinitely postponed. The proposition was rejected. Dr. Collineau then spoke in favor of the contagion theory

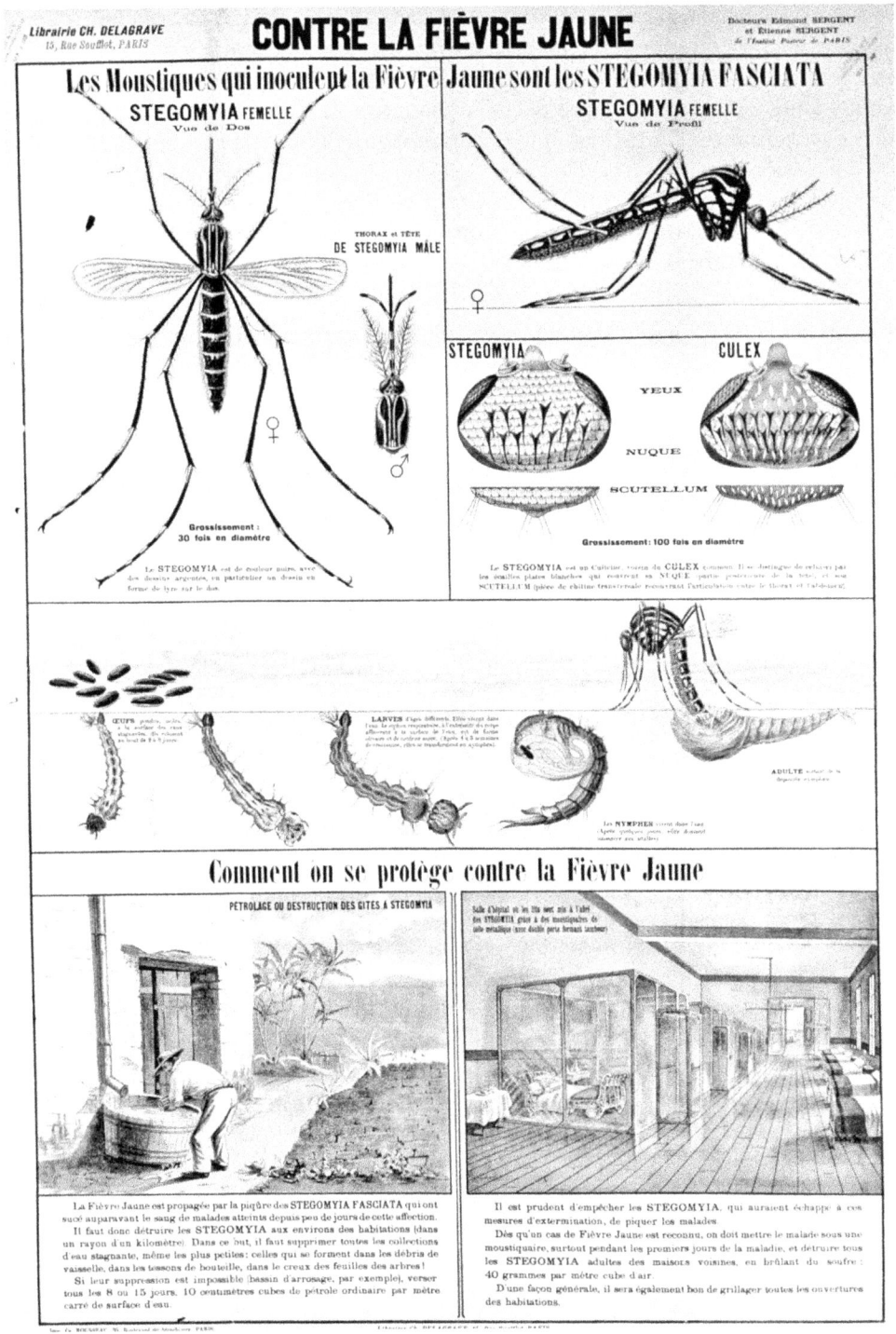

One way to inform the public how to combat yellow fever was by displaying posters on city streets and passing them out to individuals. This illustration from Paris, circa 1907, depicts the life stages of the mosquito and offers suggestions on how to contain their spread (courtesy National Library of Medicine).

by offering data taken from the epidemics at Cadiz. His arguments proved unconvincing as the academy considered the disease "as *infection* and not contagion."

The matter was no clearer in England. In a discussion on the "Report on the Quarantine Laws" (1826), John Smith declared they were "a mass of absurdities and contradictions," noting that in 1824 two physicians of great eminence had completely disagreed on the nature of yellow fever. The matter was settled on political and economic grounds when Mr. Huskisson remarked that "it would be highly injurious to our commerce, if a notice should get abroad that we were disposed to pay no attention to the regulations which other countries thought fit to observe on this subject."

Dr. Daniel Osgood of Havana spoke in plainer terms when writing on the subject in 1826. When asked whether yellow fever was contagions, he began by stating, "A disease is acknowledged to be contagious if it produces, in the person sick with it, a poison, which, being communicated to well persons, generates in them the same disease." That point made, he discussed the contagionist argument purported by Dr. Blane concerning the outbreak of yellow fever in a squadron in the West India station. Blane believed that the shipboard disease appearing on the *Warrior* and *Royal Oak* was introduced by new recruits who had been brought from England aboard the *Anson* and were then sent to the *Namur* before being permanently assigned to the *Warrior* and *Royal Oak*. Osgood wrote, "It is remarkable that the ships that brought them from England were not affected by them," thus proving the noncontagious theory. He also dispelled the argument that yellow fever was imported into Cadiz from Havana (particularly in 1800) by remarking that there was seldom a year when yellow fever did not rage in Havana and yet it was only in some years and not others that the disease appeared on the southern coast of Spain.

His theory of cause was less persuasive. Like most of his generation, he felt yellow fever was brought on by "exhalations, produced by a high degree of the heat of the sun, and the atmosphere, from water, when somewhat stagnant," adding that pure yellow fever "exclusively prevailed in the vicinity of some extensive body of water, when the heat of the weather has been great, and where vegetable substances are not abounding." Furthermore, he believed the malady had not been seen on the seacoast of the North of Europe because the winds conveyed the exhalations from the shore away from land. As far as preventing the disease, he advocated fumigation of ships and fires on shore where the air was suspected to be infected. When the atmosphere had become extensively infected, however, the situation could only be changed "by an alteration of the weather."[23]

Another writer in 1829 suggested that the cause of the fever consisted "exclusively in the alteration between heat and moisture—in the transition from a hot mid-day to a cool, damp night, followed by a foggy morning." He suggested persons avoid being overheated and to shut doors and windows at night so that closed rooms would retain the dry air of the day. The suggestion, of course, would have seemed to effectuate positive results, not for the reason of maintaining dry air but from the fact sealed egresses would prevent mosquitoes from entering the dwelling.[24]

Even closer to the truth was a letter signed only "H," published three years earlier in the same newspaper as the above (*Washington* [DC] *Daily National Intelligencer*) on November 24, 1826. After discussing the idea that doctors acknowledged yellow fever originated in dark, moist places, polluting the air, he expanded on that theory by asking, "May not certain small insects be produced by rotten vegetables, on board a ship or in a cellar?" Noting that locust and "Chintz bugs (or black insects not larger than a pin's head)" overspread the land, he continued: "Why, then, may not the atmosphere be filled with these deleterious insects [and thus communicate the disease]?" By way of experiment he suggested letting "condemned criminals have the option of execution or of a trial of the disorder to be endeavored to be created. There would be no cruelty in this."

Pursuing that idea, "H" stated that yellow fever generally appeared only on seacoasts where the holds of ships were opened "and there the exhalations from marshes, wharves, &c. may be favorable to the existence of the animalculae. They do not, I believe, fly high, and therefore persons in garrets and elevated situations escape." Convinced that "the cause of the black vomit may be generated in any confined place with insect producing vegetation," he concluded that insects living in the holds of ships were transported to foreign ports. "Sick men shipped to Havana will not give the disorder at Cadiz but a bad cargo will." He concluded by asking for Congress to form a committee to investigate yellow fever so that "much confusion would be prevented."

Prophylactic and Curative Views Upon Yellow Fever

While not exactly a prophylactic or a cure, the following story is just too good to ignore. Under the title "New Orleans Thirty Years Ago: Adventures of a British Officer," the well-traveled tale was first published in the *Boston Transcript* and then in the *Concordia Intelligencer* before making its way to the *Grant County* (WI) *Herald* September 26, 1850. Purported to be true and written in the first person by a member of the Peerage from the "house of "H____t," it recounted the story of a major, late of the British Army, who then resided at Beal's Hotel around September 1820.

Having dined with a young Scotsman named Cameron for several days, the officer was surprised to see his friend absent from dinner. Upon the officer's inquiring his whereabouts, the proprietor took the major into a back parlor where he beheld the corpse of his friend, already resting in a magnificent coffin. The proprietor, Mr. Beal, explained the man had been struck down by yellow fever then raging in the city. He added that as the fever killed in a matter of hours and mortification immediately ensued, it was the policy of his house to have coffins made for all lodgers in case they should fall victim. Apparently unaware of the soldier's distaste for the idea, Beal showed him a coffin that had been designed for him bearing the major's own family crest. Determined to leave the city where coffins were made before men died and graves were dug beforehand, the major demanded his bill. Seeing that it included $150 for the coffin, he indignantly refused to pay.

The landlord seemed perfectly agreeable, observing "the coffin was made in pursuance of a rule of my house. Had you remained a week, you would most probably have needed it, and as we bury strangers before they are quite dead, your aristocratic body would have been sent to the trench in a pine box." Do not pay for it, he added, but the first pauper who dies will be buried in this coffin bearing your coat of arms. Finding that too much for his ancestral pride, the major "threw down the sovereigns, made a bonfire of the coffin, and the same evening hired a barge to carry me from a city where such dreadful customs prevailed."

In 1826 the Chevalier Feureau de Beauregard presented to the Royal Academy of Sciences in France an extract from a memoir dated December 31, 1823, and entitled

Physical and Medical Topography of Florence and a Part of Tuscany. Similar to what others were presenting to newspapers and learned societies across the world, but of a wider scope, Beauregard discussed the history of yellow fever epidemics, concluding that "beyond a certain distance from the sea it loses its contagious faculty." Citing the epidemic at Leghorn in 1804, he reminded his listeners that those who fled to Florence, Sienna and Pisa were spared. According to research confirmed by Dr. Louis Valentin, of Nancy, the author determined that a distance four or five leagues from the sea was adequate to provide protection. Expanding his theory, he added that "the banks of the river where the waters of the sea make its presence felt, are to be considered sea-shore, so far as regards the contagious quality or propagation of the Yellow Fever." The idea of a limited field of sickness was put into operation as far back as 1793 when New Jersey extended quarantine only 15 miles above Trenton, where the tide ceased to be visible in the river.

Asking whether the authorities could rely on persons interested in their own and their families' preservation to remove to a safe distance on their own accord, he answered his own question with the blunt, "Of course not." In order to ensure compliance, he argued for a coordinated system of transportation to carry those infected away from the source of the disease. Describing what could be considered today as the design for a modern hospital he advocated private rooms, the proper placement of windows, and a system of ventilation and suggested how outside gardens might be constructed as well. He took great pains to plead for the removal of the French hospital constructed on the island of Ratoneau. Acknowledging it as a "perfect model" for yellow fever victims he worried that it was "build in the midst of the sea atmosphere."

Observing that the question of nomenclature often obscured medical discussions he explained that Dr. Valentin used the expression "focus of infection" as a substitute for "contagion" and that he used "collective atmosphere" to indicate a class of diseases including yellow fever and typhus that were caused by "the accumulation of patients in places deprived of sufficient ventilation," meaning those areas in close proximity to the sea.

In October 1817, while practicing at Florence, he began using "the ratanhia (called *ratacina* in Peru—*Krameria triandra*)." The plant extract was commonly employed against hemorrhage. Beauregard found it effective in yellow fever, which he considered a hemorrhagic disease, especially in its later stages. Mixing an extract of ratanhia with two ounces of common vinegar, he administered it in three doses two hours apart, "which always succeeded." His project "was favored by the discovery of a peculiar acid in the ratanhia, which received the name of *Krameric acid*." Interestingly, and with modern parallels, he was dissuaded from promoting this acid "because of its dearness, in the treatment of yellow fever." It was not until six years later that he decided he could no longer withhold this cure from the public.[25]

A review of this book published in the *Washington* (DC) *Daily National Intelligencer* (December 2, 1826) offered the reviewer's own private warning:

> The facts in relation to the non-contagion of yellow fever seem to have been collected with great care, and communicated in a spirit of modesty, respect, and truth. This branch of the subject alone is of the utmost importance to the medical faculty of the United States: for her medical history, in relation to it, will be remembered with sorrow, if not reproach, for ages to come, by all, whether physicians or not, who are friendly to the advancement of science. And, however mortifying, still truth impels the remark, that, although the conflict commenced some thirty years since, time has had little other effect than to lessen the high degree of asperity which originally existed.

In relation to temperature affecting the cause and spread of yellow fever, an idea purported in 1821 held a fascinating allure, if not for a cure, for the well-being of the general population: air conditioning. Based on the fact the first cold weather put an end to epidemics, a Mr. Vallance proposed to change the atmosphere in a confined space, thus rendering it (and presumably everyone inside) free from infection. If this were possible, one reviewer noted, "it may be set down as one of the most useful discoveries of modern times."[26]

Using the technique of Professor John Leslie to make ice "under any climate, at any time of year" (developed in 1810, producing ice by evaporation in an air pump),[27] Vallance proposed that "by condensing air, caloric is squeezed out of it: as may be conceived by supposing a wet sponge squeezed in the hand. On liberating the air from the condensation, it will imbibe a quantity of a caloric, equal to what has been pressed out; as may be conceived by supposing the hand which has squeezed the sponge dry immersed in water, and the sponge then liberated. Combine, therefore, these two principles; squeeze as much heat as we can out of air; cool it in this condensed state to below the freezing point by means of the ice Leslie's method enables our producing; and then admit it, either by itself, or mixed with the hot air of the atmosphere (according to the temperature required), into the place to be cooled: and by doing this in proper proportion, it is *indubitable* that any building may be rendered of such temperature as we please, *under any climate!*"

This idea would resurface again in 1832 when Jesse Remington, of Baltimore, patented a device "for the purifying of the foul atmosphere of the holds of vessels, between decks, cabins, state-rooms, &c. The atmosphere generated by the apparatus can be made many degrees colder or warmer than the temperature of the ordinary atmosphere." Benefits included "disarming" the dreadful malady of yellow fever on board ships by the decomposition of pestilential miasma.[28]

If yellow fever did not actually give rise to the widespread use of air conditioning, it did have a significant effect on the importation of "Rhenish wine" into England. After English physicians affirmed that Rhenish wine was a "preventative, or cure, in cases of yellow fever, and other malignant fevers in the tropical countries," the trade in this article soared from 998 Ohms in 1824 to 1,750 in 1825.[29]

On a slightly more far-reaching scale, in 1827 M. Labarraque, a chemist in Paris, discovered a material "to disinfect places and objects of the offensive and deadly vapors inherent in putrefactive masses; and also in confined and infected situations." His formula consisted of a combination of chloride of soda and chloride of lime. The latter was well known for its usefulness in the purification of lazarettos, infected ships, hospitals, manufactories, sewers and on the persons of soldiers and sailors, but the chemist believed that by adding soda, the remedy would aid in healing wounds, arrest mortification, modify cancerous and other disagreeable tropical complaints, including yellow fever, and divesting "the dissecting room of its noxious qualities, preventing those severe cases of typhus fever which are found among the students of anatomy who thus fall a sacrifice to their love of science by constantly inspiring an atmosphere loaded with pernicious exhalation." Further testing of Labarraque's formula proved it to be a true fumigation by chlorine, only less violent.[30]

Further testimony on the efficacious nature of chloride of lime and soda came in 1829 when the French government sent a deputation of physicians (including Dr. Pariset) to Egypt and Asia Minor to investigate the character of the plague. By numerous experiments there they determined the chlorides acted "not only as preservatives from that dreadful disease, but even as capable of removing the causes which generate it." The text, taken from the *Journal of the Philadelphia of Pharmacy*, went on to state that Dr. Pariset "has not the least doubt that not only pestilential disorders, but also *varioloid*, measles, typhus, and even yellow fever, may be arrested by means of the chlorides."[31]

Chapter 14

"All the evils which hell may contain"

The Board of Health.—A countryman walking along the streets of New York, found his progress stopped by a close barricade of wood. "What is this for," said he to a person in the street.—"Oh, that's to stop the yellow fever."—"Ay, I have often heard of the Board of Health, but I never saw it before."[1]

Throughout the decade of the 1830s yellow fever was a companion of many southern cities, especially those along the major inland waterways. During the summer of 1832 Cincinnati and Frankfort, Kentucky, were especially hard hit, but as usual New Orleans seemed to be the favorite belle of malignant diseases. This dire reality prompted the *Société Medicale de Nouvelle-Orleans* to promote another board of health (the fourth) and to support sanitary and quarantine regulations, with an emphasis on the epidemiology's mortality list.[2]

Yellow fever prevailed "very generally" in New Orleans during the summer of 1830, but it was not considered as malignant as formerly, considering there were fewer deaths in August. But for the week ending September 18 the number of deaths reached 121, while the number of sick in hospitals up to that date was 239, with no abatement of malignancy. A letter written September 12 warned those planning on visiting the city that seven cases of yellow fever had been diagnosed, four of them terminating fatally. The very warm weather of the previous ten days was said to have produced it, and with showers occurring daily, followed by a scorching hot sun, physicians feared the disease might become epidemic. The rains persisted throughout the month and by September 29 "a great number of individuals who were not acclimated" had perished; reports of interments in the two cemeteries (Protestant 71 and Catholic 121) indicated that 192 persons had been buried in the final week, having died from a combination of yellow fever and cholera. The *Mercantile Advertiser* of October 1 stated that the "city was more sickly than it has been, at this period, for the last three years." This opinion was seconded by the *Argus*, which also noted "some Creoles and acclimated persons have been attacked." By October 20, the *Advertiser* downgraded its opinion: "There has not been as much sickness as then existed, since the year 1822."

Calls for the city council "to take into consideration the suggestion of the board of health, and "adopt such measures as will enable the public to obtain the information" of death tolls and causes (yellow fever and cholera) such as had been attended to by every other city in the union would satisfy "the curiosity of the public, which is always eager for such intelligence during the prevalence of epidemics."[3] Beginning October 29, one letter writer warned, "We are sorry to state, that the number of deaths have increased to an extent unheard of in the history of our country." He continued:

> There were 133 interments yesterday; or rather so many were taken to the burying grounds. We doubt whether all were interred, as the night before there were 13 bodies left over in the Protestant ground, part of them without coffins. The panic is now so great that it is almost impossible to get coffins made, graves dug, or the dead buried in any way. Five dollars per day is not a sufficient inducement.... Thus far the ravages have been confined principally to the laboring, indigent and intemperate class, together with many negroes. Nevertheless, a good many temperate, regular, acclimated citizens, both male and female, and even little children, have been carried off in a few hours. There appear to be none safe.

In the Catholic burying ground the above writer noted there were 125 exposed coffins; some were piled together in stacks of ten or twelve; others had been split open and their contents exposed. Continuing to paint the horrific picture, he added that church authorities did not pretend to dig separate graves but had large ditches dug, 50–60 feet long and 8–10 feet in depth, into which coffins were placed three tiers deep, which brought them nearly to the surface. The price of grave digging was put at $6 a day and that of nurses $10 a day. Speculation ran high that the city council would recommend the bodies be burned, as it was "impossible to bury them, and the stench is already so great at the grave-yards, that it is almost impossible for persons to remain there."

People resorted to burning tar outside their doors, keeping bonfires going in the streets and firing off guns and cannon until late at night. On November 8 the *Bee* reported "ten thousand pounds of powder were shot off on Saturday" alone. Untended or over-large fires often got out of hand; one conflagration spread below the market, while the sound of fire bells continued to peal their ominous warning that other parts of the city were also threatened. The death toll for November 1 was placed at 177 and as many more were expected the following day. A letter dated November 4 warned, "The deaths for the last ten days, by Cholera and the Yellow Fever, have been about 300 a day." Mortality estimates for the first week of November eventually reached 1,070.

A private correspondence dated November 12 put the final death toll from cholera and yellow fever at 4,000. The writer added, "When you take into consideration our present population, not much over 40,000, you discover that the mortality has been much greater here than in any part of the United States." The *New Orleans Courier* summed up the horror of death and uncertainty of diagnosis in one grim paragraph "The dreaded epidemic which fills our unfortunate City with mourning and desolation, and which by some is designated as the *Cholera,* by others the cold plague, and which many call a *compound of all the evils which hell may contain,* finds no obstacle to check its destructive course. The rich and the poor, the temperate and the intemperate, equally fall victims to its baneful influence."

By December 13, another letter, published in a Charleston paper, indicated that the diseases went as suddenly as they came, leaving behind carnage beyond precedent.[4]

Matters were not destined to get significantly better. The *New Orleans Courier* of August 3, 1833, indicated that the health of the city was very bad from yellow fever of a "more malignant type that [has been seen] for a number of years." Some hope appeared on August 31 when one newspaper noted that although yellow fever was extending its operation and cases were on the increase "the complaint, from becoming better understood, was more easily subdued by medical treatment." That hope appears to have been premature, for on September 7 the directors of the Charity Hospital published the following: "*Resolved,* That during the prevalence of the present epidemic, the doors of the Hospital *be thrown open to all persons requiring its aid,* and that although unprepared to accommodate the numerous applicants that have and may present themselves, every exertion shall be made to succor them as far as possible. All destitute persons may accordingly present themselves directly at the Hospital, without applying for a ticket of admission."

The threat of yellow fever was so great that by the second week of September it was said that 20,000 persons had absented themselves; by the 12th, death tolls had reached 12 per day. On September 20 there were 29 deaths; on the 21st, 81 deaths and on the 22nd, 89 deaths. Estimates of total mortality for 1832 and 1833 were placed as high as 10,000, or one-fifth of the permanent population.[5] The year 1835 proved to be less harrowing. Reports in the *New Orleans Union* from October 5 indicated that yellow fever had been present for the past few weeks but not in sufficient numbers "to amount to an epidemic." The cases that did occur were of a milder form than had been witnessed for years, but strangers were still advised to stay away for two or three more weeks. The same held true for 1836.[6]

As incredible as it seems today, a comment from 1837 noted that the number of deaths from yellow fever in September "is not much less than fifty per day; when we take into consideration the addition to our population since 1833, which was the last period we think that the yellow fever was epidemical, the number of deaths is small.... Our present population is not much less than seventy thousand persons, therefore if this disease continues at the same rate of mortality for the next thirty days, the deaths would be but about two of every hundred of the whole population.... The time was, when the deaths in our city amounted to two hundred and fifty to three hundred per day out of a population of about forty thousand."

The fever was exacerbated by a week of heavy rain during the end of September, rekindling the disease that had begun to diminish, leaving one account to state, "The truth is, that the epidemic is as bad as ever; it only lacks subjects. Let, then, strangers keep away from the city till frost." Unfortunately, the advice came too late to save passengers aboard the *Nestor,* which left New York on August 23. While at New Orleans, 162 out of 212 passengers had died by October 4, chiefly of yellow fever, and on the 19th, "ONLY TEN *out of the whole number* survived."

Natchez citizens also fell victim to the resurgent disease. On September 20, reports indicated that it raged with fatal violence. For the week ending November 4 yellow fever continued to prevail, with 28 deaths (black and white); the previous week the total had been 23.[7]

The year 1838 proved to be a healthy one for the Crescent City. Summing up the state of affairs on October 5, the *Bulletin* informed its readers that as it was well known the disease first made its appearance at the Charity Hospital and up to that point there had been but few cases, "New Orleans is now as healthy as any city of its size in the United States." This was a fortunate coincidence for one London manufacturer, who the same year published an ad that began this way: "Yellow Fever in New Orleans.—Intelligence has reached the British College of Health, that the above malignant malady is entirely cured and prevented by copious doses of the Vegetable Universal Medicines. Surely this must go a long way to prove the utility of purgatives in Fevers generally!"[8]

"Sauvé qui Peut!"

The above quote, roughly translated as "Save himself who can," headlined an article on yellow fever in New Orleans in 1839.[9] As early as June 17, after a week of unusually warm weather, five cases were reported, creating enough fright that departing steamboats were filled with passengers. Two days later the *Bulletin* denied the presence of the fever; by July 30 the *True American* repeated that confirmation, dispensing news that although a "few sporadic cases" had appeared there was no apprehension of an epidemic. Oppressive heat in August radically altered the picture. On the 9th the *Bee* warned that a considerable number of cases had been admitted to the Charity Hospital and almost every physician with a moderate practice had attended more than one patient afflicted with yellow fever. Bemoaning any official confirmation, on the same date editors of the *Bulletin* informed readers that since August 3 there had been 25 yellow fever deaths at the Charity Hospital, 8 of which occurred on the 8th. This prompted the paper to urge authorities to establish a board of health "in order to get from them the *whole truth*." Noting this idea was supported by the two medical societies, the writer added, "The only astonishment is that there should be a moment's delay. What earthly ground can there be to hesitate?" The fourth medical board was convened and created sanitary and quarantine regulations.

Adding to the general terror, the *Courier* warned that medical remedies used successfully in 1837 had little effect in 1839 and added, "Candidly speaking, we believe the yellow fever is destined to afford now and hereafter, as it has done formerly, cause of wonder as to the inefficiency of medical skill, whenever it seriously attacks people whose blood and habits are foreign to warm climates." Between August 10 and the 17th 143 victims of yellow fever were buried in Potter's Field. In response to the growing epidemic, the Council of the First Municipality appointed two physicians and two druggists in each ward to attend gratuitously on indigent people suffering from yellow fever. In the midst of a sustained period of rain physicians warned that when they ceased and northwest winds prevailed, the change in weather would bring "certain death to the sick," raising apprehensions "that the effects of the pestilence will be still more awful." On August 19 the *Louisianan* urged "cautious strangers and others" to leave the city.

In some cases, this was easier said than done. The ship *Richmond*, bound for the Havre, was forced to put back to New Orleans after Captain Winship died of yellow fever off Tortugas. For those steamboats plying the inland waterways, yellow fever continued to prove a threat. The *Wheeling Times* reported that both the *Marmion* and the *Fusileer* arrived at the mouth of the Ohio with yellow fever aboard, the former 4 cases and the latter 11. The victims were all buried at the mouth of the river. On the subject of nautical matters, a paragraph from the *Washington* (DC) *Globe* on August 29, 1839, touched on another matter affecting not only New Orleans but the country at large: "We are told there is a ship now lying at our Levee, the crew of which (not the captain or mate) are all black men or mulattoes. There is some difference of opinion among the knowing ones, which time will best settle, as to the liability of the black and brown mariners to an attack of yellow fever. At any other season, we believe not a few might be disposed to inquire, whether another danger did not exist—that of a few of our slaves being enticed away by the darkies."

In an eleven-day period (August 18–28) 198 yellow fever victims were buried in Potter's Field, while interments in the Protestant and Catholic cemeteries averaged three per day, making the average deaths per day about 30. According to the *Courier* of August 29, notwithstanding the death toll, more than 600 strangers including boatmen, mariners and passengers had arrived at New Orleans. In attempting to explain how this could happen, the paper speculated "indifference to life, or the love of gain, must be strong indeed, when facts like these stare us in the face."[10]

Matters continued to worsen. On September 8 the *Picayune* observed, "Not a cheering sentence, not a word of hope have we to offer, relative to the epidemic. It is still unsparing in its attacks and deadly in its design—insidious and mortal." On the 5th there were 46 interments and on the 6th there were 37 deaths from the fever. On September 10 the *Bee* reported that during the week ending the 8th, 140 new cases of yellow fever were admitted to the hospital; of these, 60 were cured, 56 died and 29 remained. For the previous week, there were 110 admissions, 84 recoveries, and 34 deaths: "The number of new cases has been greater, the recoveries in less proportion, and the deaths more numerous than since the announcement of the disease.... But hospital practice is no longer a safe and unerring guide to the sanitary conditions of the city. The hospitals are no longer the exclusive receptacles of the indigent sick."

Yellow fever struck Natchez on September 8 and lasted until November 20. During that period the total number of deaths was 234, of which 69 occurred in September, 135 in October and 31 in November. Of these, about 180 were reported as cases of yellow fever and the rest were unspecified. Very few of long residence were affected. Compared to the epidemic of 1837, a total of 244 died during September and October. In estimating the comparative fatality of the two outbreaks, those who could do so fled Natchez in 1839, which was not the case in 1837.

At New Orleans, for the week ending October 6, thirty-nine deaths were attributed to yellow fever. As this was considered an abatement of the disease it signaled a renewal of business, and the number of visitors arriving on steamboats rapidly increased. By the 16th the *Bee* announced the epidemic had subsided almost entirely and interments were down 50 percent. In the previous 8 days only 20 deaths were attributed to the fever and the newspaper waited only for the frost to state the pestilence no longer existed.[11]

As testimony to the fact that historical data is difficult to compile and frequently contradictory, the following table, which does not quite square with newspaper and personal accounts of the decade, was taken from George Augustin's *History of Yellow Fever*.

Deaths from Yellow Fever in New Orleans, 1830–1839

Year	Number of Deaths
1830	117
1831	2
1832	18
1833	210
1834	95
1836	5
1837	412
1838	17
1839	452[12]

"The melancholy task..."

"The melancholy task has at last devolved upon us of announcing to our readers and the public, the arrival of this dreadful disease in our town." The disease was yellow fever and the town was Memphis. According to local reports, the first case of 1832 was brought to Memphis on board the steamboat *Experiment* from Louisville on Sunday, September 14. The patient, Mr. Kendrick, had been returning from Philadelphia homeward to St. Francis County, Arkansas Territory, 40 miles from Memphis. Upon arrival he complained of a slight indisposition and retired. By midnight he was violently attacked and died at 10:00 a.m. On Thursday the steamer *Constitution* passed down from Trinity, having on board a dozen cases; it reported seven deaths during the short trip. On Sunday the 21st, the *Freedom*, also from Trinity, touched at the landing with another seven cases and a reported 8–10 deaths.

Slight outbreaks persisted throughout the first seven years of the decade but it was not until 1838 that death tolls once again became alarming. The Mobile Board of Health reported on September 13 the existence of two cases of yellow fever, but it hoped the malady would not assume a very malignant form. The major concern lay in the introduction of the disease from New Orleans and Charleston, and officers of the port were enjoined to keep strict watch on all vessels arriving from those cities.

Charleston first reported "fever" on August 5, 1838, and the first death occurred the following day at the Marine Hospital, although by this point many deaths from bilious fever had already been reported. News spread rapidly to outside cities—at times, it was avowed—with exaggerated notices. The *Charleston Mercury* began one article with this opening paragraph: "STRANGERS' FEVER: The fever, we are sorry to say, has increased since our last notice of it; but it is not one tenth as bad as represented by presses out of State. Instead of fifty per day, the deaths from fever have not been one hundred per week. It does not attack, indiscriminately, natives and old residents as well as strangers. It is bad enough, however, to keep away the latter until a frost." Historically, however, more deaths were reported in 1838 than in most previous seasons and it was feared that with the unfavorable weather the malady was far from over.

Deaths from Fever in Charleston

In 1817 by September 14	144
In 1819 by September 15	105
In 1824 by September 12	68
In 1838 by September 9	111

Duration of Fever Season in Charleston

In 1817	July 27 to October 12
In 1819	August 8 to October 20
In 1824	August 9 to November 20

Doomsayers were correct. In the two weeks ending September 8, 1838, there were 81 deaths, or about 40 per week. Nor'easters and rain from the previous week did not have the desired effect of creating "a better atmosphere," and the temperature rose to 88°F, 8° higher than the previous week. "Great gloom was spread over the city by the large number of funerals on yesterday's week." While Washington, DC, remained healthy in 1838, reports from Charleston indicated "the epidemic was unquestionably the yellow fever, and it is more severe than had been known for 20 years." Other reports stated that the vessels had drawn out into the harbor to escape the contagion. By the time the epidemic ended on October 31 the death toll was placed at 352, of which 345 persons were white and 7 were black. The greatest mortality during any one week was that ending September 19, when there were 65 yellow fever deaths.[13]

The epidemics of 1839 were more widespread. As early as June 18 the mayor of Charleston released an official communication stating that several cases of yellow fever had occurred among the crews of Eastern ships lying in harbor. A letter dated August 27 from Augusta noted that yellow fever prevailed to an alarming extent: "None have recovered who have been taken, and many die in from three to five days. Some of our oldest residents, even of 20 years' standing, have fallen victims to the fell destroyer. Young and old, strangers or residents—all are subject to the devastating calamity."

In Charleston 14 deaths were registered for the week ending August 18 and 16 more from the week ending the 31st. For the year ending October 31, there were 456 patients admitted into the Marine Hospital, of which 35 died, 397 were discharged cured and 24 remained. Yellow fever patients numbered 93, of which 29 died and 73 were discharged. At the same time, however, the *Charleston Mercury* named the disease "Broken Bone Fever," adding that it was not considered malignant and yielded readily to medical treatment. (Also known as "Dengue fever" and "breakbone fever," it is an infectious tropical disease transmitted by several species of mosquito within the genus *Aedes*. The cause, however, was not known in 1839.)

Under the date of September 1, the Board of Health of Augusta announced five deaths from yellow fever during the two previous days. By September 12 the disease had become a "prevailing epidemic," with a number of deaths occurring daily. Two days later the *Journal of Commerce* reported that all the older physicians were dead or down with the fever and that the sheriff and marshal had also succumbed. Deaths were estimated at 8 to 12 per day, "though there are not 1,500 persons in all who sleep in town."

News from Florida revealed a dichotomous situation. In September the *Pensacola Gazette* stated that for the previous six months there had been only three deaths from yellow fever. Information from St. Augustine on October 17, however, indicated that nearly two hundred cases of yellow fever had broken out in that community. Furthermore, information was given on Commander Mayo of the U.S. steamer *Poinsett*, who went into the Everglades with 50 men. The bilious and congestive fever was "prevailing there," although of a manageable type, with a fatality ratio of 30 or 40 deaths among 500 cases. Among those who died causes were attributed to neglect of early symptoms, relapses brought on by imprudence of diet or in over exertion.

For the first time, major newspaper exchanges carried news of yellow fever in Texas. Early notices from September indicated that the disease had broken out at Houston, where deaths averaged 8–10 daily. By the 16th the disease was also reported at Galveston. The following day the *Houston Intelligencer* noted several cases of black vomit and lamented the loss of some of the oldest and most respectable citizens. Not surprisingly, a great deal of news from Texas reached the outside world via steamboat. The *Columbia* reached New Orleans on November 11 with news dated the 7th. Gleaned from the local newspapers delivered, the *Bee* advised that "mortality, in proportion to the population" of Houston and Galveston, "was very considerable" and added that 26 deaths had occurred at the former town during the 5 days the *Columbia* remained in port.[14]

September brought an even greater calamity to Mobile. One letter dated the 5th began as follows:

> The disease seems to be confined to no particular section of the town, nor to any distinct class of people. Indeed, it is somewhat surprising that the widest, cleanest and most pleasant street in the city (Government street) should have suffered the most....
>
> It is astonishing to see the difference of opinion prevailing among the physicians relative to the

true character of the existing epidemic. One says it is yellow fever; another pronounces that he has not seen a single case of yellow fever, but that the prevailing disease is infinitely worse. I believe, however, that all physicians view it as something greatly more severe and fatal than any of the fevers peculiar to the climate which they have before seen. Do not suppose that I exaggerate when I tell you (for my own impression is I do not come to the reality) that, out of a population of eight or nine thousand, the number supposed to be now in the city, it is estimated by those well informed that *one-half* are confined with the *epidemic*. Instead of forty or fifty dying in a week, there are that many daily. The scenes of distress and mortality now existing in Mobile are unequalled in the history of epidemics in modern times.

On September 7, the *Mobile Register* noted, "We are unable to note any change for the better; on the contrary, sickness and gloom appear on the increase. Most of the stores are closed, the Post Office is not opened in the afternoon; the banks will continue business only two hours in the day [11:00 a.m.–1:00 p.m.], and some of the papers have concluded to publish weekly.... Since Sunday, the interments number 100; yesterday 23 were reported; the day previous 18."

On the same date, the *Chronicle* reported a notice from the magistrates indicating that during the prevalence of the epidemic, duties in all civil cases were being suspended. On September 10 the *Advertiser* advised that since the first nine days of the month 149 persons had "been consigned to the tomb." On the 12th, the *Register* cried, "GOD only knows where the pestilence may end! Our friends are falling around us like the leaves in autumn, and we write each paragraph with but a faint hope of indicting another. The interments for the past two days number about *thirty-two,* comprising many of our most worthy friends and several females."

By September 17, the *Advertiser* had counted 249 deaths since the first of the month, sadly noting that while for the past several days the numbers had been down it was from a want of subjects rather than a true abatement of the disease. Three days later the *Journal* added that "the common enemy—which is unequivocally yellow fever," was being treated by several physicians from other places who, "with a highly creditable spirit and philanthropy, have come among us ... but the number of sick is still greatly too much for all the medical force in town."

Comparative Report of Interments in Mobile

In the months of	1839	1838	1837
August	139	44	64
September	380	52	96
October	120	68	204

The *Register* of October 23 stated that business in Mobile was beginning to revive, but added, "The HEALTH *is not one iota better,* nor has the disease lost a jot of its malignity. Six interments were made yesterday, and four the day previous."[15]

Little news of yellow fever was seen during the decade of the 1830s on the eastern seaboard. From the *Boston Daily Advertiser* in 1835 there was one mention of the disease stemming from "foul atmosphere" on Central, Rowe's and other wharves, attributed to "the presence of hides and other animal substances, which, thought out of sight in cellars or sheds, are poisoning the air." Apparently the New York newspapers played up the story to such a degree that the Boston papers countered by reworking familiar standbys such as "The city is deserted—grass grows in the streets, and very good oats on the side walks" and "If you wish a ride you may always find a hearse at hand ready to carry you" with humorous effect.

In 1839 a notice of yellow fever in New York indicated that one or two persons had died and that all cases were traced to vessels at quarantine from West India ports. Perhaps the most interesting notation indicated that the old Potter's Field, which contained, with few exceptions, all the destitute who had died from yellow fever between the years 1798 and 1822 (estimated at 50,000 persons) had been converted into the "finest pleasure ground" in the city, known as "Washington Parade."[16]

"In a Nutshell": The News Compressed into Sharp, Pointed Paragraphs

Reports from Mexico were typically spotty and incomplete, often reported in paragraphs titled "In a Nutshell" to American readers. Such news primarily relied on eyewitness accounts of businessmen and maritime officers who habitually traversed the coasts along the Gulf of Mexico. A report from late 1829 indicated that at Tampico, Mexico, it was feared two-thirds of the Spanish soldiers stationed there had perished from yellow fever. Another report, this one from 1833, linked Tampico and Vera Cruz to outbreaks of yellow fever and cholera. At the latter, yellow fever prevailed to a great degree that it was feared the disease would prove more fatal than in any season for the past six years, while at the former, death tolls were said to reach between 80 and 90 per day: "This atmospheric plague had also extended its polluted breath to the shipping in port lying five or six miles below the town."

A letter from Vera Cruz dated June 15, 1833, supplied information on Santa Anna and the war for independence, adding, "Business here is very dull. The yellow fever has carried off about one-eighth of the population of this place within forty days, ending the 10th insta.… The cholera is shockingly bad at the two Tampicos, and we fear it will ere long visit us." By early September the fever was subsiding at Tampico but cholera was making great ravages in the interior, particularly Mexico City, "the deaths being estimated there at about *fifteen hundred per day.*" A brief "nutshell" from 1835 mentioned that yellow fever was reported epidemic in Sonora, Mexico, and in 1836, after providing information that the Mexican authorities were unsuccessfully attempting to collect contributions in its war against Texas, a report incidentally mentioned that yellow fever had made its appearance at Tampico.[17]

Information from Cuba was equally incomplete and typically linked to how local diseases affected business. In 1835, Her Majesty's frigate *Forte* arrived at Halifax flying the yellow flag that signified disease aboard. The vessel had put out from Jamaica, but her last port of call had been Havana, where yellow fever was believed to have been contracted. No less than 80 crewmen were ill and the ship was forced to anchor in Bedford Basin, near Stevens Island "no intercourse between the town and the vessel had prudently been allowed."

In July 1837 another "nutshell" indicated yellow fever prevailed to some extent at Havana among strangers and the shipping in the harbor "and has assumed a malignant character." The following year, 30 or 40 American vessels were reported in port at Havana, "and the yellow fever prevailed among persons not acclimated." The "business news" also included information that five or six vessels from the coast of Africa had arrived within the fortnight and "succeeded in landing their slaves on the coast of Cuba."[18]

The year 1837 turned out to be a deadly one for residents of Sierra Leone. Reports from June 30 indicated the ravages of yellow fever were "frightful," with 40,000 persons afflicted. Consequently, the governor-major and General Dundas escaped the contagion by sailing for Sunderland. A number of Europeans connected with the military as well as private establishments also fell victim, while mortality on board Her Majesty's ships *Buzzard, Dolphin* and *Scout,* cruising off the African Station, "had been considerable."

The health of the region had not improved by March 7, 1838, when reports indicated the terrible loss of life from yellow fever, and the black vomit continued at Sierra Leone. British crews also continued to suffer: the *Buzzard* was ordered to have no contact with the shore, while the *Etna* lost 27 crew members, the *Bonnetta* lost her commander and 13 others, the *Forrester* lost her commander and 18 others and the *Raven* lost 10, making a total of 70 causalities.[19]

British interest in the West Indies also centered on military losses. In a letter dated October 11, 1837, from a correspondent to the *London Colonial Gazette* (December 1, 1838), he noted that while the barracks at St. Joseph's (the old capital of Trinidad) were the most beautifully situated in the world the facility had been established close to a great marsh. Consequently, the inhabitants as well as the garrison were "frequently nearly annihilated" by yellow fever. A detachment of the 89th Regiment lost two officers and 36 men in July, and another officer and 29 men perished in three weeks. The survivors were withdrawn and a company "of the black corps (1st West India regiment) sent out, but so virulent was the poison, that two of the white serjeants immediately fell victims; yet strange to say, the black troops remain quite healthy." He added that Tobago, Dominica, Grenada and Guadaloupe had also had epidemics in the worst form. Making a distinction between diagnoses, the reporter noted "no *Bulam fever* was ever more severe," but the five islands noted above were "the only ones in which the *yellow fever* prevailed."

The article continued, observing, "We hear nothing of its contagious nature, but we have our own suspicions, after what occurred in British Guiana last year." While not advocating strict quarantine because "all our inter-island trade would be destroyed," the writer argued that if "*true yellow fever*" prevailed to any extent, such measures would be necessary. To emphasize the point, he added, "During the prevalence of the *fever* in Demerara [on the north coast of South America, known as British Guiana from 1838 to 1958] last year, and at Trinidad this year, while the white inhabitants were falling by hundreds, *scarcely a black or coloured person became its victim;* or though many of them had the fever, and some very severely, very few died." To further drive home the point of danger to British troops in the West Indies, a medical officer reported that in 30 years more than 30,000 soldiers had perished from yellow fever and other epidemics peculiar to the islands: "Consequently in this short space of time more than four times the whole force has been cut off by disease alone, and the average duration of every soldier has been only seven years and a half."

In 1839 a report dated July 16 from Demerara (British Guiana) offered a heart-rending account of the condition of the 76th Regiment. It stated there were only two officers fit for duty and not enough soldiers to bury the dead. Black troops were employed for that purpose: "We hardly get coffins made fast enough." In consequence of the yellow fever, the commandant was prevailed on to move the troops, leaving only 50 men at headquarters.[20]

A History of Yellow Fever in Antigua

On July 4, 1853, Dr. Thomas Nicholson presented a paper—"An Essay on Yellow Fever, Comprising the History of That Disease, as It Appeared in the Island of Antigua, in the Years 1835, 1839 and 1842"—to the Epidemiological Society of London. He contended that true yellow fever was absent from the Leeward island between 1816 until 1835. On August 12, 1835, a severe hurricane struck St. John's; before that time the inhabitants were reasonably healthy, but afterwards "a great quantity of marine organic matters and vegetable rubbish" was deposited about the wharfs and precincts of the town bounded by the harbor.

By October 10 Dr. Nicholson treated the first case of yellow fever, with the last fatal case occurring toward the end of December. In total he "attended 220 cases, of which 75 were Europeans [12 died], 65 white Creoles [none died] and 80 coloured [2 died]." In June 1839 the epidemic broke out again, primarily striking young men who had arrived on the island after 1835. In September 1842 a third outbreak occurred and lasted until the middle of November. During this period he treated 22 Europeans, 20 white Creoles and one person of "mixed or coloured race."[21]

Observations on the Healthy and Diseased Properties of the Blood

This text, written by the English physician William Stevens and published in 1832, became one of the prime topics of consideration throughout the decade. Stevens' pronouncement was summed up by one sentence in the preface: "It is now, I believe, generally admitted, that the blood is endowed with vitality, and, if this be granted, it then follows, that this fluid, like everything else that possesses life, must be subject to disease."[22] As fundamental as it seems today, his development of this theory (also purported by Dr. Clanny) was groundbreaking for its time and set the course of medical research in a new direction. With nearly 20 years' experience treating fevers in the West Indies, Stevens believed the proximate cause of yellow fever was to be found in the changes which the blood undergoes, and that the true remedy for this and other fevers consisted in opposing by proper means those changes. Stevens described the changes the blood underwent in the following order:

(1) The blood loses its solid parts and becomes thin
(2) It loses its saline principle and becomes black and vapid
(3) Its preservative elements are now dissipated and it goes fast to decay, the more rapidly as no new blood can be formed
(4) It loses its vitality and is incapable of supporting life

Having found in yellow fever victims the quantity of saline matter below that which belongs in the blood in a state of health, he turned to the practical purpose of administering saline medicines. Treatment consisted in allaying the excitement of the blood, if any existed, during the first 24 hours by venesection, mild purgatives and sponging the body with cold water. The saline medicines which he considered the best agents for preventing the decomposition of the blood were then exhibited in small and repeated doses.

Those usually preferred were Rochelle salt and the carbonate of soda, potass and ammonia. In speaking out against any treatment using emetics, calomel (mercury), or antimony, opium, or acids, he noted that "those patients left to nature have a better chance of recovery" and they "increase the evils they are meant to relieve, and add greatly to the mortality of fever in hot climates."

Passing through New York in 1832 on his way to England, Stevens spoke of his theories, earning praise for "a novel and simple" treatment using the saline remedies that produced the "most fortunate result" in several hundred cases of West India fevers. One letter to the editor concluded, "When this surprising success, so little to have been anticipated, is considered, it may not be amiss to give the plan a fair trial in this hitherto intractable affliction."

In 1839 Dr. Jordan R. Lynch attempted to summarize the current theories: "Dr. Clanny has shown that the blood is altered in composition, as well as appearance. Mr. Searle has abely supported the same proposition. Dr. Stevens has confirmed the opinions of both writers, and pointed out the nature of the changes which take place in the blood, which, he thinks, is the primary seat of the infection, called yellow fever, in which it [the blood] is always black, whether examined during life, or taken from the heart after death, and always wanting the saline matter which it is said to contain. And as many neutral salts, with earthy bases, possess the property of changing healthy black venous blood into a bright arterial colour, he determined upon trying what effect they would have on the living body, and was so successful that out of 343 cases in Trinidad, lost not a single patient."

In response to the discussions generated by Stevens and others' work, it did not take long for "cures" to reach the market. By 1836 the British College of Health advertised "Hygeian Vegetable Universal Medicines" both in England and the United States for treatment of "Impurity of the Blood." By 1839, however, it was "Dr. Warburg's Vegetable Fever Drops," which promised it had "never been known to fail, even in the most malignant Fevers." Interestingly, in 1843 P. Cunningham of the Royal Navy wrote that Article 8 of the Naval Medical Instructions directed that a drachm of Peruvian bark in a gill of sound wine be administered twice daily to all employed in wooding and watering in tropical climes as a fever preventative. He then observed that Warburg's drops "have been found equally effective by medical men in curing the miasmatic Mediterranean fevers." Consequently, he suggested quinine as a miasmatic fever preventative and Warburg's drops as a curative.[23]

Stevens' work did not change everyone's outlook. "Diocles," writing in Washington D.C.'s *Daily National Intelligencer* (September 4, 1832) persisted in claiming "the same cause that produces cholera modified by a remote and probably existing state of the atmosphere, produces yellow fever, typhus fever, bilious remitting, and all other diseases of a similar character." By the end of the decade, Dr. Laidlaw persisted in the same idea: "The whole of the Pyrenees is, from time to time, guarded by French soldiers, whose duty it is to arrest the progress of the yellow fever, and while the poor Spaniard would be slain as the mortal aggressor, the invisible vapour of disease, like an unclean spirit, might pass by unseen; for a military cordon cannot impede the passage of a miasma."

As far as cures went, there remained no consensus. Dr. Chabert of Vera Cruz, Mexico, advocated a plant called "Huaco," also known as "Guaco" in South America, as being effective in cholera and yellow fever. In commenting on this, a writer from Bogota noted the plant was known primarily as a preventive and a cure for snake bites but had no larger applications, concluding the idea "ranked among the other evidences extant, that the spirit of quackery and of credulity is not yet extinguished either in the old or the new world." Henry Congreve, in his book, *The Medicine Casket* (1836), advocated everyone's favorite cure—wine—be "taken in moderation" for treatment of yellow fever, the blue stages of cholera and in all cases of debility, for monarchs and peasants alike. According to the book, white wine was stimulating, port and red wine were both stimulating and astringent, Champaign with a little brandy agreed with weak subjects, and hock and Rhenish wines were the least powerful but best calculated for hot weather. As a preventive, Thomas Johnston of Glasgow suggested charcoal be used as a substitute for stones in filling drains to purify all stagnant water.[24]

An observation by Thomas Jefferson, taken from Tucker's *Life of Jefferson*, serves as an apt conclusion for the decade of the 1830s:

> When great evil happens, I am in the habit of looking out for what good may arise from them as consolations to us, and Providence has in fact so established the order of things, as that most evils are the means of producing some good. The yellow fever will discourage the growth of great cities in our nation, and I view great cities as pestilential to the morals, the health, and the liberties of mankind.[25]

Chapter 15

The "Dead Book"

> *The New Orleans Times publishes the details furnished by the Dead Book kept by the Board of Health, in which the whole number and the names of the victims of yellow fever the present year are given.*
> Whole number of deaths (1848): 680
> Of this number there were American born: 78
> Of the 602 foreigners, the number of Irishmen was: 222[1]

On August 14, 1841, one report from New Orleans (*Albany* [NY] *Log Cabin*) stated the following: "The health of the city is still good; not a single case of yellow fever has been reported by the Board of Health.—The report of the Board for the week ending last Saturday exhibits a considerable improvement upon the preceding week. I hope we shall 'steer clear' of the epidemic, but fear we shall not." On the same date, the *Washington Globe* noted, "Several cases of yellow fever have occurred in New Orleans, and the disease is spreading."

Such is the difficulty of accurately ascertaining historical data. The matter was apparently cleared up with an August 24 article from the *New Orleans Bee* that stated 15 deaths had been reported to the board of health in the previous 48 hours. In the Charity Hospital on the 23rd, 12 fresh cases were admitted and 5 died from the fever. For the week ending August 30, seventy-two were reported dead, with the appendage, "the epidemic is greatly on the increase." On September 1 twenty more had perished. This time the newspaper warned, "The mortality is said to be very great for such an early period of the season."[2]

Yellow Fever in New Orleans, September–November 1841

Date	Mortality
Sept 6 & 7	38
Sept 9	35
Oct 21	9
by Nov 11	a total of 497 deaths
by the end of the season	a total of 1641 (288 natives, 1,055 foreigners and 298 origins unknown)

At a sermon preached in New Orleans, the Reverend Clapp noted that during his 20-year residence in the city he had witnessed eleven yellow fever epidemics and two cholera epidemics, "carrying to the grave never less than three thousand human beings and often five thousand." While this was clearly an exaggeration, it is not difficult to believe that for one living through such calamities the numbers must have appeared staggering.

Another story that, if not totally accurate, presents a vivid picture of the times is from the *Louisville Journal*, which reported that after officials were advised of 300 newly arrived emigrants below the city at Balize they sent a deputation warning the travelers of the fever and offering to provide subsistence until the epidemic passed. Having heard that there were jobs paying $3 a day in the city, the foreigners moved on to New Orleans, "and at last date, it is said, that not one of them was living."[3]

In 1842 yellow fever was considered by the local newspapers to be "epidemic" but of a mild character. The year 1843 proved to be more deadly, spreading to Balize and along the Mississippi towns of Natchez, Rodney (forty miles upriver) and Vicksburg. By the end of September the situation was so critical at Rodney that the inhabitants had all fled, and "even the apothecary—doubtful, we suppose, of the efficacy of his own drugs— is now 'not at home' to his customers." The western part of the state was also afflicted, with the paper published at Lafayette, Jefferson County, reporting that "scarce a breeze passes by, or a day dawns, but brings to our ears the melancholy tidings of the departure of an immortal spirit." By the end of the season, the *New Orleans Republican* published the nationalities of those who had perished.[4]

Yellow Fever Deaths in New Orleans by Place of Residence, 1843

Germany	227	Spain	3
Ireland	205	Denmark	3
United States	128	Nova Scotia	3
France	67	Poland	2
England	22	Prussia	2
Scotland	12	Sicily	1
Italy	7	Canada	1
Switzerland	5	Unknown	132
Sweden	4		
Total			824[5]

Believing that yellow fever first attacked the poor and indigent living and working along the docks, residents of New Orleans typically assigned the start of the yellow fever season to the first fever admissions to Charity Hospital and used mortality lists from that institution to gauge the severity of the outbreak.

Statistics from the New Orleans Charity Hospital, 1839–1843

Year	Admitted	Discharged	Deaths
1839	1,085	634	452
1840	None	1	1
1841	1,113	520	690
1842	410	214	211
1843	1,090	175	467 (through November 25)[6]

In addition to statistics, there were often "heart rending" accounts of personal tragedy that put a face to the countless victims of this terrible disease. In 1843, one such story told of a father, mother, two daughters and a son newly arrived from New York. Stopping in the city to await passage to St. Louis, the husband was taken sick but from ignorance of the symptoms failed to call a doctor. He soon died, followed by his wife and daughters, leaving only a "blue-eyed, ruddy-cheeked boy" of ten years. The little fellow was taken into the cabin of a packet ship at the levee and the captain promised "to place him in the hands of affluent relatives." The tale concluded, "God bless the orphan!"[7]

The 1844 season began with a warning from Her Majesty's consul at New Orleans, noting that yellow fever was "singularly destructive of life amongst emigrants arriving from Europe," and urging those contemplating the trip to avoid leaving Great Britain during the months of June through September. For this year, at least, the disease was "unusually mild—so much so, that it is comparatively harmless." Good luck held through 1845 and 1846, infrequent cases appearing late in the season of both years.[8] The year 1847 would prove to be a horse of a different color.

"...the very centre of an epidemic"

After three relatively healthy seasons, inhabitants of New Orleans anticipated a resurgence of yellow fever and in 1847 their worst fears came to fruition. In the last week of July, 150 cases were reported, with 47 deaths. Authorities reacted quickly. By August 2, noting the city was "on the eve of an epidemic," the board of health announced the fever's existence in an official bulletin, warning the unacclimated "to absent themselves in time, and avoid such exposure and imprudence as may increase their susceptibility to the disease." Numbers climbed quickly. A day later, the *New Orleans Delta* stated there were "at least 87 cases of yellow fever patients under treatment in the Charity Hospital." For the week ending August 9, deaths had increased to 133.

Complicating matters was the evolving Mexican War. Notices began appearing in newspapers as early as mid–August "entertaining great fears" for the volunteer soldiers passing through the city from the various states. With a view toward avoiding the danger of contagion, the army gave orders to have "means of transportation ready at Baton Rouge, Natchez or some other healthy point, for all the volunteers who are ordered or to be ordered to Mexico, during the present state of health of New Orleans, and who, in their progress to the seat of war, must pass down the Mississippi by that city."[9] By August 18 the *Delta* calculated that a continuing escalation of deaths would eventually reach 448 per week, a number picked up and widely distributed throughout the country as fact. An editorial of the same paper (reprinted by the *Weekly Wisconsin*, September 8, 1847) offered a tragically poetical view of the city:

> One may look upon the broad, populous streets, that during other seasons are crowded with the brave, the beautiful and the fashionable, and yet now could scarcely find anything to relieve the eye. Cast your gaze from St. Peter up Chartres st.—instead of finding the street filled with all that is redolent of life in New Orleans, you find a blank. Here you see a solitary citizen, who, through his business, is obliged to remain tugging at his desk; and another who from some cause or other pulls his occupation after him, in the same manner that a dray horse pulls his load.
>
> The Levee is deserted and the forests of masts that skirted it have dwindled down to almost nothing. The streets that in winter time were filled with all sorts of happy, joyous persons, are now almost desolate, and in fact the whole appearance of our city is sadly against the prevalence of health. It is useless to conceal the fact—we are now in the very centre of an epidemic.

Less dramatically but with equal power, the *Bee* observed, "We have never experienced an equal dullness and desertion of the city, to that which exists at present.... The Levee is deserted by ships, steamboats and animal life, and the noon-day sun pours down its burning rays upon lifeless tranquility."[10]

As was typical during such epidemics, a correspondent for the *St. Louis Republican* wrote on September 2 that there were 3,000 new cases of yellow fever in New Orleans, noting that not half of the deaths were reported. He added that "the Board of Physicians have called a meeting to determine what to call the prevailing epidemic—some say yellow fever, some say vomito and some a combination of yellow and ship fever." To make it worse, the reporter added, "The fever has commenced at Pass Christian, Biloxi and Bay of St. Louis, while the Board of Health at Mobile have declared an epidemic and fever raged at Pensacola. The physicians," he concluded, "have declared this to be the worst epidemic ever known in this city."

Notices did not improve, as yellow fever deaths reached 52 on August 29 and between the 29th and 30th there were 52 more. While national headlines centered around General Winfield Scott's "Attack and Defeat of the Mexicans!" near Mexico City, four of New Orleans' daily papers, the *Times*, the *Bee*, the *Bulletin* and the *Courier*, were forced to publish only three times a week while the fever continued. Patrons at the great St. Charles Hotel often found themselves alone in the dining room, while those foolish enough to travel by steamboat experienced terrible tragedy. After reaching New Orleans, the *Hard Times* out of St. Louis lost her captain, first clerk, several other officers and nearly 30 passengers to the fever.[11]

On September 29 the *Weekly Wisconsin* published a notice stating, "The Pestilence at New Orleans seems to be more terrible than ever. It mows down the population with the sharpness of a scythe. Death seems literally 'to walk in darkness.'" The present population, it added, was between 50,000 and 70,000, with the usual number around 150,000. With mortality so great, local newspapers began comparing statistics. The *Delta* reported that between August 1 and September 1 yellow fever had claimed 1,128, the largest death rate that ever occurred in August.

Death Rates in New Orleans from All Diseases During Epidemic Years for the Month of August

Year	Mortality
1817	489
1819	292
1820	299
1822	165
1833	410
1837	483
1839	619
1841	562

Death Rates in New Orleans from All Diseases During Epidemic Years for August, September and October

Year	Mortality
1822	1,262
1833	2,758 (yellow fever and cholera)
1837	2,239
1839	1,554
1842	2,231[12]

While the *Picayune* was pleading with northern editors to "dissuade those in search of employment from coming here too early,"[13] the *Courier* was arguing with the statistics published by the *Delta*. That newspaper claimed 1832 was more deadly than 1833, noting that "bodies accumulated in large heaps in the hospitals, and the only way of disposing of them was found to be burning!" After supplying other mortality lists, the editor wisely noted, "All these figures were no doubt exaggerations; but the mortality was awful beyond any that was ever experienced in an American city." The text continued:

> It was a very common thing to hear announced in the streets—"There were three hundred deaths in the last twenty-four hours," or five hundred, or six hundred, and one occasion the number rose in the popular fear (always inclined to exaggerate danger) to upwards of seven hundred. Indeed, we know individuals then residing in New Orleans, and now living, whom it would be difficult to convince that the number of deaths in that never-to-be-forgotten epidemic did not sometimes amount to seven hundred in twenty-four hours.

The *Courier* added, "The epidemic of the present season, is sufficiently fearful, without any pretensions to equal, or even to come near that of 1832."[14] The epidemic slowly faded and on October 22 the *New Orleans National* pronounced that between July 5 through October 17, a period of 107 days, the total number of deaths was 2,544.[15]

In 1848 Dr. Luke P. Blackburn was appointed city heath officer and was influential in establishing a quarantine against the yellow fever outbreak in the Mississippi River Valley. Outbreaks that year proved less devastating but by the end of the season the *New Orleans Times* reported 666 deaths. By October 5, 1848, the board of health officially announced the disappearance of yellow fever and advised strangers and the unacclimated that they might return in safety. In late June 1849 the disease broke out in Havana and fears were entertained that it would soon be imported, but by August 25 the city remained healthy and newspapers reported "there is not the slightest apprehension of the appearance in New Orleans this season of the yellow fever to any extent." That proved to be wistful thinking, for the board of health reported 769 deaths from yellow fever, 416 of them coming in the month of October 1849.[16]

Deaths from Yellow Fever in New Orleans, 1840–1849

Year	Number of Deaths
1840	3
1841	594
1842	211
1843	487
1844	82
1845	2
1846	146
1847	2,306
1848	808
1849	769[17]

Proving that even in the most harrowing circumstances Americans could find some humor, a reporter from the *St. Louis Reveille* recounted a story told by Mr. Bradbury, the "ex–French editor of the Cincinnati Sunday News" concerning Dennis Corcoran, then (1847) the Irish editor of the *New Orleans Delta*. Apparently (and the author purported "to believe every word of it!") during the epidemic of 1841, Corcoran was thought to be dying of yellow fever. While friends and the attending physician were in an adjacent room preparing for his funeral, the patient got up in search of some alcoholic drink to imbibe before he died. Finding "an old fashioned junk bottle on the mantle-piece," he gulped the contents and hurried back to bed before being found out. Moments later he began throwing up the "black vomit," a sure sign the end was near. Passing into a sort of sleep, the victim woke in an hour, cured of his fever. After confessing his "crime" of downing a drink, the doctor retrieved the empty bottle and inspected the label. It read:

Superfine Record Ink
Manufactured by
HOGAN & THOMPSON
Philadelphia

This became "undoubtedly the most extraordinary case of 'black vomit' on record," and Corcoran continued his work on the newspaper, "but he is very careful that the bottles he has occasion to use are not labeled 'black ink.'"[18]

Yellow Fever Throughout the United States, 1840–1849

Yellow fever prevailed throughout much of the south during this decade but outbreaks were considered mild when compared to those of New Orleans. Scattered reports from Mobile in 1842 and 1843 mentioned few causalities. Key West was said to suffer from the ravages of the disease in 1841 and 1843, but numbers on the death lists were low. In 1843 a report typical of the decade noted, "Several cases of yellow fever have made their appearance at St. Louis, but they are said to have created no apprehensions, as scarcely a summer passes without them." In 1844 several papers carried stories that the malady had appeared at Galveston, but physicians indicated the attacks were "less violent, and for the most part yield[ed] readily to medical treatment," although one newspaper reported 200 had perished during the four weeks ending August 14.[19]

On a lighter note, at the dawn of the California gold rush, the *Vox Populi* (Wisconsin, February 5, 1849) published the following: "CALIFORNIA: There are great reports astir, in relation to California Gold, &c. Many of our citizens have got the *yellow fever,* and will start in the Spring, we almost wish the yellow fever will get them before they can get back again to this peaceable community."

Much excitement occurred at Rondout, the port of Kingston, New York, in August 1843 when two persons engaged in unloading a cargo of salt off the schooner *Vanda* sickened and died of yellow fever. Reports indicated the *Vanda*, out of Point Petre, Guadaloupe, arrived at Staten Island but was permitted by Dr. Vanhovenburg, the physician of health, to leave quarantine after two days and proceed up the river, even though he was aware the captain had died of the disease onboard and that one of her crew was infected when the vessel reached New York. The board of health convened on Sunday, August 27, and sent a deputation to investigate the incident. The following day a proclamation was issued declaring a "non-intercourse" order between Kingston and New York City.[20]

In early September 1848 four cases of yellow fever were reported at the Marine Hospital and by mid-month, in consequence of Dr. Whiting's communication to the board of health that yellow fever had prevailed at Staten Island for ten or twelve days, the Common Council passed a nonintercourse act with that place. They "*resolved*, that all ferry and other boats or vessels, are hereby prohibited from touching at, landing or taking up passengers, at either of the docks on Staten Island, known as the Stapleton and Quarantine docks, until otherwise ordered." This "excited the deepest dissatisfaction among the

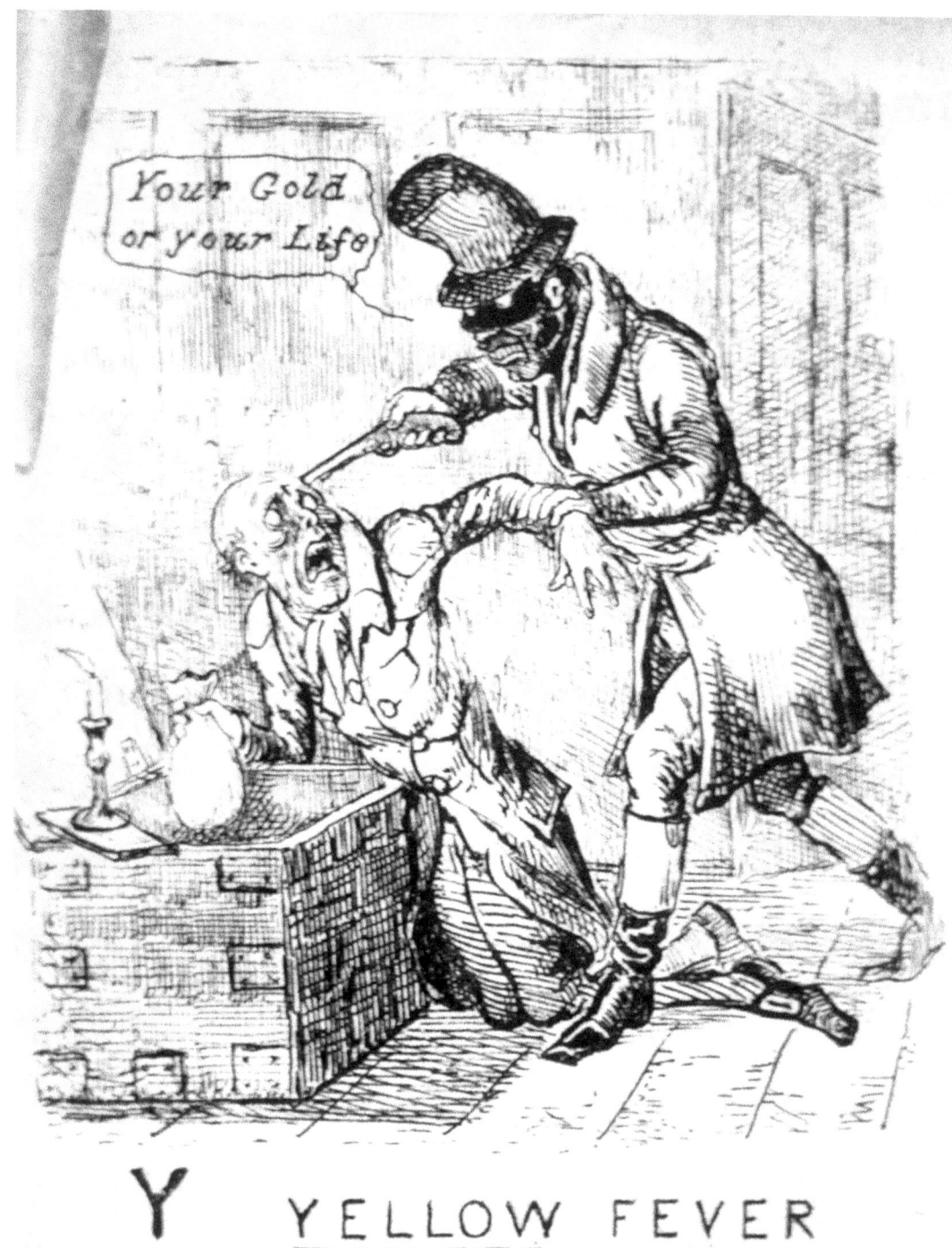

In the mid–1800s the term "yellow fever" often had a dual meaning. Not only did it represent the deadly epidemic disease but it was also playfully used to reflect the lust for gold (courtesy National Library of Medicine).

thousands ... in the habit of resorting to the quarantine grounds" for holidays. The infection was traced to a vessel from New Orleans and subsequent reports indicated that 50 cases occurred, seven of which terminated fatally.[21]

Mexico and the Mexican War

Isolated reports of yellow fever in Mexico occasionally made the newspapers in the United States but they were often vague and passed through many exchanges before reaching the East Coast. Typical of the times were such notices as the following: "The *Civilian* of the 20th says, 'We received a letter from Corpus Christi on Wednesday, which says that at last accounts people were dying of yellow fever at Matamoras at the rate of 30 per day'" (*Bangor Daily Whig & Courier,* December 9, 1841); "A late Mexican paper states that the yellow fever prevailed to a frightful extent in Guayaquil. Many distinguished persons have fallen; among them are the sister of President Rocafuerte, Alena, and Saenoz, the two Espantoses, and others" (*Washington* [DC] *Globe,* February 8, 1843).

Most of the Mexican yellow fever news filtered through New Orleans or was transmitted by private letters. In the early 1840s information concentrated on Santa Anna, Mexico's internal political matters and the country's relations with Texas, adding epidemic notices as space permitted. One exception that found its way into a number of papers was the "Mexican Cure for the Yellow Fever." According to the *New Orleans Tropic,* which passed the recipe along to the *Globe* (October 16, 1843), the sure-cure consisted of a tumbler two-thirds full of olive oil, mixed with the juice of two lemons and a teaspoonful of fine table salt. Interestingly, an almost identical notice appeared in the *Adams* [PA] *Sentinel* (October 30, 1843), but the mixture called for limes instead of lemons.

In 1844, besides news suggesting that Santa Anna's invasion of Texas had been abandoned "on condition that Mexico shall have the right to renew the war whenever we offer ourselves to the United States," it was reported that yellow fever raged at Matamoras and "the American consul and several others have fallen victim to the epidemic." Two years later, an American named Dr. Charles Davis, a longtime resident of Matamoras, wrote to the *Washington Union* stating that yellow fever had occurred only twice at Matamoras and both times came after the river overflowed its banks in the month of August.

Interest in Mexico altered considerably in 1846 at the start of the Mexican War. The *Charleston News* informed its readers that yellow fever did not extend inland more than 60 miles from the seacoast; consequently, "the enemy will not be vomito, but wide deserts, devoid of the means of subsistence for an army." By contrast, the *Journal of Commerce* ran a short notice stating that when General Almonte was in Washington as minister of Mexico it was believed his country "would have nothing to oppose the overwhelming power and force of the United States. General Almonte replied—'It is a mistake, we have the 'vomito,' alias Yellow Fever.'"

On the warfront, General Zachery Taylor was quoted as saying fewer than 5 percent of those afflicted with yellow fever died. This statement proved politic as the *New York Herald,* addressing those who might volunteer for military service but feared yellow fever, promptly reported that the troops under Taylor and General Winfield Scott were in good health, noting that only the area around Vera Cruz was infested. The article added that no yellow fever had appeared among U.S. soldiers along the Rio Grande in 1846 and no outbreaks were expected in 1847. The paper helpfully added, "The fact may be attributed to the perpetual excitement in which the men were in, which, as it is supposed, has a counteracting effect upon a sickly climate."

In a letter dated June 16, 1847, Lieutenant Cady wrote home, stating he arrived at Vera Cruz on June 13 after a passage of 12 days from New Orleans and encamped four miles below the city to avoid the yellow fever and vomito, "which is doing its work terribly—some 50 are buried daily. And the destruction by the fever is not confined to the citizens and soldiers, but the natives are dying—which is something unusual." After going into the city on business, he found "the most horrible stench that was ever snuffed.... Every other building is converted into a hospital, and dray loads of coffins meet you at every turn." A significantly different picture was presented in an official report by Dr. E.H. Barton, a surgeon in the U.S. Army and president of the board of health:

Yellow Fever Mortality at Vera Cruz, 1847

Victims	Number of Deaths
Soldiers	27
Quartermaster's Department and other Americans	17
Mexicans	6
Total	**40**

The following year, a correspondent from the *New Orleans Crescent* stated that at Vera Cruz new yellow fever cases amounted to about 40 per week.[22]

"The latest intelligence": Yellow Fever Around the World, 1840–1849

The ravages of yellow fever were considered uncommonly malignant in Havana and St. Jago de Cuba during 1841; during June at the former city 424 persons died in hospitals compared to 76 the previous June. The malignancy of the fever was also seen throughout the West Indies, although undoubtedly the good news was that sugar crops were favorable. Similar accounts without specific details were printed throughout the decade without indicating any major epidemics.

Two items from England, however, were especially relevant. The first concerned the "imposing military force" maintained by the government in the West Indies. The author questioned its necessity, noting, "It cannot be said that [the colonies] are in danger of being wrested from us by a *coup-de-main*—a buccaneering expedition set on foot by any other nation without previous warning.... While the negroes of these colonies were slaves, a large military force was required to guard their masters against occasional insurrections; but that state of affairs is altered." He concluded the reason was that "our rulers have so many regiments that they are at a loss how to dispose of them, and therefore send a certain number to the West India and other colonies, in order that they may be out of the way, or may appear to be doing something."

He added that, while this was unfair to tax-paying people, it was "a wanton inhumanity to the soldiers. It is a certain sentence of death to a proportion of the soldiery which can be estimated within a fraction. A tropical climate tries the soundest constitution of a white man, even when varied and interesting employment contributes to keep him alive; but it is sure to enfeeble the constitutions of all whose time is not fully occupied, or whose avocations are monotonous and merely mechanical ... [and] the truth is that no white man can with impunity discharge military duties in tropical climates for any length of time."

The second subject concerned the submission of a report to Parliament on "Quarantine and Sanitary Regulations." It concluded "there was little or no generic difference between epidemics [plague, influenza, cholera, yellow fever, scarlatina, typhus] and the second, that they were not transmissible after any such fashion as that combatted by the institutions of quarantine." In discussing the prevailing theory of contagion by merchandise, the subject was concluded by the remark that if this were so "the human race could scarcely have survived the ultimate consequences of such conditions."[23]

Medical Reviews and Cures, 1840–1849

A summary of the decade revealed little original thinking and a general disagreement as to the origin of yellow fever. In 1840, Dr. Clott's text, *Contagion and Non–Contagion*, offered his opinion: "The non-contagious nature of that epidemic is admitted by nearly all the physicians of the American hemisphere. Honor and glory to *Dr. Chervin*, who has, with an ability and perseverance above all praise, most contributed to the adoption in Europe of the same truth." On the subject of lazarettos, cordons, quarantines and isolation, Clott considered them "useless measures" but acknowledged that the state of public opinion precluded the immediate and utter abolition of them. Clott (also known as "Clot" and "Clot-Bey") was a Frenchman who spent many years in Egypt studying the plague and became inspector general of the civil and military medical service of Mehemet Ali and president of the General Board of Health of Egypt.

The same year, Dr. Chervin read his paper on the origin and nature of yellow fever to the Academy of Medicine and afterward announced his intention to emigrate to New Orleans in order to practice his theories in that theatre.

Josiah Clark Nott, a man destined to become one of the leading southern authorities on yellow fever, wrote his first paper in 1845. Published in the *American Journal of the Medical Sciences* and titled, "On the Pathology of Yellow Fever," his text stressed "*facts derived from the bed-side and post-mortem observations.*" Nott argued there was a great variety in the different epidemics of yellow fever and in the symptoms he had observed in his practice at Mobile. He stressed the fact that not all disease could be viewed as originating from inflammation, and each epidemic required modifications in treatment. Based on autopsy work, he correctly determined that black vomit consisted of blood acted upon by the stomach's secretions. He concluded yellow fever was a poison received through the atmosphere, probably working on the nervous system and the blood in some way that altered its normal state. In his opinion, this generally ruled out bleeding: "The *rule* is, beware of the lancet."[24]

In 1847 a discussion entitled "Autumnal Fevers" by E.B. West supported the theory purported by Dr. Wilson that "yellow fever is the product of the combined agency of gasses evolved by the humid decomposition of vegetables of *a woody fibre*, with some more general causes." This opinion was based on the fact that the disease "often breaks out in its most violent forms on board of ships, and in other situations on land, remote from any of the usual sources of paludal [plant, animal or soil living or existing in a marshy habitat] exhalations; while it has been maintained by nearly *every* writer that it owes its origin to decomposition of *some* kind, in connection with certain other atmospheric conditions." The importance, then, was to entirely remove timber "from all lands previous to their being overflown."

Also in 1847 an article published by the *New Orleans Delta* on the subject of "Fever" described it as being caused by "cold applied to one of the most important organs of the body, viz the skin—by which its office becomes for a time more or less destroyed." In condemning the use of alcohol, the author wrote, "Good God! Scotch ale and London porter to a man raving with acute fever; as if it were necessary to send him reeling drunk into the presence of his Maker!" The writer also noted the use of quinine in acute fever "is contrary to common sense, contrary to sound science, contrary to all experience, and contrary to the constant practice of the most accomplished physicians of the day." (Most physicians accepted the prevailing theory of the "unity of fevers," meaning all fevers originated from a common source and what worked for one fever should work for the rest. The theory was incorrect and while quinine was of great benefit when treating malarial infections, as this authority stated, it was useless when treating yellow fever. It was not until after the New Orleans epidemic of 1853 that quinine was largely abandoned as a treatment for yellow fever.)[25]

In 1848 one British authority called for the use of common salt dissolved in bath water and hot water bottles next to the body when in bed. This, he stated, "has been found highly beneficial in the yellow fever in the West Indies." In *An Account of the Origin, Spread, and Decline of the Epidemic Fevers of Sierra Leone,* by Alexander Bryson, the author takes great pains to discredit the work of Sir William Pym (*Observations of the Bulam Fever*). In explaining his own ideas, one particularly interesting section dealt with what Bryson called the "bread and butter system" of construction for intertropical steamships that created "pest-houses"

> In these vessels there are two layers of plank separated by an interposed layer of felt. From the peculiar construction of these vessels, their want of strength to resist vibration soon converts the interposed felt into a source of disease. The vessel, from its extreme lightness of planking and the frail mode of its fastenings, necessarily ships water as soon as the external planking is loosened,—and this takes place immediately the engines begin to work, causing the ship to leak more or less from stem to stern. This water is rapidly, by the chemical action, induced not less by the construction of the ship, (which is a perfect galvanic arrangement), than by the accident of climate and the heat, inseparable from a steamer, decomposed and fills the ship with a loathsome and deadly combination of gasses, not only amply sufficient to generate or aggravate disease under a tropical sun, but also capable of exercising the most baneful effects upon the health of the crew, in a temperate latitude.[26]

Also in 1848 Josiah Nott published his most significant article on yellow fever, entitled, "Yellow Fever Contrasted with Bilious Fever Reasons for Believing It a Disease Sui Generis; Its Mode of Propagation—Remote Cause—Probably Insect or Animalcular Origin, & c." (*New Orleans Medical and Surgical Journal* 4). Arguing against the "unity of fevers" concept, Nott declared yellow fever to be *sui generis* (of its own kind/genus), unlike malaria (which was supposed to arise from miasma) and bilious fevers. Nott intended to offer "reasons for supposing its specific cause to exist in some form of Insect Life." His biographer, Reginald Horsman, concluded Nott's use of the word "insects" referenced "microorganisms, invisible to the naked eye that had usually been described as 'animalcules,'" as opposed to insects such as mosquitoes.

Citing Christian Gottfried Ehrenberg's *Insuforia* (1838) and influenced by Sir Henry

Holland's *Medical Notes and Reflections* (1839), which included an article on "insect life as a cause of disease," Nott concluded that the "morbific cause of Yellow Fever ... accords in many respects with the peculiar habits and instincts of Insects." Noting that during the yellow fever epidemics in Mobile during 1842 and 1843, wind and weather had no impact on the manner in which the disease spread, Nott concluded there was a "perfect analogy between the habits of certain insects and Yellow Fever." He also suggested various marsh fevers might actually be different diseases caused by different insects.

Nott refuted the arguments of Nicolas Chervin, who believed yellow fever and marsh fevers were the same, by stating yellow fever developed independently of meteorological changes and miasmic influences, agreeing only that it spread more rapidly in dry than wet weather and adding that insects were impeded by rains and frost. (A later story, recounted by Nott's friend Dr. Stanford Chaille of New Orleans, told of Nott's comment during an autopsy: "Chaille, I'm damned if I don't believe it's bugs.") Nott also wrote, "Vegetable matter is *certainly* not a cause of Yellow Fever." He believed the disease was not contagious, if that meant "a morbid poison" generated in one body could be passed on by contact. He did consider the possibility "the germ or *materies morbi*" might be transmitted or transported from one locale to another by ships, but he saw no purpose in quarantine, falling back on the old argument that "commerce is one of the *greatest necessities* of society." He ultimately concluded his article by stating is was "highly probable" that animalcules not only caused yellow fever but other diseases as well.[27]

In 1843 Dr. Nott began experimenting with creosote, "a substance in the nature of the volatile oils, discovered in 1830 by Dr. Reichenbach in the products of the distillation of wood." Initially it was used externally for the treatment of wounds and ulcers and internally for arresting nausea, vomiting and seasickness; in overdose it acted as a poison.[28] As it was also known to be an antiseptic, Nott hoped it might exert a positive influence on the morbid poisons of yellow fever. Using a mixture of creosote, alcohol and *spititus mindereri*, his first two experiments were on local prostitutes. When they recovered after its application he used it on a larger scale with success. He ultimately concluded creosote was a valuable remedy but not a specific, or absolute, cure.[29]

Finally there were the advertisements. In 1845 under the heading, "Botanico Medical Notice," Dr. T.S. Ripley of the "Botanic Fraternity" offered to cure everything from consumption and the King's Evil (scrofula) to yellow fever with his vegetable medicines, hoping to follow "the venerable Dr. Rush, of Philadelphia" that "the only outlet of life might be that of old age." And not to be overlooked were the venerable "Brandreth Pills" (advertised in Indiana in 1846), which "saved valuable lives in those regions where the DREADFUL YELLOW FEVER was prevailing" and in Pennsylvania in 1847, where it was claimed they "removed all impurities from the body" and were "not only the most proper medicine, but generally the only medicine that need or ought to be used."[30]

Chapter 16

New Orleans: A City of Desolation

On the 2nd [August] inst. the city was one vast hospital. For two days not a steamboat has arrived from any other port, but over fifty have left during the last six days, all loaded with passengers—each boat containing from 400 to 1,000. Business of every kind was suspended, except such as was carried on in the retail way for supplying families with the necessities of life, and nothing was talked of but means for alleviating the distressed and dying, and burying the dead.[1]

In 1850 the "Dengue Fever, called by some the broken-bone fever" was prevalent in New Orleans but by mid–October the city was declared healthy and all danger passed. Deaths in 1851 were too slight to make the newspapers, but the disease did appear at Mobile starting around the middle of October. The board of health warned strangers to stay away, but by mid–November after three or four severe frosts the risk was considered over.

In a bit of Americana, in 1851 when Grant Thorburn—widely known as the hero of John Galt's *Lawrie Todd; or, The Settlers in the Woods* (1830) and a man who considered himself under the care of a special Providence—was rewriting his autobiography for the *Home Journal,* he mentioned the yellow fever epidemic of New York in 1807. Upon observing a driver pass by with a cartload of corpses, he said, "O for the chisel of Powers, or the pencil of West, for now would I sketch a second edition of Death on the Pale Horse!" The statement was remarkable from the fact Mr. Powers (the cited artist) was a child at the time, far removed from fame and fortune.[2]

The yellow fever season began in the first week of September 1852 at Charleston, with 12 deaths being registered by the 4th of the month. By October 14 only one death was reported within 24 hours and it was felt the disease was rapidly disappearing. After three more inhabitants perished on Thursday the 16th the mayor declared Friday "a day of humiliation and prayer." On September 20 the board of health reported 15 more deaths between Friday and Sunday, the mortality being attributed to the weather. For the week ending the 29th, 43 more were added to the mortality list. Similar numbers were registered through November 22 but the local newspapers reported that "passengers from the North can pass through that city without danger from the yellow fever. Whenever the Wilmington or New York steamers arrive too late extra trains are run to prevent the necessity of passengers staying in the city over night."

Deaths in New Orleans for 1852 were scant enough not to merit much national press until October, when 26 cases were reported in early in that month. Thereafter, mortality numbers remained low through the end of the season.[3] Such fortune was destined to come to an abrupt end the following year.

Yellow fever came calling nearly two months before its usual time in 1853. On Friday, July 22, the New Orleans Charity Hospital accepted 27 admissions, discharged 44 and registered 48 deaths, 43 of them from that dreaded malady. For the last week of July, as the *Delta* spoke of the epidemic as "worse than ever before," the hospital reported 130 (or 190) deaths, depending on which exchange was consulted. Deaths were "confined mostly to the poorer classes in the hospitals," but "mostly" carried wide latitude. On August 5 the death notice of Colonel Bliss, a Mexican War hero and son-in-law of General Taylor, was said to have occurred at Pascagoula (near Baton Rouge), Mississippi. During one 48-hour period ending on the first day of August, 253 yellow fever deaths were reported and for the week the number reached 660. For the week ending August 7, a staggering 950 deaths were said to have resulted from the epidemic.[4]

The New Orleans Charity Hospital and Temporary Infirmaries

While many patients feared being taken to the hospital, as it was considered nothing better than a death house, the New Orleans Charity Hospital, charged with the care of those unable to pay for medical attention, received glowing reports from contemporaries inspecting the premises and judging its staff. Even those fearful of "the uncertainties" and "neglect of private attendance" were willing to pay $3 per day to secure accommodations "little better than those extended to the poor." With as many as 1,000 patients collected inside the walls and, during epidemics, facing 60–80 daily admissions, a well-regulated system provided for prompt care and attention.

When yellow fever raged, it was not uncommon to see a line of cabs and dark-covered wagons supplied by the corporation lined up at the gate. They each reported to the clerk who stood outside taking down the name, age, country of origin and occupation of the afflicted. Each patient was then given a ticket and when called either walked or was carried to the first floor. There the warder received the ticket and indicated to which section the sufferer should be taken.

The hospital was divided into wards, each containing 30–40 patients, with a physician and nurses assigned to it. Upon reaching the ward, patients were required to stop and bathe in warm water. Their clothes were removed, labelled and stored. They were then dressed in a long, cotton, sack-like sheet and put to bed. The nurses were all from the Sisters of Charity or those acting under their direction, each wearing their "sombre habits" and performing work of "restraining the violent, cleansing the filthy and offensive, and ministering in a thousand ways to the relief and comfort of their fellow beings."

The only drawback to the system was the congregation of the sick, the dead, the dying and the convalescent, all in the same room. "This," it was observed, "is unavoidable but very injurious…. In no disease are the destructive effects of fear more palpable than in this." Everything that could be done was attended to "but alas! this mysterious disease is the especial enemy of the poor and ignorant. Science and philanthropy essay in vain to arrest the effects of neglect, exposure and ignorance. Few of the very poor escaped. In every Ward we could see the sheets doubled up over inanimate bodies, to conceal the dead from the view of the living."

The patients were generally quiet, orderly and submissive, but "now and then the quiet of the room would be disturbed by the sudden burst of delirium of some fevered patient, who would leap from his bed and commence to shout or cry with maniac violence, but a stout porter would soon seize the disturber, and, if it were necessary, strap him or her down to the bed by broad leather belts." In the hall stood another porter holding a bier. When summoned, he would tightly wrap a body in a sheet and hurry down the stairs.

The dead house was a low brick building 30 feet long, divided into three apartments, the smallest of which was allotted to the corpses "from the pay department" and a much larger one "to the commonalty of corpses ... aristocracy in a dead house." In the main area a long table covered with bodies stretched the length of the room, with their names printed on their breasts; the table being too crowded, other bodies were placed on the brick floor. Chloride of lime was sprinkled on the floor to "keep the atmosphere free from odor." The observer noted, "To see so many human beings, who a few days before, had been full of life, of passion, of joy and of hope, now folded up, as so many packages of merchandise, and labelled to be sent abroad—sorted, counted and arranged—was certainly as depressing an exhibition of human mortality and littleness as we have ever witnessed."

Bodies were stripped of their sheets and their shirts or sacks "with little ceremony or decency" and placed in wooden coffins of cypress and pine and deposited in carts, three at a time, for delivery to the hospital cemetery. The only break in the gloomy scene came from the chapel, 50 yards from the dead house, where the Sisters of Charity made their devotions: "If any religious feelings lurked in a man's bosom, such a spectacle would certainly draw them forth in all their earnestness." Disturbing the solemnity was a carpenter, "solacing a dreary employment with snatches of a popular Ethiopian melody." When asked to be quiet, he smiled grimly and remarked, "But a man who made as many coffins as he did had little other comfort but singing."

When it became obvious that the Charity Hospital would be unable to accommodate all the sick, authorities established four infirmaries in different parts of the city, under the joint care and direction of the board of health. One of these was placed in the Globe Ballroom, a "fine airy room in the old Third Municipality. Among the loose, floating and dissipated population of New Orleans, the Globe Ballroom is a famous place. In the winter it is the scene of the wildest and most reckless revelry—where rowdies and bawds assemble in masks to indulge in every species of dissipation and vice." "The stirring strains of music," the writer added, "have been succeeded by the low voices of nurses and physicians, and the elastic tramp of dancers by the heavy steps of stout porters bearing biers, on which lay the newly-arrived sick or the freshly dead. Beauty is no longer visible through that sallow, yellow mask in which the Pestilence has vested it, and the gay and rich ornaments of fashion and taste have surrendered to the simple garb of the hospital, or the scale toilet of the tomb."[5]

The Misery Continues

The charitable Howard Association (chartered in 1839) published the following in the *New Orleans Bee,* noting, "Reader, this is no fancy sketch":

Imagine a woman lying on a dilapidated pallet, in a building which flattery could hardly dignify with the name of hovel—without a solitary friend to assist her—in the most dangerous crisis of fever—

scarcely conscious—tossing wildly on her wretched couch, burning with this insupportable thirst which seems unquenchable, without a drop of water by her bedside. Imagine this woman the mother of two children—one of whom is just old enough to comprehend the terror of the scene, but as yet incapable of helping her parent, while the other, an infant, hangs on its mother's breast, striving to draw nourishment from an exhausted fountain.

Private telegraphic dispatches indicated the city was in a "universal panic," with business suspended and houses and stores closed. The writer implored people of the East and North to send aid as soon as possible, as many perished from want of medical help and "the want of physicians is painfully felt." This and other similar pleas were apparently heard, for a report of August 15 indicated that $13,000 had already been given by the people of New York City. Another report indicated that the Howard Association had received $25,426 from New Yorkers to be distributed to yellow fever sufferers, while H.W. Hill, a New Orleans planter, pledged $100 a week to the Howard Association for as long as the disease lasted. Ironically, Mr. Hill died on November 17 from yellow fever (leaving property estimated at $1,600,000). By mid–July to mid–August, the Howard Association had ministered to the wants of 3,000 unfortunates and they expected soon to add another 1,000 at a cost of $10 each. Interestingly, at the same time, it was noted that contributions to the Washington Monument at the Crystal Palace had reached $1,411.54.

Getting personnel and supplies to the city proved more difficult than merely sending money, however, as firms found it impossible to man crews to New Orleans ports, and all ships departing there were strictly quarantined as news spread that several steamboats destined for St. Louis and Cincinnati reported heavy losses from the disease.[6]

Scenes from a New Orleans Hospital

In one room I visited there were about forty females. They are placed in cots on either side of the room, with just enough room between the cots for the attendants to give the poor sufferers their medicines. On one cot was a mother who had just died of the black vomit; in the next cot the daughter was not only suffering with the fever, but what must she have suffered in her mind on seeing the lifeless body of her mother! On another cot was a young woman from Tennessee (the *only* American in the hospital.).... On one side of her was a woman raving mad, with the black vomit, and *lashed down* to her cot....

In the room below were about forty men in the various stages of the disease. There were some three or four tier of cots, in this room. Many of the sufferers had the black vomit, others were raving and lashed down to their cots. Some were groaning, others cursing, and a few quite quiet. How any of the patients can ever get well, surrounded as they are with the dead and dying, and obliged to see every dead body as it is removed, is truly surprising. No doubt many die from fright, and others, no matter how calm they may be, most lose all hope and give up in despair. As soon as life is out of the body, they are put into a rough box made by the prisoners in the workhouse. This box is painted black with lamp black. The Corporation carts back up to the Hospital, the boxes or coffins are taken into them— say from three to four at a load—and they are thus taken through our streets, without even a cover to the cart, or anything covered over the coffins.[7]

In addressing the high mortality among foreigners, Professor DeBow of Washington, D.C., stated that between 1844 and 1850 total admissions to the Charity Hospital were 60,000, of which only 700 were citizens of Louisiana, 10,000 were from other states and nearly 50,000 were foreigners. In 1849 admissions to the Charity Hospital were 18,680, of which 248 were citizens, 1,500 were from other states and over 15,000 were foreigners; in 1850 there were 9,680 deaths in the city, of which only 1,000 were citizens. The annual average medical expense was $60,000; the state paid between $15,000 and $20,000, or nearly 30 percent, while its share of patients was slightly over 1 percent. For 1853 DeBow estimated the death toll could reach 7,000 and require charity for 30,000 cases, "half of which will be necessities, $100,000 from all sources."

Yellow fever showed no abatement. For the third week in August the board of health reported that out of 1,580 deaths, 1,350 were from the fever. With so many bodies brought for burial, fights broke out among families and friends claiming precedence. In consequence, the mayor and the recorder were obliged to send a large force to many cemeteries to keep order. Nor was Natchez in any better condition, as steamers from New Orleans were supposed to have brought up the disease. Although its population was only 5,000, mortality there had reached 200 by mid–August. Vicksburg was also said to be in a similar condition, while physicians at Mobile blamed cases there on ships arriving from New Orleans with yellow fever aboard.

In the same vein, the *New York Tribune* ran an article, "Will the Yellow Fever Be Brought to New York?" It warned that bodies from the Charity Hospital were being put into coffins naked and their clothing sold to the highest bidder. In order to disguise the origin of the clothes, these rag speculators put the soiled items in casks and shipped them to other states, where they were sold. With an eye toward money rather than human misery, the newspaper feared that if the rags caused an epidemic, "It would be a terrible calamity there—as it would disorganize the business of the whole nation—for New York is now the king ruler of American commerce." When word of this report on rags reached New Orleans the newspapers, including the *Crescent*, denied and ridiculed the charge, the latter expressing great indignation that the city was reported as a community of "Yahoos."

Also from New York came a quarrel between the *Daily Times* and the *Evening Post*. The latter published a story on August 15 stating that 10–12 cases of yellow fever were then at the Quarantine Hospital. The former sent a reporter to check the report's verity and discovered there were no cases at the hospital but that two weeks earlier a ship from New Orleans had some deaths on the voyage up. Charging the *Post* with having an "evil eye of omen" and being alarmist, the *Times* concluded there was nothing more than the "ghost" of yellow fever in New York.

For the 48 hours ending August 22 the New Orleans Board of Health reported 469 deaths from yellow fever. While Nashville was sending $3,261 to the relief fund and the New York Life Insurance Company sent $250 to the Howard Association, private dispatches indicated that tar cans were burning through the streets and cannon were fired in an attempt to break the chain of disease.[8]

Mortality in New Orleans, 1853

Week Ending	Other Deaths	Yellow Fever	Total
May 28	139	1	140
June 4	141	1	142
June 11	150	4	154
June 18	146	1	147
June 25	158	9	167
July 2	152	25	177
July 9	129	50	188 [179]*
July 16	149	201	344 [350]*
July 23	188	429	617
July 30	188	692	880
August 6	105	1,033	1,186 [1,138]*

Week Ending	Other Deaths	Yellow Fever	Total
August 13	163	1,369	1,252 [1,532]*
August 20	109	1,365	1,535 [1,474]*
Total	2,004 [1,917]	5,201 [5,180]	7,208 [7,097]*[9]

(*addition corrected)

Charity Hospital Report for Five Weeks

Date	Admissions	Deaths	Yellow Fever Deaths
July 29	570	218	207
August 5	547	218	307
August 12	592	282	286
August 19	198	372	214
August 26	271	168	157

Total interments from May12 until August 27 were 8,591, of which 6,442 were attributed to yellow fever.

Charitable Contributions to the Howard Association, August 23, 1853

From the Citizens of Washington	$2,000
From the Mayor of Washington	$1,300
From the City Council of Charleston	$2,000
From the Citizens of Savannah	$1,000[10]

Receipts for the Washington Monument as of September 1853 were $2,158.30.

The Plague City of the West

"The Plague City of the West" was the title editors of the London paper *Nonconformist* gave to an article on New Orleans on September 7, 1853. After giving a summary of the yellow fever epidemic with statistics, entries from private journals, and notices from select Crescent City newspapers (noting that the *Delta* did attempt to describe the horrors in words but it was "too repulsive for quotation"), the article contained one circumstance that "frightfully illustrates the moral condition of this city of vice and slavery"

> No sound was there of sorrow within that wide Gehenna. Men used to the scent of dissolution had forgotten all touch of sympathy. Uncouth labourers, with their bare shock heads, stood under the broiling heat of the sun, digging in the earth; and as anon they would encounter an obstructing root or stump, would swear a hideous oath, remove to another spot, and go on digging as before. The fumes rise up in deathly exhalations from the accumulating hecatombs of fast coming corpses. Men wear at their noses bags of camphor and odorous spices—for there are crowds there who have no business but to look on and contemplate the vast congregation of the dead. They don't care if they die themselves—they have become used to the reek of corruption. They even laugh at the riotings of the skeleton Death, and crack jokes in the horrid atmosphere where scarcely they can draw breath for utterance.

On the subject of interments, rumors persisted that, due to the increasing number of dead, conditions were desperate enough that burning bodies in mass bonfires had been resorted to. While the papers indignantly denied those reports, others were reminded that in Imperial Rome, burning the dead and preserving their ashes "was *the* mark of honor. Inasmuch, too, as burning adds to the health of those who survive, there are many considerations which could show that the ancient fashion was more appropriate than the decaying form with clods of earth."

Mortality in September began to reflect a gradual diminution. While the number of yellow fever interments for the week ending August 27 were 1,352, by the first week of September that number had been reduced to 767. Reports of deaths among steamboat passengers, however, continued to appear with some regularity. The *H.D. Bacon* arrived in Iowa with a number of clerks suffering from the disease. The *Michigan* arrived at St. Louis with 24 cases aboard, not counting six of the crew and one passenger who were left at Natchez (which was still suffering as many as 22 deaths per day) when it was discovered they were infected. Both vessels had departed New Orleans and concerns persisted that the epidemic would spread along the waterways with increasing fatalities.

There was cause for concern. At Vicksburg it was estimated there were 250 cases in mid–September and many of the planters on the river refused to sell wood to the steamers because they were afraid of going aboard to collect their bills. At Warrenton, Hard Times, Fort Adams and Rodney the locals remained free of disease but those towns were used as dropping-off points for steamboats ridding themselves of the sick and the dying. At Grand Gulf one-half of the residents "had been taken down," with 13 deaths in six days. At Port Gibson, eight miles from Grand Gulf, yellow fever was considered more malignant than at New Orleans and a chapter of the Howard Association was formed to help those in need. Fayette, an inland town, was considered under the influence of an epidemic. Nor were the plantations along the waterways immune; those within a radius of 8–15 miles from Port Gibson reported as many as 13 cases.[11]

For the week ending October 8, there were 58 yellow fever interments in New Orleans and the board of health ceased issuing daily reports.[12] That did not mean all was well, however. In a reflective editorial from the *Logansport* (IN) *Journal* of October 1, 1853, the writer observed that between 1830 and 1840 the population of the city increased from 46,310 to 103,193, being a greater rate of increase than Cincinnati and twice as that of great as Boston, Philadelphia or New York. From 1840 to 1850 the scourge of yellow fever operated as a serious check on population growth. While Boston added 43,000, Cincinnati 69,000, Philadelphia 150,000 and New York 203,000, New Orleans added a mere 17,000.

A few healthy seasons restored confidence and from June 1850 until July 1853 the city added as many to its population as the whole preceding ten years: "But on a sudden the pleasing anticipation of its citizens are nipped in the bud; the pestilence comes down on them like those terrible visitations of the plague." The editorialist concluded, not without justification, "There must be stronger inducements than those of ordinary success in business, to induce men to face the horrors of the *black vomit*."

Charity for the Sufferers

The outpouring of money for the sufferers of the 1853 New Orleans epidemic was a tribute to the generosity of the nation. On September 12 the Howard Association issued its latest report, stating the amount of contributions received from those in New York and the surrounding areas. Among the largest donors were the Crystal Palace ($1,823), Niblo's Garden ($1,207) and the Ladies of Newport ($1,028). Numerous churches and individuals were also cited, bringing the total to $5,147.00.

With the Howard Association's name appearing in so many papers, people were curious to know more about it. J.O. Harris, a member of the association, offered additional particulars in a September 26 article. He explained that the body, chartered by the state, was composed of 30 members, all of whom worked without salary. It had been in existence under the present name for 16 years; before that it had been called the "Samaritan Society." Their mission was to devote their time to the indigent sick whenever the board of health declared the existence of an epidemic in the city. They received no funds from the state but were entirely dependent on the generosity of charitable people. By 1853 the Howard Association had established charter offices in numerous cities around the country that were called into action whenever an epidemic struck.

Although the New Orleans City Council neglected to elect a board of health at their meeting in May, the Howard Association organized for duty on the 27th of June. The next week a board of health was elected, a majority being selected from the Howard membership. Up until September 26 Harris estimated the number of sick taken in charge by the association to be 10,000, at a cost of $14–15 each. Of this number, 2,000 died. The association maintained five infirmaries, each with two physicians and nurses, and two convalescent hospitals, although Harris estimated that most of their patients were taken care of in their own residences. The association also ran three orphan asylums. During the epidemic, local representatives were maintained in the outlying cities of Carrollton, Jefferson City, Gretna, McDonoughville and Algiers.

At the termination of the epidemic, the Howard Association distributed its surplus funds to city institutions, including the Orphan's Home ($7,600), Camp Street Female Orphan Asylum ($3,400), St. Mary's Catholic Orphan Asylum ($4,000) and the Hebrew Benevolent Association ($400). Contributions from San Francisco to the sufferers in New Orleans amounted to $10,000, which reached the city after the epidemic had ended. The major distributed the money among the various orphan asylums and other benevolent institutions.

New Orleans was not the only city to receive charitable contributions from across the nation. The total subscription for those suffering in Mobile reached $9,232, of which $3,146 came from New York and $5,982 was received from local companies and citizens.[13]

Yellow fever struck Mobile in early July 1853, traced to a ship that had sailed from Portland, Maine, to New Orleans and then to Mobile Bay. By the second week in August newspapers believed the disease was of the mild type but by the end of the month it had reached epidemic proportions. Beginning August 21 the mayor ordered burning tar, pitch and rosin, but these measures proved to be of little worth. By the week ending August 26, thirty-seven were dead; the following week, that number rose to 156 and the week after that 194 died.

One of Mobile's main hotels, the Battle House, closed the first week of September and that same week the major ordered a day of humiliation and prayer. Nothing helped and by the second week in August the disease had spread from the center of the city to the outskirts. In a significant observation, Dr. Nott later wrote, "I have many times seen my little children lying in a trundle-bed covered by mosquitoes...." In fact, the *Mobile Register* of May 14, 1853, noted mosquitoes were "pests and plagues of each man's home." Although mosquito netting was frequently used around beds, it was not typically used to cover open windows, creating easy access for the disease-laden insects.

The year 1853 proved to be the worst for Mobile. By Dr. Nott's estimate, from the beginning of August to the middle of December almost 1,200 people had perished out of a summer population of little more than 12,500.[14]

Coffee (Again), Fresh Dirt and Humor

Proving that old theories faded but never disappeared, residents of Fulton, situated on the Ouachita River in the interior of Louisiana, blamed the presence of yellow fever in their midst from a consignment of coffee, shipped direct from Rio by way of New Orleans. Another theory reappearing in 1854 pertained to the contamination of soil. The *New Orleans Picayune* of October 10 carried a story from the *Bayou Sara Ledger* remarking that yellow fever had broken out there. The crux of the article, however, was contained in the concluding sentence, beginning with the fact the weather was quite favorable for health, "but no matter what beneficial results might arise from a pure atmosphere, we think all can be very easily counteracted by the fresh dirt that is now being hauled in to level our sidewalks."

Substantiating another truth that humor could be found in the grimmest situations, the *New Orleans Crescent* published a story on August 29 under the heading, "A New Cure for Fever." According to the story, "an empyrical physician" was called to treat a Frenchman who was dying of yellow fever. Demanding as his last wish a dish of herrings and molasses, the doctor supplied him with this food. "Strange to tell the Frenchman got well, in spite of his physician and the molasses and herrings." The doctor wrote in his notebook, "Herrings and molasses good for yellow fever in the case of a Frenchman." The doctor was then called upon to treat a Dutchman; straightaway he ordered herrings with molasses sauce. The man promptly died and the doctor wrote in his book, "Herrings and molasses *not good* for yellow fever where the patient is a Dutchman."

In typical New Orleans fashion, under the heading of "The Ruling Passion," the story was told of a noted gambler in the city whose favorite expression was "I'll bet you." When told by a doctor that he was dying of yellow fever and had but three hours to live, he remarked, "I'll bet you my funeral expenses, that I will live *six* hours, just double what you assign me." The doctor accepted the bet and the gambler lived through the six hours. "While chuckling over his triumph, [he] was seized with the spasm and died." A second bit of humor had to do with a stage manager from New Orleans who went to Paris in search of *"prime donne* and other melodious attractions." He made an offer to Mme. Cabel and was on the verge of signing the "treaty" when her husband expressed concern over the yellow fever then raging in the city. He was not worried for himself, he avowed, but was afraid his wife might be stricken. The manager quickly reassured him by remarking, "The fever never seizes any body but men." The contract was never signed.[15]

Yellow Fever, 1854: The Southern Disease

Reports from New Orleans as early as June 1854 indicated a sickly city. The primary disease was cholera, taking over 50 souls a week; the last week in the month over 220 were reported dead. Complicating matters, by July 3 yellow fever had made its appearance, with three reported dead. Dr. Luke Blackburn was again involved in establishing quarantine for the city, but the disease spread quickly and by early September, convinced that an epidemic was in the making, the Howard Association commenced taking care of patients.

Mortality in New Orleans, 1854

For the Week Ending	Number of Deaths
August 13	66
August 20	118
August 27	187
September 10	78
September 17	340
September 24	341
October 1	269
October 8	202
November 5	42
November 19	169

According to the board of health, final mortality reached 2,425.[16] Complicating matters, on Sunday, September 10, a political riot broke out in New Orleans "between the citizens and watchmen. The latter are mostly Irish, and the cause was taken up by the countrymen of the latter." The American party assembled in front of city hall and marched to the foreign quarters, "where the battle raged violently." Irregular fighting spilled over into Monday and Tuesday, muskets being fired on both sides, and the mayor ordered out the national guard. The toll for the unrest was at least seven dead.[17]

News dated May 24, 1854, indicated yellow fever had been "raging" for several weeks at Key West, "several" people having fallen victim. The disease was considered of local origin. By July 22 it was considered to have entirely disappeared but the situation altered on September 12 when the *Edwin Flye,* en route to Liverpool, arrived "in distress," as yellow fever had broken out two days after it left New Orleans. Captain Hitchcock and five of the crew had died onboard and it was said the ship would proceed under the mate once the crew had been replaced.[18]

By the end of August yellow fever had broke out at Charleston; reports indicated all but three of the victims were foreigners. A week later, as "great uneasiness was manifested," authorities made plans to open a yellow fever hospital should the disease become epidemic. Fears were confirmed, for in the week ending September 11 seventy-six deaths were attributed to the malady; between September 15 and the 17th an additional 29 deaths were reported. By the end of the month the fever was said to be abating.

Total Mortality in Savannah, 1854

Month	Whites	Blacks
August	235	22
September	541	55
October	108	79

Early in an epidemic causes of death were often ascribed to other diseases, so actual mortality from yellow fever was likely higher than given.

Yellow Fever Mortality in Savannah, 1854

Month	Whites	Blacks
August	132	22
September	381	9
October	67	4

The epidemic at Savannah commenced August 3; by September 12 conditions were said to be "horrible," as deaths from yellow fever continued to mount. Business was at a

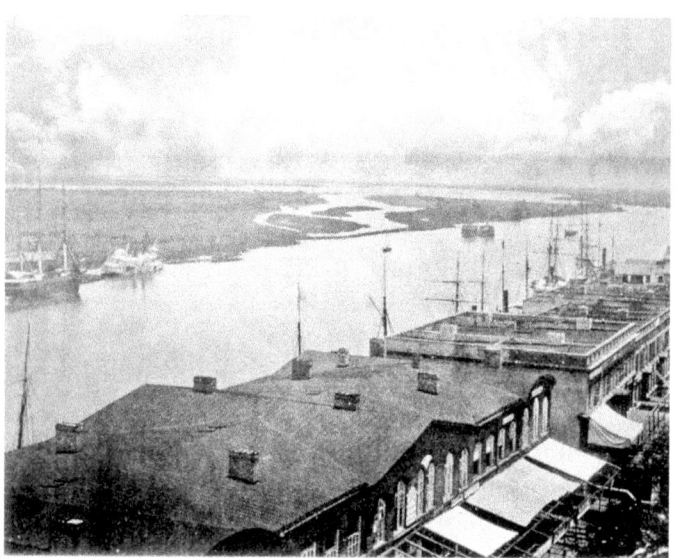

Savannah, Georgia, was often host to yellow fever epidemics. Plentiful swamps and hot summers provided breeding grounds for the *Aedes albopictus,* or yellow fever mosquito. Before 1900, most states had strict quarantine rules against those cities and ports identified as harboring yellow fever cases. To prevent the introduction of the disease, those states prone to infection also established lengthy quarantine periods of up to two weeks for passengers and cargo arriving from infected ports (National Park Service).

standstill and "there were not enough hands to bury the dead." By September 19, $1,030 had been collected in charitable contributions from the people of New York and by mid-month total contributions had reached $10,000. By September 23 (some sources place the date as late as November) "Yellow Jack" was "killed" when frost made its appearance. Other cities suffering epidemics were Augusta, Staten Island (between 40 and 50 at the Quarantine Hospital in late September), Galveston and Montgomery, Alabama.[19]

On a side note, the New York hotels were filled with southerners escaping the various outbreaks. One correspondent reflected on the old adage "circumstances alter cases," referring to the eagerly awaited frost in the South that would kill the yellow fever, while New England farmers "look solemn and sad" at an early frost because it killed their cranberries.

On the issue of quarantine, an interesting editorial was written in the *New-York Daily Times* (April 11, 1854) concerning a case of yellow fever aboard the *Empire Steamer*, which left Havana on March 29. Apparently a passenger was taken aboard "in health" but developed symptoms soon afterward. The ship arrived at New York on April 4 and the officer of quarantine took the captain's word "that the vessel had been entirely free from sickness on her voyage" and allowed the ship to come up without inspection. The sick passenger died the next day. A coroner's jury was convened, and the officer of quarantine was quickly censured. The editorialist noted that when ships were entering port it was not uncommon for the sick to scrape their tongues, take tonics and "walk the deck" to deceive health inspectors, not wishing to be the cause of detaining passengers and cargo in quarantine. As the captain had sworn there was no sickness aboard, the reporter also noted it was typical for officers to accept the captain's word rather than go to the trouble of a full inspection. He politely concluded that at best all parties were deceived and at worst it represented a serious dereliction of duty. On a further look at quarantine, during September the United States mail steamship *Florida* arrived at New York from Savannah, where yellow fever was raging. The ship was detained at Staten Island, but the mail was permitted to be sent into the city without delay.[20] This time no comment was made about a breach of quarantine.

Chapter 17

"To the manor born"

It is now 9 o'clock p.m. and I have just got back to my office, after being necessarily engaged since 5 o'clock this morning. I have seen and prescribed for over one hundred patients today and every moment new calls are made upon me, and the most urgent [pleas] used to [summon] me to see a father, mother, brother or other friend. But I can go no further. I am completely exhausted, and must have a little rest to enable me to resume the duties of the morrow, if, perchance, I am spared in health.

I am no alarmist, and have no disposition to exaggerate, and certainly no wish to harrow the feelings of any one by the mental scenes of distress, but it would sicken anyone to know what is now transpiring in our town. Whole families are down, without the ability in many cases to procure a drop of water to cool their fevered lips. Alas, alas for poor Portsmouth. Oh God, how long.[1]

Yellow fever made an extremely early appearance in 1855, with the first cases reported at New Orleans and Vicksburg in late April. This elicited fears of a severe visitation and authorities in towns along the inland rivers took steps, "so far as human means can do," to prevent what many suspected would be an epidemic year. One of these steps included quarantine and in May the *Picayune* expressed pleasure to see all the necessary arrangements and measures pushed forward.

The reappearance of the disease again brought into question its origin. The *Commercial Bulletin* deduced from the prevailing medical reports issued by the sanitary committee and opinions issued by the medical community that in New Orleans, it was "eight to two against the theory of importation. If the question then is to be determined by the weight of numbers, it is no longer a moot point. Yellow fever is endemic to New Orleans," or "to the manor born," and was likely to persist in spite of boards of health and quarantine regulations.[2]

This argument was taken up by the *New Orleans Bulletin*, which argued that quarantine to prevent its introduction or importation was useless. In support, the newspaper quoted the *Medical News and Hospital Gazette,* which offered the fact that the first official case appeared on May 3; the victim was an Irishman who took sick coming down the river and had no communication with shipping. The next case appeared June 15, forty-three days after the first. The man named Draugod was a German who emigrated through Liverpool and had worked in a beer saloon ever since his arrival six weeks earlier. There was no evidence of his "having caught" the disease from any person or bale of goods. In the cases of several more Germans and Irish, most were new to the city and in no way exposed to the fever, leading credence to a local source of infection.

The *Commercial Bulletin* of August 8 took the argument in a different direction, pointing out a peculiar feature of yellow fever its regularity and uniformity of duration. During its presence in New Orleans, there was always a gradual rise to a culminating point and then a corresponding decline and fall, with the average duration of an outbreak averaging 60–70 days.[3]

Mortality in New Orleans, 1855

Date	Total Deaths	Deaths from Yellow Fever
July 8	160	32
July 15	187	44
July 22	240	119
July 29	275	73
August 19	517	394
August 26	471	357
October 14	120	24[4]

One report indicated that from the beginning of the epidemic to September 9, a period of nine weeks, 1,649 of the unacclimated perished from yellow fever.[5] A second noted that during the month of August 1,599 deaths occurred from yellow fever:

Nationality of Yellow Fever Victims, New Orleans, August 1855

Native Americans	170
Irish	424
German	386
Unknown place of birth	349
French	151
English	27[6]

By October 16, newspapers advised that absentees could now return without danger. Of significance, the *Delta* also reported that in more than 3,000 cases during that season, inoculation for yellow fever "has been tested, and with entire success." On the economic front, the president of the Vicksburg, Shreveport and Texas Railroad Company announced the contractors Messers. Fannin, Grant & Co. had "a large force of negroes coming out from Georgia, so soon as the yellow fever subsides on the Mississippi." And for those wishing a cure for fever and ague, there was "Dr. W.T. Owen's Pills." The manufacturer did not claim "miraculous and wonderful cures in ALL diseases" but did promise to offer suffering humanity a "safe, sure, and speedy remedy" not "composed of cheap ingredients and made by machinery, for the purpose of making money" but consisting of "costly and pure drugs" that could not be sold "at such prices as are generally set on patent pills."[7]

Perhaps the ultimate expression of yellow fever was carried in the newspaper exchanges in 1857: "In New Orleans, it is said, that 'it requires three persons to start a business firm; one to die with the yellow fever; one to get killed in a duel, and a third to wind up the business."[8] In 1859, the joke was slightly amended: "It takes three editors to start a paper in New Orleans—one to get killed in a duel, one to die with the yellow fever, and one to write an obituary of the defunct two."[9]

The "Other" Epidemic of 1855: Portsmouth, Virginia

Americans had grown to expect yearly visitations of yellow fever at New Orleans and Mobile, but in 1855 they were stunned and horrified to hear how that disease ravaged

Portsmouth and the surrounding environs. The tragic set of events began innocently enough. On July 25 the newspapers reported 18 cases of yellow fever at Portsmouth, thought to have been brought there by the steamer *Benjamin Franklin* out of St. Thomas. At this point, the disease was confined to the Navy Yard (Gosport Shipyard; the name was changed to the Norfolk Naval Shipyard in 1862). By August 27 two deaths had occurred and three new cases diagnosed. One day later, the dead reached 18, with 34 new cases, all traceable to Gosport.

Not atypically, the *Richmond Enquirer* denied the presence of yellow fever, claiming the disease to be no more than "some few cases of ship fever." The state, it claimed, was "as healthy now as at any former period." Unfortunately, the newspaper's sources proved to be incorrect. By August 3, the sanitary committee indicated that within the previous 24 hours there had been 10 new cases and 8 more deaths. "Quite a panic prevailed," stores were closed and "without exaggeration, one third of the citizens of Portsmouth had left the place." By August 11 newspaper exchanges reported one-half of the population had abandoned the city, leaving behind the Sisters of Charity to care for the sick. The Norfolk pest-house contained 60 cases and was soon overrun, forcing authorities to place tents outside to accommodate the sick. When this proved inadequate, they procured the Race Field building. To alleviate overcrowding, the secretary of the navy gave the Sanitary Commission of Portsmouth permission to send the sick from that city and Gosport to the Naval Hospital, which quickly admitted 40 patients.

Relief for the afflicted was quickly organized. On August 13 a subscription begun at Baltimore raised $2,200 and it was expected to reach $3,000, while a Howard Association, similar to the one in New Orleans, was organized to aid the sick and distribute the collected funds. Members of the New York Corn Exchange forwarded $2,500 to Virginia. Money was also collected from Washington ($1,000) and Philadelphia ($3,600), while $3,116 was received from local Norfolk businessmen.

By August 23 the local Howard Association was paying $600 per day for provisions and there was "no falling off" as many waited their turn to be served. One estimate put the number dependent on charity at 600 families. The association, however, expected quid pro quo, asking those able to work to serve as nurses or carry out other assignments "Those unwilling are sent about their business. The consequence is that the number of nurses is daily increasing."[10]

In addition, women from as far away as New York volunteered as nurses. Miss Andrews, from Syracuse, wrote of her service at Norfolk: "Deaths are occurring all around us, new cases are multiplying hourly, and our means of treating them are hourly diminishing. This you will more readily understand when I tell you I am doing the duties of two physicians (Drs. Schoolfield and Maupin) besides my own, which are sufficiently numerous and onerous to occupy me unnecessarily, and God knows how long I shall be able to do what I am doing. I shall continue at the laboring oar until I fall."[11]

By August 18 deaths at Portsmouth averaged 8 every day out of the remaining population of 2,000, while at Norfolk 30 new cases were reported in one day, with 9 deaths. As a means of preventing the disease from spreading, the secretary of the navy ordered that no workman who left the Portsmouth Navy Yard (the force being reduced from 1,800 to 600 since the start of the epidemic) be employed in the Washington Yard. This action was expected to delay the construction of two frigates and various other public works.[12] A correspondent from the *Baltimore American* (August 23) offered a commercial point of view from Norfolk:

> **CHOLERA AND YELLOW FEVER.**
>
> Malarial Miasmatic and contagious or Epidemic Diseases, and many ailments attending change of climate, food and water, may be entirely prevented by wearing a Cuticura Plaster over the pit of the stomach, with frequent changes, whenever exposed to these affection. A cure by absorption is effected by it when all other plasters fail. It is the best plaster known to physicians and druggists. At druggists, 25.; five for $1.00. Mailed free Potter Drug and Chemical Co., Boston.

The idea of wearing a form of cummerbund or a plaster around the stomach was an often-used practice to prevent yellow fever, primarily because many doctors and laymen believed the disease had a digestive or intestinal origin (*Shelbyville* [Indiana] *Evening Democrat*, **July 3, 1885).**

> A Sabbath stillness prevails, broken only by the rattle of the doctors' chaises, and the rumbling of the hearse and sick wagon. Scarcely a store is open on Main-street, Market square, or Broad Water street, the business portions of the city. The apothecaries have removed with their pills, plasters and drugs, to their residences, and *mirabilis dictu!* so have the brokers! There is not a quorum of directors in either of the Banks; only two or three of the city fathers are in the city; preachers look around their churches in vain for their parishioners, newspapers daily accumulate on doorsteps and on porches for want of readers, gaunt poverty stalks abroad with downcast look and tearful eye; the wail of the widow and of the orphan startles the solitary passenger, and all its gloom and grief, almost without hope.[13]

Dr. J.C. Nott of Mobile wrote in 1855 that he had predicted there would be an outbreak of yellow fever at Norfolk and thought it probable the disease would break out in New York either that summer or the next. Nott originally believed yellow fever was not contagious, but in 1853, when that diseased raged in Mobile, he brought a patient from the city to Spring Hill, where his family stayed during the epidemic. Although he was never positive this victim introduced the disease to Spring Hill, the fact remained that soon afterward yellow fever broke out, eventually taking four of his own children.[14] This prompted a slight alteration in his views on quarantine. In an article published in the *National Intelligencer,* he wrote the following:

> Although my mind leans at present toward a belief in the contagiousness of *this* disease in certain instances I still doubt, and my judgment is in suspense; but with regard to its *portability* by vessels from place to place, and by railroads, I do not see how any human being familiar with its history can doubt, and *I should advise our Northern friends to quarantine rigidly against it. The disease has gone to every port within a certain distance of the Gulf which was frequented by steamboats and railroad cars,* and I believe would have entered New York in 1853, had it not been stopped at the Quarantine.[15]

According to Nott, since the fever's first appearance at Rio Janeiro in 1850, it traveled along the Caribbean Gulf and Atlantic coasts until reaching Norfolk, "which is about the boundary of the yellow fever latitude." He believed it was essentially the same disease that occurred at Philadelphia in 1793 and subsequently appeared with different grades of violence afterward. He reiterated that bleeding and active purgation or emetics were "worse than useless," while cold drinks and cold sponging were refreshing but had "no specific virtue in controlling this Herculean disease."[16]

The New York City Committee for the Relief of Norfolk and Portsmouth met on August 25, having collected $3,000 for yellow fever victims, which they resolved to transmit to the mayor of Norfolk. Another $1,000 was collected from the officers at the Navy Yard, while Niblo's (by this time a major New York music center) donated 200 tickets for the Teresa Parodi concert to be held August 28. (Parodi debuted at the Astor Place Opera House November 4, 1850, in *Norma*. By August 1855 she was in the middle of her highly successful operatic tour. Accompanying her in the benefit were her touring companions Maurice and Amalia Patti Srakosch; joining them were Aptommas, Bernardi, Julius Siede and Allan Irving, among others. On October 6, the Pyne/Harrison troupe, with Bristow conducting and with the full participation of Niblo's forces, donated a gala performance for the yellow fever victims.)[17] The citizens of Baltimore collected $44,889, Frederick County, Virginia, sent $1,360 and the Odd Fellows of various lodges in Virginia added $1,642. By September 18 Simon S. Stubbs, mayor of Norfolk, wrote that good Samaritans from abroad had placed at the disposal of the Howard Association $100,000. This helped cover its expenses, which averaged $2,500–$3,000 a day. President Franklin Pierce's cabinet contributed $325 to the cause. For his part, Pierce permitted the commandant of the Gosport Navy Yard to close the yard and advance a month's pay to all employees who wished to leave. How-

> **BOSTON MUSIC HALL.**
> —A—
> **GRAND CONCERT**
> —OF—
> **Vocal and Instrumental Music!**
> Will be given under the patronage of
> **His Excellency the Governor**
> AND
> **His Honor the Mayor,**
> On MONDAY EVENING, the 16th Oct., 1876, in aid of the suffering people of Savannah and other cities of the South, now terribly afflicted by the yellow fever scourge. It is intended, and its projectors promise to make it one of the most pleasant and entertaining Concerts to be given in Boston this winter. The talent and attractions to be presented ought to be sufficient of themselves alone to fill any Hall in Boston, but when the proceeds are to be devoted for a most worthy and charitable object, and the price of admission placed within the means of all benevolent persons, it is hoped and expected that every ticket will be disposed of. The tickets will be placed at the low price of fifty cents each, so that all can aid in this philanthropic and worthy object.
> Full particulars will shortly be announced.
>
> **STEREOPTICON ENTERTAINMENTS**

Americans were generous people, and it was not uncommon in the 19th century for people in distant states to collect money for the relief of suffering countrymen. This was especially the case when cities were beset by devastating epidemics. One specific method used to raise funds was through the performing arts. Actors held benefits, circus performers passed the hat and concerts were offered, all with the aim of collecting funds to be used to buy food and medicine and pay for doctors' services (*Boston Globe*, September 30, 1876).

ever, he turned down the request of the Norfolk Committee to use Fort Monroe as a refuge for the locals because of the time required to remove the troops and there being no suitable place for their reception.[18]

Many physicians and nurses also volunteered their time at Norfolk; of the fourteen who arrived from Philadelphia, seven were stricken by the fever and three died. Those still able to attend the sick gathered at the Crawford House, the principal hotel of Norfolk and headquarters of the sanitary commission, to discuss cases and compare observations. Lacking a universally agreed-upon system of practice, methods often varied widely and with different degrees of success; the only point upon which they could agree was that good nursing was indispensable.

While Mr. Merriam of Brooklyn proposed by scientific operations "to get up artificial frosts to kill off the yellow fever," the weather remained "close, humid and suffocating, with an average temperature of 80°." No peculiar odors were observed but a stretch of marshy ground was believed to be an inciting cause of the malady. A peculiarity of the fever was that soon after the attack "the skin of the *white* patients takes on a yellowish tinge similar to that of a lemon or orange. *Black* patients undergo a similar metamorphosis—their hue changing to bronze. In all cases, the progress of the fever is very rapid and very often fatal."

Dr. Stone of New Orleans declared the fever to be similar to that seen in New Orleans in 1853, given the name *la peste* by the Creoles. However, in his opinion the present epidemics differed from the "old type of yellow fever in manner of attack, in treatment required, and in the celerity with which the work of death is performed—many of its victims dying within a few hours of their attack." He suggested wrapping the patient in ice, followed by hot mustard applications, the object being to produce perspiration. Very little internal medicine was required, except for a slight tonic.[19]

One member of the Ward Visiting Committee at Norfolk noted the following: "Many families have shut themselves in with but a scant supply of provisions, waiting in terror for an attack of the fever, and when attacked they have been in some cases without assistance or even the common necessities of life, and know not where to get them, having completely shut themselves off from the outer world. Indeed, gossiping has even been at a stand still in Norfolk among the lower classes, some not even allowing any one to speak to them for fear that their breath may be charged with the pestilence." The same correspondent added that some estimated the number of death to be 2,000, while others believed the number closer to 1,500. In either case, out of a population of 6,000 he considered the mortality of greater proportion "than has ever before occurred in the ravages of a pestilence within the bounds of civilization."[20]

Adding to the despondency, the weather continued unfavorably and Mr. Ferguson, the president of the Howard Association, died of the disease. On another note, during a day of thanksgiving in Richmond for sparing the city, "the Roman Catholic Bishop, McGill, availed himself of the occasion to insinuate that the cities of Norfolk and Portsmouth were desolated by the yellow fever as *a judgment of Almighty God* to punish their inhabitants for voting the American ticket last spring. Unfortunately for the Bishop's 'argument,' the Mayor of Norfolk, when the fever broke out, was a Catholic, and was one of the victims of the fever. Besides, how happens it that Richmond, Fredericksburg and Alexandria, all of which gave the American ticket large majorities, have not been visited by the yellow fever."[21]

A different view of Americana of the mid–19th century came from John Wise, the famous aeronaut. In order to dispel the miasmic atmosphere of Norfolk and Portsmouth he suggested exploding gunpowder from cannons "to produce atmospheric waves that would travel hundreds of miles." Aided by large fires, this would "put the atmosphere in motion, driving the infected air off, and receiving the pure from abroad." He also recommended fumigating infected houses with chlorine gas or chloride of lime.[22]

The Strange Case of the Crescent City *and the Ire of Baltimore*

The *Crescent City* arrived at New York on Thursday, September 13. After the ship surgeon informed the health officer yellow fever had prevailed during the passage, the steamer was ordered into quarantine for 30 days. Applications from the ship were immediately made for the purpose of bringing the vessel into the wharves of the city, which were refused. On Saturday, in violation of quarantine, the ship weighed anchor and steamed into the city. On Sunday morning the health officer issued a warrant for the captain's arrest. Fernando Wood, the mayor, met with the board of health at 6:00 a.m. Monday to reiterate the order for the *Crescent City* to complete 30-day quarantine.

Although protesting his innocence, Captain Croswell was arrested and required to post $5,000 bond. Meanwhile, bargeman John Wiley took the ship to quarantine. By 3:30 p.m. two tugs went down from the city filled with passengers and cargo. The men ignored the order of the health officer, Dr. Thompson, and the vessel was loaded and quickly departed. A card (letter of explanation) was issued by the steamer's agent stating that within six hours of her arrival, all passengers had been discharged and her cargo broken ("to break bulk"—to discharge cargo), delivering only a consignment of cotton to quarantine. The agent denied there had ever been yellow fever aboard and concluded with the defense that as the steamer had a contract to deliver United States mail, the post office "forbid the idea of her remaining at Quarantine thirty days."

The idea of the *Crescent City*'s "bravery" in ignoring the order for quarantine ran rampant through the business section, forcing local newspapers to weakly comment that the action was "as generally condemned by the people as the press."[23]

Concurrently, an incident that garnered louder and greater protestations was the action of the New York Board of Health in passing a regulation that all ships from certain southern ports, including Baltimore, be inspected from the present time until November 1 for the presence of yellow fever before being allowed to enter the harbor. On September 15 J. Hincks, the mayor of Baltimore, wrote a scathing letter to Mayor Wood, calling the action "entirely uncalled for" and threatening to retaliate by "subjecting all vessels from New York to the strictest quarantine."

The *Baltimore Patriot* went further, scoffing at New Yorkers' "attempt to defend this outrageous measure, this gross violation of the amenities which should always exist between neighboring cities." Adding it could not "find language sufficiently strong to express our reprobation," the newspaper accused the city of "shamefully promulgating a regulation of quarantine" for no other reason than to steal the trade of Baltimore. In more conciliatory terms, the *Baltimore American* noted a more likely explanation stemmed from the fact the board of health had, "in a moment of timidity, given too credulous an ear to the interested statements of others, and adopted [the act] without sufficient consideration."

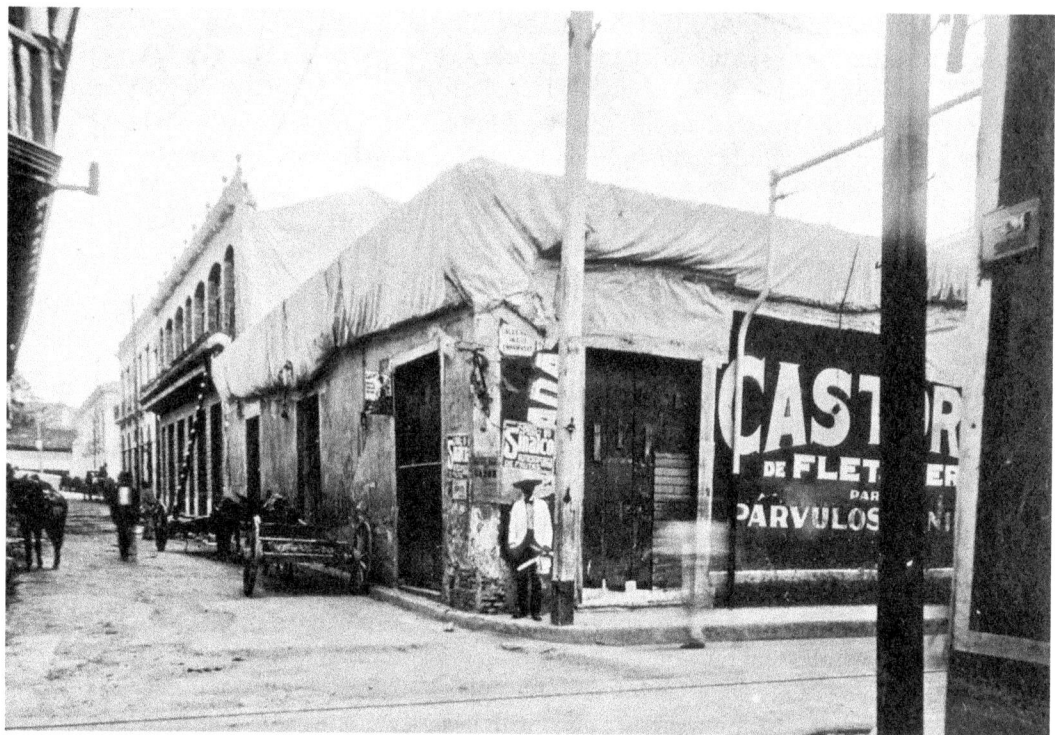

Fumigation was one way health authorities had for killing off deadly yellow fever–carrying mosquitoes. A photograph of Santiago De Cuba from 1908 demonstrates how an entire city block was covered to prevent the insecticides—and the insects—from escaping the deadly gas (courtesy National Library of Medicine).

In a rather smug rejoinder, the New York papers claimed the step "was purely one of precaution—one of self-defense, intended not to injure any other city": "But what is this terrible tax we inflict upon vessels from Baltimore? Simply this: Each vessel from that port, as she arrives, is boarded by the Health Officer; if there is no sickness on board she comes directly on—having suffered a detention of some ten minutes!" The editorial concluded: "[T]he temerity of those responsible for the *Crescent City* outrage becomes fearful, the indignation of the Baltimoreans an indecent opposition of their commercial interests to the safety of our lives; and the thoughtful prudence of our Board of Health commendable in the highest degree." The writer then asked why "railroad trains" were not quarantined and answered: "It is not personal contact that conveys the infection, nor the infected clothes of occasional passengers. Yellow fever spreads from port to port almost exclusively by means of vessels and their cargoes. The crews of quarantined vessels, after being properly examined, and when due attention has been paid to cleanliness and fumigation, are not prevented from coming on shore. If our seaboard is well guarded, we are safe."[24]

An indication of the confusion that still existed was an article in the *Times* of August 23, 1855, less than a month before the above incidents, which remarked that there remained in the city one "dangerous spot, where the disease will be most likely to fasten itself, and spread its desolating influences, [and that] is on the opposite side of the river in Brooklyn." The reporter added this:

Brooklyn is ill-prepared to resist the ravages of a pestilence. It is a large city, and it has no sewers. Each house has attached to it two disease-breeders, in a cess-pool and an out-house, and the filth thrown into the streets has festered there, creating a foul and offensive stench. Under the beautiful Heights are long ranges of warehouses, in which are stored hides and bags of guano, which render the air so offensive that one cannot walk with comfort throughout the streets that lie parallel with the Heights. A city which so abounds in fine churches and magnificent streets of private dwellings ought not to be destitute of such essential aids to health as drains and sewers. If the yellow fever manifest itself in this City next year, its ravages in Brooklyn, we believe, will be much greater than on this side of the river.

"New York: The health of this city..."

"New York: The health of this city engrosses more of the attention of those who are obliged to remain in it under the August suns than any of the public matters of the nation." This opinion, expressed by the *North-China Herald* (Shanghai, November 1, 1856, adequately summed up the situation in 1856.

By August nearly 120 vessels were anchored in the bay undergoing quarantine. All passengers from these ships were obliged to land at the health officer's wharf and from there pass out of the gates into the village or come up to the city as they desired. In consequence of these loose arrangements, one or two fatal cases of yellow fever occurred among the locals.

At Castleton Village, Staten Island, which was in the immediate vicinity of the Quarantine Marine Hospital, residents charged that their lives were in danger from the spread of yellow fever and demanded strict measures to protect their safety. Dr. Thompson, the quarantine health officer, declared there was no threat to local residents and assured them that no person coming from any vessel under quarantine was permitted to pass until he and his baggage had been made free from infection by washing and fumigation. The citizens were issatisfied, and a deputation of workmen under orders from a vigilante committee constructed a barricade "consisting of boards ten feet long, placed in perpendicular position, and so arranged as to make a semicircular enclosure of the gateway, reaching about twelve feet from the center of the gate and extending to the wall some fifteen feet on either side."

Complicating matters were the large number of hides brought in; because they were thought to be "especially favorable for spreading yellow fever" lighters (small vessels) were in short supply and some lightermen refused to work for fear of the fever. Concurrently, by the end of August yellow fever had broken out in Brooklyn but the actual number of victims was difficult to determine, as the city inspector declared there to be seven deaths while the board of health announced only "a few cases of bilious fever had come to their attention." One writer noted, "'mum is the word' at the Marine Hospital, but at Fort Hamilton and Yellow Hook," where the first victim was struck on July 26, there had been no fewer than 58 deaths, "in consequence of the large number of infected vessels anchored nearby, in Gravesend Bay." He concluded, "As yet, I am glad to say, there is but little 'Jack' in the city and as August is about over, we begin to hope to escape, altogether."

On September 2 a meeting was held by the residents of Castleton and the county of Richmond at Tompkinsville, under the chairmanship of Ray Tompkins. Among other things, the attendees resolved that, inasmuch as the population had grown since the establishment of the quarantine grounds and in light of the "utter impossibility of preventing" yellow fever from infecting the inhabitants, "humanity dictates the necessity of the removal of the whole Quarantine establishment to a much greater distance from the City for the greater protection of a million of peoples." Their choice was Sandy Hook, but unfortunately "the promontory known as Sandy Hook [lies] within the territorial limits of the State of New Jersey," and those residents were not about to harbor New York's quarantine problems.

Saratoga was harboring those well-to-do citizens fleeing New York City, but one newspaper sneered, "Saratoga has but a short time to fleece the New Yorker" during the yellow fever outbreak. The Norfolk Howard Association offered to send nurses and other assistance to Fort Hamilton, "as some acknowledgment of the services extended to the sufferers at Norfolk last summer."

By September 2 the outbreak had run its course and the disease assumed very mild characteristics. George Hall, the mayor of Brooklyn, was presented with a handsome brick dwelling and lot on Livingston Street for his part in containing the yellow fever in that city.[25]

Chapter 18

The "Quarantine War" and the "Quarantine Armada"

Health Statistics, like many other good things, are liable to misappropriation and abuse. The papers inform us that the Mutual Life Insurance Company of New York has, for some months past, been engaged in collecting statistical material with a view to ascertain the relative mortality of different portions of the United States; and that the results as compared with New York or Baltimore, the risk of life in New Orleans is more than 2 to 1. As a consequence, we are informed that the Life Insurance Companies will feel bound, in duty to their own customers, to enhance their rates on lives south of Richmond, Virginia.[1]

The Mutual Life Insurance Company of New York was apparently very industrious when it came to calculating risk. The following discussion and statistics were compiled for that company and presented in 1857. In the southern states, their agent determined that for the health of the acclimated (those used to the climate and likely to have been exposed to and survived endemic epidemics), the advantage favored the city, while for the unacclimated, the country was safer. The most prevalent diseases for city dwellers were listed as yellow fever, cholera (intestinal affections), heat, moisture, filth, bad habits, insufficient drainage and general negligence in policing; for country residents, cholera (bilious fever and intestinal diseases), intemperance, exposure to undue heat and moisture, malaria and aberrations in general and personal hygiene were primary causes of ill health and mortality.

In discussing the relative mortality between natives and strangers (American and European), reference was again made to the acclimated and unacclimated. The following table was derived from "the liabilities of each nation and people, foreign and domestic, and from the different latitudes," made from data furnished during the 1853 epidemic at New Orleans.

The Life Cost of Acclimation or Liability [Susceptibility] to Yellow Fever, as Derived from or Influenced by Nativity, Per 1,000 of Population

New Orleans and the State of Louisiana	3:58
Arkansas, Mississippi, Alabama, Georgia, South Carolina, North Carolina, Virginia, Maryland, Tennessee, Kentucky, and of this class of States, the largest mortality existing	13:22
among those coming from TN and KY	30:09

New York, Vermont, Mass., Maine, Rhode Island, Connecticut, New Jersey, Penn., Delaware,	32:83
Ohio, Indiana, Illinois, Missouri	44:23
British America	50:24
The General Average in America	**29:11**
Great Britain	52:19
Ireland	204:97
Denmark, Sweden, Russia	163:26
Prussia and Germany	132:01
Holland and Belgium	328:94
Austria and Switzerland	220:08
France	48:13
Spain and Italy	22:06
The General Average from European Countries	**146:45**

The total liabilities in passing through the acclimating process in New Orleans in 1853 was to their respective populations 60:56. In relation to America, the tables indicated that the liabilities to yellow fever existed "pretty much in proportion to latitude." With regard to Europe, this was "modified by climation [sic] and their cold moisture, so dramatically opposite in its effects on the constitution to warm moisture," and to "their personal habits of crowding into cheap and filthy dwellings and the immigrants being of a low class." The comparatively small mortality in Great Britain was attributed to "these immigrants being of a higher class of subjects." In regard to the proportion of deaths between the male and female population in the southern and southwestern states, the agent placed the marked difference at 6–13 males to 1 female.[2]

Lastly, in regard to insurance companies, one agent suggested that contagion from yellow fever was frequently communicated by old clothing or bedding thrown from infected vessels into "New York Bay." He proposed constructing a boat as a floating furnace where infected articles from vessels could be consumed by fire. This would eliminate dangers ashore "and at the same time [purify] the air by combustion."[3]

New Propositions For and Against Quarantine

Since the site of the quarantine station was first established on Staten Island, the population grew up around it "as dense as that of many of the upper Wards of this City. For the most part this is made up of gentlemen doing business in New-York, who are daily passing through the atmosphere of the Quarantine grounds…. Thus, for all practical purposes, the laws of Quarantine have become ineffectual for the protection of the public health." In response to demands by those living near the grounds, the legislature passed "an Act for the removal of the Quarantine Station" on March 6, 1857. This act called for three appointed commissioners (George Hall, Egbert Benson and O. Bowne) to select a site for a permanent quarantine hospital, and to remove the present hospital from its situation and second to provide temporary accommodations "upon or near Sandy Hook." This proved remarkably difficult to achieve.

Opposite: **This map of New York Bay, published in** *Harper's Weekly* **(V1, p. 234), May 23, 1857, depicts the site of the old quarantine hospital and the new fever hospital. New Yorkers fought bitterly over quarantine sites and on several occasions took to vigilante law, burning hospitals and outbuildings, callously leaving the sick and dying exposed to the elements, in an effort to preserve their property rights and prevent the spread of disease (courtesy National Library of Medicine).**

18. The "Quarantine War" and the "Quarantine Armada"

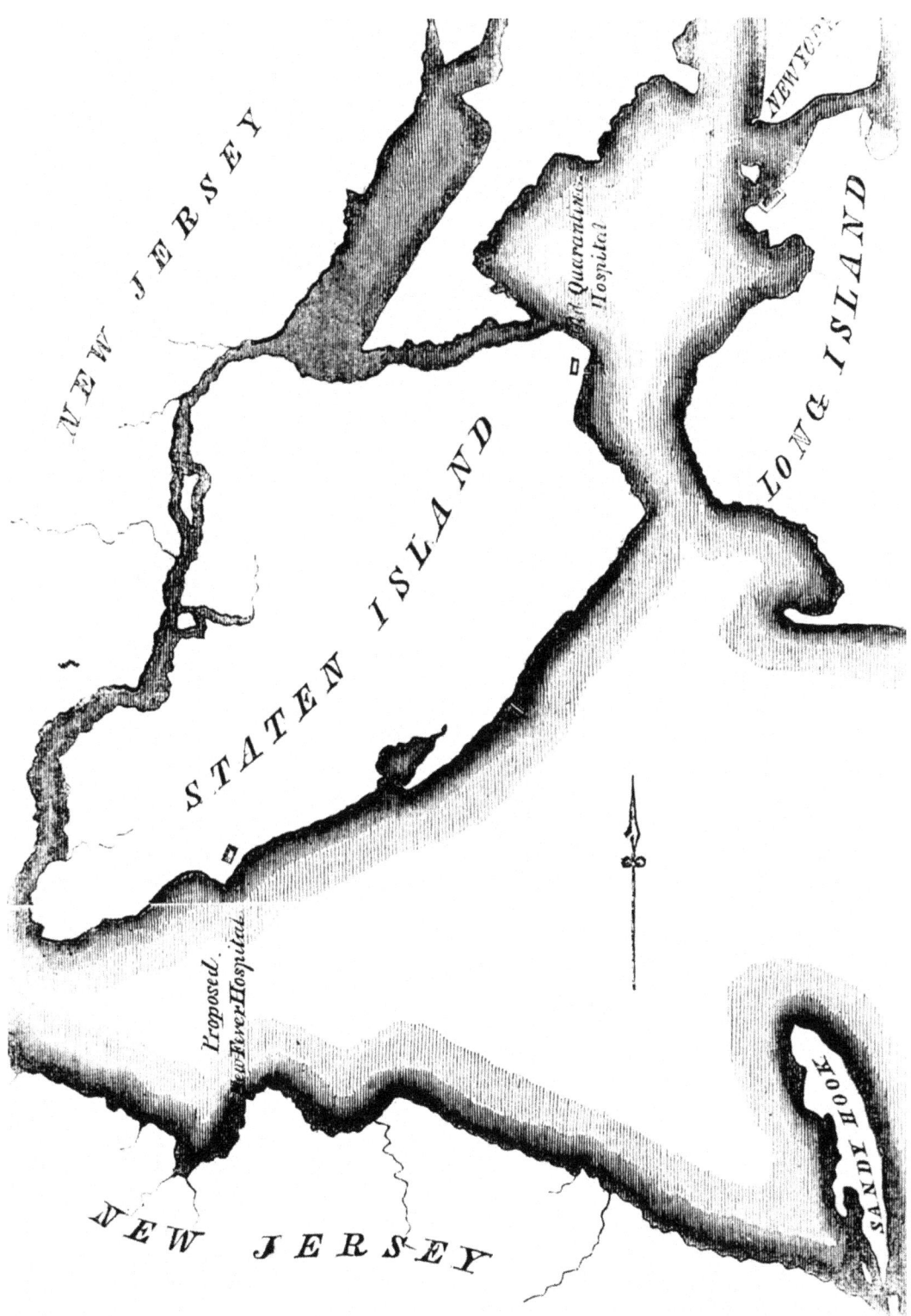

Negotiations were immediately entered into with representatives from New Jersey to either buy or lease Sandy Hook. New York's neighbor had no desire to harbor its yellow fever victims or cede jurisdiction to another state and that idea, however practicable it may have seemed to New Yorkers, went nowhere. The second choice was Coney Island, but the title to the desired land belonged to the people of Gravesend and "they would not consent to the proposed location at a favorite bathing resort." Other choices included the Dry Romer, the West Bank, a hulk in the lower bay and the neck of land at the Great Kill.

This compelled the commission to fall back on the loose wording of the 21st section of the act by stretching the word "near." They selected a piece of land 10¼ miles from Sandy Hook in the town of Westfield, New York, on the south shore of Staten Island adjoining Seguine's Point on the east. It contained 50 acres and was purchased from Thomas R Lush of Brooklyn for the sum of $23,000. The project was approved by Governor John A. King, Lieutenant Governor Henry R. Seldon and Comptroller L. Burroughs. Their approval immediately prompted "very singular stores" and "unpleasant imputations" that King had seen little or nothing of the spot, "though his Secretary may have known it a good deal better. It is remarked as a curious coincidence, that friends of Mr. Thurlow Weed evinced a singular desire for country residences on Staten Island just before the bill passed for the removal of Quarantine." Or, as the *Herald* (June 2, 1857) noted, "We know it must be very hard for the ardent republicans who bought the land at Seguine's Point before they went to Jersey to negotiate for Sandy Hook, and who had laid out their purchases in village lots in the hope that their new fever depot would prove a nucleus for a village—we know it must be very hard for them to see their little speculation thus baffled at the eleventh hour. But what can be done? One cannot risk a hundred lives in order that these operators may make fifty thousand dollars."

Just as quickly, opponents pointed out that the locale on Seguine's Point was "nearly as far from Sandy Hook as the present Quarantine station," thus violating the "spirit and letter of the act." It also incurred the fury of the oystermen of Prince's Bay, who violently complained a quarantine station there would jeopardize their livelihood, taking little comfort in Dr. Thompson's promise that "he [would] not molest them except in unusual seasons." By May 26 the *New York Herald* wrote, "Meanwhile, we hear little or nothing about the Quarantine war; it is surmised that the Commissioners have had the manliness and nerve to acknowledge the unanimous condemnation their choice has met with from the press and the public, and to take steps to avoid a collision with the poor—but very plucky—fishermen of Prince's bay."

The temporary solution became an "armada" of fever ships fitted out by the police commission for the reception of passengers off infected ships. Unfortunately, they could not be sent down to the ground at Seguine's Point for want of funds to get it underway. On May 31 the wharf prepared for the reception was burned in the same manner as farm buildings in the area had been consumed by fire. Blame was placed on the oystermen of Prince's Bay and a detachment of men under Captain Walling was sent to protect the region.[4]

While a reporter for the *Times* indicated (June 15, 1857) those opposed to the new quarantine at Seguine's Point had determined to offer no opposition until the new hospital was completed and then planned to "burn it to the ground," the ringleader, Ray Thompkins, son of former governor Thompkins, openly warned he was prepared to apply a torch to the present quarantine hospital. To prevent "accidents," Thompkins went so far as to qualify for the position of deputy sheriff and was ready to assume the position of sheriff in case of sickness.

The inhabitants of Staten Island were not the only ones opposed to quarantine. Businessmen complained there was "not proper discrimination made between vessels perfectly healthy and those that are infected." In any case, an organized system of pilfering was carried on in boats that "float carelessly down stream in the afternoon, their occupants crying, 'Old rope!' but bring up alongside of vessels in Quarantine, where they drive a brisk trade, and put off with their plunder before daylight." At Yellow Hook and all along the shore, great profits were derived from "the fruits of this contraband trade."

Additionally, there was a decrease of 10–15 percent in cargoes of sugar and molasses from vessels anchored in the Lower Bay. Clandestine cargoes were sent off in lighters to other eastern ports where they would not be subject to quarantine. After unloading their goods at New Haven, New London, Newport, Providence, New Bedford, Boston, Portsmouth and Portland the lighters returned for another round trip. The expense of freight from these ports to New York, where they would ultimately be sold, would "not generally exceed the charge for lightering" from the main vessels. To prevent this type of deception and to crack down on the unlawful practice of visitors onshore being rowed out to quarantine ships, the legislature passed a law on April 18, 1857, changing the fine for such transgressions from a mere $10 to a misdemeanor that carried a fine of $100–500 or imprisonment for not less than 3 months.

Ultimately, there were no epidemics in New York during 1857, leaving matters to be settled at another time but not necessarily by other men. On May 13 delegates from Boston, New York, Philadelphia, Baltimore, Norfolk, Charleston, Savannah and New Orleans met in Philadelphia to discuss the possibility of drawing up a uniform system of quarantine laws for general adoption that would supersede "the uncertain character of the regulations now in force." While the concept was an excellent one, it was not destined to succeed.[5]

The Great Quarantine Question Culminated

On March 8, 1858, the *New-York Times* reported as follows: "The receipt lately of anonymous letters by the Health Officers and Commissioners of Emigration, announcing that an attempt would be made to burn the Quarantine buildings at Stapleton, Staten Island, and warning them to remove the sick outside of the inclosure, has renewed some of the excitement of last Summer."

While authorities waited to see what would happen, matters took a dangerous turn on April 15, 1858, when the United States steamer *Susquehanna* arrived from Jamaica after a five-day passage. Aboard were 155 cases of yellow fever among the crew, 15 of which ended in death before arrival at the port. Twenty-one men were immediately removed to the Marine Hospital by the health officer, Dr. R.H. Thompson, and the vessel was sent to the lower quarantine anchorage to ride out her probation of 30 days. In consequence of "formalities" between the New York City Health Department and the secretary of the navy, two months were allowed to pass before orders were finally issued to disinfect the ship by scraping, fumigation and ice.

As tensions simmered and questions lingered on the cause of yellow fever, Dr. Thompson complicated the issue by warning it was "a singular and well attested fact" that coal brought from St. Thomas to Liverpool and "discharged in large quantities on the wharves, emit[ted] a gas which favor[ed] the generation and spread of the infection of yellow fever."[6] Complying with a request from the commissioners of health, Thompson presented statistics comparing the present year with that of 1856.

Number of Infected Vessels, 1856 and 1858, from the Period April 10 through August 1

	1856	1858
Number of sickly vessels	43	47
Number of sick in their port of clearance	98	27
Number of deaths	51	16
Number of sick on their voyages	115	39
Number of deaths	39	34
Number of sick on their arrival	33	41
Number of sick subsequent to arrival	57	18

In 1856 vessels from Havana (25) were the most commonly infected; in 1858 vessels from Havana numbered 27 but were surpassed by those from Kingston at 41, which was absent from the 1856 list.[7]

On September 1, 1858, what should have been an unthinkable act of barbarity was committed by vigilantes. The explanation—not the justification—was summarized by the *New-York Times* on September 2:

> The recent spread of yellow fever outside of the Quarantine walls, the excitement growing out of it, the agitation respecting the stoppage of the ferry boats from making their landings at the Quarantine dock, (made for the purpose of allaying excitement,) the passage by the Castleton Board of Health on Thursday [September 2], of a series of ordinances striking directly at the efficiency of the administration of quarantine affairs, and the application by the New-York Commissioners of Health for an injunction to restrain the Islanders from interfering with the Health Officer and his prerogatives, all taken in connection with the too bold and repeated threats to burn the buildings strongly warrant the belief that the deed is at least done.

And so it was. The large hospital buildings, the wards of low buildings and Dr. Thompson's private residence were all reduced to ashes. Around 9:00 p.m. a large party, disguised and armed, assaulted the place on two sides, "removed the patients out of the buildings, carrying them bodily upon their mattresses," and deposited them on the ground. The smallpox hospital suffered the same fate. Frank Mathews, a stevedore who was shot on the morning of the attack, died on Saturday. On Friday night Ray Tompkins was arrested. The following day Charles DeForest, Justice William Muller, Matthew Carroll, Jacob Vanderbilt, Thomas Garrett and John C. Thompson were placed in custody. They were quickly released on bail.

Temporary shelters were erected for the sick, and twenty convalescents were conveyed to Ward's Island during a pouring rain. Those in tents or placed in the barn "were very uncomfortable," and their groaning could be heard at a distance of 300 yards. The situation was later deposed by J.P. Cumming and William Jellenghaus, members of the Voluntary Committee of Inspection on Staten Island: "It almost seems to have been the idea of the lawless mob to see the sick perish between the two burning buildings. In the most barbarous country, inhabited by the wildest savages, hardly could men have acted in a more atrocious way." In denouncing the acts, Governor John A. King's proclamation stated the perpetrators acted in "total disregard and contempt of the laws," committing "crimes of the highest infamy." The governor declared the County of Richmond "in a state of insurrection."[8]

Proving how divisive the issue played out in the newspapers, the *Tribune* pleaded "extenuating circumstances" for the arsonists, and the *Herald* blithely observed, "It is not worth while spending time in vain regrets. The hospital is gone; and on the whole, however it perished, New York is a gainer by the loss.... For years it has been so cruel and shocking a nuisance to the most pleasant suburb of the city that the people of the locality must have been long suffering indeed to have borne with it so long." The *Times* offered the only sane and sentient observations: "The disgraceful outrage which was committed at the Quarantine grounds on Wednesday night, was the most diabolical and savage procedure that has ever been perpetrated in any community professing to be governed by Christian influence. For pure senseless ruffianism it is without parallel."

In another wanton act, Mayor Powell of Brooklyn appointed 100 men to patrol the wharves and shore as far as Bay Ridge for the purpose of preventing anyone from Staten Island reaching the city, while the Castleton Board of Health adopted an ordinance prohibiting the quarantine authorities from burying those who died of infectious diseases in the hospital burying ground.

On September 24 the quarantine commissioners presented arguments at Albany for the creation of floating hospitals only after being "assured of the impossibility of obtaining the only site on land which will satisfy the public—Sandy Hook." Noting each application to New Jersey for Sandy Hook had been refused, "in terms more and more emphatic," they added the state acted in a "sort of retaliatory" way by making it a high crime for a sickly vessel bound for New York to touch at Sandy Hook or stop in any waters of New Jersey.[9]

The Quarantine and Sanitary Convention

During the Quarantine and Sanitary Convention held in late April 1858, day two revolved around this question: "Have Quarantines secured the object for which they were originally intended?" Dr. McNulty of New York called for total abolition of quarantine. Dr. Guthrin of Memphis noted it did little for those places where yellow fever was indigenous but for those places where it existed only upon importation it was absolutely necessary. Dr. Tuthill brought out the point that as "commerce is king" the public considered quarantine as unnecessary. Dr. Griscom presented statistics indicating sanitary regulations were more useful than quarantine. Dr. Bell of Brooklyn advocated for protection for his city, and Dr. Elisha Harris, former marine physician, argued that as imperfect as it was the present system had prevented pestilence from sweeping New York.

Dr. Alexander H. Stevens of New York proposed the resolution that "in the absence of any evidence establishing the conclusion that yellow fever has ever been conveyed from one person to another, it is the opinion of this Convention that personal Quarantine of yellow fever cases may be safely abolished." Further discussion achieved little consensus and the matter was postponed. Day three began with more debate on contagion. A paragraph summary by Dr. Stevens perhaps best summarizes the discussion: "[He] was sorry that a little more of his eloquent friend's remarks were not pertinent to the subject. He was old enough to be very skeptical of what he had not himself seen. He hoped prudent men would rely more on their own observations than upon the rigmarole stories of men who lived in the past and were too much blinded to look at things as they were." Stevens challenged the attendees to name one case where the disease had proven contagious by contact but no one accepted.

Ultimately, by a vote of 70 ayes to 4 nays, members finally passed a resolution very similar to the one earlier proposed by Stevens: "*Resolved,* That in the absence of any evidence establishing the conclusion that yellow-fever has ever been conveyed from one person to another, it is the opinion of this Convention that the personal quarantine of yellow-fever cases may be safely abolished, provided that fomites of every kind be rigidly restricted." In essence, the resolution stated that healthy persons arriving on infected ships were to be allowed to land, their baggage and exposed clothing only being delayed. Persons arriving sick of yellow fever, having been carefully washed and their clothing changed, were also to be allowed to return home or enter a city hospital, "and that there is not the shadow of a foundation for alarm on their account." As carefully debated and resolved as it was, the resolution carried no weight and was promptly ignored. The May and June meetings of the Academy of Medicine, New York, went over the same subject but achieved no consensus.[10]

The appropriations bill passed at Albany set aside $50,000 with which the quarantine commission was to "provide temporary accommodations for persons arriving in our port sick with yellow fever or other pestilential diseases." By late June the old steamer *Falcon* (late of the gold rush days) was outfitted as a yellow fever hospital and anchored at Red Hook. Arguments immediately ensued over who was to pay for the upkeep of the ship, who was to assume care of patients and what would happen if the city were to receive a deluge of immigrants, all sick of yellow fever.[11] Such questions were argued in the legislative halls and through the newspapers, ultimately without resolution as the decade ended.

CHAPTER 19

Deluge of Yellow Fever in the South and Worldwide Epidemics

It is a great mistake which some men make, counting as experience all that they have said. Some, before whom the greatest dramas of the age have been played, are as ignorant of the points made and the lessons taught in them as if all the while they had been shut up in cloisters or locked within thick-walled cells. Judgment must assort and memory sift the facts that daily pass in review, to make them of service in after life.[1]

As early as mid–May 1858 newspaper exchanges were already carrying articles under the headline, "Apprehensions of Yellow Fever at the South." The fear was that the coming summer would be a very sickly one based on the fact "the long continued freshets, at this particular time, are likely to breed febrile diseases." Nearly one-fourth of the land on the Mississippi, from Vicksburg to the mouth of the river, had been waterlogged for weeks, "until all the swamps, bayous and lagoons at the South are gorged with stagnant water. In the interior of Mississippi, Alabama and Georgia, the freshets have been unprecedented."

One month later a more serious article titled "Deluge of the Lower Mississippi" warned that another disastrous crevasse had occurred at the Yazoo Pass, which was feared to submerge the entire valley of the Yazoo River. While such inundations left rich, fertile alluvial soil ideal for the production of cotton and sugar, the levees or dykes gave way, causing the turbid floods to sweep away towns and plantations. "There are not wanting those," the article added, "who hold that the location of New Orleans is altogether a mistake, and that the great commercial and shipping town for the Mississippi should be St. Louis." The article concluded: "It will require the profits of several fortunate years to repair the damage of the present flood."[2] The year 1858 was not destined to be one of those years.

Early reports were spotty. At New Orleans "the scourge appear[ed] to be confined to those of dissipated habits; the disease [was] prevailing on the gulf shore of Louisiana, and causing not a little uneasiness." Deaths, however, were slow in being reported.

The Epidemic of Yellow Fever in New Orleans, 1858

For the Week Ending	Yellow Fever	Other Deaths	Total
June 27	2	128	130
July 4	8	134	142
July 11	9	139	148
July 18	20	107	127
July 25	25	162	187

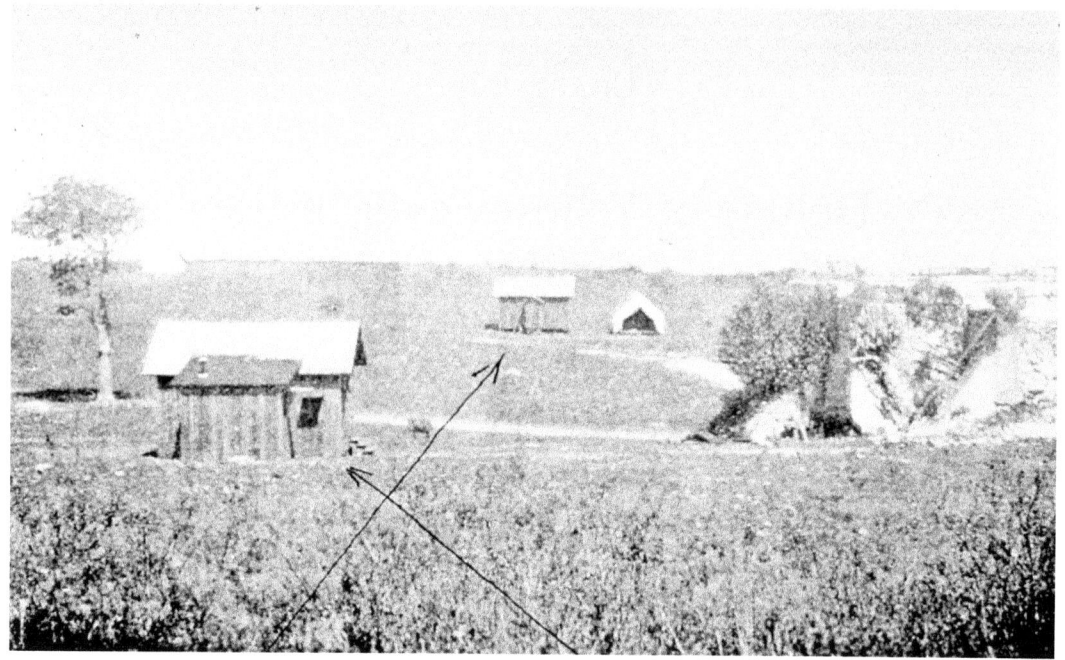

Camp Lazear (?) (1898), well isolated from populated areas, consisted of several buildings used for isolating yellow fever individuals (courtesy National Library of Medicine).

By July 27 there was some hope the fever would not become epidemic as the season was too far advanced; others, however, feared the worst was yet to come, "as it has two or three months to work upon a country that has been so submerged in water as to render it necessarily unhealthy, when the water retires." By the first week of August deaths were thought to come principally from shipping, but by August 14, as mortality continued to climb, the intensely hot weather did not bode well for remission and most people felt another week was likely to determine the direction the disease would take. It did not take that long; by August 17, the disease was declared epidemic and the Howard Association began active operations for the relief of the indigent sick and quarantine was established at Mobile. For the week ending August 1 the New Orleans Board of Health indicated only 4 of the 70 deaths were natives, while 10 were from France, 8 from Italy, 11 from Ireland and 18 from Germany.

For the Week Ending	Yellow Fever	Other Deaths	Total
August 1	70	120	127
August 8	140	166	306
August 15	286	171	457
August 22	312	165	477
August 29	402	184	586

On September 4 the *Crescent* reported that the yellow fever was "characterized by a new development—that of attacking creoles and old acclimated people whose birth and continued residence in New Orleans have always exempted them from its attacks. In this respect, the fever is worse than it was in 1853." While the weather continued to be oppressive, the *Bulletin* reported "where delirium and the death rattle drive men from the abode of misery, there is found woman." The women of the city, those "educated" and the "ornaments of society," took to the streets, devoting themselves to care for the sick "with a courage, a zeal, and a faithfulness that would astonish those who know nothing of their labor of love."

For the Week Ending	Yellow Fever	Other Deaths	Total
September 5	449	197	646
September 12	472	164	636
September 19	474	188	642
September 26	444	175	619

By October 9 the Howard Association felt it their duty to inform the country that the prolonged existence and great mortality of yellow fever was "solely owing to the influx of strangers, who rapidly fall victims," and promised to give "timely notice" when the epidemic had abated. In confirmation, the *Picayune* announced that between the first appearance of fever in June until October 9 the death toll had reached 3,875, noting, "This is within one hundred of the mortality in Boston from all causes, during the year 1857." Adding to the problem, it was reported that a physician's fee in tending a yellow fever case was $100, "more or less, kill or cure.... One, two and three thousand dollars is no uncommon amount of fees for a good yellow fever physician."

It was not surprising, then, when on October 20 the *Delta* carried an appeal from the Howard Association stating that at the outset of the epidemic they had $37,000 on hand. Relying on that fund they refrained from soliciting donations, but as "the demands upon their resources have surpassed all reasonable expectation" they found themselves with an exhausted treasury and were thus compelled to ask for monetary donations.

For the Week Ending	Yellow Fever	Other Deaths	Total
October 3	380	160	540
October 10	390	147	537
October 17	308	182	490
October 24	266	144	410
October 31	174	164	338

By early November the *Crescent* complained that but for the ingress of unacclimated strangers the fever would have ceased to be epidemic two weeks earlier:

> In vain does the associated press telegraph all over the Union, warning strangers to remain where they are until the danger has passed. Hundreds and hundreds have come, hundreds have died, and hundreds and hundreds will come, to share the same fate, only to be succeeded by reckless thousands. We ought to have a quarantine to compel the absence of fresh, healthy, unacclimated strangers. They nourish the fever, stop business, and put our people to the labor and expense of nursing and burying them. Instead of doing any good they kill themselves and injure us.

For the Week Ending	Yellow Fever	Other deaths	Total
November 7	136	133	269
November 14	66	164	230
November 21	17	172	189

Two stories, both printed in the *Delta*, highlight the pathos and the hearts of New Orleans residents, both human and animal, during the heartrending fever epidemic of 1858. The first concerned an infant who lost its mother to the dread disease. Adopted by the family nanny goat, the "quadrupedal wet nurse" quickly placed her teats "at the service of its thirsty lips" whenever the baby cried. The second concerned a boy wandering the streets. When found by a stranger, the child stated, "God sent for mother and father, and little brother, and took them away to his home in the sky; and mother told me, when she was sick, that God would take care of me.... He will come, won't he?" The man was compelled to reply: "Yes, my lad, he has sent me to take care of you."[3]

The population of Louisiana, taken in 1858, was 529,796, "with some allowance based on the absence of thousands of citizens during the prevalence of the yellow fever," at which time the census was taken. Even so, this showed an increase of 113,114 over the total of 1850. Of the 1858 number, 211,217 were white (an increase of 55,726); 18,005 free colored (increase of 623); and 300,574 slaves (increase of 55,765). The population of New Orleans was placed at 117,224.

By the first week of June 1859, early reports of yellow fever were announced and by mid-month 4–5 cases per day were reported. However, by early July physicians indicated the city would escape a severe visitation. Contrary to previous beliefs, the New Orleans Medical Review came out in defense of the theory that "the long continued overflow of the Mississippi river" served as a preventative of yellow fever, with the idea "daily becoming stronger in the public mind." On August 4 the board of health officially announced the city clear of yellow fever.[4]

Deaths from Yellow Fever in New Orleans, 1850–1859

Year	Number of Deaths
1850	107
1851	17
1852	456
1853	7,849
1854	2,425
1855	2,670
1856	74
1857	200
1858	4,845
1859	91[5]

"Blood and thunder" in Charleston, 1858–1859

Charleston health officers declared a yellow fever epidemic on August 23, 1858, after 28 deaths were registered for the week; of these, 13 victims were from Ireland, 11 from Germany, 3 from New York and one a native child. For the week ending September 4 there were 73 deaths and for the week ending on the 18th there were 103 yellow fever deaths, of which 77 were white adults, 22 white children and 4 colored persons. At the same time, the Howard Association of Charleston acknowledged the receipt of $500 in aid for the sick. For the week ending September 24 there were 81 deaths, with similar numbers appearing through October, finally compelling the mayor of Charleston to declare October 23 a day of fasting and prayer for the alleviation of the disease.[6]

On the eve of the Civil War, politics and yellow fever became inextricably combined. In April 1859 Governor Hammond of South Carolina wrote a letter to the Cotton Planters Convention at Macon, Georgia, expressing sympathy with southern efforts to secure direct trade with Europe and thus bypassing the major northern shipping centers. In his message, Hammond saw only two drawbacks to such a scheme: the shallowness of southern waters to accommodate the "mammoth vessels" of the age, and the prevalence of yellow fever at the ports during the four summer months. The governor suggested the difficulty of yellow fever might be readily gotten over "by a heroic determination on the part of Southern merchants to do all their business in eight months," and, as the *New-York Times* of April 23, 1859, sarcastically noted, "fly from the malady in the remaining four."

Another method of addressing the problem of excessive heat and malignant fevers came a year earlier when the *New-York Times* (June 21, 1858) published a tongue-in-cheek article, "An Invention for the South," noting, "A Britisher has recently invented a machine which not only makes ice by the square mile, but possesses the valuable property of reducing a given temperature to the healthy point. The inventor proposes to use it in Southern Hospitals.... Here then is a ready way to grasp the commerce of New-York. Put a few machines into Charleston, import a quantity of great coats and then for Independence and France. The healthfulness of a place has a great deal to do with its prosperity, and it may now be freely confessed—the remedy being at hand—that all that is needed to make a Southern port rival a Northern is a fair balance of vital prospects" (see Chapter 13 for a discussion on ice-making and its application to disease).

"Blood and thunder" prophecies were also aroused in July as preparations for the Democratic National Convention at Charleston to appoint a presidential candidate elicited threats against Senator Stephen A. Douglas's delegates. With cries of mob violence, the probability of being "shot in the street" or "carried off by the yellow fever," there seemed little prospect of achieving a unified goal. But as one writer noted, "It is scarcely credible that by way of fighting off the Douglas men, the Southern Fire-Eaters should have both mob and yellow fever at hand. But we shall see what we shall see." In a slightly more humorous vein, one joke making the rounds of the exchanges went like this: "A Yankee with the yellow fever may very properly be called a Northern man with Southern feelings."

"Feelings" were indeed high, even between northern newspapers. In August the *New-York Herald* carried on the theme of yellow fever by warning it would be unsafe for delegates to visit Charleston in June "as they would be running the risk of being carried off by the strangers' or yellow fever." Coming to the defense of New York's "sister city," the *New-York Times* called this a slander, vowing it was as safe in Charleston in June as in New York or Philadelphia.[7]

Yellow Fever in South America: The 1850s

Yellow fever struck Pernambuco in late 1849 and by January 1850 it had begun to affect shipping. Reports of January 22 indicated that mortality "is represented as frightful, and unless it soon disappears it will seriously check business, and prevent produce from coming to the city." Unfortunately, matters were destined to get worse.

While the capital of Brazil had been known as one of the healthiest places on earth, yellow fever struck Rio de Janeiro in the middle of December 1849, occurring simultaneously in the harbor and city. At first it was believed to be an aggravated form of "Polka Fever" (so called from the circumstance that the new dance and the new disease made their appearance at much the same time),[8] which had prevailed three years before. But by mid–January, the ravages were so great those who could escape fled to the mountains.

Although it was commonly held that yellow fever had "never appeared on the coast south of the equator," by February 14, 1850, the disease had spread along the eastern coast of South American from Bahia to Rio. At first, Danish, German and Swedish shipping suffered most, but in short order it spread to American and English vessels. By March 25 conditions had deteriorated, the fever raging "worse among the shipping and the lower classes. Many natives have died of fright. Several of the foreign mercantile houses were closed owing to the universal sickness among the inmates." Typically there was no agreement among medical men as to the actual cause, some considering it to be "the kind of fever that prevails on the coast of Africa, from whence the contagion probably came." In the same week, a British vessel reported "mortality amongst the blacks had been very great, and accounts had reached Rio that the malignant malady had manifested itself at Rio Grande, where many deaths had likewise taken place." The epidemic even reached the town of Petropolis, 40 miles from Rio and between 2,000 and 3,000 feet above sea level. A correspondent of the *New York Post* wrote from Rio on April 4:

> There have been times, for a week at a time, that there were not seamen enough in health to man half the vessels in port. What number of seamen have perished here during the few months past I have not as yet had an opportunity of knowing. The number, however, must be very great.
> Scores of vessels have lost every soul on board. Many have left with a new crew, and in a few days returned again with only men enough to get the vessel back, and frequently bereaved of the captain, and one or more subordinate officers. In the city and its various suburbs the fever has been equally, if not more fatal.... Entire families have been swept away in a few days. California [bound] vessels, from Europe and America, stopping here, have suffered much. Passengers exposing themselves by going ashore, have taken the fever in a short time, and found a grave long before reaching the gold region.

The government prohibited the ringing of church bells and the interment of the dead in niches of churches and other public buildings: "For a long time no report of deaths was made; but now an official report has been made of the aggregate mortality since the commencement of the epidemic, and it amounts to between 12 and 14,000. Probably about 14,000 deaths of this fever in the harbor and city, in the last 3 or 4 months. The estimate is now 300 deaths daily, and no abatement either on shore or in the harbor." The death tolls eventually lessened but the fever reappeared again at Para in late summer "with great virulence."[9]

Yellow fever was already raging at Cayenne, French Guiana, by December 1850, having taken 60 French soldiers out of 460, or about 1/20 of the white population. The fever was unusually prevalent among the "higher ranks of life," and the governor and vicar-apostolic were among the victims. To reassure the troops, the acting governor, M. Vidal de Lingendes, issued a "curious order" in January 1851: "In an epidemic such as the one which strikes us, there are necessarily victims. It is as in battle. Some are hit, others respected by the balls. You would not quit the field of battle; then don't fear the combat with the epidemic." He added that when their hearts would sink they should "look up at the tricoloured standard" and be brave.[10]

In 1851 advices from Rio to April 15 stated that during the past 10 days, 1,156 persons had died of yellow fever and at least five times that had fallen victim in the provinces and along the coast but Pernambuco remained almost disease free. Yellow fever was also believed to have spread to Oporto, Portugal, on ships originating at "the Brazils." By April 4, 1852, yellow fever at Pernambuco was confined to shipping, but at Rio "its ravages [were] described as heartrending." Another report from Rio announced "out of a shipload of colonists from the Azores, 270 in number, all had died" but 37, while out of 17 workmen who went out from England on the last packet (to work at the New Gas Company) only 6 remained. In keeping with the times, a report dated December 28, 1852, noted that the dread yellow fever still prevailed at Rio: "[On shipboard] 1000 negroes had been landed at Santos about 200 miles from Rio, and sold for 800 reals ($100 each). That is a low price comparatively to what they now command in the Southern States." At Demerara in 1852 it was stated that influenza had become epidemic and fevers were extensively prevalent, but "on the principle that two maladies cannot co-exist in the same locality, we hear scarcely anything now of yellow fever."

Intelligence from 1853 through 1859 contained similar statements, with most of Europe's attention drawn to the problem of yellow fever among sailors. Captain Edward Robinson of Sunderland, commander of the English ship *Raleigh*, wrote in 1858 that of those vessels in the waters around Rio most had lost captains and officers. Out of 1,609 registered deaths, fully 600 were attributed to sailors. Calling the condition of Rio "a disgrace to civilized people," he added, "all manner of filth is to be met with in most parts of the town. Dead animals and filth I cannot describe, meet your eye and offend your senses almost everywhere. It is laughable, yet sorrowful to see the walking water-closets— that is, negroes carrying large tubs in the streets giving an odour more peculiar than [dis]agreeable as they pass along, to empty the tubs in the river opposite the shipping." Looking past sanitation to other causes, authorities at Monte Video ordered the gas works, from which the city was lighted, to be discontinued, "believing that the introduction of gas is in some way connected with the existence of yellow fever!"

A private letter, written from Rio in 1857 summed up the decade: "[T]he yellow fever is carrying away from twenty to thirty foreigners daily, besides leaving several hundred sick in the hospitals, you will agree with me in thinking that it would be a pretty poor speculation for any company to insure my life; and, as my occupation keeps me out of doors, exposed to the sun, you may expect before long to see my obituary in the papers."[11]

One fact of political note did distinguish the decade. In 1856 charges were made that French prisoners, including members of secret societies, old criminals and those sentenced by the Republic, were to be transported to Cayenne to serve their time. Approximately 320 were among this group, reduced in October to 180 by escapes, liberation and 52 deaths from yellow fever. Foreign journals picked up the story of these "calumnies" and it became an international scandal. In response, the French *Moniteur* presented the government position, retracting previous accounts of the deadly climate by stating that, "in the establishment of Cayenne, it was justly considered that the convicts in the bagnes, encumbered in France within confined and unhealthy spots, might be much better treated in a colony." To the *London Times* and the rest of the world, however, this was, "a sentence of death—death lingering and horrible—death to which a file of musketeers or the guillotine would be mercy."[12]

Yellow Fever in Portugal, 1857

Yellow fever at Lisbon was believed to have broken out on September 16, 1857 (the young King Pedro II's birthday); reports dated September 25 indicated the disease was "supposed to have been brought from Rio in a vessel laden with hides." The situation quickly deteriorated and by October 1 the minister of the interior called together a

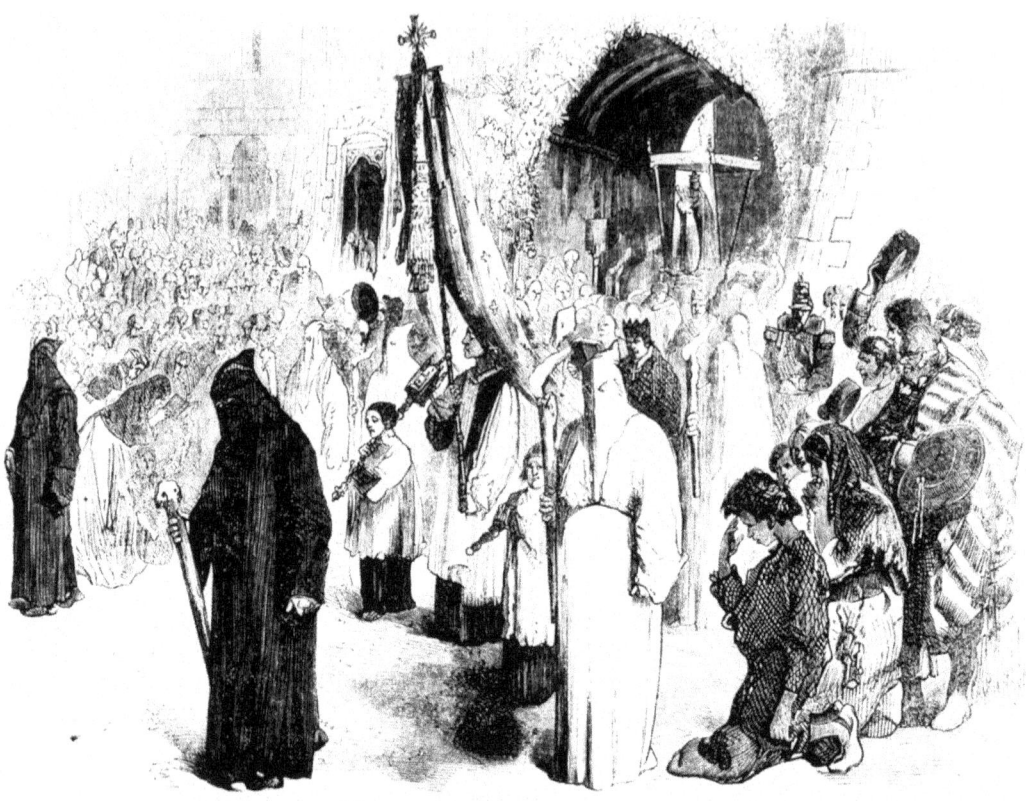

Yellow fever was as mysterious as it was deadly, and when all known scientific efforts to prevent its reoccurrence failed, people looked to religion for succor. The "Penitential Procession at Lisbon," published in *Harper's Weekly* (Vol. 2, p. 109), February 13, 1858, represents one community's effort to ward away yellow fever (courtesy National Library of Medicine).

sanitary commission. Members were of the opinion that "the prevalent fever was of a typhoid character, but that many actual cases of yellow fever have occurred.... It is a remarkable fact that the Custom-house appears to be the focus of the disease, and many of the employees have fallen victims to it." By October 19 the disease had spread from the parishes of the Se and Magdalena. No life appeared in the city, "no business, the shops are shut up—no carriages wake the echoes of the silent streets." The government provided encampments in the squares for the gallegos, or water-carriers, who could not afford attention to cleanliness. Published accounts indicated an average mortality of 60 daily.

Dr. Robert D. Lyons, the British authority on the pathology of diseases of the army in the East, left for Lisbon on November 27 for the purpose of investigating the symptoms and progress of the disease. The government of France also sent two commissioners, but the English government "has not yet moved in the matter." These experts had no lack of material to study, as an official statement from Lisbon reported that as of November 17 there had been 10,556 people attacked by yellow fever, of whom 3,350 had perished. The report also indicated the number of new cases reported daily ranged between 150 and 200, having been as high as 229. In its own report, the *Medical Gazette* of Lisbon asserted that "all the persons of that city who reside in houses lighted by gas have escaped the yellow fever."

Between September 16 (some accounts place the date as September 9) and December 24 there were 13,482 cases reported, with 4,759 deaths. Yellow fever was not limited to Portugal, however, and in 1858 recent ravages of the disease in Lisbon "roused the Legislature" to pass a law for sanitary improvement in the capital. A loan of £225,000 was obtained from the Bank of Portugal to pay for the work.[13]

Yellow Fever in the West Indies and Cuba During the 1850s

During the warm months of 1852, news from the West Indies typically reflected the deaths from yellow fever of British seamen and French soldiers. Martinique, Port-au-Prince, Jamaica, Barbados and St. Thomas were all reported as infected, with most deaths associated with shipping. In England, death lists of passengers who died on the voyage from the West Indies were printed in most newspapers along with reports on the status of the sugar, coffee and pimento crops. Occasionally stories of individual passengers caught the fancy of editors and became prominent news. One such involved "Madame Carregeot," a French woman of about 22 years of age who died of yellow fever aboard the *Magdalena*, which arrived at Southampton in January 1853. Apparently, Madame Carregeot met a wealthy young Mexican merchant in Paris who "became enamoured" and took her home to Mexico City with the intention of marrying her. His friends determined she was not of the proper class and paid her $3,500 plus passage to England. After her demise aboard ship, it was discovered "Carregeot" was an assumed name and that "she had an extensive correspondence with the frequenters of theatres, and many of the gay ones in Paris." The pay-off she received from her former lover's friends was found in the form of a draft drawn on one of the first Mexican mercantile houses in Paris.[14]

Admission into the Military Hospital at Barbados
September 4, 1852–January 14, 1853
All Deaths from Yellow Fever

Regiment	Admitted	Died
34th Regiment	80	7
69th Regiment	168	36
Royal Artillery	33	7
Total	281	50

Admission into Hospital and Deaths from Yellow Fever
Aboard Her Majesty's Ship *Dauntless*

	Admissions	Deaths
Officers	22	15
Men	136	64
Total	158	79

By January 14, the epidemic was considered over.[15]

The yellow fever epidemic at Bermuda dated from a storm on August 20, 1853, which "disturbed the accumulated corruption of years in which the *Thames* convict ship had been embedded. Miasma impregnated the ship. Twenty-five percent of the convicts were destroyed." Early in September the garrison became infected. The 56th Regiment had 106 cases and the Sappers lost ⅖ of their strength. Between September 1 and 18, the 56th had 225 cases and lost 70 men, 13 women and 6 children; the Sappers lost 19 out of 34 cases. An English commission appointed to inquire into the origin of this outbreak issued a report in January 1855, stating their belief the yellow fever was "engendered at Bermuda" and was not imported by outbreaks onboard the *Tenedos* convict hospital hulk off Beaz Island or from any cases occurring on the *Thames* convict hulk.[16]

Yellow fever outbreaks in the West Indies were reported throughout the rest of the decade, causing the most dread among those in the shipping trades. "Sailors," it was stated, "have a horror of 'Yellow Jack,' as they call the fever. They dread it far more than they do the cholera. This arises, no doubt, from the former prostrating the mental powers more than the latter does." This concern was especially important to England as Royal Mail steamers were capable of leaving one of the Caribbean Islands and reaching that country in as few as 13 days. Their fear was tempered somewhat by the fact most fever victims died within a week of leaving an infected port. Thus, even when a ship entered British waters flying the yellow flag indicating there had been disease deaths aboard, rarely were these vessels quarantined; when it was refused pratique, it was usually for a brief period.[17]

Throughout the West Indies, the question of sanitation was usually foremost in European minds. In 1858 the *London Daily News* (May 19, 1858) described conditions of the harbor of St. Thomas, reporting it had a narrow entrance not affected by the tides or sea breezes: "A number of ships are always there, and a great deal of refuse from them is thrown into it. The sewage of the town is also emptied into the harbour. When a paddle-wheel stirs the water there a stench arises. The floats of the paddle-wheels of steamers also which are painted red become black after being some time immersed in the water of the harbour."

After St. Thomas was conquered by the Danish in 1666, the Dutch West India Company established control, dividing land into sugar cane plantations requiring vast numbers of slaves to make them profitable. The slave trade was abolished after the 1848 Danish Revolution and the sugar trade began a slow decline. The port continued to play a prominent role in the shipping trade, however, although the frequent appearance of yellow fever and other tropical diseases played havoc with unacclimated seamen.

Similar to outbreaks in the West Indies, yellow fever appeared in Cuba throughout the 1850s. In 1853, on this island where slavery was legal, thousands of recently introduced Africans were killed by a "terrible kind of diarrhea" that rapidly extended throughout the interior. The following year "the only topic of news was the terrible devastation by the yellow fever.... The *Grey Eagle* slave ship has been given up to a mixed commissioner to whom she belonged by right of capture. Several arrivals of American vessels with slaves were daily looked for."

Conditions were little better in 1855, compelling authorities at New Orleans to quarantine vessels out of Cuba, while in 1858 one notice warned, "It is not the yellow fever which prevails at Havana, but the African fever which is still more fatal, as it takes off even the Creoles."[18]

In two divergent reports, in 1850 the city of Canton, China, and neighboring towns were afflicted by a malignant fever commonly called typhus. Some European physicians, however, were of the opinion the disease was "akin to the yellow fever of the West Indies; others think that it resembles the plague which desolated London two centuries ago." In 1855 a letter dated February 2 from Constantinople stated that at Scutari Hospital "a new sort of yellow fever has been on the increase, and from all accounts it seems to resemble the yellow fever of the West Indies. It not only attacks the men in hospital, but the staff officers living at Scutari."[19]

The State of Yellow Fever in the 1850s: Theory and Cures

Most of the medical articles emerging in the decade of the 1850s repeated what was already known or supposed to be true. In 1853 the respected New Orleans physician Dr. McFarland sided with the prevailing theory that two or more diseases could not coexist, declaring, "All the filth in and around New Orleans has never created one single case of yellow fever, and cannot create one, but, on the contrary, that the local *malaria* arising from these and other causes, is calculated to retard the existence of that disease—and that it has done so and held it in abeyance to such an extent as to have exempted us from yellow fever, as an epidemic, for five or six years past."

One method of "cure" spread from the West Indies to London and New York. Devised by an old woman named Mariquita Orfila, it consisted of crushed Verbena leaves mixed with water, strained and combined with coarse salt and administered every three hours. It became very popular in 1853 but quickly fell out of favor when physicians at St. Thomas used it without success.

In 1854 Dr. William B. Carpenter of London asserted, "*Intemperance* is one of the most powerful of the agencies which determine the development of the Cholera-poison in the human body." Extending the evils of drink to yellow fever, he cited Dr. Drake, an American physician, "who informs us, too, that it is well known to the physicians of New Orleans and Mobile, that the victims of Yellow Fever are chiefly those who drink freely; and this statement has received a most fearful confirmation in the recent epidemic of that disease." He noted New Orleans had 1,127 dram shops in one of its four districts. The same year, at a meeting of the Medical Association of St. Louis, Dr. Linton of New Orleans attributed the cause of yellow fever to "excessive eating—on the sensible theory that the heavy food which the Northerner eats in a warm climate, acts as so much unnecessary fuel, in producing the fire of fever." His observation was strengthened by noting the disease "rarely occurs in the prisons of New Orleans." He concluded, "*The mode of life,* in a word, is the principal incentive to the disease called yellow fever."

In an 1857 discussion on "Disease in Animals," Dr. Rene LaRoche, in his work, *On Yellow Fever,* expanded the theory that "the epidemic constitution of the atmosphere during the prevalence of yellow fever" not only affected humans but animals. Offering research that extended back to 1798, he stated that flies were found dead in great numbers in the unhealthy parts of New Orleans. In June 1805 cats and dogs were fatally affected, while in 1806 the disease struck cats, rats, fish and oysters. In 1819 and 1833 cattle, sheep and hogs died with rotten tongues. Another study pointing to the same cause was promoted by a New Orleans paper that claimed there "can be no doubt that the poison producing yellow fever is fungi diffused through the atmosphere, just as the odoriferous particles of a rose or other fragrant flowers are diffused through it." Believing the danger crept in during the night, it was admitted that neither chemical analysis nor the microscope was able to detect the "exceedingly minute particles that produce yellow fever."[20]

Two interesting topics were developed, albeit briefly, in the 1850s. The first dealt with vaccination to prevent yellow fever. Based on the success of that procedure against smallpox, a German practitioner, 36-year old William Lambert de Humboldt (whose medical education was said to be "imperfect"), developed this technique for yellow fever after observing "that galley-slaves brought from Mexico to Vera Cruz, who had been bitten by some viper on the way, always had decided symptoms of yellow fever." Over the course of nine years of work in New Orleans he inoculated 1,438 patients, of whom only 7 were attacked and 2 died. His injection consisted of venom of a serpent (later identified as Crotalus Horridus) that caused fever "which has all the symptoms of the yellow fever, but with very feeble effects," along with a syrup of Mikamia-guaco, the well-known antidote for snake bites. Reports indicated the patient vomited blood on the third day, which Humboldt inferred made them safe from further attacks of yellow fever. In October 1854 Humboldt wrote to Don Jose de la Concha, the governor of Cuba, notifying him he had discovered a preventative for yellow fever. Concha invited him to Cuba and turned over a wing of the military hospital for his private use. Subsequently, several high Mexican functionaries and five hundred soldiers were inoculated.

Following this success, in 1855 *La Cronica,* a Spanish paper published in New York, indicated the government of Cuba ordered the inoculation of 1,000 newly arrived troops with "the greatest success." While in Cuba, Humboldt made the acquaintance of Dr. Manzini. Sharing the same conviction that epidemic, remittent fevers of tropical countries and yellow fever were identical, varying only in degree, the two worked together on further research. Unfortunately, later that year it was reported "Wm. De Humboldt," inventor of the "Preservative Inoculation against yellow fever" had been given "some poisonous mixture, which had driven him mad. It is believed to have been done through the jealousy of certain medical men in Havana. A physician and two other persons have been arrested for this crime." Humboldt later died at Vera Cruz.

Manzini abandoned his medical practice to study the "immense scientific question" of using venom, ultimately inoculating over 2,000 patients. When those who had been treated subsequently developed yellow fever, he treated them with bleeding from the feet and administered large doses of quinine and calomel, which he claimed cured them in 12–48 hours. Senor Bastareche, chief Military Health Officer in Cuba, also made experiments on the technique and by the end of 1855 pronounced inoculation "a total failure."[21]

In 1857 the *Gazette Medicale* reported that Dr. Lucien Papilland had "performed no less than 2,477 inoculations on persons living in districts ravaged by yellow fever, and with the most satisfactory results. Only 288, or 10 per cent. of the number inoculated were subsequently attacked by yellow fever, though exposed to its influence; 68 ... of the total number, or 2 ½ per cent. died; and 2,247, or 90 per cent. were altogether protected." Papilland's work was based on that of "Dr. G. Humboldt," who discovered that the inhabitants of Central America were liable to be bitten in the foot and legs by a reptile of undetermined species. Those who survived remained free from the ravages of yellow fever, prompting him to introduce the venom as a preservative. Papilland's serum was derived from the diluted poison of the reptile, "which he irritates until it bites a piece of sheep's liver, and the juice of the latter, thus impregnated, is the material employed for inoculation."

The second incident concerned "The Case of Transfusion." During 1858 Dr. Benedict of New Orleans resorted to the so-called heroic measure of treating a young woman in the last stages of yellow fever by injecting one of her veins with blood taken from a volunteer who had just recovered from yellow fever. The success obtained with this and other patients likewise treated prompted the *Delta* to speculate that it would not be surprising if transfusion should become as popular as phlebotomy once was."[22]

At the end of the decade, an interesting argument arose between two prominent physicians. Sir John Forbes, in his work, *Nature and Art in Disease,* stressed the point of "superiority of nature over art in the cure of sickness," condemning the art of the physician "as an idle and even dangerous fiction." Assuming the opposite position in his book, *Art Versus Nature in Disease: A Refutation of Naturalism,* Dr. A. Henriques undertook to prove "man possesses no inherent power in his constitution able to cure diseases;—that, in fact, nature unaided never cures." Ironically, neither point could be carried in the case of yellow fever, where studies revealed "every patient has recovered under every form of treatment," while on the other hand, "all methods of treatment" proved fatal. Henriques himself was a homeopath, part of a growing number of converts who opted for Hahnemann's system over conventional allopathic medicine.

Another developing treatment during the 1850s was that of hyrdopathy, or the water cure. The wealthy had access to luxurious resorts where bathing and massage were incorporated into dietary regimens; the middle class was more likely to visit a private physician's office spa, the so-called Hydropathic Establishment, while those of more limited means found numerous publications including those of the Fowlers (famous for their phrenological readings) where the benefits of home shower baths were lauded. Typical of the times, an advertisement by R. Wipprecht of Galveston promised the successful treatment for "all Acute Disease, including yellow fever," with his Water-Cure. At Vicksburg, the water cure "gained an unexpected triumph" when a patient in the last stages of the disease threw himself into the Mississippi. Contrary to the expectations of his physicians, once he was pulled out, the patient improved rapidly from his "plunge bath" and yellow fever.

With these new ideas coming into prominence, physicians began taking a closer look at the drugs they prescribed. An ad for Carter's Spanish Mixture noted, "Fever and Ague cured without using Quinine, Arsenic, Mercury, Opium, or any of the poisonous drugs, or dangerous compounds generally resorted to by sufferers." This played nicely into a rash of articles dealing with cases of insanity brought on by treatment of yellow fever with quinine. The *New Orleans True Delta* (1853) advised that physicians noted a tendency to insanity from the over-use of quinine, while "public opinion" attributed "not a few of the many yellow fever deaths" to the unwise use of that drug. The following year, a Mr. Donnell of Brandon, Mississippi, committed suicide by throwing himself in front of a train; his insanity was attributed to "a severe attack of yellow fever last summer."

As opposed to the old "Fatal Medical Practice" of "bleeding, emetics and *drenches of Calomel and Jalap,*" the manufacturers of Radway's Ready Relief and Regulators notified readers that yellow fever was easily, safely and successfully treated with their modern nostrums. From a different perspective, the *Philadelphia Ledger* (1857) announced that "all the yellow people—especially the yellow children who are supposed to be turned yellow by fever and ague," could be returned to the "clear white" nature intended by teaching wives, daughters and cooks "to keep the pearlash out of their bread." Noting that bad bread killed about as many people as bad rum, the article lamented that pearlash, "under the name of 'saleratus,' is King." Remove it and dyspepsia and yellow skin coloration would be resolved. (Pearlash, or potassium carbonate, was derived from wood ashes and used as an inexpensive leavening, most commonly between 1780 and 1840; Saleratus is chemically similar to baking soda.) Finally, on the economic front, Mr. Letcher, from the House Committee of Ways and Means, reported passage of a bill extending the time for the Norfolk and Petersburg Railroad to pay the duty on its iron, "in consequence of an embarrassment of its finances" occasioned by the late yellow fever epidemic.[23]

Beating the Drum on Quarantine

During the 1850s there was no end to the discussions on quarantine. The point would seem to have been settled with the report of Dr. James Gillkrest, the inspector general of army hospitals in Great Britain: "Yellow fever is not contagious under any circumstances, not even in the case of crowding, in this disease, whether of the dead or of the living; that the removal of the individual from the influence of the local causes which produce this affection is the fittest means of preventing its extension; and, lastly, that the cordons, called sanitary, and quarantine measures, far from arresting yellow fever, on the contrary favour its extension by confining the population within the influence of the local cause which give it birth." This report was presented to the French National Academy of Medicine in January 1852. That body concluded, "Dr. Gillkrest's work places beyond a doubt the inutility of quarantine, as applied to arrivals from countries where yellow fever prevails."

Supplementing this was the second report on quarantine respecting yellow fever presented by the General Board of Health to Parliament in April 1852. They concluded as follows:

(1) Yellow fever breaks out simultaneously in different and distant towns, often under circumstances where communication with infected persons is impossible

(2) Epidemics are usually preceded by sporadic cases

(3) Epidemics are limited as to the space over which they spread

(4) Epidemics do not spread by gradual progression but often ravage certain localities

(5) Epidemics are often strictly confined to a particular house or street

(6) In general, only one or two individuals in an infected house are stricken

(7) Rigid seclusion of an infected locality affords no protection

(8) The dispersion of the sick to healthy localities is the best measure to prevent the spread of epidemic

(9) Such dispersion of the sick is not followed by transmission of the disease, nor between hospitalized yellow fever victims and those not infected

(10) Yellow fever is local or endemic in origin

(11) Conditions which influence the localization of yellow fever are the same as those causes of cholera and all other epidemic diseases

(12) When localizing causes are removed, yellow fever ceases to appear or recurs at more distant intervals

(13) Besides external localizing, non-acclimation is a predisposing cause

(14) Quarantine and sanitary restrictions are not the means of protection; removal

of localizing conditions is the only answer, supplemented by temporary removal of individuals

The board concluded, "We have not found a single fact or observation clearly ascertained and authentically recorded opposed to the general tenor of such evidence. We have met with no exceptional cases."[24] In plainer language, in an article entitled, "The Yellow Flag and Yellow Fever," the editorialist stated the following:

> The oldest of the "old world politicians" cannot stand before the advance of the new system of locomotion. Railways, and steamers must in the long run beat prejudice, jealousy, the passport officers, and the Custom-house *douaniers* out of the field. People who have whirled along at the rate of twenty miles an hour up to a frontier will not endure to be detained for the sake of some frivolous ceremony or some official exaction for hours and days on the wrong side of the invisible barrier.
>
> Among the barriers whose frivolous and vexatious character is fast becoming recognised are those erected, ostensibly for the purpose of health, to avert the supposed danger that plagues should be propagated in one country by visitors from another. Every traveller who has cruised along the shores of the Mediterranean knows how increasingly his business or pleasure have been interrupted by the operation of the quarantine system and has esteemed himself lucky if he can succeed in escaping a dreary incarceration, sometimes lasting for weeks altogether, within the noxious and foetid prisons over which the yellow flag was kept waving. And the system was capricious as it was annoying. There was no scientific diagnosis by which to identify the particular diseases that should be deemed infectious, and so condemn their possible bearer to the penalties of quarantine.... Much suffering has been inflicted, and many acts of cruelty and absurdity committed beneath the sanction of every flag—but none so great or so continuous as under the yellow flag.[25]

None of these arguments ended the debate. In 1853 when discussing the British ship *Agamemnon*, which was considered "rank with a contagious fever," *Lloyd's Weekly Newspaper* (April 3, 1853) noted, "We do not now propose to open so very large a question as that of general quarantine; but supposing that a reasonable doubt upon the subject prevails in the minds of well informed men, it is clear enough that the Agamemnon is in as piteous a case as any vessel upon which yellow fever as declared itself." The same year after a man died of yellow fever aboard the *La Plata* a few hours after her arrival at the Southampton Docks, the *Weekly News and Chronicle* (June 4, 1853) complained, "The desirability of permitting yellow fever cases to be introduced into the port in summer time is much questioned."

The *New-York Daily News* (March 17, 1854) took the *McAllen* (TX) *Edinburg Review* to task for declaring quarantine regulations "were relics of an ill-informed age—urging that they should be entirely dispensed with as unnecessary and grievous hindrances to commerce." Arguing "the balance of late opinion has seemed to be in favor of the contagious theory of yellow fever," the writer urged strictly enforced rules. The same argument was made in New Orleans, where a rigid quarantine was proposed at Belize for the entire yellow fever season to protect "the entire southwest, as it always appears in New Orleans first, and spreads from thence over the country." In keeping with the universal theme of commerce, the article concluded with this: "A great amount of country trade has been diverted from New Orleans to New York on account of the sickness of the last two summers."

Two additional stories serve as a look at how yellow fever affected commerce. The first involved a law case brought before the U.S. District Court in June 1854. In *Francis Leland vs. William Agnew et al.* the plaintiff sought to recover the freight on 116 hogsheads of tobacco brought from New Orleans to New York aboard the *President Fillmore* the previous August. The ship had to be discharged at quarantine and the tobacco was placed in lighters there and brought up to the city. "The defendant claims to deduct the expense of lighterage from the amount of freight, the bill of lading mentioning that the tobacco was 'deliverable at Tobacco Inspection Wharf,' which the libellant insists by general usage is satisfied by a delivery at Quarantine."

In the second instance, *The United States Mail Steamship Company vs. The Bark "John Potter"* involved a case of salvage brought by the steamer *George Law*. The bark *John Potter* sailed from Havana bound to New York but during the voyage the master and mate died of yellow fever, leaving the ship without a navigator. It fell in alongside an English vessel that could not spare a navigator but advised the crew to follow her. On August 22 the *George Law* came alongside and sent over her third mate, Mr. Wendell, to navigate the ship to New York. This was done and the owners of the *George Law* claimed salvage on the *John Potter* in the amount of $16,000. The judge acknowledged the service rendered was technically a salvage, but noted the *George Law* was only delayed half an hour and only slightly inconvenienced by the loss of the third mate. Consequently, he awarded $1,000 in the case, of that amount $700 going to Mr. Wendell; $65 to the captain of the *George Law*; $35 to the first mate and $200 to the owners.[26]

CHAPTER 20

The American Un-Civil War Period, 1860–1866

Almost the only fixed and undeniable fact connected with this disease [yellow fever] is that its prevalence is simultaneous with the heats of summer, and that frost is its deadly enemy. From these frank acknowledgments it may be understood how exceedingly limited is our knowledge of the subject. Although most deeply interested in it, and although for half a century the most prominent and learned physicians have bestowed labor and investigation upon it, they have failed to establish beyond contradiction and controversy a single fact that would prove of clearly practical utility in guarding against the approach of the destroyer, or in cutting short its ravages.[1]

In June 1860 the Quarantine Commissioners of New York met to discuss their proposed investigation "touching the destruction of property at Quarantine," and to address the presentation of claims for losses incurred due to the arson. At the same time, the new physician of the Marine Hospital, Dr. J.H. Jerome, presented a letter to the Commissioners of Emigration warning that the public would hold them "to a strict accountability if pestilence should reach us unprepared."

In the same month, the Fourth Annual Convention of the Sanitary Reform Association met at Boston. One of their main topics concerned whether heat or cold was best employed as a disinfectant. Reaffirming the resolution of the last session that declared yellow fever "not to be infectious," they resolved to appoint a committee of five to obtain maps from the various cities with an aim of determining necessary sanitary measures to be presented the following May at the next convention. Not surprisingly, in a letter to the *New York Times,* one of the delegates complained that of those who accompanied him to Boston only one *"attended the Sanitary Convention, and he only as a part of the first day of its session. It was currently reported in Boston that a large majority of this party spent their time, from the moment of their arrival, in carousing and visiting houses of questionable repute; or, in other words, they had a jolly good spree upon the money* [$2,500] *filched from the City Treasury."*

By mid–July, New York was considered "never healthier," attributed, in part, to the new health officer, Dr. A.H. Gunn, and his creation of an affidavit he required all captains to sign before vessels could be brought up to the city. The old steamer *Falcon* was still used as a floating hospital, having been moved from Gravesend Bay to five miles from the New York side of Sandy Hook. Due to the loosening changes in quarantine, the board of health stated that under the new regime of ventilation and observation, ship owners saved hundreds of thousands of dollars in towing, lighterage, stevedoring and fumigation.[2]

Two preludes to the coming strife were noted in 1860. The first came on May 19 when the Senate took up a message from President James Buchanan. It noted the capture on April 26 of the slaver *Wildfire*, by Captain Cragin of the steamer *Mohawk*. Aboard were 507 Negroes who were carried to Key West, Florida, on April 30. In consequence of the increased activity in the slave trade, it was suggested the president be authorized to make a general agreement with the Colonization Society. Until that time, an expense of $12,000 had already been incurred, "but worse than this, the yellow fever is likely to come to Key West." The marshal urged their removal at an early date.

The second, from the *Raleigh* (NC) *Register,* reissued a warning first sounded in 1859, that South Carolina, in her clamorous demands for disunion and her cherished hopes to "become the great Southern port," ought to remember "that the harbor of Charleston is far less capacious than Beaufort, has less water upon her bar, and that for three months in the year, she is subject to the yellow fever."[3]

The War Between the States

On April 13, 1861, the Federal garrison at Fort Sumter surrendered to Confederate officers and all the firebrand talk of secession became a reality. Although most of the fighting was done on Southern soil, yellow fever did not play a major factor in the war. Most of the early mentions of the disease from Northern papers were similar: yellow fever seemed "specially inviting" in Charleston. "Down South" they had nine months of the year devoted to mosquitoes and the other three to yellow fever; those who could were fleeing New Orleans because they expected an attack from United States forces, and yellow fever was expected to be of an especially violent type. (In fact, by late May the first three cases were reported at Charity Hospital and on August 3 the *New-York Times* reported the disease had broken out among the troops and civilians. Actually, a letter published in the *London Standard* of August 20, 1861, was far closer to the truth when the writer stated he could not remember "a season when there was so little sickness in the Southern countries as this year."[4]

Deaths from Yellow Fever in New Orleans During the Civil War Period, 1860–1865

Year	Number of Deaths
1860	15
1861	0
1862	2
1863	2
1864	6
1865	1[5]

Although residents of New Orleans attempted to scare the Federal troops by "irritating epithets" inviting the soldiers "to come and be measured for their coffins, as Yellow Jack is waiting for them" and telling stories "either to drive us out or scare us," even the *Picayune* reported, "the Yankees don't scare worth a d—m."

Ultimately, Northern newspapers attributed the success in combating yellow fever in New Orleans to General Butler's sanitary regulations and general administration. Southern-leaning papers were more likely to consider "Butler had as much to do in keeping [yellow fever] away as the Tycoon of Japan." At Vicksburg in August 1863, diarrhea was the principal disease. To guard against yellow fever, chloride of lime was thickly spread over the town and suburbs.

By mid–August 1862 yellow fever was reported as "raging" at Key West, the report noting a vessel from that city arrived at Boston with 30 cases aboard. By early October conditions had not improved with two ships, the *St. Lawrence* and the *Huntsville*, having lost significant numbers of crew to the disease. Attempting to prevent yellow fever from being transported from Key West to South Carolina, General Hunter, the Federal officer in charge, established a rigid quarantine at St. Helena Sound (below Charleston, between Beaufort and Colleton counties), requiring every vessel to anchor, be inspected and receive a permit from Surgeon Crispell to proceed. A gunboat was stationed near the lightship at the entrance of the harbor to notify ships of the sanitary restrictions. In July 1864 reports again indicated yellow fever was raging at Key West and no communication was had with that port except for the exchange of mail at a point five miles below the city. By September 27, the *Wilmington* (NC) *Journal* reported the dreadful scourge was at Jacksonville, Florida, and extending its ravages along the coast,

Isolated reports from 1862 indicated yellow fever was at Charleston, but there were no major outbreaks, despite the fact that on July 7, 1862, Union medical reports indicated the soldiers were nearly overcome by "clouds of mosquitoes" and little peace was available "for men without netting to protect them at night." Soldiers of the 7th New Hampshire arrived at Hilton Head on August 29, 1862, carrying yellow fever with them. This caused an outbreak of the disease that proved deadly, although it was generally confined to the island. Houston and Sabine Pass, Texas, also suffered outbreaks but there were no major epidemics.

The most significant reports came from Wilmington, the disease supposed to have been brought there by the crew of the *Kate* or some other vessel that had recently run the blockade. By mid–September, 30–40 cases had been reported and "the most active exertions have been made to cleanse the town and prevents its spreading." On September 15, a correspondent ("Worrell") wrote that the symptoms were the same as in 1821: a pain in the back and head with scorching fever and ending with the black vomit. He added, "There is much alarm of its spreading, principally from one thing, the steam-mills and distilleries have stopped operations. The health of the City heretofore has been chiefly attributed to them."

General Beauregard sent several physicians from Charleston and the mayor sent nurses to attend the sick. On October 20 the *Wilmington Journal* reported that a sudden change to cold "had a deadly effect on 500 pending cases," with new cases reaching as high as 53 per day and 18–20 burials. Dr. Choppin also arrived from Washington, declaring the fever to resemble "ship or Asiatic fever." Worrell added in a September 29 report, "It seems as if the atmosphere is so intensely poisoned, that no matter what kind of sickness a person is taken with, it is certain to terminate in the 'prevailing epidemic.'"

Losses in the war required Confederate authorities to move Federal prisoners from one location to another. Many from Andersonville and Libby were eventually sent to Charleston. During the last of September or the first of October 1864 yellow fever broke out at in the city. Although daily mortality among the civilian population was described as "quite large," Federal captives later reported they "were singularly exempt from the scourge." In order to protect their own troops, however, the Rebels were compelled to send their prisoners to Columbia, South Carolina. Yellow fever outbreaks were also reported at Savannah, with the worst reports coming from Newbern, North Carolina. A report from November 1 stated, "The number of deaths from fever will not exceed 2,000, consisting mostly of citizens and refugees. The fever originated from the ship at the foot of Craven St. in Newbern [where the dock] was filled up last June by Capt. Bradley with manure and barrels of rotten meat." Interestingly, cases of yellow fever were reported at Bermuda (not extending beyond the island of St. George's), where it was believed to have been introduced by Southern blockade runners.[6]

In one concluding paragraph on the war, in an article titled, "Geographical Knowledge as Developed by the War," the *Indiana Herald* of March 8, 1865, observed that little was known of Charleston, Mobile and Savannah before the conflict except that those cities "had quite a wide-spread reputation for oranges, yellow fever, [and] sharp-billed mosquitoes."

Ultimately, yellow fever struck with limited violence during the Civil War, summed up by the *Castle* (IN) *Courier* on September 15, 1864:

> We have not heard of the malaria in any of the swamps except in the Chickahominy, nor of any death-winged fevers at the west and in the low lands of the southwest, nor of that dreadful scourge the yellow fever, in the southern parts.... We all remember with what glee our Northern armies were welcomed by the rebel press to the pestilence which walked in the Southern noonday, but hitherto their wicked welcome has been all in vain. They should try to see the Providence in so remarkable a fact.

The "Yellow Fever Plot": A Case of Bioterrorism

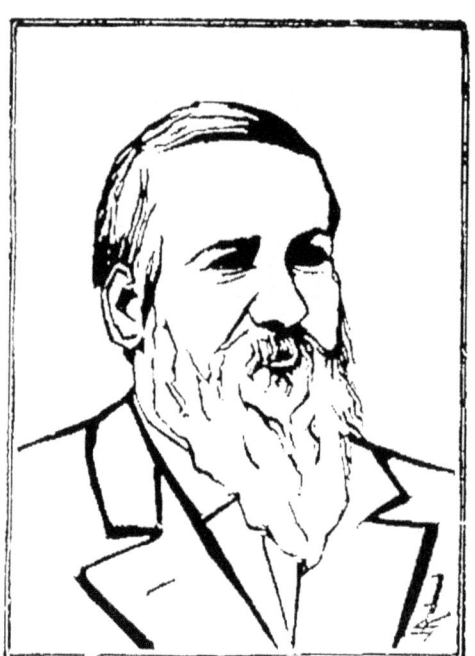

Two assassination plots—one successful, the other not—occurred in 1865, both having their roots in the Civil War. On the evening of April 14, 1865, John Wilkes Booth shot President Abraham Lincoln. The 16th president died the following day. While the nation was still in mourning, news of a different plot—one aimed to destroy the lives of hundreds, if not thousands of Americans—was revealed.

The story, as developed over several months, was often confused, occasionally con-

John Hood, who later became pastor in a Presbyterian church, volunteered to serve in the Union Army during the Civil War. On May 3, 1863, he and 1,365 other Yankees were captured at Rome, Georgia, and sent to Libby Prison, where Hood was confined for twelve months. Afterward, a grueling trip took the prisoners from Danville, Virginia, to Macon, Georgia, and then to Charleston, South Carolina. There Hood and his companions were placed in the line of fire when Union soldiers bombarded the city. After yellow fever broke out among the prisoners, Rebel authorities determined that, to prevent the spread of disease to their own soldiers, the prisoners were to be sent to Columbia, South Carolina. Along the way Hood and a companion escaped. With the help of the "colored people" who gave them food, clothing and red pepper to put on their shoes to prevent the bloodhounds from tracking them, they eventually made it to safety (*Cedar Rapids Gazette*, May 16, 1885).

tradictory, and ultimately unsettled. The main character in what became known as "The Yellow Fever Plot" was Luke P. Blackburn (June 16, 1816–September 14, 1887), a physician born in Kentucky who in 1847 moved to Natchez, where he established his practice and became friends with Jefferson Davis. (During investigations into the plot, a letter from Davis, addressed to the "Senate Chamber, 14th March, 1849, Secretary of the United States Treasury," endorsed Blackburn as "being well known to me as of the highest respectability and intelligence.") The doctor subsequently practiced at New Orleans, serving as the city's health officer in 1848 and successfully implemented quarantines in 1848 and 1854.

Blackburn, described as a rabid secessionist, was asked by Mississippi governor John J. Pettus to travel to Canada to collect provisions for blockade runners there. At one point he was aboard a blockade runner en route from Halifax to Mobile with a shipment of ice when the vessel was captured by the Union navy. Assumed to be an innocent civilian, he was released and returned to Canada.

In April 1864 yellow fever broke out at Bermuda, a strongpoint for Confederate smugglers. Fearing the disease would hamper operations Blackburn traveled to the island and was instrumental in treating victims. In mid–July he briefly went back to Halifax but returned to Bermuda in September 1864 to continue his work, remaining there until mid–October when the disease abated. For this service he received £100 and a commendation from Queen Victoria.

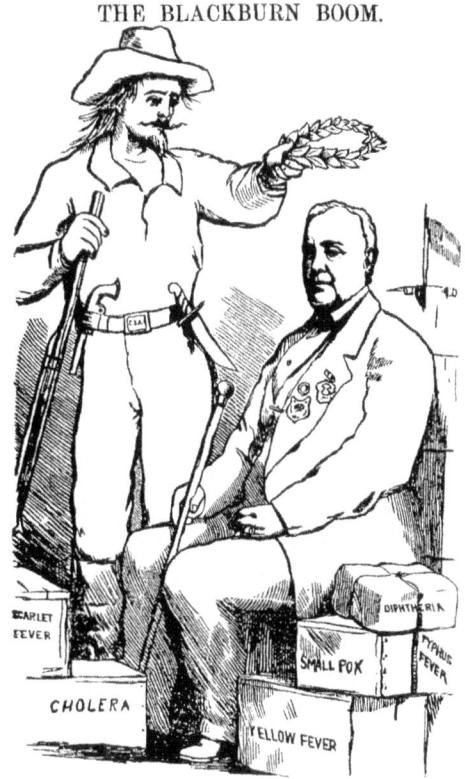

In many Northern states, Luke Blackburn was considered "The Wickedest Man in the World" for his alleged role in biological warfare during the Civil War. In this political cartoon, all the transmittable disease evils in the world—scarlet fever, diphtheria, cholera, smallpox, typhus and yellow fever—were laid at his feet, while a Confederate soldier prepares to place the laurel wreath of heroism on his head (*Indianapolis Journal*, October 29, 1879).

According to testimony taken in May 1865, while in Bermuda Blackburn attended "several yellow fever patients at Hamilton hotel and at Mrs. Slater's. Some of them died under his care. He collected their bed-clothing—including a large quantity of woolen clothing which, in one case at least, he had ordered to be piled upon the patients in order to receive the infection, packed it in trunks, and sent it to the house of Edward C. Swan, to be kept by him till an opportunity offered to send it North. Blackburn then left for Halifax."

When authorities were alerted that Swan was in possession of infected clothing, the trunks were confiscated. Swan testified that Blackburn had given them to him and advised him to "call on the officers of the Confederate Government for money." Other witnesses swore they had been paid $150 per month to assist Swan in the business. One of the trunks had a shipping label marked "St. Louis hotel, Upper town, Quebec," and the other, "Clifton house, Niagara Falls, Canada side."

On April 24, 1865, Captain Smith of the brig *J. Titus* arrived in New York from Bermuda with news that Blackburn "had collected four bales of infected clothing, consisting of sheets, shirts and other refuse matter, from the hospitals, which he intended to ship to New-York for the purpose of spreading the fever in the city." Authorities burned the bales on quarantine two days after Smith left. Meanwhile, the investigation held at St. Georges implied Blackburn had visited Bermuda "ostensibly on a philanthropic mission, in connection with the causes of yellow fever. The evidence showed he collected infected new clothing with orders to ship them to New York in the spring. "One witness testified that Blackburn identified himself as a Confederate agent, whose mission was the destruction of the Northern masses. It also shows that several persons connected with the agency of the Confederate States were cognizant of these facts.... Blackburn is well known in these provinces [Canada] as a leading ultra rebel."

On April 26, the preliminary examination at Bermuda resulted in the committal of a resident of the island named Levan on the charge of having conspired with Blackburn, who made "liberal promises" to him, provided the contract to ship trunks was fully carried out. Funds were to be supplied "freely from the Confederate Exchange, and meanwhile Blackburn himself was to retire to Halifax and watch the progress of events until the opening of spring, when the session would probably be more favorable." On May 10 the magistrates at Bermuda decided to send the case to the attorney general for prosecution before the Court of General Assizes or Quarter Sessions. Swan was remanded for bail in £50 with two sureties for £25 each.

Understandably, news of the plot was not well received in the United States. The *Philadelphia Inquirer* noted the following:

> That it is possible to introduce a pestilential disease into a community by means of infected clothing is a well-known fact. That any human being should be so diabolical as to originate a plan to disseminate pestilence by wholesale in any community would, until lately, have exceeded the limits of belief.... It will be recalled that there is no love for the Union in Bermuda. That island has participated in the gains and excitements of blockade running, and the feeling of the residents has been strongly manifested in behalf of the Southern Rebellion. It must have been a shameless and exceedingly wicked combination of circumstances which would have incited the Bermudians to reveal the treble sinfulness of their "friends".... There developments were only needed to convince mankind that the spirit which ruled the Secessionists has never been exceeded in fiendish attributes by anything known to civilization.

The *New York Tribune* added, "If hellish malignity can further go than the assassination of the late President, it certainly seems realized in the scheme of a Dr. Blackburn."[7]

Dr. Blackburn was bound over for trial in Toronto on May 25, 1865 on $8,000 bond on a charge that read as follows:

> ... that LUKE P. BLACKBURN and one GODFREY JOSEPH HYAMS and divers other persons unknown, did at the said City of Toronto, on or about the 15th day of April, in the year of our Lord 1864, combine, conspire, confederate and agree among themselves to commit the crime of murder in the United States of America, by importing and introducing from Her Majesty's dominions into certain cities of the said United States of America, to wit: the City of Washington, in the District of Columbia; the City of Norfolk, in the State of Virginia; and the City of Newbern in the State of North Carolina, one of the said United States of America, and there disposing of, to and amongst the inhabitants of said cities, divers large quantities of shirts, blouses, coats and other articles of clothing, infected with the virus of yellow fever and other deadly poisonous and noxious substances, calculated and liable to produce said fever, for the purpose of creating and spreading the said disease amongst

the said citizens by means of said yellow fever and the poisonous, deadly and noxious substances aforesaid. And that in pursuance of said conspiracy, combination, confederation and agreement, the said LUKE P. BLACKBURN, to wit, the 1st day of June, 1864, did cause to be exported and sent from the said City of Halifax, in the Province of Nova Scotia, divers, to wit, tea-trunks containing such infected clothing into the said United States, and did cause the said infected clothing to be disposed of and sold in the said Cities of Washington, Norfolk and Newbern, to and among the citizens thereof, for the wicked and unlawful purpose, and with the wicked intent aforesaid, and that by means of the said infected clothing, so imported in and disposed of as aforesaid, in the cities, in pursuance of said conspiracy, the death of divers persons in said cities to the informant unknown, was caused and procured.

Hyams was the principal witness against Blackburn, testifying that the physician matured his plot in Canada and at Clifton, on the Canadian side of Niagara Falls, consulting with other villains "who were pretending to be engaged in the celebrated 'Peace Conference' at which Horace Greeley was so sadly befooled." The plan was to sell the clothing at auction in areas held by the Federals "so they would take sick and death be caused by the fever, and that they would easily be driven from the Confederate territory held by them." For Hyams' services, he was promised $100,000. Blackburn advised him to smoke strong cigars and chew camphor to protect himself against the fever. He traveled under the name J.W. Harris and said he shipped the goods to Boston and took one valise to his hotel, "as he was ordered to be sure and make a present of it to President Lincoln." He expressed other trunks to Philadelphia and from there to Baltimore.

Hyams (accused of being a double agent and paid for his testimony) continued his recitation by stating he heard some of the clothes had been sold in Norfolk and he saw by the papers that yellow fever had been there. Later, when seeing Blackburn, he was asked if he left clothes at Washington and he replied yes, "to which the doctor replied that he was glad of that, as its contents would kill at sixty yards." On cross-examination by Mr. M.C. Cameron, Hyams "contradicted himself in several important points, including the fee he was promised. He stated he was an American citizen, "but that as the Federal soldiers had broken his furniture and insulted his family, he was bound to have revenge. He had not taken the oath of allegiance, however, to the Confederates."

In reaction to statements at trial showing that yellow fever had been introduced there ("which carried off some thousands" that summer) advances from Newbern on May 5 "caused the utmost horror." President Johnson pardoned Hyams on June 22, 1865. Counsel for the defense "admitted the evidence" of subsequent witnesses W.W. Cleary and Edwin J. Hall—who made similar statements—but "contended that there was no decided authority in support of the prosecution for conspiracy to murder in a foreign country, and that it was not punishable by the common law in England unless it was contemplated to murder the head of a government." In October 1865 the court dropped the charge of conspiracy to commit murder on those grounds and further acquitted him "on grounds that the trunks of garments had been shipped to Nova Scotia, which was out of the court's jurisdiction." Blackburn was "admitted to bail on his own recognizance, his sureties being discharged."[8]

Although Blackburn was acquitted, historical reevaluation has not always been so kind. Edward Steers Jr. in his book, *Blood on the Moon,* believed in the doctor's complicity and also implicated Confederate authorities as high as Jefferson Davis. On the charge of attempted assassination of President Lincoln, he wrote, "The small valise of gift shirts designed to infect Lincoln with a deadly disease show that he was a target of the Confederate operation in Canada."[9]

Several interesting side-notes on Blackburn appeared in the years immediately following the Civil War. In January 1866 the *Toronto Ledger* was reported as publishing a series of medical articles by Dr. Blackburn, "the person charged with attempting to introduce yellow fever and small-pox among the United States soldiers during the war." In June of the same year the *Atlanta New Era* contained an article noting that Robert Bruce Blackburn, of Blackburnsborough, Scotland, and one of the wealthiest manufacturers in Europe, had died, leaving an estate of $2,000,000. Heirs included the late John Blackburn of South Carolina and another brother who settled in East Tennessee. The estate was represented, in part, by Dr. C.C. Blackburn of Atlanta and perhaps by another brother living in Texas or Arkansas. The notice concluded, "Can this lucky Dr. Blackburn of Georgia be the man who took so much trouble to give us the yellow fever in 1864, importing several packages of it duty free?"

In April 1867 reports indicated that Luke Blackburn had applied to the attorney general for permission to leave Canada and return to his native land. The attorney general announced he had no authority to grant the request. On September 4, 1867, Blackburn wrote to President Andrew Johnson asking permission to return home and treat victims of a yellow fever outbreak in New Orleans. Johnson never answered. On September 17, D. Thurston, U.S. consul in Toronto, sent William H. Seward, the secretary of state, an affidavit containing Blackburn's oath of allegiance. Seward returned it on September 25 with this comment:

> The affiant is understood to be the person who is called Dr. Blackburn. Nothing is known by the Department concerning him has having directly or indirectly participated in the late rebellion. All that is known, is that he lies under the charge of felony, in this, that he conceived and put into execution within a foreign jurisdiction, a plot to disseminate contagion and pestilence in this and other cities of the United States, by clandestinely transmitting for an unsuspicious market here, masses of auction clothing taken from the corpses of persons who had died of the yellow fever in the tropics. It is not easy to understand how an offense of that character which is a detestable crime against mankind, can be supposed, even by the felon himself, to be entitled to be regarded as an act of insurrection, rebellion, or civil war. The President's proclamation offers no immunity in this case.

Ultimately, Blackburn risked arrest and prosecution to return without permission, arriving at Louisville on September 25. After treating patients in New Orleans, he and his family moved to an Arkansas plantation owned by his wife. Blackburn was never charged in the United States and ultimately was elected governor of Kentucky in 1879, despite having been nicknamed "Dr. Blackvomit" by out-of-state presses.[10]

Another infamous character associated with attempting to introduce yellow fever-infected clothing into Northern cities during the War was Jake Thompson. After his death in 1885 Secretary Lamar closed the Interior Department and ordered the flag lowered to half-mast in Thompson's honor. In one of many responses, the Ohio Republican platform condemned Lamar, causing ripples of approval or anger throughout the nation. The *Philadelphia Press* defended the Ohio Republicans by arguing, "The attempt to shield the memory of this dastardly traitor shows how thoroughly the Copperhead Democracy sympathized with his peculiar efforts to aid the rebellion, and a yellow shirt, emblematic of the loathsome disease he endeavored to introduce, should be the flag of his defenders." The *Des Moines Register* added, "Does any fair man want to know the real character of the new administration...? If he does, let him size up" two factors: lowering the government flag in honor of Jake Thompson and the fact it did not lower the standard on the anniversary of the death of Abraham Lincoln. The *Goshen Times* (April 2, 1885) added,

"When the National flag was lowered last week on account of the death of the fiend Thompson, the red flag of small pox and the yellow flag of yellow fever ought to have been raised."[11]

Warnings Ignored, 1866

Ironically, Galveston and New Orleans, the two cities destined to suffer horrific yellow fever epidemics in 1867, had divertive views on the subject in 1866. Although "old citizens" of both places predicted major epidemics in 1866, they were a year off. In Galveston one civil leader named T.J. Heard suggested that quarantine (to which "the masses of the people look for protection") was of little value. Dividing the population into two categories—those who knew nothing and moved about as automatons, and the far less numerous class of those, "well-defined on the subject,"—he urged the latter to carry out a system sanitation to keep yellow fever at bay. In a refrain that sounds as fresh today as it was nearly 150 years ago, he acknowledged his advice of making Galveston one of the healthiest cities on the continent would cost a great deal, and any such plans would run counter to those "whose great aim and ambition" was to make, rather than to spend, money.

He suggested a barrel of salt be cast into old privies and the privies covered up, that backyards be cleaned up and the earth saturated with salt, excrement be removed from stables and ventilation improved. Heard was also head of the committee appointed to report on the sanitary arrangements of Galveston, by order of the secretary of the United States Treasury. The report of this group called for the appointment of a board of health and acknowledged yellow fever to be of local origin, thus making quarantine "powerless for good," especially when sanitary measures were not implemented. The group called for the drainage of ponds, called attention of the municipal authorities to "the habitual and almost universal violation of the rules conservative of health, on the part of the negro population," and the application of "anti-septics" (salt, lime and copperas) as disinfectants.[12]

In New Orleans, one writer offered the peculiar opinion that as yellow fever was not indigenous to the city many expected it to run its course and wear out "as it has done in other places, where after returning periodically, it finally disappeared." The season began late in 1866, with most notices of mortality coming in October. By the 17th of the month the death toll had expanded from five to eight per day and by the end of the epidemic official records placed the total at 185.[13]

Yellow fever outbreaks throughout the South were limited in 1866, giving the editor of the *Mobile Advertiser* the liberty to recount the story of "Straight-back Dick" and his joke upon a northerner who had recently departed off an upriver boat. Spotting the stranger walking up Dauphin Street, carpet sack in hand, Dick ran up to him, ordered that he stand straight and began measuring him. When he worked up his nerve to ask the meaning of Dick's action, "Straight-back" replied that he was the city undertaker and was sizing him for a coffin. Immediately terrified, the man protested he was not dying but Dick declared he would be dead by morning from yellow fever. He suggested he return to the boat, swallow a gill of brandy and get under the covers until perspiring freely. The "Hoosier" followed Dick's instructions to the letter and vowed he would never forget the kindness of the tall man in Memphis who gave him such good advice.[14]

Chapter 21

Holding On Until the Other Jack (Frost) Says "Enough!"

A New Orleans letter, dated the 23rd ult., says that, owing to the yellow fever, "the city is a vast hospital. It is believed that there are ten thousand cases now under treatment. You hear of it everywhere and in almost every house. It is in all our crowded orphan asylums. The good Sisters are stricken down. Language fails to depict the misery and distress existing here."[1]

The first identified cases of yellow fever at Galveston were announced on July 24, 1867, followed by further information that five deaths had occurred from the fever and two from black vomit. The mayor ordered the free use of disinfectants but stated there were "no fears of the disease becoming epidemic." By August 4 the local newspaper stated that *if* there was yellow fever in the city (as reported by a team of physicians from Houston who reported 130 cases and 25 deaths) the disease did not originate locally but was imported from places "with which we are in communication." Two days later, the Mortuary Report indicated 7 confirmed deaths; numbers quickly escalated to 12–20 per day. Although local newspapers continued to downplay the severity of the epidemic, they also reported that 6,000–8,000 citizens had fled the city, leaving behind 15,000, of which 10,000 were unacclimated.

Deaths in Galveston, 1867

Month	Date	Deaths
August	10	24
	11	21
	12	20
	13	28
	14	29
	15	29

By August 15 over 1,000 cases had been reported, putting a great strain on the local chapter of the Howard Association. Sending out a desperate call for money, groceries and blankets, the association supplied 30 nurses to tend the growing number of sick.

Among those exposed to the danger were numerous Union troops stationed in the environs under the command of Major General Phil Sheridan. On August 19 he wrote to Washington, notifying his superior, General U.S. Grant, that the situation was becoming dire:

> General:—The yellow fever has abated but very little. On the coast of TEXAS at Galveston and Indianola it has been very bad, and has interfered to some extent with the public service from the stampede and flight of employes [sic].

For the week ending August 24 another 187 persons perished. The following week 241 were listed dead, with an additional 100 deaths at Corpus Christi through August 16. Heeding the call for aid, contributors from New York and Boston put together $4,000 by August 30 to be sent to the Howard Association, as its expenses had reached $200 per day in Houston alone. N.B. Yard, president of the Galveston Howard Association, acknowledged an additional $500 from New Yorkers and also asked for donations of mustard, limes and lemons.[2]

On September 1, J. Holstein, a member of the Jewish community, wrote to the *Cincinnati Israelite* asking for assistance during the epidemic. He noted that at the commencement of the plague, there resided in Galveston "nearly 300 Jehudim," of whom half had fled to escape the disease. Placing the total number of dead at 707, he stated the Jehudim had lost 33, among whom were old residents of the city. He stated the Hebrew Benevolent Society had done good and noble work, its funds were exhausted and he hoped others would lend a helping hand.

By September 22 yellow fever appeared to have run its course, leaving 999 dead. However, on September 23 a quarantine was established for Brazoria County prohibiting "all Steamboats, Railroad Cars, Sail Vessels or other Craft, or all persons traveling by public or private conveyance" coming from places infected with yellow fever, especially Houston and Galveston, from entering the county until they had been absent from those areas for 15 days. The concern may have been justified, as a report from the village of Charenton, on the Teche, indicated that by October 9 out of a population of 99 whites and 24 Negroes, 14 whites and 2 Negroes had died, while on the opposite side of the stream, 11 Indians had perished from yellow fever, which was believed "probably never [to have] had a precedent."

The yellow fever subscription fund in New York was closed in November on the discontinuance of the disease, between $80,000–$90,000 having been raised for Galveston and New Orleans.[3]

Lovers, Croakers and Grunters

During the 19th century it was extremely rare that newspapers published anything negative about victims or the nurses caring for them. That makes the following articles all the more interesting:

> The epidemic brings to light some cases of very unhappy incident. One that we saw on Friday night showed a phase of life unfortunately too common. Passing a low frame house on our way home, we saw a commotion with a policeman at the door. He related that it was a house kept by a degraded and drunken woman; that within an hour a man had died therein who held a responsible place in a public office—that he was a gentleman bred, a man of education and unusual ability—that for four or five days he had been spreeing, and finally took the fever and died in that den of infamy. The woman was bewailing his death, saying that he was her "lover." Finally she became so noisy that the police took her to the station.

The second incident concerned "Croakers," or those who spread gruesome details about the fever. It concerned a "fair lady," on her way to convalescence, who was visited by a croaker who "came in with a bucket of horrors, and rehearsed them all in her hearing. In one hour the lady was in her coffin, killed by a croaker." The third story concerned "a female imposter whom we reported yesterday as collecting money on a fraudulent pretext of having a dead child [who] must have received more than fifty, and perhaps one hundred dollars." The newspaper cautioned everyone against bestowing charity and recommended giving, instead, to the Howard Association. The fourth account is the most shocking: "We regret to be compelled to allude to the report of a nameless outrage said to have been committed on the body of a deceased female. The crime is so unnatural that we can not believe it, and the witness so respectable that we can not dispute their recital. Therefore, we must wait until the case is heard before a proper tribunal, hoping, in the meantime, for the sake of decency and humanity, that there will be found a mistake." Finally, a report from the Houston *Telegraph* stated, "Our yellow fever Hospital has been shamefully imposed upon by incompetent, and, in some instances, rascally nurses. Those in charge of the Hospital have been helpless because the best nurses were all employed by our noble Firemen's Association, and paid in specie, while the Hospital nurses were given less prices, and had to look to the city for pay. Hence the Hospital had to pick up nurses whom nobody else would have. Some of them would drink a glass of brandy sent to a patient the moment he or she was out of sight."

On a slightly more humorous vein were those "on the grunt," or people who complained about their illnesses. Inspired by the 19th century humorist Artemus Ward, one story concerned the wooing of a lady, Betsy Jane, while under the influence of hot whisky punches. She ordered her beau to "come in you old fool, to-morrow you'll be going around complaining about your liver." One newspaper offered this addendum: "On behalf of convalescents, we protest that it is Yellow Jack, and not 'whisky punch' that is bothering their livers."[4]

Dry Tortugas

Dry Tortugas was a small island in the Florida Keys. Originally planned as the permanent site for Fort Jefferson, the structure was never completed and during this period was used as a prison. Its most famous inmate was Samuel Mudd, the physician who treated John Wilkes Booth's broken leg after the assassination of President Abraham Lincoln. Yellow fever (alternately called "backbone fever") broke out on the island and after the post doctor became ill Mudd treated the sick prisoners "very successfully." It was ultimately estimated that one-tenth of the entire island, including soldiers and prisoners, died from the disease. In October, soldiers at the fort unanimously signed a petition and sent it to Washington, asking the government for Mudd's release in consequence of his "great exertions in attending the yellow fever cases." On the exertions of his lawyer, Mudd was eventually pardoned on February 8, 1869.[5]

New Orleans, 1867

Outbreaks of yellow fever began in late July, with the last week of the month registering 5 deaths to cholera's 17. The first week of August the ratio reversed: 9 deaths from yellow fever and 8 for cholera. By August 14, due to apprehensions that the disease might become epidemic, instructions from General Grant's headquarters informed officers absent from their posts at New Orleans and Galveston to extend their leave until the 15th of October. The precaution was well taken: between the 19th and 20th of August 87 persons died. Numbers continued to escalate and on August 29 there were 26 reported deaths. On September 3 yellow fever deaths reached 28 per day and the board of health declared an epidemic but described it as "mild." The Howard Association immediately reorganized but announced it was without funds.

The disease spread quickly, especially along the waterways. Late in August, 30 crew and 4 officers aboard the ironclad *Mahaska* were stricken and removed to the hospital. Four soon died: "They had remained cooped up on board until the vessel had almost become a pest house." Matters worsened by importations from other southern states: by September 8 the tow-boat *Mohawk* arrived from Memphis with 7 cases, one of whom died on the wharf. The mayor placed a physician with medicines onboard and ordered the boat to leave for President's Island, where quarantine had been established.

News of the quarantine was not well taken by the local press. The *Picayune* decried it as locking the stable after the horse had gone, bemoaning the fact "lowering the gate at the mouth of the river" locked out their only summer business with the Gulf ports. The point was well taken as death tolls escalated; for the week ending September 8, a total of 249 persons had perished. Quarantine was also placed around Mobile, prohibiting any vessels from New Orleans into the city. In anticipation of that city's becoming infected, General Spinner, the U.S. treasurer, ordered the removal of all government funds deposited there and placed in cities further north.

Reports dated September 19 indicated that there was "almost an utter stagnation in business, the up-river boats keeping away through fear…. The funeral corteges are too numerous to employ even the muffled drum, and the bands of mourners that daily go to our cemeteries with the loved and lost, have no ears to enjoy a band of music. The radical press of this city lays the blame of all this on Sheridan."

Another indication of the polarization and fears that remained in the country after the Civil War were two reports, the first a September 26 insert in an Indiana paper: "One of the beauties of the President's amnesty proclamation is that the notorious Dr. Blackburn, of yellow fever notoriety, is about to visit New Orleans, having obtained leave to do so." A second report came from the *Memphis Post* on October 9, 1867: "Dr. Luke Blackburn, better known as 'Yellow Fever Blackburn,' was in the city the day previous, on his way to New Orleans. He attended the meeting of the Board of Health, and made some remarks on the subject of yellow fever. The scoundrel has been denounced as an outlaw by Secretary of State Seward, and yet he seems to be traveling through the country at his leisure."

One thousand, two-hundred deaths by yellow fever were reported by the end of September, the majority of which were attributed to foreigners and children. As an example, of the 59 dying on September 19 two were from the north, 41 were foreigners and 15 were of southern birth, while the *New Orleans Times* indicated that no fewer than 40,000 inhabitants had the fever during the present epidemic, attributing that to "the neglect of the public authorities to keep the city in good sanitary condition."[6]

On October 15 a letter sent by J.F. Caldwell, secretary of the New Orleans Howard Association, was received in New York, advising that the yellow fever epidemic was declining and asking that no more donations be solicited. As new cases continued to decline, Dr. Warren Stone advised the board of health on October 30 to suspend quarantine; the motion was opposed and referred to the Committee on Health. Ultimately, the board of health declared on November 5 that the disease was no longer epidemic. More cautious than New Orleans, the New York Board of Health announced that quarantine against certain southern ports would remain in effect until November 21.

Ultimately, newspapers reported that over 3,000 persons died from the "Bronzed John" in the 1867 New Orleans epidemic and the official total was placed at 3,107. It was estimated that the disease cost New Orleans $3,000,000,000 in actual expenses and, indirectly, from loss of trade. Galveston was said to have suffered a similar economic disaster. On an interesting side note, the *Commercial Bulletin* noted that of the 60 workers engaged in laying the Nicholson pavement—covering the wood blocks with tar—on St. Charles Street, not one was attacked by yellow fever.[7]

Yellow Fever in the United States Through the End of the Decade

The year 1868 was adeptly characterized by a paragraph in the *Galveston Daily News*, August 13, 1868:

> The Savannah papers are piping over one of those reports which leave one in doubt whether they betray more malice or ignorance. After stating that the report of the existence of yellow fever in Savannah, and of seven deaths, had been obtained from a friend "who had just left," the publication goes on in the usual style;
> > It is reported on our streets that this fearful disease is on the increase in our neighbor city, but we hope it is not true.
>
> If everybody who reads that will at once set it down that there has not been a single case of yellow fever at Savannah this season, and that it was because there had not been a single case, and was not any expectation of the disease, that the report was started, he will hit the nail precisely on the head. And what we say of this report will always be found true of similar ones.

Two more notes of worth close out 1868. The Medical Department of the University of Louisiana ran an ad for their fall classes with this addendum: "In case an epidemic of yellow fever should occur during the summer, students may nevertheless have no hesitation in coming to the city in the time here designated. During the thirty-one years of the existence of the Medical Department no student has been known to die of yellow fever during attendance upon lectures." The second, given in the Report of the Secretary of War, 1868, stated that of 48,081 men in the army as of September 30, deaths in the army were 1,621, of which 452 were from yellow fever and 228 from cholera. Total expenses for the Medical Department were $842,120.[8]

Nor was yellow fever a factor in the United States during 1869. In New York, the newly erected hospital quarters on the West Bank were opened to receive patients from plague ships. Designed to hold 1,000 persons over a strip of several acres, only a small number were on hand (between 50 and 100), and the sick were removed to the hospital ship *Illinois* anchored just below the eastern end of Staten Island in the lower harbor.

Cuba and the West Indian and South American ports where the disease raged were considered the most dangerous, and on June 22, 1869, Major General Canby, in command at Richmond, ordered quarantine regulations at Hampton Roads for vessels lately departing those ports or with yellow fever aboard. The fever did not make inroads ashore and by October 8 the season, thus consequently the danger, was considered at a practical end.[9]

The official mortality for New Orleans in 1868 was 5 and for 1869 the total was 3. One of the few mentions in the South came in the form of "inland yellow fever, or 'Addison's fever,'" which prevailed in the vicinity of Columbus, Mississippi. It had "all the characteristics of the Gulf yellow fever, termination with black vomit." Addison's disease, named for the British physician Thomas Addison (1793–1860), was actually a disease of the adrenal glands, although symptoms of weakness, nausea, vomiting and increased skin pigmentation resembled yellow fever.[10]

Chapter 22

I Am "writing from the city of the dead": Yellow Fever Around the World During the 1860s

> *Curious to think that desks and chairs kill people, but they do. Taken in large quantities office furniture is fatal as yellow fever. We sit and write ourselves away. Sedentary habits produce constipation; that begets dyspepsia; rheumatism and kidney trouble follow in their train, and death ends the chapter. You whose lives are passed over desks and the confined air of offices ought to keep Dr. Kennedy's "Favorite Remedy" always at hand for the stomach and brain.*[1]

St. Thomas, in the Virgin Islands, was destined to make more news than other islands in the vicinity during the 1860s. Ironically, St. Thomas had long been established as the depot of West Indian commerce, serving as late as 1860 as the "rendezvous of the largest fleet of commercial steamers in the world." It was also one of the unhealthiest islands and when disease raged there it affected the entire shipping community.

Between 1840 and 1867, a total of 1,524 persons died of yellow fever on St. Thomas out of a resident population of 12,500 and the "floating population" (seamen) of 30,000 that touched at the island annually. By comparison, during the same period cholera (which first appeared in 1853) killed 2,435, smallpox 355. Other diseases claimed 12,193, chiefly striking "the black and colored population." The average number of ships that visited the harbor in the course of a year was 2,184, with a total tonnage of 451,600, while 20 of the largest steamers in the world were often in harbor on the same day.

Arthur B. Forwood, managing director of the West India and Pacific Steamship Company, indicated that in 1866 his company dispatched upwards of 50 vessels to the West Indies, double the number of voyages performed by the Royal Mail Company. To safeguard the crew, new regulations were adopted:

Prevention of Shipboard Yellow Fever on the West Indies Route

(1) Maintaining premises near the entrance to the St. Thomas Harbor where there was a free current of air

(2) Prevent the crew from being exposed to the sun, prohibit sleeping on deck at night and changing clothes when wet

(3) Well-ventilated forecastles and cleanliness aboard ship

(4) Permit no drinking-water aboard from St. Thomas or put it through the distilling apparatus before use

(5) Distribute diluted doses of quinine every morning to the crew

(6) No liberty (shore leave) permitted

After instituting these regulations, the company reported only four cases of yellow fever for the entire year.[2]

Outbreaks in Cuba across the decade typically resulted in high mortality. In April 1862 alone, out of 91 cases of yellow fever 47 died, or more than 51 percent, while the radio of deaths from smallpox was 606 cases to 79 deaths, or 19 percent. During this period it was observed that although some long-term foreigners never took the disease, "it [was] generally considered to be a tribute that all must sooner or later pay to the climate." Those particularly susceptible were the Spanish troops, among whom it was estimated nearly one-third died of the *vomito negro*.

As disease raged through the island in 1867 the sanitary report for July indicated 1,219 cases, 226 perishing. By comparison, 134 deaths resulted from smallpox. Although horrifying to contemplate, one correspondent for the *New-York Times* (August 15, 1867) wrote that masquerade balls and festivals went on with "unusual brilliancy." Perhaps, he concluded, this was as it should be, "as joy is a great promoter of happiness and destroyer of sickness, and therefore masquerades may be considered as a partial preventative of the black vomit." A less effective method was the "juice of the female verbena leaf" that was promoted in Havannah the same year. The year 1869 also proved deadly when yellow

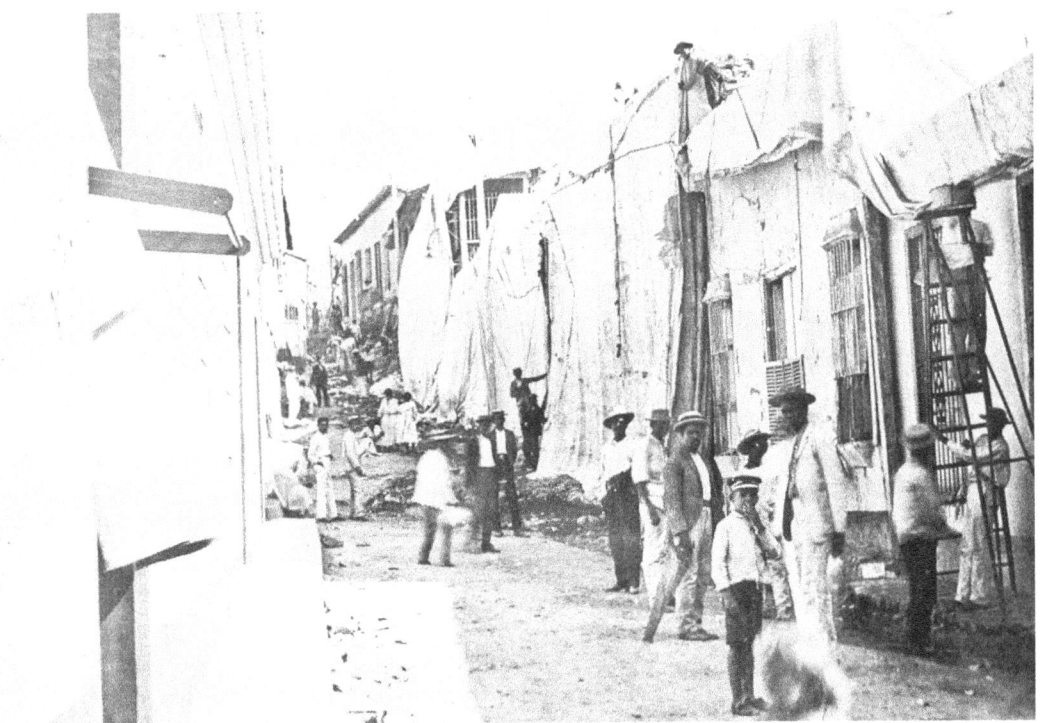

The fight to control yellow fever continues: covering buildings at Santiago, Cuba, January 1908, prior to fumigation (courtesy National Library of Medicine).

fever virtually shut down business in "Porto Rico." Those most susceptible again proved to be the Spanish troops and nationals, all of their houses being "marked with a red hand," while circulars were distributed saying all who were able were fleeing the island. By November the three most dread diseases—cholera, yellow fever and smallpox—struck Santiago de Cuba, where it was reported more than 300 had died within a one-month period.[3]

On the economic front, an interesting feud appeared in the newspapers of January 1862 concerning passage between the Atlantic and Pacific oceans. Various enterprises were in play for this lucrative business, the most common of which had been the natural passage through the Strait of Magellan. Because this route was difficult to navigate, the obvious answer had been an overland route through Panama. In 1862 those with a financial interest in the latter angrily noted, "Speaking of the opening of additional routes of commerce, it is a little singular that every new project finds it necessary to depreciate the Panama route as its opening wedge of success. The Tehuantepec-Squiers'-Honduras scheme, and the Chiriquí, all have their dig at the *unhealthy* Panama route." A new British prospectus also promoted the Magellan route, alerting passengers that this would "shun the Isthmus, where the yellow fever is a permanent institution."

In defending their interests in the Panama route, proponents warned those taking the Magellan route would be much more likely to suffer from disease fever, as those ships touched in at Rio de Janeiro, where "the dreadful African fever" attacked passengers and crews in 1849 and 1850.

Despite protestations by authorities to the contrary, yellow fever was present in Panama, particularly in 1867 and 1868. In 1867 the *New York Sun* published allegations against the Pacific Mail Company of suppressing the epidemic, warning its readers "the constant passenger traffic by way of Panama exposes our city to especial peril from this terrible and fatal disease." The concern was not unjustified, as numerous reports from San Francisco indicated passengers crossing the overland route brought the disease to their city. By December the "Panama, New Zealand, and Australian Royal Mail Company" failed to make payment of dividends because of the effect yellow fever had exerted on the traffic between the West Indies and the Australian colonies moving via the Panama route.

In 1868 physicians could not agree whether yellow or bilious fever raged in Peru, but the disease, not present since 1854 and 1856, wrought high mortality numbers. By May burials at Lima amounted to 30 per day and rapidly increased to over 200 among a population of 125,000. Commerce was paralyzed, and schools and all public places were closed. Newspapers suppressed accounts of the disease for fear of creating a panic, but as the fever spread to Islay, Callao, Rivas and Nicaragua death tolls continued to rise. In 1869, the city of Tacna, Peru, containing 10,000 persons, suffered causalities of nearly 3,000, causing another 6,000 to flee the city. The same year, a serious visitation of yellow fever struck Rio, attributed to "the unusual prolongation of drought and the very hot season."[4]

Yellow Fever in and Around Africa

The *London Lancet* reported on December 3, 1860, that one of the most fatal explosions of yellow fever on record occurred at Fort George, an English military station,

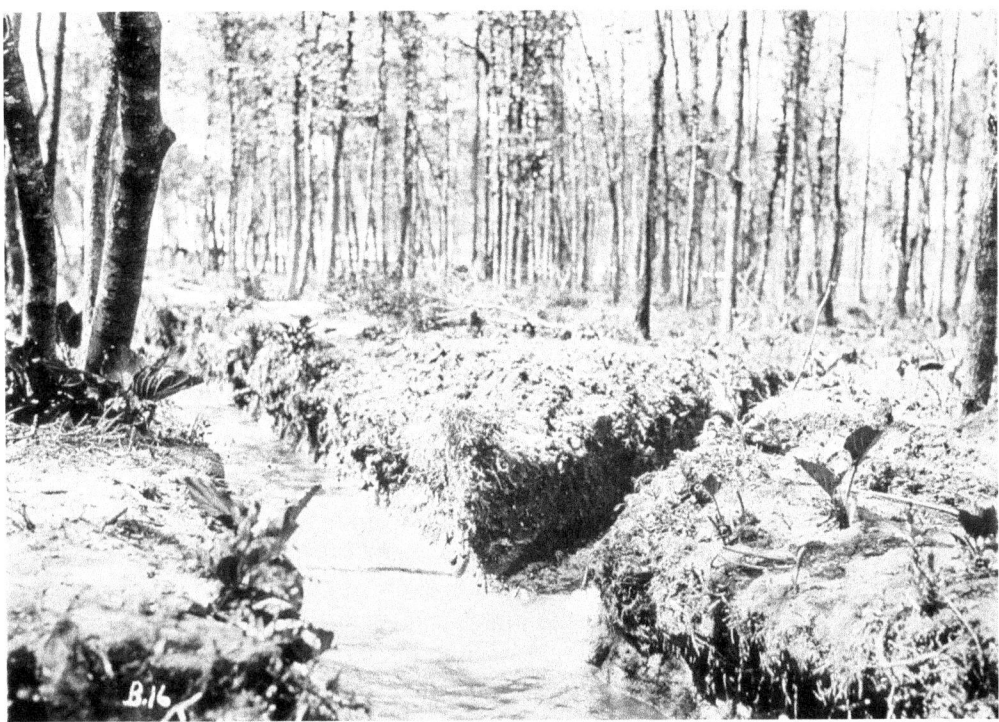

The correlation between swamps and yellow fever was long suspected, but it took centuries before researchers proved the connection. This photograph, taken in 1910, shows a swamp that is being drained in an effort to rid the area of yellow fever and malaria-carrying mosquitoes. Without such herculean efforts, finishing construction of the Panama Canal would have been impossible (courtesy National Library of Medicine).

about two months earlier on the west coast of Africa: "In the Island of McCarthy [180 miles from the mouth of the Gambia River], the malady suddenly broke out without any traceable cause, and attacked all the inhabitants, not one of whom recovered except Captain Frazer, a naval officer, in command of the station."[5]

With an eye toward commercial interests, in June 1862 English newspapers reported the worst case of yellow fever known on the west coast of Africa for the previous 36 years. The disease broke out at Bonny, where reports indicated that out of 140 whites 75 died within a month, not only natives but also foreigners. Seamen were also affected, a circumstance attributed in part to the "prevalence of easterly winds, which blow directly across the swamps." Advices dated November 3 stated that yellow fever continued to rage at Sainte-Croix de Teneriffe; out of a population of 13,000, three-fourths were in flight and wandering the country. Of the 3,000 remaining, 50–60 deaths were reported daily.

On the east coast of Africa, the island of Mauritius was severely attacked by yellow fever.

Official Returns of Yellow Fever Deaths from Mauritius, 1867

Month	Mortality
February 10–28	2,061
March	6,433
April 1–17	5,070

A change of temperature on April 14 brought relief, but quinine, used to treat victims, had advanced to the enormous price of £12 per ounce. Unfortunately, the weather did not hold and by May 29 mortality escalated. A correspondent to the *London Standard* (May 30, 1867) wrote that "accounts are very sad of the sufferings of the poor people; business completely stagnated, the government offices and mercantile houses denuded of their clerks. The railways have stopped their trains, and banks close at one o'clock."

Discussions in the British Parliament confirmed the magnitude of the disease; reports indicated that at Port Louis, mortality reached 200–250 per day, "and to have amounted on the 17th of April to 17,000, which out of a population of 300,000 was very alarming. *This was the first time that yellow fever had been known to pass eastward of the Cape.*" A "gentleman holding an official position in the colony" indicated on May 6 he was "writing from the city of the dead," where 10,000 persons were carried off in the last month; every engine-driver at Port Louis had the fever and of his entire staff 112 were absent from the same cause. During this epidemic, he added, sufferers often went through three or four attacks, each one weakening him for the next.

When the subject was broached in Parliament again in early August, the ravages of yellow fever were confirmed. However, circumstances "were not sufficiently known to justify the government in asking parliament for a vote of public money on the subject. Such votes for the relief of the population in distant colonies were very rare, almost the only exception being in the case of the distress in the West Indies." Gentlemen sympathizing with the colonists were advised to donate to private subscriptions.[6]

The Russian Epidemic

In September 1864 an unknown disorder struck St. Petersburg, Moscow, Odessa, Perm and New Archangel (Russian America), baffling physicians as to its identity.

Various Names for the Russian Epidemic of 1864–1865

Bilious typhoid fever	Revenante
Das recurrirende Fieber (in German)	Spotted fever
Fèvre à rechute (in French)	Synocha
Febris recurrens	"The illness" (common usage)
Military fever	Typhinia
Plague of the old "black death" type	Typhoid
Relapsing or famine fever	Typhus recurrent
Remittent fever	Yellow fever
"Remittent fever of warm climates"	

Various theories were offered as to the origin of this fever. Some believed it appeared in the autumn of 1864 in the northeast and southwest corners of the Russian Empire and spread from there. Symptoms included cold and shivering, intense fever, headache, debility and occasional nose bleeds. These lasted five to six days and recurred at short intervals several more times. Quinine was said to cure the fever and delirium but had no effect on the progress of the disease. The proportion of deaths to attacks was 1:6 and from August 1864 to January 1865 more than 8,900 individuals suffering from this illness were received into hospitals. The cause of the fever was almost universally attributed to the starving condition of the poor and dram drinking. By April 1865 the fever had reached the Prussian frontier, depopulating entire villages.[7]

England and the Yellow Fever Threat

The famous case of yellow fever at Swansea in 1865 occurred in September when the barque *Hecla* arrived at the port from Cuba with a cargo of copper ore for the Cobre Mining Company. Rumors immediately circulated that there was a case of yellow fever aboard and that the victim had died the day after the arrival of the ship. The mayor ordered every precaution to be taken and the deceased man's clothing was burned and the vessel fumigated. Subsequently 10 more deaths were confirmed as resulting from the fever.

On October 6 the Privy Council sent Dr. Buchanan, physician to the London Fever Hospital, to Swansea. After inspecting the scene Buchanan confirmed the diagnosis and participated in a town meeting. Inasmuch as sailors suffering from yellow fever had frequently arrived at Swansea from other ports, it was decided to appoint a medical officer at a salary of £100 per year to oversee the port. No other action was deemed necessary "because, as a rule, the atmosphere is such that 'yellow fever' cannot live here, and the weather is cooling." In the returns of "Births, Marriages, and Deaths" for 1865, the official report indicated that 29 cases occurred and 15 died, but the disease did not assume the proportions of an epidemic disorder.

On November 12, 1866, the Royal Mail Company ship *Atrato* arrived at Southampton from St. Thomas, carrying yellow fever aboard. In all, there were 35 cases, of which 14 were fatal. On December 1 yellow fever was reintroduced by the *Seine*, which had recently arrived from St. Thomas, losing two men on the voyage and carrying 8 others who were infected. She was ordered to fly the yellow flag, although her mails were unloaded after being exposed to the fumes of nitric acid for half an hour. A worse case at Southampton occurred two weeks later when the *Tasmanian* arrived from St. Thomas with 96 cases, 5 of whom died at the island and 21 perished on the voyage home.[8]

Of paramount importance to Great Britain in the 19th century was the strength of its navy. In 1859 the total mean force afloat was 52,825 of all ranks and ratings. The number of cases of disease and injury was 81,325, while the total number days of sickness in the navy was 1,145,529, meaning 3,138 out of 52,825 on the sick list per day. The number invalided was 1,994 and died 886, in the ratio per 1,000 respectively of 37.7 and 16.7. As compared to previous years the numbers reflected a decrease, although in 1859 the number of wounds received in service in China and the cases of death from yellow fever in two vessels on the west coast of Africa had the effect of making these proportions greater than would otherwise have been the case. In the North American and West Indies station for 1860 there was a mean force of 2,250 men, with 56,357 days of sickness and 4,011 cases of sickness, with an average number of 154 men sick each day per 1,000. Fever and pulmonary complaints produced the greatest number of complaints but yellow fever was the predominant cause of death.

One area of concern addressed in the 1860 annual report was directed toward the yellow fever outbreak on the *Icarus* in September. The report noted, "In hot countries it is well known that yellow fever and cholera morbus are the most dreaded enemies to life, and it has long been doubtful (and the point is still contested) whether these diseases are or are not catching." It was held that several persons were infected while on shore at Belize, where the disease was prevalent. Returning aboard they became ill and several died, "but not before they communicated the fever to others" who had not been on shore. "To check the disease the vessel ought to have proceeded to a colder latitude, but she sailed to Jamaica," eventually infecting the crews of the *Imaum*, *Hyrda* and *Barracouta*. Eventually, out of 640 men there were, in 6 weeks' time, 160 cases of yellow fever, of which 70 were fatal. Quinine wine was served to crews as a preventive against "telluric miasma."

A parliamentary return for 1866 indicated the number of seamen who died in the British merchant service was 4,866. Of these, 1,219 drowned by accident, 1,717 drowned by wreck, 131 by falls from aloft, 146 from yellow fever, 8 from murder, 15 from sunstroke and 24 from scurvy. An 1866 report from the British consul at St. Thomas on the subject of yellow fever indicated, "It is noticeable that British shipping suffered more with fever than any other vessels, which I ascribe to the facts that the forecastle accommodation is generally insufficient and badly ventilated, the crews very intemperate, and too much exposed." In consequence, the Merchant Shipping Act went into effect January 2, 1868, providing for the supply of proper medical supplies, including lime juice. It also dictated space to be allowed each seaman and apprentice of not less than 72 cubic feet and 12 superficial feet for his own use on deck. The act also provided for seamen to collect their wages if off duty for want of good food, medicine or sufficient accommodation.

During a meeting of the Royal Mail Steam Packet Company in 1867, the financial report indicated "a falling-off in the passengers and goods carried. The yellow-fever was only a temporary drawback, but it had naturally diminished the number of passengers." The report also indicated "it was a mistake to suppose that St. Thomas was peculiarly affected with yellow fever; on the contrary, it was under ordinary circumstances healthy. Strange to say not a single passenger died of yellow fever on board any of the company's ships. In six years and three-quarters there have been 15 deaths from fever, 14 from general illness, and 14 from accidents."[9]

International Quarantine, Theories and Cures

An article from the *London Morning Chronicle* of December 5, 1860, opened the decade with a discussion that holds nearly as much relevance today as it did over 150 years ago: "In this age of 'movement' almost every nation is doing its best towards the promotion of traffic and travel. It has become a sign of civilization to extend, in every available way, the facilities for commercial intercourse and personal locomotion. To this end physical impediments are conquered, and fiscal restrictions removed. With this object we have witnessed the inauguration of new railways, new lines of mail steamers, new systems of 'through' traffic, and new tariffs." "But amidst this universal recognition of the advantages arising from the free and easy transit of persons or of commodities," the article continued, was the "old semi-barbarous system of obstruction," known as quarantine.

In order to assess international quarantine regulations, in 1860 the Association for the Promotion of Social Science prepared and presented a report to the British House of Commons concerning the quarantine regulations of the different nations of Europe. Two points of interest stand out: plague was the only disease requiring universal quarantine and yellow fever was classed in the same category as cholera.

At Stockholm the existing law came into effect in 1849 and no vessel had been quarantined for several years. For known plagues, susceptible cargoes including rags, hides, feathers, hair, woolen and silk goods, cotton, flax and hemp were purified by airing, washing, heating and fumigation. In Sweden, shipboard cases of yellow fever required detention only until the sick were removed and their clothing and bedding cleansed. By a royal ordinance of March 1852, quarantine "on account of yellow fever and cholera existing in ports of departure" was formally abolished in all Danish harbors. If sickness was aboard, the quarantine physician, without going aboard, would provide medicines at the expense of the ship.

At Dantzic and Stettin quarantine regulations dating from April 1847 referenced chiefly arrivals from the Mediterranean and Levant. Vessels leaving ports where yellow fever was present were not quarantined if no sickness was aboard within ten days of her arrival; otherwise, the ship must remain in station until that period had expired. By law, the only quarantine allowed in Prussian ports was observation. No inspection was ever made of the sanitary conditions on either arriving or departing vessels. Prussian rules applied equally to Russian ports. Vessels having foul or suspected bills of health performed quarantine at Kanso before proceeding to Cronstadt, Helsingfors or other Russian ports.

In the Finish provinces, no legislation on quarantine had existed since the Imperial letters of November 2, 1819, and December 11, 1827. Quarantine regulations in Holland and at Rotterdam were "considered almost a dead letter." The most recent law concerning quarantine in Belgium was issued June 1851 and only nominally enforced; vessels with sickness aboard were held for three days, after which, if no disease remained, the vessel was released. In France, quarantine regulations were reformed in 1849 after the academy's report on plague published in 1847. The length of quarantine was reduced and in certain circumstances abolished. Until this time, defensive measures were organized only on the seacoast, but it was "now deemed to be both more simple and more logical to extend the surveillance over the countries themselves where the disease took its origin. This was done by the nomination of resident physicians by our Government in Turkey and in Egypt, to examine into the sanitary conditions of those countries, and to fix the bills of health to be given to vessels on their departure."

After the International Sanitary Conference of 1851, the French embodied its recommendations and conclusions and an Imperial decree was issued in 1853. With respect to yellow fever, clean-bill arrivals were admitted at once to pratique while foul-bill arrivals were subject to up to seven days of quarantine. Sanitary laws of 1855 required ships from Egypt and all ports of the Ottoman Empire to undergo observation of 8–10 days, while those from the Gulf of Mexico or the Brazils were to undergo a 7-day quarantine.

Great Britain and the northern United States generally required three days' quarantine from ports where sanitary measures were not strictly enforced. Arrivals with foul bills of yellow fever were not admitted into any ports of Spain but were sent to Vigo or Port Mahon, where they were quarantined for 10 days. It was said that "no country is so vigilant and strict a surveillance kept up, at all times, over every part of the world as in Portugal." Arrivals of ships from a port infected with yellow fever required an 8-day quarantine.

At Cagliari, all arrivals from the Levant and America were at all times subject to sanitary measures. Sanitary measures in Sardinia and Leghorn were "the most oppressive," holding ships up to ten days. At Naples, where the sanitary board was independent of the government, a country was considered infected not only when one of the three major contagious diseases (plague, yellow fever and cholera) were present, but also if they existed in territorial dependencies. Places were also considered infected if they were in free intercourse, either by land or sea, with infected places or areas where sanitary precautions were not enforced.

Quarantine Nomenclature for Plague

Rigor:	Quarantine was to be performed at a regular lazaret.
Observation:	Quarantine was to be performed onboard or at a regular lazaret.
Clean bill of health:	A ship was considered clean if 30 days had passed since the last case of disease. The ship, crew and cargo were admitted at once to pratique.
Doubtful bill of health:	No cases of disease had occurred in the previous 15 days. The ship was liable to quarantine for 10–15 days, according to how it was laden or in ballast (empty).
Foul bill of health:	Cases of disease had occurred in the previous 15 days. The ship was liable to quarantine for 20 days if laden and 15 if in ballast.

Days of quarantine were adjusted by the various nations depending on disease (yellow fever or cholera) being present.

In the United States, each state enacted its own regulations respecting quarantine. "The result has been a general want of uniformity, and on several points a notable discrepancy in the system pursued, or at least in the laws promulgated.... That such a state of things, which was at any time liable to hamper commerce and freedom of intercourse without affording any reliable protection to the public health, stood in need of reform, has long been felt by the leading medical men in the Union, as well as by others whose interests were more immediately concerned." Nevertheless, the British Association's report concluded, American laws were never so vexatious and oppressive as in most countries in Europe.[10]

On the subject of land transportation, George Catlin, the American author, painter and traveler, took extreme exception to the development of subterranean railways in London, writing to the *Morning Post* (September 20, 1865):

> When her underground railways are completed, London will have ready for yellow fever, the plague, or other epidemics the most extensive accommodation ever designed for such diseases, and that too, with three millions of human beings over them ready for destruction. The fact is universally known that in all districts infested with yellow fever the malaria predominates in the lowest localities, such as in the cellars and vaults of houses, and in the holds and bilges of vessels.... The yellow fever occasionally takes weeks to travel from the cellar of one house to the cellar of another, or from the hold of one ship to the hold of another lying alongside of her; but the underground railways of London are long levels in which there are few or no obstructions, and are therefore formed to convey a disease that may break out at one end of them with celerity and certainty to the other; and as malaria will thus obtain possession of the whole tunnel, its ravages will extend alike to all parts of it.

He suggested instead that all railways should be built on solid masonry, with sewers being the only exception to underground structures. Conversely, in 1866 proponents of Panama took pains to enumerate the benefits of becoming the terminus of several lines of steamers scheduled to run between that country and the various ports on the western seaboards of North and South America. "During the months of October and November," they stated, "there is a good deal of malaria, but not usually of a dangerous character; yellow fever has not been known there for many years."[11]

Discussions on the geographical dissemination of yellow fever were argued in the newspapers of Galveston in 1867. The point seemed to be carried that in climates where frost was unknown, mild winters indicated an epidemic the following year because that "which it depends for resuscitation has not been destroyed." A follow-up letter observed,

"If it be once admitted that yellow fever does not originate in any portion of the United States, and can therefore only exist in this country by that peculiar condition of the atmosphere which spreads the infection as soon as received, the inference is that medical science in this country should direct its efforts to ascertain the cause which produce that atmospheric condition, and to the proper means of preventing it." This led back to the idea that around seaports "malaria generated from damp and confined air under the buildings, combined with the effects of the decaying sills and sleepers next to and often partly under the ground." The answer, then, was to raise buildings to provide better ventilation.

From an 1866 article published in the *Scalpel* and reprinted by the *New-York Times,* "The Cholera—What Is It? Yellow Fever and Other Infectious Diseases—What Are They?," the author opines that "yellow fever is the product of closely confined warmth and moisture. It originates directly from those two conditions; united, they produce a vegetable fungus, of microscopic size, which is inhaled by human beings, and thus produces the disease." By 1869 the idea that "mould" (mold), "whether eaten in cheese, or mouldy bread, or other food, or breathed in the infinitesimal spora that are diffused from it in the atmosphere—seems to be the source of a great variety of very serious diseases." As a corroborating fact, when houses and streets were kept clean in New Orleans, no outbreak of yellow fever occurred, making the conclusion "almost proof positive that yellow fever is caused by mould, or at least by decomposition, with which mould is always associated."

Dr. Warren Stone of New Orleans lectured at Bellevue College in New York on yellow fever, beginning with this comment: "Nothing more definite could be said than that it was a disease incident to warm climates, and induced by a poison totally intangible and disconnected from any known causes of disease. There was no combination of filth—no combination of circumstances calculated to deteriorate health and excite typhoid or typhus fever, that had anything to do with the generation of yellow fever. This remarkable fact was not generally known." As for some federal officers during the Civil War having taken credit for keeping yellow fever out of New Orleans, the claim was false. The weather happened to be cooler and there was less rain, "but there was no material difference in any other respect."

Stone believed yellow fever was not imported in ships, but "wafted through the atmosphere in waves or cycles, and always made gradual and regular approaches; so that in New Orleans they knew it was coming by its prevalence in islands in the Gulf." "[Furthermore,] [i]t fixed upon a place and ran its course, increasing in a definite ratio, declining in the same way, and finally disappearing, but for the time being affecting all who were exposed to its influence." As far as contagion was concerned, he stated categorically, "beyond all doubt or hesitation, that personally it is not contagious; I *know* that it is not."

As far as treatment went, Dr. Stone recommended that the patient lie perfectly quiet and be properly nourished. That and nothing more was required. He felt ice to relieve headaches was not advisable because it offered only temporary relief and if the patient suffered from acidity in the stomach small doses of bicarbonate of soda combined with 1:32 of a grain of morphia often had an excellent effect. He concluded, "It must be remembered that yellow fever patients are wholly irresponsible, and though they may talk reasonably, they do not appreciate their own condition."[12]

Two physicians from Texas offered simple, no-nonsense advice. The first, from Galveston, noted three errors that contributed to death from yellow fever: neglecting to

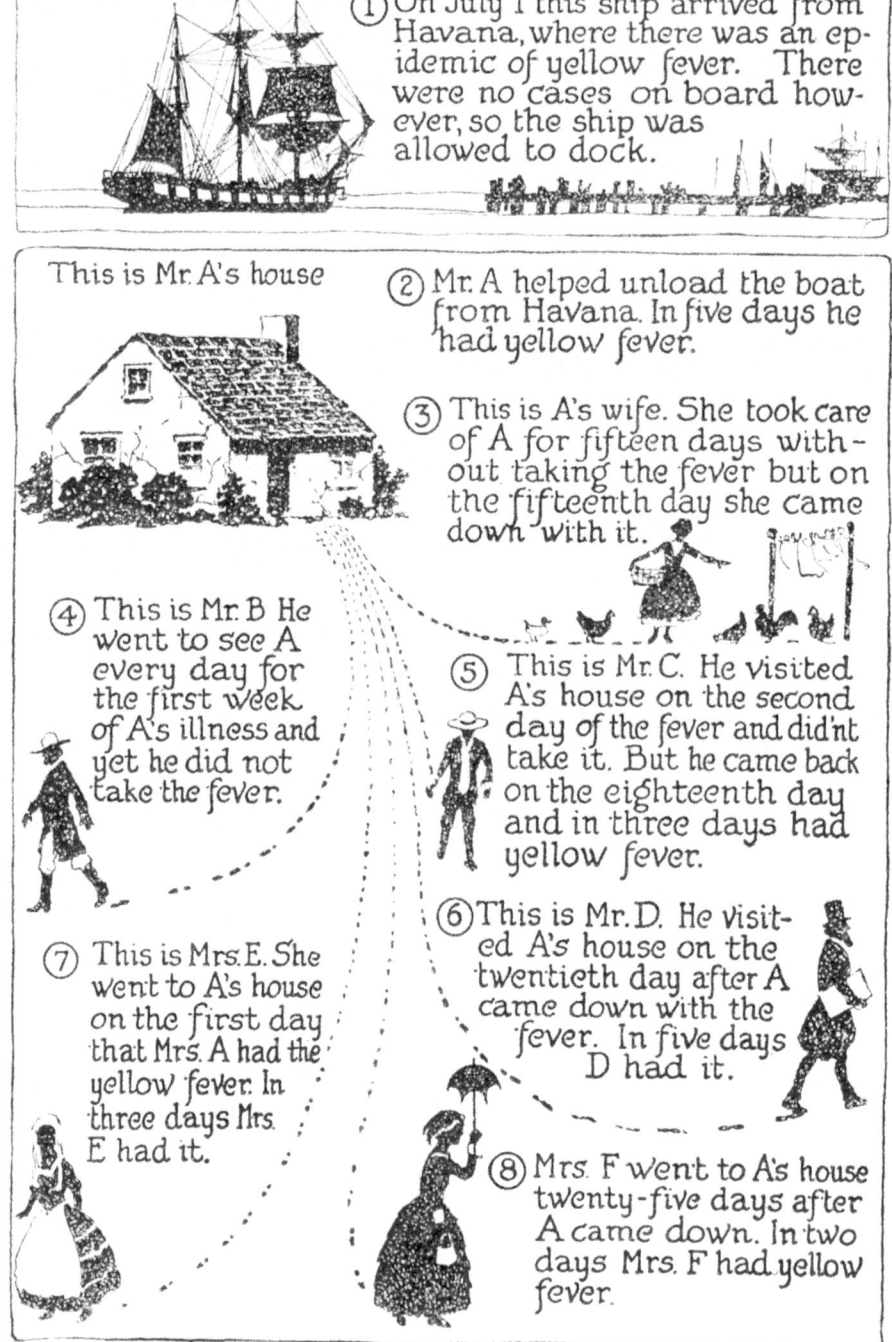

This simplistic line illustration tells the story of how yellow fever was transmitted. It answers the vexing question of why some people were exposed to yellow fever victims and did not contract the disease, while others, visiting the same patient, became victims themselves. Discovering the incubation period was what proved to be the key that linked mosquitoes to the deadly disease (author's collection, from *Health Heroes*, 1926).

acknowledge and treat early symptoms of the disease; admitting visitors into the sick room; and presuming to be cured too soon. "If there were no violations of these established rules," he wrote, "the mortality of every epidemic would be reduced at least one-half, if not a great deal more." William McCraven of Houston stated that yellow fever was a *blood* disease, belonging to the *zymotic* class. "It's cause—whatever that may be—is supposed to produce a kind of fermentation in the blood, which corrupts the whole circulating mass, so as to unfit it for building up the various tissues of the body." In acknowledgment, he offered his own rules: avoid too active medication; enforce diligent and skillful nursing; and feed the patient a light, nutritious diet, emphasizing, "*He must eat or die.* It is the one thing needful."

Under the category "Something New in Medicine," several ideas from the last decade were reintroduced. In 1864 freezing Yellow Jack out of infected ships was recommended. Alternately, two years later, Commodore Chandler of the U.S. steamer *Don* suggested that disconnecting a joint of the steam heater and filling the ship with steam for two hours would serve the same purpose. In 1869 Dr. Humboldt's theory of curing yellow fever by scorpion poison was put forth as a "powerful alternative" to other treatments. On the other hand, an unnamed doctor from Galveston warned against using the South American Remedy for yellow fever, as it was "poison."[13]

One of the most debated subjects of the decade occurred in 1867. Beginning in Jamaica with numerous "letters to the editor" of the *Gleaner* and ultimately traveling around the world, the topic concerned "an entire change in the treatment of yellow fever," as introduced by Alexander Fiddes. His approach consisted of "the internal administration of Sulphurous Acid, combined with the external application of Iced Sheets around the body when the skin is hot and dry, or with an occasional Vapour-bath when the skin is dry without being very hot." Calomel, quinine and all other medicines were set aside "as being not only useless, but positively injurious; the only medicine recommended being a full dose of Castor Oil at the beginning of the disease." "Sulphurous Acid" was classified as a *sulpho-salt*. Sulphur was used medically as a laxative, diaphoretic and resolvent, typically in affections of the respiratory organs.[14] Fiddes claimed he used it as a preventive remedy against fermentation of the blood, while the wet sheets and vapour-baths "were potent agencies for withdrawing or abstracting poisonous matter from the body without weakening the vital powers."

Fiddes claimed he had been using this acid since 1850 when its properties were pointed out to him by a chemist named Mr. Hoffman but only recently had come to employ it in yellow fever cases in the form of Sulphite of Magnesia or of Soda. Over the course of a year the efficacy, ownership and origination of the treatment were argued, at times with great vehemence, reaching from the *Lancet* to the *Galveston Daily News,* and from Kingston, Jamaica, to Edinburgh and Brooklyn. In the final analysis, the great remedial properties of sulphur were considered a potential "panacea," with credit for its discovery being given to numerous ancient and modern researchers, which ultimately satisfied no one.[15]

Three articles, each with its own degree of poignancy, round out the 1860s. An excerpt of the first, "How It Feels to Have the Yellow Fever," was written by a fever patient on the fifth day after being taken ill. "It caused a relapse," the *New Orleans Bulletin* observed, "which came very near costing him his life":

The writer of this has had a glimpse of purgatory, and the way it came to pass was this: Tuesday morning "Yellow Jack," so called, introduced himself unceremoniously, and at once proceeded to break every bone in this poor subject's body. He was left helpless and prostrated. Now appeared an army of little devils, who commenced prowling, prodding, and digging, to satisfy themselves that not a bone was left unbroken. But in spite of all the devils, the skull remained unbroken. They made a detail to keep constantly beating the subject on the top of the head, and downward, toward the neck. They had a kind of Greek fire, which at regular intervals they poured down the spine of the subject.

The second, from the *New Orleans Times*, entitled, "The Cost of Living and Dying in New Orleans," is written in a humorous style, but the sentiment is in earnest:

> When a person is attacked with yellow fever, custom demands that a physician be sent for forthwith. The fee per patient is fixed by Dr. Highprice at from $75 to $100, and Dr. Worthless, though the veriest quack in existence, scorns to take less than Dr. H. He knows that the profession is shielded by secrecy; that the value of the services rendered cannot be accurately gauged, that the prescriptions are made out in mystic characters, and he concludes that the more he charges the more highly will his skill and energy be prized.
>
> It is well known that there is no disease on which "doctors agree," so much as on yellow fever, and experienced nurses have long since arrived at the conclusion that in the most of cases they can get along better without a doctor than with one. But this trouble stares them in the face; should the patient die no burial certificate can be obtained, and great blame will rest on those who employed the nurse and assumed so unwonted a responsibility in the premises. Indeed, to die, "without the aid of a physician" is regarded not only by the profession, but by a large portion of the public, as criminal in the extreme....
>
> When the pulse is stilled and the certificate obtained there are still extraordinary expenses which make New Orleans a hard place to die in. A box for the poor remains costs $10 or $50, though its actual value is not over $10 or $15, and the hole in which ashes are consigned to ashes and dust to dust, costs $50 more!

The final entry concerned M. Le Compte, sent by the Zoological Gardens to the Falkland Islands for the purpose of collecting sea bears and penguins. He captured eight sea bears and sent four to England; but on the voyage a passenger was taken ill with a chest disease and "it was imagined that there was yellow fever on board, and the doctor ordered Le Compte to throw all his fish over. The consequence was the sea bears gradually died" of starvation. The same fate befell 60 penguins "on account of the difficulty of procuring food during the sea transit."[16]

Chapter 23

Quarantine and Avarice, 1870–1873

> PEDDLERS *around and about Natchez, Miss., make it a point to report that three or four deaths occur daily in that city from yellow fever, for the purpose of keeping the country people at home, so that they may reap immense profits by the sale of their wares.*[1]

The decade of the 1870s started out well for the Crescent City when an April announcement in the newspaper stated, "A Great Reform in New Orleans: The city of New Orleans is about to undergo a wondrous improvement by the adoption of the earth closet." Details indicated that "little doubt can be entertained that the periodical epidemics of yellow fever and cholera that have so desolated that city in former years" were to be eliminated by removing the "feculence which there was no system of sewers to remove."

Reform was apparently too little or two late, for by September yellow fever was reported in the city to such an extent that on the 14th the health officer at Galveston ordered a 25-day quarantine of travelers arriving in vessels that had departed from New Orleans or Berwick's Bay. However, mail, hardware, agricultural implements not in cases, sugar, coffee, flour, salted provisions, corn, oats and hay were permitted to come into the quarantine station and be taken by lighter into the city and then depart without detention. Officials in New Orleans promptly complained, threatening Galveston officials that they were likely to "produce a serious interruption of a very valuable and important trade" to both communities. Ultimately, from the inception of the yellow fever season up to October 19, when the epidemic ended, 385 deaths were reported by the *New Orleans Times*. Official reports from the board of health placed the mortality figure at 588.[2]

The big news in New York during 1870 was the quarantine trouble between health officer J.M. Carnochan and officials in Brooklyn, who bitterly debated enforcement and efficacy. Adding to their problems were merchants who avoided quarantine altogether by unloading their imported stock at Perth Amboy, New Jersey, and delivering it to New York, where they easily cleared the custom house. By September 12 local newspapers played up the situation by headlines declaring, "Ambitious Amboy Versus New-York—The War of the Merchants Against the Health of the City." Two days later the triumphant *New York Herald* noted "government authorities have listened to the protestations of New York against the wholesale importation of yellow fever and smallpox, via Perth Amboy," notifying the collector at the port to refuse entrance at the custom house of such vessels coming from that city: "This ought to effectually stop the disease smugglers, and consequently desolate the aspiring port of Perth Amboy."

When yellow fever ended in New York, Dr. Carnochan announced a total of 349 vessels arrived from suspected ports and were quarantined in the lower bay. Upon these vessels were 450 cases of yellow fever and 103 deaths. Eighty-three additional cases were received on Governor's Island, of which 31 were fatal.[3]

As fever spread throughout the South, descriptions of causalities became terse and to the point:

Yellow Fever in Brief, 1870

Aug. 23	185 deaths up to Saturday at Memphis; 36 from Saturday to Monday
Aug. 25	34 new cases and 8 deaths at Memphis. Death of Gen. J.B. Hood at New Orleans
Aug. 26	29 new cases and 7 deaths at Memphis; 2 new cases at St. Louis quarantine
Aug. 27	25 new cases and 10 deaths at Memphis. Gen. Hood's daughter sick. The Howard Association put 25 more nurses on duty and gov. of Tennessee asks for aid for Memphis. Houston quarantines against Galveston
Aug. 28	9 new cases and 4 deaths at Memphis
Aug. 29	22 new cases and 10 deaths at Memphis

During August, a case of "undoubted yellow fever" at Dayton, Ohio, led physicians to suspect the victim had come into contact with refugees from Memphis. On September 10 in Philadelphia the board of health adopted a resolution that, as yellow fever was prevailing "to an alarming extent" in New Orleans, vessels arriving from that city were required to stop at the Lazaretto "for the treatment prescribed by section four of the health laws of 1818."[4]

One of the more interesting observations to make for the year 1870 was the frequency in which articles appeared across the country pitting avarice and greed against public health. One of the earliest (*New York Herald,* June 30, 1870) set the tone for the rest:

MERCHANT'S POCKETS AND THE PUBLIC HEALTH.—As an evidence of the extent some of our merchants regard the public health when their pecuniary interest is likely to be affected the case of the bark Fyen clearly shows. The vessel came direct from a port where the yellow fever is raging. Two of her crew were attacked with the disease, and when she arrived in this port she had no bill of health to exhibit. Messrs. J.L. Phipps & Co., and Funk, Edge & Co., who claim, we presume, to be respectable merchants in this city, but with residences elsewhere, contend that she should be allowed to come direct to the city and discharge her cargo of coffee. It might be a little too severe to suppose for a moment that any of the above named merchants were actuated by mercenary motives in making their demand that the Fyen should be relieved from quarantine duty, but there is a singular circumstance connected with it, and that is that at present there is a good market for coffee and gold is declining.

On July 16, 1870, fixed rates for lighterage service were set by the New York Commissioners of Quarantine, in conjunction with the health officer, the mayors of New York and Brooklyn and the president of the board of aldermen.

Rates for Lightering, Stevedoring and Cooperage

Sugar—Hogshead	$0.75	Logwood—Ton	$1.50
Tierce	0.53	Hemp—Bale	0.40
Box	0.39	Coffee—Bag	0.18
Barrel	0.24¼	Flour—Barrel	0.11⅓
Molasses—Hogshead	0.75	Hides (dry)—Each	0.05
Tierce	0.53	Hides (green)—Each	0.07
Barrel	0.30	Cotton—Bale	0.80
Cigars, M	0.10	Wool—Bale	0.60
Tobacco—Hogshead	1.50	Rice—Tierce	0.43¼
Bale	0.22½	Resin—Barrel	0.10[5]

By September 30, 1870, the threat from yellow fever became the prime factor influencing the New York market:

THE GENERAL MARKET

The day opened with fair prospects for a brisk business, but ere long the report that a death from yellow fever had occurred had spread through the entire business portion of the city, and the interior merchants who had previously been operating made immediate preparations for leaving the city.... Business will be prostrated should the disease spread to any extent, and only the local demand for consumption remains to be supplied. Prices during the day exhibit no material changes, the tendency of some classes of goods having been slightly to weakness.[6]

The "Quarantine Issue" between Galveston and New Orleans turned into an outright "war," residents of each city accusing the other of destroying trade and interfering with the accumulation of the almighty dollar. A particularly sharp salvo defending quarantine against the naysayers of New Orleans came from the *Galveston Daily News* on September 20, 1870:

QUARANTINE AND TRADE

This is the characteristic title of an article in the *New Orleans Bulletin* assuming that trade is absolute every day in the year and all the year round—a piece of impudence which nobody but a worshipper of money and business will tolerate. Like everything else in this world, trade may be modified by circumstances; and we cannot conceive of any circumstances by which it may be more justly modified than those which enter into the quarantine. Nor is there anything more absolutely disgusting than the assumption of the New Orleans papers, that they are the unerring judges of a question of this kind, after having permitted Ben Butler to make the Crescent City ridiculous and himself immortal by a little energy and carefulness in sanitary and quarantine measures.

In the worst years the mortality from yellow fever epidemics at New Orleans exceeds that from any disease which has ever raged in any civilized community; and yet, a New Orleans paper thinks itself justified in talking of "medieval ignorance and superstition," where there is no place in God's world where such ignorance and superstition are more prevalent than in that same New Orleans...

The *New Orleans Bulletin* is perfectly willing that something that the devotees of red tape would call quarantine should be established, and be as vigorous at one time as another, because not intended ever to be anything more than a sham and a sinecure. But when common sense and energy determine that the question of the importation of disease shall be fairly tested, or that efficient measures shall be used on proof of importation already furnished, the prophets of business are always ready with their platitudes about "destructive and damaging intermeddling with the freedom of trade and travel."

It is as plain as anything can be that our last great epidemic was imported from Vera Cruz, by way of Indianola, and that the importation was caused by the position taken by our city authorities, whom the *New Orleans Bulletin* would probably have regarded as men after its own heart—as men who were properly influenced by the great maxims of commerce, and fully emancipated from the "traditions of medieval ignorance and superstition"—although, in fact, ignorance was never more completely personified in any public functionaries that the world has ever seen. They could not quarantine against a Texas port—they did not believe in quarantine anyhow—what was to be would be—and certainly, to interfere with trade was to violate some revelation which they could not designate or present to anybody else, but which was law and gospel to themselves. The result was, that we had yellow fever for about four months, and buried some 1200 victims of the disease, besides sending it through a large portion of the interior.

Yellow fever does not originate in this country. At one period there was an interval of thirty-seven years during which there was not one case of yellow fever in the western world; and in almost every instance its commencement among us can be traced to intercourse with the western coast of Africa. It is an African disease—fit only for negroes. There never has been a yellow fever epidemic in Galveston unless it was introduced from abroad, or revived from a previous year.

The "war of words" was not only directed toward New Orleans. Turning the sword on itself, the same newspaper attacked its own men of commerce in a September 28, 1870, edition:

> The ingenuity of man is great when money is to be made. The yellow fever in New Orleans is to be turned to a source of profit. Provisions are somewhat dear in Galveston. Therefore, the quarantine is to be evaded by direct shipments of flour and produce from St. Louis to Galveston, the produce to be landed at a point twenty miles above the city of New Orleans and placed on board the steamship Agnes to come over without touching at New Orleans. A prominent Galveston flour house originated the enterprise, but it is now probable C.A. Whitney & Co. will monopolize the venture. People will have to be satisfied that the goods do not come from New Orleans. This done, the venture cannot fail to be profitable.

A month later the issue of quarantine laws was resurrected in both New York and Galveston. At the former city, the *New York Herald* (October 4, 1870) cried that the outbreak of yellow fever on Governor's Island was "doubtless directly due to the steady evasion of quarantine laws by avaricious owners and officers of vessels from infected ports." The same day, the *Galveston Daily News* began an editorial as follows:

> The enforcement of a quarantine brings out quite strongly that selfishness which is inherent in the soul of every earthly sinner. We have watched the progress of opinion within the last fifteen days with considerable amusement. When Dr. [George W.] Peete [the Galveston health officer] first turned down the legal screws and announced the quarantine New Orleans was very indignant. There was no fever there, and if we had credited half the good things said by the papers of that city we would have made a solemn affidavit that the health-giving spirit in whose waters Ponce de Leon sought to find eternal youth was located somewhere about the head-waters of Bayou St. John.... They accused us of perpetuating a Yankee trick in the endeavor to forestall New Orleans and steal her trade.... Self interest blinded the judgment and obscured the understanding. Men were honest in their opinions, no matter how absurd they were.

"Let us have a quarantine law which shall defy evasion, or else let us have none at all," the paper concluded. Unfortunately, the argument—and the avarice—were far from over and the cost of yellow fever in treasure kept rising. A note of November 1 indicated the city of Mobile estimated a one million-dollar loss by the recent epidemic of the disease.[7]

In light of these arguments, it is significant to note the actual deaths attributed to yellow fever. In 1871 there were 27,000 deaths in New York City, of which 7,006 were children under the age of two years.

Cause of Death, New York City, 1871

Accidents and negligence	2,294
Diarrheal diseases	1,880
Other zymotics	954
Scarlatina	646
Cholera morbus	444
Croup	357
Whooping cough	350
Measles	300
Typhoid	169
Diptheria	199
Suicide	105
Typhus fever	82
Homicide	64
Smallpox	10
Cholera	4
Yellow fever	2

Of these, 16,366 were natives of the United States.[8]

Pet Crazes: Yellow Jack, 1871

The year 1871 began as the previous one had ended: with quarrels between New Orleans and Galveston over quarantine. On January 21 an editorial in the *Galveston Daily News* began as follows: "We presume that public journals are permitted to enjoy a pet craze. Right certain it is that the *New Orleans Picayune* is stark staring mad on the subject of a quarantine." On January 14 Dr. Peete and James A. McKee, members of the Merchant's Committee to draft the Galveston city charter, reminded members that section 57 of the proposal failed to provide for a board of health to supervise and control sanitary and health regulations, arguing that "the enforcement of wise sanitary rules, and strict regulations against the introduction of yellow fever will reasonably exempt us from epidemics."

Similar concerns were taken up by the United States Congress. A joint resolution was introduced on February 20:

> Whereas, Experience has proved that the present system of quarantine on the Southern and Gulf coasts is inefficient to prevent the ravages of yellow fever in the cities and towns of that section, therefore:
> *Be it resolved by the Senate and House of Representatives of the United States of America in Congress assembled,* That the Secretary of War be, and he is hereby directed to detail one or more medical officers of the regular army, who shall, during the coming season, visit each town or port on the coast of the Gulf of Mexico, which is subject or liable to invasion of yellow fever, and shall confer with the authorities of such port or town, with reference to the establishment of a more uniform and efficient system of quarantine, and who shall ascertain all facts having reference to the outbreaks of this disease in such ports or towns, and the proper means to prevent such outbreaks; and shall also make a detailed report on this subject to the Secretary of War, through the Surgeon General, on or before the assembling of the second session of the Forty-second Congress, in December, eighteen hundred and seventy-one.

On August 4, 1871, the *New York Times* published an article crediting General Benjamin Butler ("whatever the Southern people may think of [him]") as having prevented major epidemics of yellow fever in New Orleans by the "intelligent application of the simple rules of modern sanitary science." As proof of this claim, the newspaper cited the yellow fever epidemic at Buenos Aires, during the first four months of 1871, where the death toll reached 26,200, but not one of the 360 grave diggers were affected. This extraordinary immunity was attributed to the fact the cemetery was located outside the infected district. Noting the sanitary conditions in the city were atrocious and that the drinking water came from the river "so poisoned" by swill and offal that the fish died, the paper concluded that yellow fever was infectious but not contagious and that both yellow fever and cholera could be eliminated by proper sanitary measures. Addressing European fears that cholera "threatened visitation," London newspapers approached the New York report by adding that many were of the opinion quarantine was of little use but they supported the idea of sanitary measures.

According to Dr. Russell, secretary of the board of health, the whole number of deaths at New Orleans for 1871 was 53; the first occurred on August 4 and the last on December 4. The largest number of deaths for any week was 12, for the week ending October 29.[9]

History of Epidemic Yellow Fever at Natchez

1853   First death July 17, last death December 6. Total 277.
1855   Last death December 17. Total 132.

1867   First death October 2, last death December 10. Total 18, although the number of cases treated was unusually large.

1871   First reported case September 18. Total through November 9 56.[10]

While Charleston newspapers were reporting "the health of the city was never better" through August 25, news leaked out that 35 cases of yellow fever had been reported by August 20 (on August 28 the *New York Herald* would comment that this omission was caused by "misdirected anxiety to prevent injuring the business prospects of the city"). On August 26 the Medical Society of Charleston issued a statement indicating the first case appeared on July 27 but the disease existed only in a mild form and did not seem to be of a character disposed to spread rapidly or widely. This was in direct contrast to a report from the board of health that was issued the same day, stating its members considered the disease to have reached an epidemic state. The *Charleston News* of August 26 opted to promote the findings of the medical society, accusing "fleeing fugitives" and word-of-mouth from spreading "frightful and ridiculous statements." Siding with the board of health, Charleston's mayor telegraphed the mayor of Wilmington, North Carolina, to report the epidemic. Through trains and sleeping cars were immediately discontinued between the two cities and passengers were forced to change cars at Florence, while all travelers coming from Charleston were forbidden to stop within the corporate limits of Wilmington.

A letter dated August 28 from J.M. Selkirk (superintendent of the Freight Line via Charleston) to Bentley D. Hasell, Washington, stated that reports of yellow fever were greatly exaggerated and advised there was "nothing to interfere with the certain and rapid movement of freights from Northern cities to all points in the South and Southwest via Charleston." This memo was subsequently distributed to merchants and shippers via freight agents throughout the South. Nevertheless, on the same date, authorities in Washington considered closing the custom house at Charleston for a period of 30 days, as the collector and his staff were unacclimated.

Not atypically, in the same newspaper (*Fort Wayne Daily Gazette*, September 2, 1871) one article noted that in Charleston "railroad trains arrive and depart with accustomed punctuality," and "the yellow fever at Charleston, S.C., seriously impedes travel in the South."

In light of the continuing reports of yellow fever, the post office at Savannah notified the postmaster general in Washington that the mails, passengers and cars from Charleston were refused admittance. To handle the situation, Charleston mails were to be sent by way of Augusta. Of more critical importance to the federal government was the passage and implementation of President U.S. Grant's three Enforcement Acts of 1871, designed to protect African Americans' right to vote. In September, as "'Dirty Work' Akerman [Amos. T. Akerman, attorney general] [was] looking up 'authorities' and preparing an 'opinion,'" the War Department was preparing to send federal troops into South Carolina to put down the Ku Klux Klan. "No troops, however," noted the *Fort Wayne Daily Sentinel*, September 7, 1871), will be sent to put down the rebellious Charlestonians until after the yellow fever disappears." On October 17, Grant suspended the writ of habeas corpus in nine South Carolina areas and sent troops to pursue prosecution of the white supremacists.

Between July 28 and September 16, sixty-three deaths were reported from yellow fever. On September 19 the Charleston Board of Health issued a report evaluating the eight wards of the city, concluding that the number of yellow fever cases did not exceed two in each ward and by November 12 the leading physicians of the city advised those who had fled to return. The city council also ordered a day of prayer and thanksgiving on the abatement of the disease. Indicative of the sporadic nature of quarantine, on November 2 the *Titusville* (PA) *Morning Herald* announced the board of health proclaimed the ports of Charleston and Key West to be infected, extending from that date until November 8, 1871.[11]

"Quarantine Quibbles"

While "eminent medical and other scientific gentlemen" in Philadelphia argued for the creation of a state board of health to oversee sanitary conditions across county borders,[12] arguments in New York City continued to be centered on quarantine. Under the heading "Quarantine Quibbles," a review of "several little difficulties" was discussed that adequately sums up the state of affairs through the decade.

James P. Pendergast, shipping merchant, complained before the Committee on Commerce and Navigation that he tried on two occasions to evade quarantine with vessels from ports infected with disease. Both carried clean bills of health but despite that they were seized and sent to quarantine. This "difficulty" cost Pendergast Brothers & Co. $320, which Pendergast thought was "about four times too much." An example of a "clean bill of health" was then introduced into evidence:

A Clean Bill of Health

The undersigned, master of the British brig Victoria, being duly sworn, deposes and says that he arrived at Quarantine from Cienfuegos, Cuba, on the 16th inst. after a passage of twenty-six days; that the day previous to his departure from Cienfuegos he received a clean bill of health from the United States Vice Consul for that port; that at the time such bill of health was granted one of his crew was in hospital with yellow fever, and that he was in consequence obliged to leave him behind; that during the voyage to this port the undersigned and six of his crew were attacked with yellow fever, and that John Olsen, seaman, died August 2 of said disease.

The article continued: "Among the grim jokes in this regard that came up was a 'clean bill of health' given to a captain of a ship sailing from Copenhagen the morning of the day he died of cholera.... The wordy rumpus ended, as the whole investigation seems likely to end, in smoke."[13]

A number of medical papers from 1872 expressed similar theories about yellow fever. While expressing the fact no one knew its origin, it was believed the disease "manifestly result[ed] from the operation of some subtle organic poison on the system through the blood" and that epidemics could not arise unless there was "a continuance day and night of a temperature of about 80 deg. farh. for a longer or shorter period accompanied by a moist atmosphere and probably by a decomposition of organic matter." Further, epidemics were "almost always confined to a dense population" where humans congregated, such as ships, garrisoned forts and cities.

In an insightful report, delivered at the medical convention at Houston by doctors S.M. Welch, D.F. Stuart and J.M. Callaway, it was argued the noncontagiousness of the disease was "established beyond all dispute." They added, "That yellow fever is portable can hardly be regarded as longer open to question. The term portability so applied is to express the idea that the germs of the disease may be transported although not produced in the bodies of those affected with it." Citing Dr. Warren Stone of New Orleans and Dr. J.C. Nott of Mobile, Welch, Stuart and Callaway stated yellow fever was a "traveling disease," moving, for example, from the Gulf of Mexico to contiguous lands frequented by vessels and railroads and no further. On the question of whether yellow fever was imported or of local origin, they deduced the two were not mutually exclusive and suggested both means were likely. Although supporting quarantine in theory, the writers pointed out that in practice historical data indicated its general ineffectiveness, particularly in light of the fact disease had multiple routes of entry beyond ships arriving from infected ports. They concluded boards of health enforcing basic sanitation laws were the best way to limit the ravages of disease.[14]

The news that gripped New York beginning August 12, 1872, was the arrival of the Spanish ironclad *Numancia,* late of Havana, with yellow fever victims aboard. Quickly dubbed the "Pest Ship," arguments arose "fast and furious" over where the huge vessel should be held, how to fumigate her and what to do with those aboard. So much interest was generated that crowds of people hourly passed up and down the bay watching "with morbid interest" everything from the yellow flag of the "floating hospital" to surveying other newly arrived "fever ships," finally causing Dr. Mosher of the Quarantine Service to observe that people would be less interested in the *Numancia* if she were a smaller vessel.

By August 19 there were six "plague-stricken crews in the Bay" and thirty victims at the West Bank Hospital. Ultimately, on August 23, port health officer Dr. Vanderpoel indicated the ships would remain at distant anchorage until all sick were recovered and ten days had elapsed after the appearance of a case of yellow fever. On August 27 the doctor announced there was "nothing now to fear," although debate continued to rage on the subject through the end of the month.[15] In the remainder of the country during 1872 no deaths from yellow fever occurred at Charleston. There were 80 cases in New Orleans, of which 40 terminated fatally, the last being on November 19.[16]

On June 6, 1872, the United States Senate and House of Representatives approved a resolution requiring a more efficient system of quarantine to operate along the entire line of the Gulf Coast. In compliance with this, the secretary of war detailed assistant surgeon Harvey E. Brown, U.S. Army, to investigate the subject of yellow fever. Brown ultimately concluded the following:

Federal Investigation into Quarantine 1873

(1) Yellow fever is imported and does not arise from local causes
(2) A system of quarantine can be organized to prevent its importation
(3) Such a quarantine, instead of interfering with commerce, will promote its interests and benefit the ports where established
(4) The present system of quarantine by the various states is defective and inefficient
(5) A national quarantine should be created[17]

At the start of yellow fever season 1873 the *New York Journal of Commerce* noted that "the usual hideous crop of yellow fever yarns is rather backward this year, like most other crops. The sensation mongers have waited for the mercury to top 80 degrees before commencing their frightful tales." Almost on cue, the *New York World* published the following: "We have no desire to excite a panic as to the probable invasion of epidemic scourges. On the contrary, we fully appreciate the disastrous influence of alarm in predisposing to disease. But in sober earnestness our duty compels us to warn our fellow-citizens that there is something more than a possibility of the importation of infectious material into New York, and that, should such a contingency occur, the condition of our city, as shown by THE WORLD's reports, is such as to insure a rapid and overwhelming extension of the pestilence."[18]

The pestilence came but not to New York. News of yellow fever at Shreveport began in early summer. Situated on the west bank of the Red River in the northern part of Louisiana about 300 land miles northwest of Baton Rouge, the city was advantageously situated for the shipment of cattle from Texas and cotton from Louisiana. After the Civil War the population was given at 4,607 of which 2,439 were white and 2,168 were "colored," but in the following decade, drawn by economic advantage, northern immigration more than tripled the number of whites. Unfortunately, these newcomers were "particularly susceptible" to yellow fever, as the disease struck down "with irresistible force those unaccustomed to tropical weather and to Southern modes of life," causing one Indiana newspaper to note, "Cholera and yellow fever in the summer and small-pox in the winter, seem to render many Southern cities cursed."

The introduction of yellow fever (locally known as "the real Spanish vomito, a high and fatal type of yellow fever") into Shreveport was attributed to the Transatlantic Circus, a strolling company from Vera Cruz, Mexico, which had traveled the line of the Texas Pacific Railway, leaving "the seeds of contagion along their route." While in Shreveport several members of the company died of the disease, and, after it left, other members who stayed behind also perished. Two other causes aiding the intensity of the disease were thought to be the unhealthy condition of the town arising from the removal of the Red River raft (thus exposing the bottom of the river to the rays of the sun) and the infected atmosphere caused by the stench of diseased Texas cattle—from the sunken steamboat *Ruby*—that had been slaughtered and left to rot in the river near town.

As death tolls rose rapidly, neighboring towns and states quickly initiated quarantine and by September commerce had ground to a halt. By September 6 trade was considered "paralyzed," compelling the United States marshal there to telegraph Attorney General Williams that local authorities on the Texas Pacific Railroad had stopped the cars by force on account of the prevalence of yellow fever. He asked that Williams compel the running of the trains but received a reply stating that the "government cannot interfere in the case of local authorities forcibly stopping the running of the trains on the Texas Pacific Railroad." The federal government did act, however, for the benefit of its own employees. The secretary of the treasury directed the collector of customs at Galveston, Key West and Pensacola to grant leaves of absence to all employees of the treasury who had not had yellow fever. On September 13, Senator West, of Louisiana, received a dispatch from the mayor of Shreveport: "The people are panic-stricken. All that could have left. The poor are nearly all on our hands. No money in the city. All pecuniary aid will be thankfully received. The fever is increasing."

Matters only worsened with a change in the weather from hot and sultry to cold and rainy. On September 14, five hundred individuals were down with the fever, with a total mortality estimated at 146. Members of the Howard Association sent money, doctors, nurses and druggists, noting in a dispatch, "No report you may have received from here can possibly exaggerate the condition of affairs. They are indeed deplorable." Quarantine only exacerbated the situation. By the 22nd, when the steamer *Gladiola* arrived from New Orleans, owners were forced to store her cargo. They were not alone, for there were already over one hundred car loads of freight bound for points west that could not be moved. In an interesting observation on the times, the *Lafayette Advertiser* (September 27, 1873) copied an editorial from the *New York World*:

> The situation of the town of Shreveport at present is a curious anomaly in a generation in which the most remarkable fact is the enormous increase it has furnished in the facilities of communication among men. No quarantine established by an ignorant Spanish municipal[i]ty in the middle ages, no seclusion of a city of the plague in Arabia, was ever more complete and rigid than that which is now practiced upon the inhabitants of that unfortunate town. By land and water alike they are made inaccessible to the outer world. By the telegraph alone we learn what their deplorable condition is.

By September 29, L.R. Simmons, president of the Howard Association, indicated that over 400 of the community in Shreveport had perished and there were still 700 sick from yellow fever. He indicated the "Howards" had opened an orphan asylum and were feeding about two-thirds of the city residents. Local physicians determined that "beyond a question" the disease had been imported from Cuba. That appeared to be all the medical faculty agreed on, for debate continued on whether the disease was "yellow fever of the most malignant type and consequently contagious" or the noncontagious "yellow disease," a malarial fever peculiar to southern swamps.

A subordinate of the Texas and Pacific Railway wrote a letter describing conditions: "Business, in a measure, is abandoned. Those that are well are nursing the sick. The depot is the only institution in town, outside of drug stores, that holds out, and, ere you get this, some of us may be down. During the [Civil] war I was in 105 battles and skirmishes, and have since been through frightful epidemics, but nothing has ever taxed my nerves like this plague." A correspondent of the *Philadelphia Press* added his own thoughts: "The old and the young, the blonde and brunette, white and black, are falling daily as victims."

AGE OF YELLOW FEVER VICTIMS AT SHREVEPORT

Children under 10 years	100
Between 10 and 20 years	94
Between 20 and 30 years	156
Between 30 and 40 years	134
Between 40 and 50 years	59
Between 50 and 60 years	29
Age 60 and above	13

Another study indicated that the severity of yellow fever varied with persons of different nationalities: "The Germans and Irish seldom have it so lightly as do the French and Spanish, while Americans and the English are attacked with medium violence." Summarizing the epidemic, Dr. D.P. Tenner, who collected statistics for the national government, gave the population of Shreveport in 1873 as 10,000 in the summer and 14,000 during the winter. The population just prior to the epidemic was 9,000; during the height of the disease it fell to 4,500. The first notable case was discovered August 20; between then and November 13, a total of 759 persons, of whom 150 were Negroes, died of the disease.

Shreveport was not alone in its misery. The city of Cairo, Illinois, was quarantined against all Mississippi upriver steamboats and in regard to reports of fever at Galveston the *Mobile Register* warned, "Texas has worked herself into a complete panic about yellow fever; to such an extent has it been carried that intercourse between even the interior towns has almost entirely stopped. It is quarantine against quarantine all over the state.

In very many instances, towns are quarantined that never had, and never will have, a case of the disease." The situation was similar in Memphis. The disease there was believed to have originated in a "low, flat district, not long ago submerged when the Mississippi was playing the part of an 'inland sea.'" The first locality affected was known as "Happy Hollow," an area just north of Market Street on the river bank, known for hovels, rudely constructed shanties and the stench of filth, "mixed up promiscuously with goats and hogs dwell[ing] near one thousand negroes and low Irish." Word first leaked out on September 12, and the following day the board of health officially announced that yellow fever had appeared in the city (later reports confirmed that at least 30 had died before the city acknowledged the epidemic). Conditions worsened to the point that bodies were said to have been thrown in the river to be rid of them and undertakers were "required to move with the celerity more becoming to merchandise transport." On the 19th the mayor ordered a day of fasting and prayer.

By October 14, a month after the first announcement of yellow fever, reports stated that at least 700 inhabitants had fallen victim to the scourge, far surpassing the last epidemic of 1867 when only 191 died during the same time frame. The Howard Association eventually sent 350 nurses (receiving $5/day salary) and its expenditures were placed at $1,400 daily. Ironically, on October 12 the *Memphis Appeal* noted, "We can hardly credit the fact now, by the baleful light of the epidemic, but that a few days ago members of the General Council, unable to comprehend the possibilities of the fever, higgled over an appropriation of $10,000, and gave vent to much feeling over the possible cost, over that amount [requested] by the Board of Health.... It is safe to say that almost $100,000 have been expended the past thirty days [by charitable organizations] and it will take another $100,000 to provide for future demands." By November 4, citizens resolved to prosecute Mayor Cicella for fraud in dealing out supplies for the poor.

One letter writer eventually asserted that during the first eleven weeks of the epidemic 1,500 persons died, with a high of 40 deaths per day. The same writer noted that Dr. Luke Blackburn was in attendance at several bedsides. On the same subject, in late October two doctors named J. Murry Ryan and E.D. Hilliard arrived from Chicago and offered their services; due to a lack of success, the ability of both was soon questioned. After being charged with interfering with one of Blackburn's patients, Ryan called him a liar and engaged him in an altercation for which Blackburn severely caned him. Whether Ryan was actually a physician remained in question, but Hilliard was said to have been a doctor in the army who fell "into bad company when he struck Ryan's path."

As in Shreveport, the medical community disagreed as to the actual cause of the plague, some citing yellow fever and others the common malarial fever of the Mississippi river bottom. Those in Memphis, out of "bravado and carelessness," termed it not only "yellow jack" but "bronze jack," "saffron jack," and even "johnny vomito." By the first week of November, as the weather grew colder, the board of health issued a "safe-return" order, although at least one local physician felt this was premature because homes had not been thoroughly aired and freed from noxious vapors.

Yellow fever was thought to have been introduced into New Orleans by J.M. Arran, a mate of the Spanish bark *Valparaiso*, which left Havana June 16 and arrived at the quarantine station June 24. He died July 8 and on the 12th the mate of a steamboat tied up for repairs at the same wharf came down with the fever and it spread from there. Eventually the death toll reached 226 persons.[19]

Statistics and Theories Concerning Fever Epidemics

In accordance with a resolution of the Senate, Dr. Frank W. Reilly, surgeon, United States Marine Service, prepared a report on the yellow fever epidemic of 1873 as it prevailed at the various ports of the U.S. This report stated that from February until November 21 there occurred 3,789 deaths from malignant and epidemic cholera. During the same period there were, in round numbers, 21,000 deaths from diarrhea, dysentery and cholera infantum. From the first case on March 23 until the last reported case November 29 there were 3,349 deaths from specific or epidemic yellow fever. During the same period each year there occurred from the group of malarial fevers an aggregate of 8,500 deaths. The last preceding epidemic appearance of yellow fever was in 1867 and from its subsidence up to the close of 1872 there had been an aggregate of 970 deaths from this cause, but during the same period there had been an aggregate of over 50,000 deaths from malarial fevers. "Year by year, such more or less preventable diseases as small-pox, scarlet fever, typhus, enteric fever, and consumption are the causes of a tolerably constant average of over a hundred thousand deaths per annum. The report states that absolutely nothing has been learned of the cause of the disease."[20]

Toward that end, a letter to the *Scientific American* from a correspondent at Fayette, Mississippi, observed that prior to outbreaks of yellow fever the rains were unaccompanied by lightning and thunder. From this he drew the conclusion that "the prevalence of yellow fever is dependant [sic] upon the electrical position of the atmosphere." The idea that "concussions of the air," either natural (thunder) or manmade (gunpowder explosions), could clear the atmosphere of malarious fevers became prevalent again in the early to mid–1870s. At Vicksburg in 1871 firing cannon and burning tar were used in an attempt to purify the air against the advances of Yellow Jack.

The same year, news that a Jacksonville, Florida, fruit grower had succeeded in clearing his orchards of the "curculio" by the discharge of gunpowder tended to support the theory that such actions also cleared the air of floating "animalcules" that caused and fed yellow fever. This tied in with the observation that during yellow fever epidemics few thunderstorms occurred. It also offered further "proof" that during the Civil War, in consequence of the repeated discharges of gunpowder, neither yellow fever nor any other epidemic disease prevailed in the South.

Concurrently, Dr. B.S. Hargis of Pensacola had no fears of an outbreak because "atmospherical electricity and ozone abundant, and, as a consequence with regard to disease, catarrhal affections are prevalent and malarial diseases absent." The theories of Dr. Pettenkoffer also resurfaced in 1870 when Dr. Merean Morris, New York City sanitary inspector, determined that upturning soil for local improvements "had much to do with generating malaria" and yellow fever, as sun-baked subsoil exhalations poisoned the atmosphere with miasmatic diseases. Another cause-and-effect theory was espoused in 1874 after the British government addressed a circular to scientists concerning the production and consumption of timber. Numerous responses dealt with the sudden appearance of epidemic diseases after the destruction of large forests, supposedly due to the suppression of thunderstorms.

J.M. Toner, MD, president of the American Medical Association, believed yellow fever "has never reached in an epidemic form any locality that is five hundred feet elevation above sea." Statistics he gave for Memphis during the outbreak of 1873 indicated fatal cases were 29.5 percent of the whole, the totals being 1,244 deaths out of 4,204 cases, while Shreveport had 3,000 cases and 759 deaths. The fact yellow fever always began near the water level and in unhealthy conditions "is full of admonition." A second report stated that yellow fever never occurred in any climate above the elevation of 2,500 feet and in the United States it had never been known to strike over 460 feet, which point it reached only in Arkansas. It concluded "that the stratum of air infected by the poison is heavier than pure atmosphere, and therefore sinks."

On the subject of carbolic acid as a disinfectant, Professor Cochran of the Alabama Medical College argued that it was "conducive to the spread of disease rather than its suppression."[21]

The Lessons of Shreveport and Memphis

The official report on the epidemic at Shreveport, as prepared by Dr. D.P. Tenner, stated, "The prevalence of the disease, it is said, is directly traced to official neglect of duty.... Complaints from the people and warnings from the press, although loud and frequent, failed to stir the officials from their criminal negligence...."[22] A resident from Memphis voiced similar complaints:

> A city whose government's only care is to be sure that no kind of business is carried on within its jurisdiction without having paid its "special tax," and that taxes the black porters in hotels $200 a year for the privilege of toting trunks, and "all other things in proportion," ought to be rich enough to keep

"Ozone Water" was hailed as a "perfect disinfectant" and "Ozone Powder" a "sure preventative" of yellow fever and cholera. Those two diseases, along with malaria and smallpox, equated to the Four Horsemen of the Apocalypse when it came to deadly diseases in the 1700 and 1800s. One case was considered an epidemic and the mere suggestion of contamination could cause entire cities to be cut off from the rest of the country (*Galveston News*, September 14, 1884).

itself clean; but alas, here, as in many other American cities, the inevitable "ring" [gang] pockets the proceeds, while the "Nicolson" [common man] rots in the streets uncared for, and the swine fatten on the garbage in the back alleys.[23]

Criticisms from around the country were swift and pointed. The *Boston Globe* (October 17, 1873) editorialized: "There is reason to suppose that the recent ravages of yellow fever both at Shreveport and Memphis were occasioned by neglect of sewerage, which, as dwellers in European and American cities have learned to their cost, is responsible for a large share of the mortality that has sometimes been under otherwise favorable conditions.... The laws of health are so well known, nowadays, that a neglect to obey them by the authorities having charge of the interests of populous districts, must be regarded as culpable." By October 18, its editors took a firmer stand: "The Government, being in the hands of mere politicians and indifferent to everything but their own self-interest, naturally declined to comply with the appeals made for cleansing the town, which would divert money from their own pockets. The connection between political and sanitary demoralization was perhaps never more clearly displayed than in the ravages of yellow fever in a place whose accumulations of filth were occasioned by official incompetence and delinquency."

Taking a more constructive stance, the same newspaper (November 5, 1873) reported that lessons should have been learned from Charleston, where 15 years earlier authorities constructed, "at great cost, an admirable system of sewers which are washed out twice daily by the tide," thus nearly eliminating yellow fever. Proving that even southern papers were not immune to the troubles of their sister cities, the *Vicksburg Herald* (carried by the *Jackson* (IA) *Sentinel* (October 23, 1873) observed, "Is it astonishing, or rather, is it not perfectly natural, that such a violation of the laws of health should be followed by a frightful epidemic?" Ultimately, the *World* (October 27, 1873) had the final say: "Every town throughout the Union should be forced, by State laws, to appoint sanitary officers, and it should be made a part of the duty of these officials to use all possible means to check the egress of epidemic diseases, not merely from house to house, but from town to town. Under some such system alone can we hope for comparative immunity from pestilence which, as in the case of cholera in our South-western cities, Last Summer, and yellow fever, are allowed to roam unhindered over the continent."

Across the country the concept of quarantine continued to be rehashed. The New Orleans Chamber of Commerce acknowledged "simple detention and ordinary fumigation" were unreliable and granted permission for Dr. Perry to experiment at the Mississippi Quarantine Station. His proposal called for forcing gascons, or volatile disinfectants, by means of steam-power blowing machines through every portion of an infected vessel's hold. If the procedure were successful, the hope was that a few hours of detention would destroy all germs, thus eliminating the need to quarantine Spanish or South American ports.

Dr. Vanderpoel, health officer of New York, offered statistics in a report issued in January 1874:

Yellow Fever Occurring in New York Harbor

Year	Cases
1864	56
1865	68
1866	7

Year	Cases
1867	43
1868	9
1869	54
1870	26
1871	18
1872	46
1873	62

He stated, "The generally accepted principle that the individual in no way conveys the disease, but that it is transmitted by clothing, certain articles of merchandise, and, above all, by conditions in the vessel itself, relieves passengers wholly from observation as soon as the period of incubation has elapsed after the last case since leaving an infected port." Noting that speed was of the essence when disinfecting a vessel, he recommended that during the voyage the captain change the bilge water daily until it returned clean and free from smell; compel the crew to bathe at the close of each day's labor and to put on clean flannel in place of clothing saturated by perspiration and animal effluvia; prevent the crew from sleeping at night on the open deck; maintain cleanliness in their quarters; and leave the hatches open as much as possible. If these sanitary procedures were followed, health authorities at port would be warranted in subjecting him to "the least possible detention." This report was lauded by the *New York World* of August 16, 1874, as demonstrating a practical reality: "the thorough guardianship of the public health with little, if any, restriction of commercial interests."

Interestingly, a false alarm led to an intervention by the federal government that brought universal praise from around the country. After hearing of outbreaks at New Orleans, Galveston, Pensacola, Mobile and other cities, Secretary of the Treasury Bristow issued a circular in which he observed that "in the absence of uniformity of the regulations of quarantine in the Atlantic and Gulf coasts" it was desirable that officers compel strict compliance with local quarantine laws. Although reports of yellow fever proved to be exaggerated, his preemptive strike to mobilize a large and well-trained force was held to be the best first step ever taken to prevent a universal outbreak.[24]

A second false alarm had equally widespread consequences, although not so positive a conclusion. In the last week of March 1875 word spread like wildfire there was an outbreak of yellow fever at Key West. Subsequent dispatches from Washington confirmed the disease "had greatly increased within a few days" and that all naval vessels were quarantined. Due to the unprecedented early occurrence, panic among those southern cities prone to the disease became widespread. The *Galveston Daily News* on March 31, 1875, berated the surgeon general for not acting quickly and hoped Surgeon General Barnes would authorize $2,000 to aid Key West in combatting the extension of the fever. On the same date, that newspaper added, "The United States steamer Dispatch [also spelled *Despatch*], sent to New Orleans to convey the Senatorial party to Mexico, was at Key West when the fever had broke out, increasing the solicitude felt here not only for the naval officers, but for the prominent persons comprising the excursion party."

By April 3, however, under the caption "The Yellow Fever Canard," the *News* began an editorial by saying they suspected "all was not right" and reminded its readers that "last fall the Treasury Department issued a sensational circular to similar purport, which turned out afterward to have been the result of some newspaper correspondent's humbuggery." The editorial went on: "It looks strongly as if the Treasure Department has lent itself to the purposes of Northern newspaper correspondents who have already been accused and suspected of attempting to divert trade from Southern cities by the publication of such matter."

The charges would only get worse. The *Chicago Times* titled its editorial, "The Sensational Scare," warning, "There is ground for suspicion that the yellow fever in the Gulf cities was manufactured out of almost whole cloth by Mr. [Simon] Cameron's mourning patriots. The suspicion may not be very charitable, but it is irrepressible. The tearful train set out from Washington with the intention of embarking at the port of New Orleans on a government steamer" for Mexico "in search of the parched graves of patriots." On their arrival they received a telegram from Tar Robeson, master of the public ships, who suggested it would be well if they "made their pious pilgrimage at their own expense to avoid scandal." Unwilling to make "pecuniary sacrifices for a parsimonious country which had sternly refused to let them raise their salaries above $5,000 a year," they "bethought them of the yellow fever. One or two cases had occurred at Key West and that sufficed."

A second newspaper put the opposite slant on the situation: the rumor of yellow fever at Key West was started "for the purpose of scaring the Mexican excursionists, who had secured a United States war-vessel for their pleasurings." In any event, the "distinguished pilgrims" went their separate ways and the early scare of yellow fever ended as quickly as it started.[25]

CHAPTER 24

"Falling Like Leaves"

> *Since the 21st of August [1876] there have been over 1,800 interments in the city, almost a decimation at the highest estimate of the remaining population, and considerably over at the lowest. Of these about three-fifths are given to yellow fever proper, the remainder to swamp-fever, congestion of the brain, and kindred affections, all of which are but thin disguises for the milder types of the great destroyer.*[1]

The year 1876 was destined to put Savannah on the national map, as it proved to be a horrific year for yellow fever in that city. Of all the newspapers, the *Atlanta Constitution* had the most spectacular headlines, a sampling of which begins with "Yellow Jack" on August 31 and progresses to "The Fever" (9/9), "Fever-Stricken" (9/12), "The Yellow Fever" (9/14), "The Death Roll" (9/15), "Pestilence in Savannah" (9/16), "The Death Call" (9/17), "The Reaper's Harvest" (9/21), "Falling Like Leaves" (9/22), "Gone to the Grave" (9/23), "Shriven in Savannah" (9/26), "Entrance to Eternity" 9/27), "The Chastening Couch" (9/28), "Decrease of Deaths" (9/29), "The Sick of Savannah" (9/30), "Running Up Again" (10/1), "Frost and Fever" (10/3), "The Seacoast Scourge" (10/5), "Pathway of Pestilence" (10/6) and, ultimately, "Fever Figures," on November 1, 1867.

"The fever was discovered to be an epidemic August 20th. The discovery [of yellow fever] fell like a thunderbolt from a cloudless sky upon the people of Savannah—it was so wholly unlooked for, as since the war Savannah had perfected an excellent system of drainage and built water-works to afford a full supply of pure water; and the police, in addition to their other duties, are made sanitary inspectors; and there had been no yellow fever to speak of since 1856," said Colonel Albert R. Lamar, former editor of the *Savannah Advertiser*. "The cause," he continued, "were the very extraordinary rain-fall in June of fifteen and one-half inches, which overflowed the rice fields near the city and remained there under a temperature of over 90 degrees for sixty days, with an easterly wind from off the gulf stream since April."[2] Another perspective came from a letter published in the *Philadelphia Press* on October 3, 1876. It was written by a Savannah resident who believed the epidemic was imported on August 21 by two sailors off a vessel from the West Indies and who came ashore and died. Beginning slowly, the fever increased until August 31 when, for the first time, the *Savannah News* admitted its existence by announcing the Benevolent Association discovered that during the ten days preceding their report there had been 39 cases of yellow fever and 9 deaths. By September 10, the writer alleged the population had been reduced to 12,000–15,000 and 5,000–7,000 having fled for safety. Other estimates placed the population at 30,000 with 10,000 having fled by November 9.[3]

One particular point stressed in the newspapers was the unanticipated appearance of yellow fever among the Negroes. On September 9, the *Constitution* noted, "It will be seen that the colored people, who have heretofore been thought exempt from yellow fever, are becoming victims to the scourge, three interments being reported among them. We would suggest to the gentlemen composing the committees of the benevolent association and of the authorities that particular attention should be given to those quarters of the city occupied by the negroes." Less charitably, the *Athens* (OH) *Messenger* (November 9, 1867) reported, "Savannah has a negro population of about 15,000, who are naturally careless and improvident, and then she has a large white laboring class who are dependent upon their daily labor for their bread. Businesses of every sort, except through cotton, is suspended, and the laboring classes are wholly without means. The disease has run through this class of ill-fed, ill-clothed and ill-lodged ones, and swept them away like chaff before a whi[r]lwind, and is now attacking the better classes."

Mortality at Savannah, August 1–November 26, 1876

Month	Total Deaths	Yellow Fever	Other Diseases	Whites	Blacks
August	172	33	139	21	81
September	783	556	2,279	575	208
October	474	287	187	301	173
November	145	64	81	91	51

The numbers were compiled by the *Savannah News*, and the reporters noted that in the early period of the epidemic the immediate cause of death was given as "congestion, convulsions, spasms, gastritis, etc." but added it was "fair to presume that they had their origin in the prevailing fever." In an attempt to prove their city should not be singled out as being unhealthy, Dr. Semmes of that city published a list of other known outbreaks.

Historical Yellow Fever, Years of Visitation Compiled in 1876 (Local Physician)

Boston	1619, 1693, 1795
New York	1702, 1743, 1748, 1762, 1791, 1793, 1795
Philadelphia	1699, 1732, 1742, 1743, 1748, 1762, 1793, 1794, 1820
Baltimore	1794, 1795
Norfolk, VA	1747, 1795, 1855
Charleston	Ten times anterior to its appearance in New Orleans in 1796, in a period of 94 years
Savannah	1820, 1854, 1858, 1876
Memphis	1873
Pensacola	1873, 1874
New Orleans	1796 and then very few years epidemically down to 1873; in the epidemic of 1853, out of a population of 150,000, 30,000 fled the city. For the four weeks ending August 28, the average yellow fever mortality was 1,211 per week. In the week ending August 21 the maximum mortality was 1,346, other causes 152. The greatest number of deaths for any one day was on August 22, when 239 died. The greatest number of deaths in any one month was 5,189 in August; added to death from other causes, the average was 201 per day, 9 every hour, and 1 every 6–7 minutes for an entire month. The Howard Association cared for 11,080 yellow fever patients, of whom 2,942 died and 8,146 recovered, at a total cost of $159,190.32, or $14 per head. Donations from all parts of the union totaled $228,077.46. In 1867 the mortality was 3,800–4,000.[4]

It is interesting to compare statistics compiled in 1876 with those researched by the World Health Organization (WHO) in 2005.

Historical Yellow Fever Epidemics

Boston	1691, 1693, 1694, 1803, 1821
New York	1668, 1694, 1702, 1734, 1743, 1745, 1751, 1791, 1801, 1819, 1821, 1822, 1870
Philadelphia	1668, 1693, 1694, 1699, 1751, 1778, 1791, 1793, 1802, 1803, 1805, 1819, 1820, 1821, 1867
Baltimore	1783, 1817, 1819, 1821
Norfolk, VA	1801
Charleston	1690, 1693, 1699, 1703, 1728, 1732, 1745, 1748, 1792, 1807, 1817, 1819, 1821, 1824, 1839, 1843, 1852, 1854, 1856, 1858, 1876
Savannah	Not listed
Memphis	1828, 1873, 1879
Florida	1811, 1823, 1829, 1841, 1867
New Orleans	1811, 1817, 1819, 1820, 1821, 1822, 1824, 1827, 1828, 1829, 1837, 1841, 1847, 1854, 1856, 1867, 1873, 1878, 1905
Mobile	1825, 1827, 1829, 1837, 1839, 1843, 1847, 1854, 1867
Galveston	1839, 1843, 1853, 1867, 1870[5]

The city of Augusta ordered quarantine of freight and passengers from Savannah, holding the former 60 days and the latter 30. Ironically, this proved to be good news for the merchants of Savannah, as one editorialist noted "all river freights will now come to this city. Heretofore considerable cotton and other freights have found a market in Augusta." Several days later it was reported that cotton bills were higher than normal and ships laden with that commodity were steaming from the city for New York. While the "Howards" and the "Nightingales" were performing humane work, their benevolence was not always contagious. Other reports indicated certain bakers, butchers and ice men refused to sell their wares to such associations except at excessive charges.[6]

On September 24 the superintendent of the Marine Hospital Service detailed surgeons with large experience in yellow fever to Savannah to prevent spread of the disease further up the Atlantic coast. While local physicians were accusing one another of "unwise treatment" of yellow fever victims, S.M. Inman, chairman of the Benevolent Association, wrote that "doctors say it is not yellow fever alone they have to contend with, but with a high type of malarial fever supervening the yellow fever. The latter is bad enough but the two combined puzzle the best skill." One doctor complained that at the bedside he "found his theories completely at fault, and he had to back upon his own perceptions and judgment."

Including September and the first week of October, the city averaged 20 deaths per diem, with nearly one-third of them occurring among children. The *Savannah News* of October 4 noted the "curious fact" that, "although the colored population is within a thousand or two of the white, but 154 of them have died since the 1st of September, or a little over a fifth." Personal observations differed, however, with one letter writer pointing out that "contrary to experience in other localities [the Negroes] die there of yellow fever in the same ratio as white people."

Total Death Average of Races, September 1–October 28, 1876

Total white	873	9½ percent
Total colored	324	2¼ percent

Census Taken October 26

Whites, including children under 12	7,853
Colored, including children under 12	11,988

Excess of white females over males	143
Excess of colored females over males	1,498

The great disparity of females was accounted for by the number of male absentees.

Martyrs

Profession	Died	Prostrated
Doctors	2	12
Apothecaries and assistants	9	
Policemen	7	¾ of force
Protestant clergy	2	5
Catholic clergy	5	8
Sisters of Charity	5	15
Staff of *Morning News*	5	28

Physicians, Patients, Physic

Number of sick	12,000
Whites who escaped	500
Doctor visits	50,000
Doctor fees on paper	$125,000
Doctor fees in prospect	$15,000
Apothecary fees	$20,000
Undertaker charges	$20,000
Rations expended	100,000

What Savannah Lost

Expenditures of refugees out of city	$500,000
Loss of sale of merchandise, 2 months	$500,000
Loss of taxes to the city	$50,000
Loss of rent and depreciation	$250,000
Bales of cotton diverted to Charleston and other points	50,000

Ultimately, the *Savannah News* published statistics in December calculating that all deaths between August and November numbered 1,574, of which 940 were attributed to yellow fever. The total number of whites was 1,058 and blacks 516.

Encouraging his fellow citizens of Thomasville to welcome victims of yellow fever from Savannah, Dr. T.S. Hopkins attempted to prove there was no local danger by citing the work of Dr. Daniel Blair, Surgeon General of British Guinea. Blair's research indicated that non-yellow fever patients at Demerara were commonly placed in beds where yellow fever victims had died, without being infected. He added that the "muco-purulent matter, which exudes from the eyes in the last stage of the yellow fever, was applied to the eyes of well persons without producing yellow fever. These human experiments were not considered at all hazardous to the subject, the only objection being on the score of cleanliness. Has the swallowing of black vomit, which has often been done by stomachs more retentive than mine ever produced yellow fever? Has inoculation ever produced it? Never!" To further his case, Hopkins added that in 1805 a Spanish physician named Don Cabeuello took his children into the Lazaretto and slept with them in the beds in which yellow fever victims had died in order to test the infectiousness of the disease. None of them contracted the disease.

Perhaps the best way to conclude the Savannah epidemic of 1876 is to relate the story published in the *New York World* of a young drug clerk who stayed to perform his duties while his friends fled. After one employer died of the disease he went to another, performing nursing services with a friend as well as dispensing medications. When his friend took ill, the clerk nursed him, as well, tragically dying shortly after the passing of his companion. The paper wrote, "We are not much addicted to what is known in the newspaper profession as gush." But, they concluded, "At a time when the national character has suffered a great deal abroad through the misconduct of officials through whom we are mainly known to other people, and the American is pictured as a hard, angular, superficial, unscrupulous personage, occurrences like this at Savannah should bring us reassurance and comfort." As a further point of significance, a decade after the Civil War, the newspaper concluded the story with the statement, "They were brave boys, were they not? Does it make any difference which side or which flag such souls fought for twelve years ago? Can't you reach out and shake hands over any distance?"[7]

As a last note on quarantine for 1876, on August 5 Dr. Kelley of Galveston received a letter dated July 31 from a medical practitioner at Houston inquiring whether yellow fever was in the city. Before denying the rumor, Kelley added a tongue-in-cheek observation: "*Dear Doctor*—Whew! the mail from Houston to Galveston on the new gauge quite outstrips pneumatic tubes and telegraph lines, for at the end of five days your letter, dear doctor, full of earnest inquiry, lies before me. A careful scrutiny of it fails to detect any unpleasant gases, nor is it marked "non-infectious," nor yet does it give token of having been handled with long-legged tongs, as it was held at a safe distance by some frightened and trembling mail clerk, yet it must have been in quarantine."[8]

Foreign News—Yellow Fever Rears Its Ugly Head

Attempting to ward off disaster, in early 1870 Mr. Childers and other British authorities issued an order to all West Indies stations that as soon as yellow fever was found to prevail, her majesty's ship captains were to run north, even as far as to touch ice-laden latitudes, to kill the disease. By March the disease broke out at Rio, first among foreigners and seamen and then extending outward; by April deaths were noted to have decreased, averaging "only" 40 per day. By September 20 Reuter's Telegrams indicated 560 deaths at Havana during the previous week.

Perhaps more interesting from a historical perspective, a London newspaper argued for a new shipping line that would require 9 days from Milford Haven to Portland, 7 days to San Francisco and 23 days to Australia or New Zealand, which had the advantage of getting intelligence from England to these territories in a little over three weeks and vice versa, as San Francisco was already connected to London by the electric wire. The existing route by Panama involved "two grave disadvantages, one of which killed the Panama and New Zealand Co. The steamer landed her passengers to cross a fever-stricken isthmus and to pursue their course through a region of yellow fever. The numerous deaths which resulted frightened the Australians, and the gain in time was unable to outweigh the danger."[9]

News of yellow fever at Barcelona began hitting the wire services around September 21, 1870, and by the following day reports indicated there had already been "1,000 attacks, and from 300 to 400 deaths" since its introduction. Sources attributed the introduction of the disease to the steamer *Maria* (also referred to as the *Maria Pla*) from Cuba. Fears of "the very virulent type" of fever spread quickly spread across the Mediterranean coast and all those who could leave the area did so. By September 25 the exodus was calculated at nearly 90,000.

First Week's Mortality from Yellow Fever at Barcelona, September 1870

Date	Attacks	Deaths
20	33	23
21	36	25
22	55	24
23	35	24
24	29	28
28	58	38

In light of the ongoing Franco-Prussian War (1870–1871), the idea of epidemic disease cutting down soldiers on all sides became a very real fear. Writers at the *Janesville* (WI) *Gazette* (October 1, 1870) were particularly concerned, noting, "It is not necessary that a disease be brought into an army by a person who has been exposed to its contagion; given the conditions favorable to its development, it will appear spontaneously. Florence Nightingale mentions the production of small pox in this way, and says that in crowded, ill ventilated hospitals, and in camps, she has often seen and smelt this disease 'while it was growing.' and before the victims had a thought of their danger."

By October the panic had spread to New York, where consignees of vessels trading between that city and the Spanish Main "in their excessive greed of gain have sought, only too successfully, to evade the quarantine regulations, in order the more speedily to receive and dispose of their cargoes." For those "fond of coincidences," it was observed that the Barcelona yellow fever epidemic of 1870 occurred on the same day as in 1821, appeared first on the same street, suddenly increased the same day and attained its maximum of victims on the same day. Proving that even the titled were affected by the outbreak, the deputation of the Spanish Cortes, charged to offer the Crown to the Duke of Aosta, were held in quarantine at Genoa because they had departed from a port infected with yellow fever.[10]

The year 1871 brought death and destruction to Buenos Aires on an unprecedented scale. Early reports of yellow fever began around January 10 but official notice was not given until January 27, when three deaths were reported. From that date until February 24 there were 250 registered deaths; on the 26th were added 37 more fatalities, "after which the death rate increased alarmingly until on the 30th of March the number during the day was 301, and on the 8th of April 749!" From that time on, numbers began to decrease, reaching 550 on April 10; 427 on April 12; 105 on April 23, 130 on April 30; and 76 on May 2. Deaths then remained stable at around 24 per day. Official returns placed the total mortality at 13,403. Typically, official returns were significantly lower than those compiled privately and in this instance there developed what became known as a newspaper war. Generally, numbers published by the British press were similar to those offered by the *Standard* and the *Guardian,* the latter published on June 7, 1871:

Mortality Figures from Yellow Fever, Buenos Aires 1871

Month	Total Deaths
January	200
February	1,000
March	11,000
April	14,000
Total	26,200

Nationality	Total Deaths
Italian	11,000
Natives	8,000
Spaniards	3,500
French	2,200
English	600
German	300
Various	600
Total	26,200

In consequence, as reported by the *New York Herald* on June 19, 1871, "at once all the native papers, as well as the Italian periodicals, opened a tremendous attack on the *Standard*, and charged it with all sorts of improper objects, in thus, as they claimed, exaggerating the facts. The newspaper war still continues," as the *Standard*'s assertion of such high death tolls was "unsupported by any evidence whatever."

Regardless of specific death tolls, letters to the editors of numerous English newspapers depicted horrific scenes:

> The appearance of the country was like that of a freshly plowed field. The graves were made as close together as possible, in rows of fifty and one hundred, At one side of the cemetery large pits were dug, about fifty by twenty five feet deep in which the poor were buried. A layer of coffins was put in, then a little lime, and then more coffins, until the pit was nearly full, after which the earth was thrown in, and one large mound was made to mark the grave of hundreds. Poor fellows, they have been crowded and huddled together in unhealthy tenements while living, and being dead, were denied solitude even in the grave!

While concern for the citizens was heartfelt, predictions about the economy in an era of expanding international trade also received its fair share of press. The *New York Herald* (May 25, 1871) carried the following warning: "'[T]he prestige of the city has been destroyed, and … the full recovery of its trade and commerce is impossible.' Great commercial cities may recover from the effects of war or other misfortunes, but not very well or soon from the destructions or diversion of their commerce through a devastating disease." Money Markets reported such items as the Buenos Ayres Great Southern Railway traffic return for the week ending April 23 showing a decrease of 1,614*l*, owing to the prevalence of yellow fever. But as the crisis died down, London papers indicated that "fortunately, the financial crash which was supposed imminent in Buenos Ayres has been warded off by the great success of the Argentine Loan in London, the liberality of the banks, and the mercantile body generally."

For those concerned with the natural sciences, a paragraph in an American newspaper gave other reason for optimism: "Another link in Mr. Darwin's chain of evidence is regarded as supplied by the report that during the recent epidemic of yellow fever in Brazil, the monkeys there were as prone to take the disease as were the human residents. Other animals were exempt from contagion."[11]

"Its name is miasma": Bad Air, Monopolies, Race and Humor

The state of medical art was aptly summed up by the *Galveston Daily News* on March 21, 1875: "Specific modes of prevention or limitation of yellow fever remain as vague and inept, medical opinion as confused and conflicting, and medical skill as baffled as ever." With that in mind, the June 1871 issue of the *Journal of Health* declared "plague and pestilence, and all those diseases called epidemic, which suddenly fall upon a whole community, such as fever and ague, chills and fever, bilious fever, yellow fever, diarrhea, and dysentery are caused by marsh miasma." (Five years later, "Its name is miasma" would be used almost verbatim to promote Udolpho Wolfe's "Schiedam Aromatic Schnapps" as a preventative for malarial diseases.) On a similar note, Dr. S.P. Hubbard of Taunton sent a scorching letter to the *Boston Journal* declaring that his son narrowly escaped death by inhaling poisonous gasses in the ill-ventilated laboratory of the Harvard medical school, adding that "a yellow fever pest house would be no less dangerous to the young men who go there."

On a slightly more scientific level, Dr. Vanderpoel's 1874 *Annual Report to the New York Commissioners of Quarantine* noted that over the past several years trade with yellow fever ports had undergone "a marked and radical change," due to the fact steamships had replaced sailing vessels. In the latter case, such ships had long passages and lay for extended periods in infected ports so that fomites had ample opportunity to reach the hold of the vessel, gaining force and virulence. In the former instance, steamers remained in port for limited periods, lessening the likelihood of becoming infected. This fact permitted Vanderpoel to be more lenient, greatly limiting the number of ships quarantined. In 1872, there were 115 lightered; in 1873 there were 112 and by 1874 only 69 were held over.

On the subject of economics, in 1876 great concern was expressed over the presence of yellow fever in southern ports delaying cotton shipments and thus keeping back some of the commercial bills until later in the season. The same year there was great anxiety over whether Savannah would be able to pay interest on its bonds as the yellow fever epidemic prevented authorities from collecting taxes. More dire for racing fans in the city, it was announced that due to yellow fever the past summer there would be no races over the Ten Broeck course in 1877.

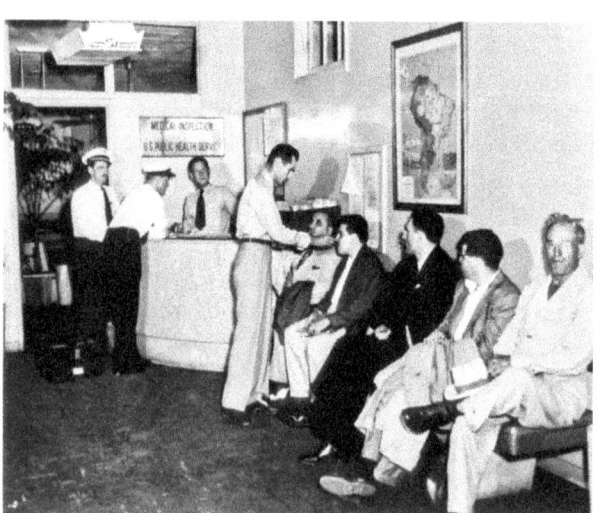

One of the more significant economic fights to emerge in the 1870s was that concerning the monopolies on quinine and calomel, two medications commonly prescribed for fever patients. In 1873 two Philadelphia laboratories supplied the bulk of quinine throughout the United States: Powers & Weightman and Rosengarten & Son, by rea-

The yellow fever–carrying mosquito is not a strong flier and has a very limited range. But once brought aboard an airplane in luggage or cargo, it can be transported thousands of miles. An infected female passes on the disease through her eggs and when these insects reach adulthood, they too become carriers. In the same manner, an individual bitten by an infected mosquito may not show outward symptoms for some time. These passengers at a Miami, Florida, airport, are having their temperatures taken in an attempt to prevent any from entering the state who may not appear ill but who have a fever, indicating the possibility they may be suffering from yellow fever (courtesy National Library of Medicine).

son of the ad valorem duty of 20 percent. As argued by the *New York World,* in 1857 the duty on quinine was 15 percent. That year a French chemist named Pelleties arrived in New York and established a quinine factory. To eliminate the competition, the two Philadelphia companies charged 20 cents less a bottle than the Paris price and by spending $800,000 in the contest, they finally drove the Frenchman out of business. Afterward they appealed to Congress to gradually raise the duty on processed quinine to 45 percent ad valorem. Simultaneously, they used their influence to eliminate the tax on the import of Peruvian bark, the principal ingredient of quinine. This permitted them to make a larger profit while at the same time eliminating foreign imports.

In 1872 the House Committee placed quinine on the free list but the two firms brought pressure to bear on the Senate Finance Committee and a compromise was effected whereby the duty on quinine was reduced from 45 to 20 percent. With free Peruvian bark, quinine could be made as cheaply in the U.S. as abroad and the duty of 20 percent ad valorem amounted to 40 cents an ounce on all quinine used. Passed on to the consumer, the duty became "a bonus paid by the invalid to the monopolist." The story was the same for calomel. A duty of 30 percent gave a monopoly to three Philadelphia firms: Powers & Weightman, the Rosengartens and Pfizer. In 1873 the importation of calomel amounted to about $2,000 a year, on which duty paid to the Department of the Treasury was $600. The total consumption of calomel (with mark-up) amounted to $150,000, on which patients paid the tax of $45,000 to the three firms.

In an early case concerning malpractice among druggists, the case of *McCubbin, Tutor, vs. Samuel Hastings* was heard in New Orleans and went all the way to the Louisiana Supreme Court. On August 26, 1867, Dr. W.G. Austin was called in to see Mrs. Ellen Leigh McCubbin, wife of William McCubbin, who was suffering from yellow fever. The physician prescribed an enema of Aqua Champhorae (camphor water), 4 ounces. The clerk filling the order made an error and issued a mixture containing camphor 300 grains and alcohol (spirits of camphor). The patient was given the treatment, began suffering immediately and died on Friday, August 30. On advice of the doctor, the husband sued and won a judgment. The case was closely followed, as the lower courts held that the employer was responsible for the acts of his employee. In 1875, after "a long and tedious litigation," the Louisiana Supreme Court ruled against the defense's contention that death resulted from the "strange idiosyncracies [sic] of yellow fever," the death certificate listed the cause of death as yellow fever, not poisoning, and the defendant was not the individual who actually prepared the medicine. In upholding the lower court's decision the state supreme court issued a monetary reward of $2,500. Public sentiment went for Mr. Hastings, who had to pay a substantial sum for the mistake of an employee, but it was also suggested that legislation, similar to that used in England, where "pharmaceutists" (pharmacists) were required to pass a rigorous examination and stand by the quality of their drugs, would better serve the public.[12]

During this period little advancement had been made on "cures." Dr. Turner of Savannah recommended the old standby Brandreth's Pills as a specific for yellow fever; French physician Dr. Stephens observed that in cases of yellow fever in the army the blood drawn was very black but upon salt being added it became vermillion and retained its freshness. He therefore treated his patients with a mixture of various salts, reducing mortality in the West Indies from 1:5 to 1:50. There was also a revival of faith in the treatment of an old woman named Mariquita Orfile, who claimed the juice of the vervain plant was a cure for the disease.[13]

In writing about the yellow fever epidemic in New Orleans in 1875, Dr. T.J. Dills quoted from a book written by Charles Gayarre, *History of Louisiana and Spanish Domination* (1867). In discussing the epidemic that broke out in August and ran through October 31, 1796, he noted "a peculiarity to be remarked in the disease is, that it attacks foreigners in preference to natives, and it seems to select the French, English and Americans, who rarely recover, and who die on the second or third day after the invasion of the disease. Such is not the case with the Spaniards and colored people."

The same year, the *Deutsche Versicherungs-Zeitung* of New Orleans published an article on the mortality of the two races taken from statistics of Dr. Chille. He stated the mortality of the colored population had always been in excess of the white except during yellow fever epidemics, "this disease chiefly affecting the whites":

> In comparing the five years of freedom from 1866–70 with the four years of slavery from 1856–60 we find the aggregate death-rate has remained the same. But when a comparison is drawn between the whites and blacks in those periods it appears that the mortality of the blacks has greatly increased. Thus, during the four years 1856–60 (1858, a yellow-fever year, being excluded) the colored death rate was about 44 to the thousand, and the white 39 per thousand; while in the four years 1866–70 (excluding the yellow fever 1867) the colored death-rate amounted to 43 and the white to only 33 per thousand.... Some of the causes doubtless lie in the greater ignorance and improvidence of this race, and in the fact that its mortality from small-pox, cholera, consumption, still-births, and diseases of children is greater.

In 1876 data on the health of New Orleans proved "the entire feasibility of confining yellow fever to the places where it first appears, by strict disinfection. The total mortality from ordinary disease is much greater among the colored than among the white population of the city—nearly double." Finally, in answer to the question whether any "full blooded negroes had died of yellow fever" during 1876, the *Savannah News* responded, "The result of our observation and inquiries upon the above subject is to the effect that the pure-blooded negro is not a subject for yellow fever. Those colored people who have died here without exception, have been persons of mixed blood."[14]

Rounding out the first six years of the 1870s is a glimpse of the humor of the times. The first comes from London, under the heading "Professionals Abroad," from the February edition of the *Cornhill Magazine*. It concerns the story of a French opera company on its way to New Orleans. By special arrangement, the impresario in charge had agreed to include only one tenor in the company and after several days of seasickness that individual went topside to exercise his voice. As he was running up the scale he heard a second tenor and then a third until it was revealed there were actually five aboard. When these angry gentlemen confronted the manager, he cheerfully explained that none of them had been to New Orleans. Upon their arrival the yellow fever was sure to be raging and he expected four of the five to be taken off during rehearsals. The one who survived would thus become his "first and only tenor." From the *New York World* came the tongue-in-cheek report that a new disease in California was termed "green fever." Their medical advisor suggested the malady "was the result of yellow fever in a patient who has the 'blues.'" Good news for certain occupations came out in 1875 when a Texas newspaper noted yellow fever, smallpox and cholera went sailing through a community "but for some mysterious reason won't hit a book canvasser or a back pay Congressman once in a thousand times." Similarly, the *Appeal* remarked that "not a single newspaper fiend in Memphis surrendered to the scourge of 1873," while the *Savannah News* noted "not a single book agent died during the yellow fever epidemic of 1876."[15]

Chapter 25

"The grim monster still on his pathway": The Outbreaks of 1878

> *There are eight hundred and sixty-four drinking saloons in New Orleans. The yellow fever did not hit in the right places.*[1]

Generally speaking, the year before a major outbreak of yellow fever was relatively mild. This was the case in 1877 when the only outbreak to make national headlines was that in Fernandina, Florida. Reports began circulating in September and by the 7th the board of health had acknowledged two cases. By the 10th the death toll had reached seven and a general panic ensued, causing the principal towns in the state to enact a quarantine against the city. By September 26, mortality had reached 52 and medical assistance was requested from Jacksonville and Charleston. Interestingly, there was some public outcry when Charleston physicians refused to go to Port Royal, Georgia, which was also suffering from yellow fever, without payment being guaranteed. They answered the criticism by saying, "We do not endorse the common notion that the doctor is merely a public servant and is bound to make a martyr of himself whenever an opportunity offers, gratis. The physician has to work for his daily bread like other men, and his life is just as dear to himself and to his family, and no one has a right to demand that he shall abandon a lucrative practice and put his life in jeopardy from merely sentimental motives." Equally ironic was the report that Luke Blackburn, the infamous physician connected to the Civil War scandal of attempting to import infected clothing into the Union, was asked by Governor McCreary of Kentucky to assist in administering to the yellow fever victims and left for Florida on October 12.

A census taken on September 21 indicated only 1,632 persons left in Fernandina: 518 whites and 1,114 blacks. Although "the colored people, so far, have escaped, in a great measure," overall mortality was 1:7, equal to 14 percent.[2]

Dateline: New Orleans

On July 24, 1878, the *Picayune* announced 14 cases of yellow fever had appeared in two areas emcompassing four squares each, of which seven cases terminated fatally. These locales were disinfected with carbolic acid, prompting the board of health to hope they had succeeded in checking the spread of disease, while the *Democrat* on July 27 announced there should be no fear of a yellow fever epidemic, as the number of cases was "far below the average of any previous year." The situation changed radically and two days later the board of health announced the total number of cases had reached 80, with 33 deaths. The board's president, Dr. Samuel Choppin, noted that at that time "it would not be proper to issue clean bills of health to vessels leaving this port."

Despite hopes for the best, by August 2 the total number of deaths had reached 195 and, as fear spread faster than disease, municipalities along the Mississippi began issuing quarantine notices. One case in point, described by the *Cincinnati Enquirer* (July 31), gives an insight into how the scare of yellow fever ran rampant throughout the country. On Saturday, July 27, Mr. William Hines, a wealthy cotton broker from New Orleans, and his wife arrived in Cincinnati to escape the contagion. He complained of indisposition on arrival and the couple took a room at a leading hotel. Convinced her husband was suffering from yellow fever, Mrs. Hines called in Dr. Reamy. He was not convinced of the diagnosis and waited until Monday to call in Dr. Minor for a second opinion. Minor decided the patient did suffer from yellow fever and in order to protect the hotel patrons determined to admit the patient to the Commercial Hospital. Those authorities became panic-stricken at the thought of yellow fever and refused to receive the patient. The doctor warned that unless they cooperated he would call out the sanitary police and take possession of the hospital. The threat worked and the administrators agreed, but upon Mrs. Hines being informed, she became hysterical, telling the physicians that in New Orleans it was considered extremely dangerous, if not fatal, to move a patient in the throes of yellow fever.

Dr. Minor remained inexorable, declaring that the safety of the many took precedence over one victim. However, the servants refused to touch the sick man and it appeared he might remain in the hotel. Finally, one colored man volunteered to help and the patient was taken to the hospital. A follow-up story dated August 6 indicated Hines was steadily recovering.[3]

As mortality climbed and the number of outbreaks increased to 28, certain features in connection with the fever became worthy of note. Among them was the observation that there was "a peculiar and unprecedented disposition ... to attack children, and it does this without any reference to their being acclimated or otherwise." Many were less than two years old and several younger than 12 months, causing speculation as to whether this was "really the yellow jack of our fathers." Similarly, the *Bee* noted, "We must acknowledge that it is difficult for us to believe that creole children, by reason of their birth and race, should be the victims of yellow fever. Can it be that we have some other malady prevalent among us?" By August 11 Dr. A. Mercer of the board of health declared he had never seen a child born in New Orleans to suffer from yellow fever and declared the proper diagnosis to be "malarial fever." Not everyone agreed, as indicated by the report that to that date 121 children under the age of 10 and 19 colored persons suffered from yellow fever. Notwithstanding, the board of health considered the outbreak "mild" and called for a quarantine of vessels from infected ports on the grounds they might introduce a more malignant virus. Simultaneously, that body resolved to trial irrigation as a means of disinfectant by use of various mechanical appliances to throw water from the Mississippi into the drains and street gutters, running night and day for a week or more until a determination of effectiveness was reached.

As "the grim monster still on his pathway" staggered the people of New Orleans, the Howard Association once more sprang into action, supplying nurses, financial aid and rations to the afflicted. On the subject of statistics, the association complained that not even half the number of cases were being reported to the board of health, minimizing the totals. The fault, it decided, was in individual physicians who purposely failed to report instances of yellow for fear fumes from carbolic acid used by the sanitary corps as a disinfectant were worse than the disease itself. Working with the authorities on matters that could be influenced, the chief of police received instructions to remove the bells from ice cream wagons and to instruct drivers to go slowly when passing localities where people were suffering from fever.

On the economic front, the Crescent City Ice Company took advantage of the presence of the fever by increasing the price of ice to $60 a ton. On the opposite side, problems with mail delivery prompted the Western Union Telegraph Company to offer free telegraphy to anyone wishing to transfer money from banks in New Orleans to New York. The obstruction of mail also prompted the presiding officers of the Cotton Exchange and Chamber of Commerce to address a communication to the postmaster general protesting quarantine measures adopted in Arkansas, Texas, Tennessee, Louisiana and Mississippi. Protecting local environs first, the Post Office Department proposed to cut chisel gashes in an X shape through the center of each letter sent to Washington and Virginia from contaminated areas and subject it to fumigation. This technique would penetrate the inside of the envelope without making its contents public.

A businessman describing a trip to New Orleans from Cincinnati stated that on the passage down, at Arkansas City, the boat was not allowed to land or coal and men stood on the banks with guns, threatening to shoot if an attempt was made. At Memphis, "not a dog, not a mule, not a negro could be seen…. Vicksburg was almost as bad as Memphis. Terror reigned all along the Mississippi. If the boat had freight for any town, it was taken on to New Orleans, the inhabitants refusing to receive it. At New Orleans things looked much better. Men were at work on the levee; business houses were open, but little or no business was being transacted. The return trip was made by rail. At Grenada not a white man was visible, only a few negroes. At Holly Springs about 200 people came aboard. Yellow fever had broken out the night before. The scenes at the depots were heartrending."

Another writer, in a description of New Orleans, observed, "It is said that a stranger visiting that city, would, perhaps, be impressed with the great diligence used in cleaning the streets and other sanitary measures, but otherwise there is nothing to arrest his attention that yellow fever is raging. There is wisdom in this beside business sagacity, because the disease makes its first victims of the despondent…. The newspapers also maintain a cheerful tone, and impress upon the minds of their readers that, bad as the present affliction may be, the city has been visited in past times by the same scourge in far more deadly form."

On August 15 Surgeon General John W. Woodworth issued a statement advising the Marine Hospital Service that although Congress had passed a resolution requiring medical officers of the service to assist local authorities in enforcing local yellow fever quarantines no appropriation of funds was made. He reiterated that "the weight of scientific evidence seems to warrant the conclusion that yellow fever is produced by an invisible poison capable of self-multiplication outside of the human organism, which it enters through the air passages. This poison germ, or miasm, is a product of the tropics…. Yellow fever can not be said to be epidemic in the United States, from the fact that in some years it does not appear…. The germ is transmissible…." His suggestion for individual prophylaxis was the internal use of small doses of sulphate of quinia and of tincture of iron and chlorate of potassa. He also recommended the nasal passages be bathed frequently with a spray of quinine.

DR. VICTOR BAUD'S
ORGANIC MEDICINES.

THE BAUDEINE,
A prompt and most efficient Remedy for
ASIATIC CHOLERA,
YELLOW FEVER,
DYSENTERY AND DIARRHŒA

No inconvenience is derived, or danger incurred by taking it. In good health it is a preservative against the epidemic, and invigorates the whole system. Dr. VICTOR BAUD was presented with a Gold Medal by the French Government as a reward for his discovery, and as a testimonial for the numerous cures he effected with this remedy in 1854, and ever since.

Large size Bottles, 11s.   Medium size, 4s. 6d.   Small size, 1s. 1½d.

Instructions for the treatment of Asiatic Cholera and Yellow Fever, in all the periods of those diseases, accompany each bottle, and bear the signature of "Dr. V. BAUD."

THE DIASTATIZED IRON,
FOR STRENGTHENING THE SYSTEM.
THE DIASTATIZED IODINE,
FOR PURIFYING THE BLOOD.

The above is in the shape of sweetmeats and pleasant to taste. By a scientific process of combining the oIron or the Iodine with Cress Seed, the valuable properties of the Iron or Iodine are fully developed, while the obnoxious parts are done away with, and the most delicate stomach can digest them with perfect ease.

Price 2s. 9d.   Sold by all the Chemists.

Sole Agent for England and the British Colonies,
CHARLES LANGE, 6, MONKWELL STREET, LONDON.
West-end Agent, London L. SCHOUVER, 21, Princes-street, Hanover-square.

Dyspepsia, Nervous and General Debility, etc.—Pepsine and Phosphate of Soda.
THE INVIGORATIVE NERVINE ESSENCE.

The most scientifically prepared and most powerful nutritive cordial ever introduced—restores to their normal condition all the secretions, on the integrity of which perfect health depends. It is a specific for Dyspepsia, Nervousness, and Debility of all kinds

ANALYTICAL REPORT OF DR. HASSALL,
ANALYST OF THE ANALYTICAL SANITARY COMMISSION OF THE "LANCET."

Having analyzed the Invigorative Nervine Essence, I am of opinion that it is a combination well calculated, from its containing among other ingredients, Pepsine and Phosphate of Soda, to prove serviceable to the Nervous, the Dyspeptic, and the Debilitated."
PRICE 5s. PER BOTTLE, OR FOUR QUANTITIES IN ONE FOR 22s.
SOLE AGENTS:—Messrs. BAUMGARTEN and CO., 520, Oxford Street, W.C., and 8, Cullum Street, Fenchurch Street, E.C., who will forward it, Carriage-free, on receipt of remittance.

Dr. Victor Baud's Organic Medicines came with instructions for the treatment of "Asiatic Cholera and Yellow Fever, in all the periods of those diseases." If nothing else, the promoters promised there was no danger in taking it. Although that codicil may sound humorous, so many "cures" proved to be worse than the disease it was as well to be reassuring as it was bombastic (*The Atlas*, London, August 10, 1867).

Mortality from Yellow Fever in New Orleans, 1878

Date	Total Cases	Deaths
August 7	351	95
August 11	466	126

Date	Total Cases	Deaths
19	1,219	355
20	1,355	396
24	1,866	577

[According to the *Picayune,* the greatest number of deaths for one day in August was 59 and the daily average was 28, with a total mortality of 877.]

Date	Total Cases	Deaths
September 1	—	77
2	—	88
3	—	83
4	—	72
5	—	81
6	—	61
7	—	66
8	—	77
9	—	87
10	—	80
11	—	90
12	—	57
13	—	58

By November 20 the yellow fever epidemic in New Orleans was considered over. The board of health calculated there was a total of 21,641 cases with a 25 percent mortality (George Augustin reported 4,046 deaths). Five days later quarantine restrictions against the city were lifted by Galveston and other places followed.[4]

According to "the best writers" the tabulation of the greatest yellow fever epidemics in New Orleans (omitting 1878, which was still ongoing), were as follows:

Year	Date of Outbreak	Deaths
1817	June 18	800
1819	July 1	2,190
1847	August	2,250
1853	May	7,970
1854	July	2,453
1855	June	2,670
1858	June	3,889
1867	June 10	3,093[5]

By the time the year ended the writers would have another tragic year to add to their list. On a wider scale, Dr. Greenville Dowell of Texas, the author of a contemporary text on yellow fever, stated that as of July 1877 the disease had appeared in 228 cities and towns in 28 states of the union and had "taken off" 65,311 people.[6]

Moving the Line: The Transportation of Yellow Fever

"Never," wrote a reporter for the *Hagerstown* (MD) *Mail* of August 23, 1878, "since the great cholera panics of 1832 and 1853, has there been anything in this country to equal the consternation and death attendant on the yellow fever, more particularly last week, in the infected portions of the Southern States. The pictures drawn of the scenes attending this terrible scourge … are truly frightful, and fill in their details columns of the city dailies." Noting that the disease had its base in New Orleans and extended down to the mouth of the Mississippi at Port Eads, he traced the epidemic along the river to Cairo and from there up the Ohio to Louisville, Covington and Cincinnati. Regarding a developing trend as the Iron Horse supplanted the steamboat as the favored mode of transportation, the writer added that it was "along the line of railroad running out of New Orleans through Mississippi, Tennessee and Kentucky to Cairo, that the mark of the scourge has been left with most appalling effect: and the town of Gredada, in Mississippi, on the Yalabusha River, a tributary of the Mississippi ... the greatest sufferer."

Although the original outbreak in New Orleans was traced to the steamship *Emily Souder* from Havana, in Grenada the disease was thought to have been "engendered spontaneously" by the opening of an old sewer. In less than a week, out of 1,200 white inhabitants the population was reduced to 200. On August 21 the Howard Association reported seven deaths, adding, "Negroes are dropping like sheep and will not help each other." A second report late the same day added, "The fever has attacked full blooded negroes. Three have died." At Vicksburg, 50–200 cases were registered daily, while at Memphis, the roofs of departing trains were covered with passengers, "as were the platforms and even the cow-catchers."

Embargoes were laid on trains either to keep them from spreading yellow fever to residents or from the dread of passengers contracting the disease as they sped through plague-stricken towns; trains stopped only when forced to by desperate inhabitants who lined the tracks imploring to be taken away. Norfolk, Richmond and Washington, D.C., took precautionary measures, but it was along the railroad leading from New Orleans to Chicago and St. Louis that the greatest excitement prevailed and it was not unusual to encounter armed citizens forcibly preventing passengers from the South from leaving the cars.

In the December 1878 issue of *Harper's* magazine, Dr. Coan advised readers that yellow fever was spread in two ways: by a slow and regular progression from house to house and by following the lines of travel. He noted that it was introduced by sailing ships: "Whether the part of the town nearest the water happens to be a clean or a dirty quarter, a rich or a poor one makes no difference.... The germs of the disease are portable, like bulk in freight, and they will take root in any soil ... [and] the poison will hide and ripen for some two months' time, and develop its fullest strength of infection."

The first well-authenticated case of Bronze John occurred in Memphis on August 13 when a woman who ran an eating house frequented by river boatmen came down with the disease. Three days later Surgeon General Woodworth ordered 1,000 canvas tents belonging to the War Department sent to Memphis, where camps outside the city were established to house the poorer classes freeing the infection. Dr. Noll, in charge of the camp, was met by a "mob, entirely of negroes," who demanded the tents be taken away. This prompted a town meeting in which the Bluff City Grays (white) and McClellan Guards (colored) were ordered to protect the doctor when he delivered the supplies. In the same report it was stated that since the white inhabitants had fled the city thefts of unoccupied property were becoming more common. While it was "not known for certain that all were robbed by negroes," blame was placed on them as *some* were heard to utter, "The d____d white-livered s___s of b_____s have left the city in our hands, and we intend to make the most of it."

On August 23 the board of health declared the fever to be epidemic and ordered all who could do so to leave the city. The Memphis and Charleston Railroad offered transportation to the refugees. Those who remained had the option of living in one of two camps, but moving there was no guarantee of safety. By August 26 three deaths were reported at Camp "Joe Williams." By August 27, of all new cases "the greater proportion are colored people, among whom the mortality is very great." Two days later, as the "carnival of death continues without abatement," the Negroes of Memphis published a card which declared it impossible for them to make a living as no work was to be found. The card warned, "They are starving for want of subsistance [sic] while plenty of food has been sent to Memphis from the north, but not given them, and unless rations are furnished a riot is threatened."

By August 29 a dispatch from the Howard Association reported on a statement from Dr. Lawrence of the board of health that indicated "a fearful condition of affairs among colored people. In some localities they are crowded together in narrow, filthy quarters and are an easy prey to disease and death, and hundreds of them have been sick for days without medical attendance." Apparently some aide was supplied. By September 7, A.D. Langstaff, president of the Howard Association, indicated, "Thousands of negroes are still in the city, kept here by free rations." He also said "no more unacclimated physicians or nurses from the North will be accepted," as their presence only added fuel to the fames of the growing yellow fever epidemic. In an all-too-familiar refrain underscoring racial tensions and misapprehensions throughout the era, the association offered the staggering sum of $10/day for nurses while bemoaning the fact that "although there are many negroes in the city, few of them can be persuaded to wait upon or even approach a sick person, while a majority of those who do hire as nurses for the big pay offered are inefficient." On the same subject, the *Logansport* (IN) *Daily Journal* on September 13, 1878, offered the following editorial comment: "The Louisville Courier-Journal, true to its brutal instincts, suggests that if "the colored people in the yellow fever districts want relief, they should look to the colored people of the North for it. The stolid inhumanity of the "chivalrous" leaders of the Southern political sentiment has seldom had a stronger illustration than this, but it is hoped that a better spirit prevails where the suffering actually exists, and the contributions of the people of the North are being distributed."

After returning to Washington from Memphis, an interview with Dr. William T. Ramsey dated September 13 informed the public that five miles out of Memphis the air was laden with yellow fever poison and as he approached nearer the stench was absolutely sickening. Staying at the Peabody Hotel, he was shown into a room "from which a dead lady had just been removed. The vessels of black vomit were standing about the room and the bedclothes had not been changed." Fever victims occupied two-thirds of the rooms and sulphur-pans were kept burning in the halls. He added that "negroes and many poor whites, for a section of 150 miles around Memphis" had flocked there, "hearing they could get something to eat," while most, especially colored women, had no clothes to wear. "The city," he concluded, "is in the hands of the colored police altogether, and while they behave very well, there is still a lurking fear on the part of the whites of some additional evil."

Determining the precise number of victims was given up as hopeless, "owing to the fact that but two physicians have reported to the board of health up to noon today [August 30]. Some are indifferent to the importance of reporting, others are too busy and one was in open defiance of the board and was never known to report a case, claiming that the prevailing disease is not yellow fever." Complicating matters, the *Evening Herald* suspended publication. On the final day of the month 120 new cases were reported, along with the grim news that the plague had extended two or three miles, "indicating that the atmosphere of the city and for miles around is thoroughly poisoned with infection." One of the more famous victims succumbing to yellow fever at Memphis was Jefferson Davis, Jr., who died October 16, 1878. His body was eventually reinterred at Hollywood Cemetery, Richmond, in April 1885, where he was placed beside his father. The bier was covered with the same silken Confederate flag that had rested on Jefferson Davis's coffin.

The night of October 28 brought with it a heavy front and the following day the board of health officially announced that refugees could safely return to the city. The Memphis epidemic of 1878 ended on December 7 when the Citizens' Relief Committee wound up its affairs, distributing the balance of its funds ($7,235) among four orphan asylums and ordering the 1,500 yellow fever tents to be burned.[7]

Dateline: The Foreign Front

The special correspondent of the *Boston Globe* in "Panama" reported on February 4, 1878, that Salta, Peru, reported that a visitation of locusts covered forty leagues and yellow fever prevailed alarmingly in Brazil. By March 4 deaths from yellow fever at Rio Janeiro for the first two weeks of February numbered forty-five. The appearance of the disease in Jamaica was hotly debated among physicians and theologians, while John A. Wegg, MD, wrote a pamphlet, *Hematogastic Pestilence*, offering 33 pages on hygienic rules for use by "the Unacclimatised New Comer or Stranger." In the same light, John Sullivan, MD, Member of the Royal College of Physicians of London, penned *The Endemic Diseases of Tropical Climates, with Their Treatment*, summing up the state of yellow fever prevention: "All causes of infection, all deleterious emanations from the earth's surface, however varied may be their effects, in every climate and under every sun, are capable of becoming, if not completely neutralized, at least greatly modified, by a due and rigid attention to the social condition of a people, and to the strict observance of the laws of hygiene."

In April 1878 the *British Medical Journal* reported—"for the first time probably in the memory of any living physician"—a case of yellow fever that ended fatally in the square of Belgravia, London. The victim was reputed to have caught the disease while aboard a West Indian steamer. "Under some circumstances and during periods of great heat such an announcement might have created serious alarm," the article concluded, "but, with the present temperature, and considering the precautions taken, there is no reason to consider it possible that any local extension of the disease should follow."[8]

Congress, Commissions, Causes, Cures and Costs

On April 29, 1878, Congress passed the National Quarantine Act (NQA), which authorized the Marine Hospital Service to make rules concerning the quarantine of vessels arriving from infected ports or ships carrying contagious crew or passengers. Two points of contention limited the scope of the NQA: no money was appropriated for its tasks and it was prohibited from making regulations in conflict with state sanitary or quarantine laws. The first major achievement of this body was to publish the *Bulletin of the Public Health*, the first issue of which was printed July 13. Later known as *Public Health Reports* it has been in publication ever since.

"A yellow fever convention is to say the least a novelty," wrote a reporter from the *Georgia Daily Constitution* (February 20, 1878), describing a gathering of prominent physicians from southern cities at Jacksonville. Brought together at the prompting of Mayor Boyd, the "Quarantine Convention" resolved to memorialize Congress to "establish a uniform and efficient system of quarantine on the Atlantic and Gulf coasts" and requested the secretary of state to issue instructions to American vessels to forward weekly reports of the hygienic condition of their respective ports. Additionally, they published the shipboard disinfectant specifications used by Dr. Robert Lebby of Charleston as being highly effective. The mixture consisted of sulphate of iron, 20 pounds; boiling water, 40 gallons; crude carbolic acid, 40 degrees, 1½ gallons or 1½ pounds of Calvert's carbolic acid, sprinkled by means of the ordinary watering cart.⁹

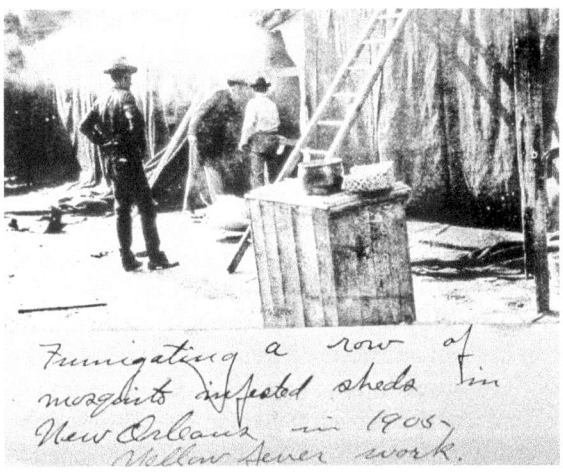

Members of the United States Public Health Service and the Marine Hospital Service stand outside a row of mosquito sheds, preparing to fumigate them. The image is from 1905 (courtesy National Library of Medicine).

What was referred to as the Richmond Health Conference, or National Yellow Fever Commission, was held in October 1878. Members of the executive committee of the American Public Health Association (APHA; president James L. Cabell; vice president Dr. John S. Billings) and concerned physicians attended. Among their requests was that Congress provide means for further study of yellow fever and the dissemination of information to "the educated classes" by circulating printed sets of questions. The commission sent experts south to investigate the origin and causes of yellow fever and presented its report in November. Their conclusions, noted the *Georgia Daily Constitution* of November 19, 1878, "should be accepted as final, at least by non-professionals. It is the latest and best information we have on the subject."

SIX CONCLUSIONS REACHED BY THE YELLOW FEVER COMMISSION

(1) No case of yellow fever was justifiably considered "as of *denoto* origin, indigenous to its locality" during the epidemic of 1878
(2) At towns of epidemic prevalence, testimony showing importation was direct and convincing
(3) Transmission of yellow fever across considerable distances appeared to be wholly due to human intercourse, carried in clothing or baggage
(4) The weight of testimony is very pronounced against the further use of disinfectants. They are useful to arrest yellow fever but the vapors are seriously prejudicial to the sick
(5) Personal prophylaxis by means of drugs or other therapeutic means has proved a constant failure
(6) Quarantine or absolute non-intercourse without exception protected its subjects from yellow fever

The report furthermore called for the establishment of "National Quarantine" under the United States government, with specific regulations dictated by the states; the federal authorities to invite foreign nations to cooperate in the establishment of uniform quarantine regulations; and sanitary measures to be adopted even at times when no disease was present. Members also offered heartfelt thanks to Mrs. Elizabeth Thompson of New York for her philanthropic contributions that enabled the commission to fund the study. In contrast, a second convention that assembled in New Orleans hosted by homoeopathists concluded the disease was "both indigenous and imported" and advocated a moderate quarantine along with "home prevention" (sanitation). The attendees also "point[ed] with pride" to the success of their methods: only 80 of their 1,600 patients treated at Vicksburg during 1878 died, while 944 of 4,361 were lost after being treated by allopathic methods.

In December 1878 the House and Senate yellow fever commission met jointly in New Orleans, electing Senator Eustis chairman. Among those present were Senators Lamar and Paddock, Representatives R.L. Gibson and General Hooker, Surgeon General Woodworth, Drs. Samuel A. Green, Samuel M. Bemis and Colonel T.S. Hardee. In an editorial directed at Lamar, the *Boston Journal* pointedly referenced the Civil War by driving home the point there was little need for a committee "unless those peculiar advocates of States rights, who now come to Congress from that section, hold that the national government, which cannot protect the citizens of the United States in these States in the exercise of their constitutional rights, must become responsible for the sanitary condition of cities and towns."[10]

In November it was announced a bill would be introduced in Congress to establish a national quarantine against yellow fever to run from May 1 to November 20 and to be enforced by the navy. In his presidential message of December 1878 Rutherford B. Hayes made reference to the subject. How it was received depended upon the political leanings of the reviewer. The following is from the *Cincinnati Enquirer,* reprinted in the *Indiana National Democrat,* December 5:

> After the customary expressions of gratitude to the Supreme Being on the ground that it is no worse than it is, and for the "general prosperity" which, though not here, is yet declared to be "within our reach," the President passes into the consideration of the yellow fever, of which the country has been blessed with one hundred thousand cases, and from which twenty thousand persons, it is estimated, have died, and which has cost the country some hundreds of millions of dollars. Even here the Republican fondness for having the Nation do every thing appears, though more harmlessly than is its wont. Here it is only a plea for a National Sanitary Administration which shall control quarantine and have the sanitary supervision of internal commerce, and hold an advisory relation to the State and municipal health authorities.

Estimates varied on the cost of yellow fever to the country. In the article "Fever Factories" from the December issue of *Popular Science Monthly,* author Felix Leopold Oswald, MD, wrote that the Mexican War cost 15,350 human lives and $123,000,000, while the total number of deaths from the yellow fever epidemic from August 5 to October 5 was 17,018, with direct and indirect losses (without any prospect of compensation) of $160,000,000. The number generally used was that compiled by A.B. Farquhar, proprietor of the Pennsylvania Agricultural Works at York. He calculated the 1878 fever epidemic cost the country about $175,000,000. Other estimates ran as high as $200,000,000 ("as great as the loss from the Chicago fire") and a total mortality of 15,000. On a smaller scale, yellow fever losses to Memphis life insurance companies amounted to $270,000. In light of the this, the House of Representatives concurred with the Senate amendment to the December holiday recess resolution, while taking time from that critical matter to approve a joint resolution appropriating $50,000 for the yellow fever investigation.[11]

On the medical front, Dr. Choppin of the Charity Hospital in New Orleans stated "physicians ought to study, by experiment, extraordinary treatment of yellow fever as the usual treatment has failed to give any satisfactory results." He developed what was called the "water cure," or "ice water treatment" (also referred to as a hydropathic treatment), which consisted of placing the patient on a fever cot designed by Dr. Kibbee (a bed filled with meshes with an India rubber receptacle for water collection beneath), stripping him naked and dripping ice water from a sprinkling can over his body for 2¼ hours. This brought the pulse and body temperature down and permitted healing.

Dr. Choppin's Estimate of the Cost of Yellow Fever in New Orleans, 1878

Estimated number of cases	25,000
Cost of 10 days sickness at $3/day	$750,000
Cost of 4,500 funerals at $25/each	$112,000
Adults, two-fifths of 4,500 victims, represent each a capital value of $1,000	$1,800,000
Remaining ⅗ at $300	$810,000
Loss of time of half the industrial population during the epidemic at $2/day	$3,600,000
Total	$7,072,000
Commercial loss	$5,000,000
Total losses	$12,072,000
Estimated profits of trade at ports during summer months where yellow fever usually prevails	$1,500,000

The difference of $10,572,500 represents the actual cost of the epidemic to the material resources of New Orleans. The figures show that trade during half a year with certain tropical ports, worth half a million dollars to New Orleans, "is held at a risk of more than twelve millions, the actual losses of 1878 from yellow fever."

Other cures were offered by physicians and laymen claiming small numbers of success. Dr. Bates suggested using chalk and cinnamon water; Cooley's *Cyclopedia of Practical Receipts* recommended chalk and laudanum; Dr. Hall suggested a watermelon diet; ammonia was supposedly the "only remedy used in Rio Janeiro"; crews of a French ship were issued a drink of brandy or whisky every morning that contained half a teaspoonful of white mustard seed to ward off yellow fever; Simmon's Liver Regulator, prepared by J.H. Zeilin & Co., "saved the people of Savannah" during 1876; and Messrs. Parke, Davis & Co., manufacturing chemists of Detroit, announced the discovery of a new remedy that was the "fluid extract of the leaves of the boldo, an alpine shrub, found on the Andes in Chile." In Jamaica, experience demonstrated that cholera, yellow fever and ague "never made their appearance where streets are paved with asphalt." In areas where yellow fever was epidemic, Dr. Fletcher argued for cremation as a preventive by eliminating the danger of decaying bodies thrown into shallow graves. Cremation also prevented the desecration of graves and he predicted that within 20 years every city would have a furnace for that purpose.

Colonel L.S. Hardee of Jacksonville, Florida, petitioned Congress in 1877 for an appropriation to test his "theory of concussion," believing that sufficient noise would charge the air, disinfect the streets and remove germs, particularly those of yellow fever. He proposed to fire cannon in the streets and explode small quantities of gunpowder in cellars and rooms in infected districts, adding that "the sulphurous acid gas" was a great agent in the destruction of spores.

Another trial that appeared to have positive results was planting the *Eucalyptus Globulus,* or "fever tree," as a means of warding off febrile epidemics. Around 1874 the tree was imported into Houston from California on the hope its leaves would absorb poisons in the air thought to cause yellow fever. Although the case sample was small, by 1878 there had been no major outbreaks of the disease and the experiment was considered a positive step forward in eliminating "the rotten diseases of the South."

Waiting for this to take hold, General Eaton, the commissioner of education, submitted his annual report to the secretary of the interior, suggesting that overcrowded orphan asylums in the South send children, many of whom were left without parents due to the yellow fever epidemic, to institutions for destitute children in other parts of the country. He also urged that Congress devise some plan for pecuniary aid to education throughout the country.

Under the wide umbrella of "odd" the year 1878 had more than its fair share. One editorial from the *Baltimore Gazette* began as follows: "It is a remarkable fact that the Chinese are exempt from yellow fever. It may be that the Mongolians are too yellow to afford any opening to the malady, but the fact remains that no yellow fever epidemic has ever prevailed in the Celestial land." Then followed a story picked up by numerous newspapers concerning Hong Chin Foo, a Chinaman who had resided in the United States since 1873. Claiming to have a cure for yellow fever, he proposed to make pipes of a peculiar construction and to provide a preparation of opium and oil, which he avowed was the real cause of Chinese immunity. A follow-up story indicated the first Chinese victim of yellow fever died in Memphis after being treated by Dr. Wow Chin Foo.

More peculiar was the case of a blood transfusion gone wrong. According to a French paper, General Yos Trebla of the Spanish army consulted Dr. Mauldew about complications from an attack of yellow fever. The physician prescribed a transfusion and a student at Bellevue Hospital offered to donate the blood. Afterward, General Trebla claimed his skin turned white, while the medical student got "a black skin as the reward of his devotion." Mrs. Trebla refused to live with her husband for fear of having mulatto children and all three sued Dr. Mauldew for damages.

Adding to the "odd" list was the fact that returns of death by yellow fever for 1878 showed that 63 clergymen died, of which 35 were Protestant, 24 Catholic and 4 Hebrew. From the newsprint perspective, "careful physicians" deduced that writing on both sides of paper will predispose the system to the yellow fever, and is one of the primary causes of that disease." One editor observed, "We trust our correspondents, especially those who write poetry and politics, will remember this." A Natchez doctor offered the opinion that "a few pet coyotes in any city will keep yellow fever away." Temperance people offered the reassuring thought that while yellow fever killed 12,000 in 1878, in the same year whiskey killed "not less than *sixty* thousand" and burdened the country with 100,000 paupers, 30,000 lunatics and idiots, 50,000 orphans, 20,000 criminals and the waste of $600,000,000.

Wrapping up the peculiar for 1878, a man arrested for being drunk and disorderly appeared before the Tombs Police Court, New York, and told the judge he had just come from New Orleans, where yellow fever was raging. The judge quickly released him, fearing the man would spread the disease to the inmates, and ordered the arresting officer to disinfect the man's clothes. And from New Orleans came the story of a "raving" Frenchwoman thought to have yellow fever. After she had been given a "vigorous course of treatment," it was discovered she was not insane but only speaking French!

Finally, under the heading "so close and yet so far" came the maddening observation that "decaying animal and vegetable matter and stagnant water have been the breeding places of the scourge."[12]

CHAPTER 26

"We are almost entirely ignorant"

About the only decided point to be gained from the report of the congressional yellow fever board is that we are almost entirely ignorant concerning this most terrible enemy. The germs of this disease lurks in chests of clothing and merchandise of all sorts.... The Yellow fever subject will bear a much deeper investigation than has yet been given to it.[1]

So went the headline and opening paragraph from an editorial from the *Indiana (PA) Democrat,* February 6, 1879. The author echoed sentiments repeated throughout the decade, and, in fact, the entire century, leaving one writer to opine, "Yellow fever is really one of the last known of all the great scourges which have afflicted mankind."

As death tolls mounted people became more and more desperate for answers but none were forthcoming. In order to expedite the situation, the National Yellow Fever and Cholera Commission, begun in 1878, was requested to continue their work. Results were generally negative, including the fact the resident physician at the New Orleans Quarantine Station, Dr. Carrington, had little if any knowledge of yellow fever; holds of vessels were scarcely ever submitted to disinfection; passengers arriving from Havanna and other quarantine areas were permitted to take their belongings ashore rather than having them burned; no one agreed on the usefulness of quarantine, and at least one authority, Dr. C.B. White of New Orleans, believed yellow fever spread at the rate of 40 feet a day.

If that wasn't hopeless enough, the *Providence Journal* noted, "It seems unnecessary to have incurred the expense and trouble of a commission to investigate the cause of the pestilence that raged during the last summer in the Southern States when astronomers tell us that the yellow fever was only a premonition of the dire calamities to be expected from physical disturbances shortly to be initiated." These included the influences of "the four great planets of the system, Jupiter, Saturn, Uranus and Neptune," reaching their nearest point to the sun. At the end of January 1879 the board of experts submitted their report recommending an international commission to develop strict quarantine rules and regulations, taking the ground that yellow fever was an imported disease. They called for a further completion of their study to determine the "duration of life or the virulence of the poison of yellow fever and cholera" and a furtherance of knowledge respecting disinfection.

On February 24 a yellow fever bill was brought forth in the Senate but it "soon became painfully apparent that much 'bay rum,' as the liquor bills in the Secretary's reports are termed, had been consumed. Points of the bill which had been thoroughly considered were taken up on mere technicalities and made the handle for speeches of a trifling character." In consequence, many senators departed and no quorum was present to vote. By March 27 the *Denver Tribune* repeated a recurring theme on the inability of Congress to act: "When the yellow fever is raging in the South next summer by reason of the failure of the quarantine bill in Congress, the able Democratic Congressmen who killed it can soothe the dying hours of their constituents by telling them that while the fever is a bad thing, to be sure, still it would have been much worse to have allowed the time-honored principles of State rights to be sacrificed to the success of the bill."[2]

On March 3, 1879, the 45th United States Congress passed a law titled, "An Act to Prevent the Introduction of Infectious or Contagious Disease into the United States and to Establish a National Board of Health [NBH]." The NBH was to have eleven members, seven of them appointed by the president, three medical officers from the Army, Navy and Marine Hospital Service (MHS, later known as the Public Health Service) and one representative from the attorney general's office. Its three major goals were to obtain information on all matters of public health; serve as a reference source and offer advice to the states; and along with the Academy of Science prepare a plan for a national health organization with special attention to a national quarantine system.[3]

"On April 1, 'all fools,' day,'" began an editorial by L.C. Fisher for the *Galveston News* (April 6, 1879), "the United States senate passed a bill appropriating $200,000 for the construction of a steel vessel to be used for the disinfection of vessels and cargoes coming from ports supposed to be infected with yellow fever and other contagious diseases." Under the provision of the bill the secretary of the treasury was to make arrangements with the London scientist John Gamgee to create a steel refrigerating vessel to be used under the direction of the national board of health: "'The mountains have been in labor, a ridiculous mouse has been brought forth'; and the unities of the farce were happily preserved in selecting the auspicious day dedicated to fools for its natal morn."

"In accordance with the custom of the Senate to appropriate money and investigate if it is needed afterwards," noted the *Dearborn* (IN) *Independent* on April 17, 1879, the funds for "the Freeze Out" system of disinfection "is a failure." Considering the "germ or the virus ... is so minute that the most powerful microscope has failed to reveal the character of the organism, even if it be an organism at all," Fisher opined, "it is not certainly known, that intense cold will destroy or render the germs of yellow fever inert for all time." Fisher had a right to be skeptical, as a well-publicized incident brought the question of disinfection by cold into serious doubt.

During November 1879 yellow fever was discovered aboard the steamship *Plymouth*, Captain Harmony commanding, while the vessel was at Santa Cruz. He was ordered back to Boston, where the ship was "thoroughly fumigated, disinfected and frozen out." With outside temperatures as low as zero degrees, all bedding and other matter were destroyed. The ship left Boston on March 15, 1879, with a clean bill of health, but about 800 miles from the Bermuda Islands yellow fever broke out again without the ship's ever having touched in at any port. "The moral is as plain as the hump on a camel's back," wrote one reporter. "No amount of freezing or fumigating can kill the germs of the fever."

Reports on the *Plymouth* notwithstanding, not everyone was opposed to the concept of using cold to destroy yellow fever and the idea of a freezer ship caught the imagination: "Every part of [Professor Gamgee's] machinery except the propeller and boilers is entirely of novel design, so as to give a maximum effect in the shortest possible time." Ships entering the Gulf of Mexico "can be brought to an ar[c]tic temperature in their interior in a couple of hours." In a commercial as well as a sanitary view "it would be desirable, as it would prevent delays of passengers and cargos, often annoying and expensive." The plan was also supported by Elizabeth Thompson, who originated the yellow fever investigations. "The sum demanded, $200,000 *is a flea bite* compared to the pecuniary losses by yellow fever and the cost of death dealing ironclads."

Gamgee's problem was finding material that would hold up under the pressure his invention generated, and he desired the government to fund his research. One editorial noted "the project looks a little jobby.... It is a poor time to experiment in gunnery on the field of battle.... Professor Gamgee's project is fishy and don't need to be meddled with." Eventually, in coordination with Samuel J. Ritchie, Gamgee obtained bits of a meteorite from Philadelphia that contained a quantity of nickel. After numerous tests they discovered that a metal containing 8 percent nickel proved sufficient for the task and, although Gamgee's freezer boat never proved successful, the incidental development of nickel-steel had far-reaching consequences for the future of transportation.

The secretary of the treasury eventually found legal obstacles to the expenditure. Perhaps the best solution was discovered under the heading "Spicilegia" (meaning "new and unfigured animals," a play on everything strange and weird), which stated, "A physician has discovered yellow fever germs in ice. The safest way is to boil your ice before using it. This kills the germs."

During debate of the quarantine act before Congress, one northern Republican angrily lambasted southern Democrats for voting against it by exclaiming, "Damn them, if they prefer yellow fever to states-rights, let them have both." The *Rushville* (IN) *Republican* (May 29, 1879) went further: "So far as 'niggers,' distilleries, Congressional and Presidential elections are concerned, the South does not believe the national government has any rights in that section which a white man is bound to respect. But whenever levees or railroads are to be built, or yellow fever fought, the States right dogma goes to the wall." That said, on June 2, 1879, Congress passed "An Act to Prevent the Introduction of Contagious or Infectious Diseases into the United States," which defined and strengthened the HBH's authority. However, it added the codicil granting the NBA a four-year charter after which it would require renewal. The political temper of the times was such that in 1882 the NBH was disbanded.

Members of the NBA worked quickly. On June 7 regulations were adopted making it the duty of consuls abroad to keep thoroughly informed of disease conditions at their stations and issue clean or foul bills of health to departing ships. At the same meeting, Sir Edward Thornton, British minister to the United States, objected to the system of quarantine in Louisiana and Texas, claiming it injuriously affected English commercial interests, especially in the case of vessels plying between Liverpool, the Bahamas and the West Indies and New Orleans and Texas ports, as well as the quarantine against Brazilian ports during the winter months in that country. Dr. Choppin explained the NBA could cooperate only with state organizations, not change their regulations, but he added that the temperature in Brazil never reached the point where the yellow fever poison would be destroyed.[4]

In 1880 Senator Harris introduced a bill to increase the powers of the NBH "in what may be called a drastic measure," as it "practically places in the hands of the President," on the advice of the board of health, the discretion to prohibit intercourse between a state in which an epidemic exists and all other states. One editorialist noted, "[W]e question whether Congress is prepared to assert for itself quite the unlimited authority involved in this measure, and still more whether it will be disposed to delegate the exercise of that authority in the manner proposed." A better proposal, the writer added, was Harris's call for an international convention interested in the spread of yellow fever. A joint resolution of Congress, passed May 24, authorized the president to call such a conference to be held in Washington City on June 1, 1881. Complicating matters, a dispatch from New Orleans to the NBH in March and later disseminated by that body announced "malignant yellow fever" was present in New Orleans. The report should have read "malignant fever" instead and created anxiety and distrust "no number of contradictions or explanations can allay."

Numerous problems continued to plague the NBH. In early July Dr. Turner, one of the officers of the board, announced his belief there was great danger of a yellow fever epidemic in the Mississippi Valley during 1880. By July 12, however, the NBH announced there was no expectation of an epidemic. Incensed by the latter, the *New York Bulletin* of July 14, 1880, asked, "Can anybody imagine what commendable purpose in the public interest is promoted by the national board of health telegraphing at intervals all over the country dispatches from headquarters like this?... One might suppose from this that if the yellow fever returns 'as an epidemic,' the public could have no possible information of the fact save through this self-important national board, which seems to be unaware that there are some fifteen hundred daily newspapers in the United States ever on the alert with the telegraph behind them, to chronicle intelligence of this kind.... It is well to be vigilant, and to exercise a wise prevision in such cases; but the frequent repetition of these alarming bulletins, without apparent justification, savor of something else.... Unless that body can find some better employment than this to justify its existence, it would not be surprising to see it suppressed ere long as something akin to a public nuisance." From a similar perspective, the *New York Journal of Commerce* noted in an article titled "Yellow Fever Alarmists" that "in the olden times, the policy of secrecy was observed [by newspapers] with reference to the earliest indications of a pestilence. The boards of health have changed all that. They take a pleasure in making public all the facts or suspicions which used to be concealed with so much care."

Perhaps the warning was taken, for in mid–September the NBH announced yellow fever had not appeared and quarantines of southern ports and rivers were to be lifted on September 15. A month later Drs. Bemis and Mitchell of the NBH issued an elaborate report indicating that between August 1 and September 10, in Plaquemine Parish, Louisiana, 100 cases of yellow fever were reported, originating from an infected vessel near the Mississippi river quarantine station. During the same period, Dr. George M. Sternberg, U.S. Army, under the auspices of the NBH, announced results of tests he had made on carbolic acid, determining that "the use of this agent as a volatile disinfectant is impracticable" and suggesting instead that sulphurous and nitrous acid gases and chlorine destroyed bacteria at once and effectively, while chloride of lime and copperas were trustworthy agents for promoting the purity of drains and sinks.

Not surprisingly, the NBH continued to encounter problems from the "persistence with which the local authorities attempt to conceal the existence of yellow fever in parts where it is known to exist," citing Key West, Florida. In 1881, when the health officer there declined to grant a clean bill of health for outgoing vessels, he was replaced, "since which time clean bills of health were granted to vessels leaving the port."[5]

Luke P. Blackburn and Memphis, Tennessee

Two specific incidents occurred in 1879: the yellow fever epidemic at Memphis and the election of Luke Blackburn as governor of Kentucky. In the first case, the legislature of Tennessee repealed the charter of Memphis, rendering its $5,000,000 bonded debt worthless. The "shame and disgrace of such a course" was caused by five writs of mandamus issued against the city by the United States Circuit Court. The city fell into debt from its inability to collect taxes, begun when the citizens were disfranchised and bonds brought only 50 cents on the dollar during the yellow fever epidemic of 1878. Added to the $8,000,000 cost of fighting the plague, even greater financial problems were anticipated should the disease reappear in 1879. Tragically, it did.

Sporadic reports of yellow fever arrived as early as February 1879 from St. Louis, New Orleans and Memphis, renewing the question of whether cold weather actually killed off the germs.

Physicians also contended that exhumation of yellow fever victims for transport back to their home cities reinvigorated the disease: "The bodies removed are mostly those of the wealthy and respectable class, who remained in the plague-stricken districts to care for worldly possessions." Removing bodies had "grown into a lucrative business" since the weather had grown colder. Undertakers were charging $20 and "negroes can be found who will remove a body for a smaller consideration by half." The cost of dying, with or without disinterment, was steep.

Post-Deathbed Expenses in New Orleans

Mahogany coffin, lined with muslin, including shroud and hearse	$75
Mahogany coffin lined with lead, shroud and hearse	$80
Winding sheet, shroud, etc.	10
Vault in Protestant graveyard	$55
Vault in Catholic graveyard	$100
Use of vault, six months	$25
Grave in Lafayette Cemetery	$20
Grave in Potter's Field	$5
Certificate of burial	$2
Each carriage with toll	$4

The expenses were greatly increased by the addition of satin linings, coffin plates, mourning scarves, rosettes and gloves, double teams and extra plumes on horses. Presumably at no charge to the dead, authorities covered Locust Grove Cemetery two feet deep with earth and had the area sown with grass, also covering all dumping grounds with a foot of lime as a precaution. In Memphis, families were urged to fill caskets with charcoal to prevent the spread of disease, while many physicians around the country advised against burial at all, urging that bodies be cremated.

On July 9, 1879, the first yellow fever death in Memphis was announced. The following day the board of health issued a statement advising citizens to "quietly remove your families to a place of safety" until it could be ascertained if the disease would assume epidemic proportions. The military was called out but as some guard units were decorative rather than useful when yellow fever threatened, "Then the citizens call on the colored troops."

By August 1 the number of victims had grown substantially, compelling the establishment of camps outside the city. Memphis was cut off from all but telegraphic communication and the "dreadful scenes of 1878 were repeated in 1879, on a smaller scale." Business was suspended and thousands were displaced. On October 25, with the arrival of frost, the quarantine of Memphis was raised. Official tallies indicated 1,537 cases and 487 deaths over the course of the summer, or almost 32 percent. Broken down by color, there were 858 white cases with 381 deaths and 679 colored cases with 106 deaths. It was estimated $100,000 in charitable contributions were received. To prevent another disaster, by 1880 the board of heath was given greater powers, and rotten wood pavement, thought to hold yellow fever germs, were torn out and replaced by stone. (This idea resurfaced in 1885 when numerous authorities linked the prevalence of yellow fever to rotting piers and decaying timber.) Not incidentally, the 1880 census revealed that Memphis was the only city in the United States to show a negative decrease in population. In 1870 the population was 40,226; ten years later it registered 33,000 people. The ravages of yellow fever were thought to account for the dramatic loss.

Statistics indicated that 15 states had some reports of yellow fever in 1879 but, peculiarly, New Orleans reported a mere 30 cases. Among the 19 deaths was John B. Hood, a Confederate general, and his wife and daughter. One obituary noted, "He was a brave officer but not a successful General." The following year General Pierre G.T. Beauregard established the "Hood Memorial Fund," selling copies of a book Hood had written for the support of his "ten little babies." A poor businessman, Hood had lost his fortune of $100,000 by investing in Louisiana State securities that collapsed from the yellow fever epidemic of 1878.

Proving that the sentiments of the Civil War were still alive, several newspapers ran similar observations: "The people of Kansas and Nebraska would lose some of their love for the negro if they realized these immigrants from the South brought yellow fever with them in their clothing." Also revisiting the past, Jacob S. West, a prominent physician of Texas, again evoked the old spectre that yellow fever germs were transmitted through grains of coffee imported from Brazil. The issue became so intense it was brought before the Galveston City Council, where arguments over the dangers of that "delicious beverage 'that excites and yet does not intoxicate the brain'" were given.

Trial Balance: Coffee vs. Yellow Fever

Coffee	*Yellow Fever*
20,000 sacks of coffee from Rio during quarantine	20,000 persons in city subject to having yellow fever
Balance to profit and loss: 1 life for 1 sack of coffee	20,000 cases of yellow fever for 20,000 sacks of coffee
20,000 sacks of coffee from Rio during quarantine	80,000 persons in cities and towns and contiguous to the railroads in the interior subjects of yellow fever

Balance to profit and loss: 4 lives for a sack of coffee, or aggregate 80,000 cases of yellow fever for 20,000 sacks of coffee.

On a more positive economic front, the "Pork King," P.D. Armour, made a fortune following the widespread yellow fever panic at Memphis. When news of the disease broke, a panic occurred in pork products, which were "largely consumed in the south." The market dropped $1.37 a barrel in two days, breaking nearly all the southern speculators. Armour cornered the market and eventually sold pork bought at $7–8/barrel for $13 a barrel, resulting in a net gain of $3,500,000.[6]

Another major event of 1879 concerned the political race for governor in Kentucky. Depending upon a person's allegiance in the Civil War, candidate Luke Blackburn was a devil or a god. The *Fort Wayne Sentinel* of May 7, 1879, summed up one view, referencing the physician's work *treating* yellow fever victims: "The Kentucky democrats nominated for governor Dr. LUKE P. BLACKBURN, the yellow fever veteran. He is one of Nature's noblemen, and eminently worthy of the distinguished honor which was paid him." From the opposite perspective, the *Goshen* (IN) *Times* on May 15, 1879, offered the opposite view, referencing the physician's work in attempting to *murder* northerners:

> [T]he Democracy of Kentucky have nominated as their candidate for Governor of that State Dr. Luke P. Blackburn, the fiend who during the war proposed to introduce yellow fever and small pox into the Northern cities by means of infected clothing and various other methods of carrying the germs of these terrible diseases. The Satanic atrocity of this blacker and more damnable than savage mode of warfare appalled even Jeff Davis, and Blackburn was not encouraged in carrying out his hellish design. Now, however, the Democracy of Kentucky, proposes to recognize and acknowledge the services offered by this demon in human form in aid of the Confederacy by electing him Governor of one of the leading States of the Union!

Blackburn was elected with a larger than ordinary turnout, and it was supposed "the Democrats of his state wished to reward him for attempting to infect Northern states with yellow fever during the war." One interesting incident occurred in October when a petty thief was arrested. After pleading guilty, the judge sentenced him to move to Kentucky, knowing of no more severe punishment than condemning the prisoner "to pass his life in the State presided over by yellow fever Blackburn."[7] To the present day, opinions are divided on Blackburn's complicity in one of the most heinous germ warfare attacks ever perpetrated on the United States.

What to Do with Havana?

In speaking before the Quarantine Commission on January 20, 1879, Dr. Vanderpoel of New York brought home the fact that between June 9 and September 30 of the previous year "there was not an interval of three days in which the bay was free from yellow fever." Repeating what he wrote to President Hayes in 1878, Vanderpoel stressed his belief the plague was introduced from Havana and "that the Government of Spain be solicited to unite with this Government in the appointment of an International Commission" to visit

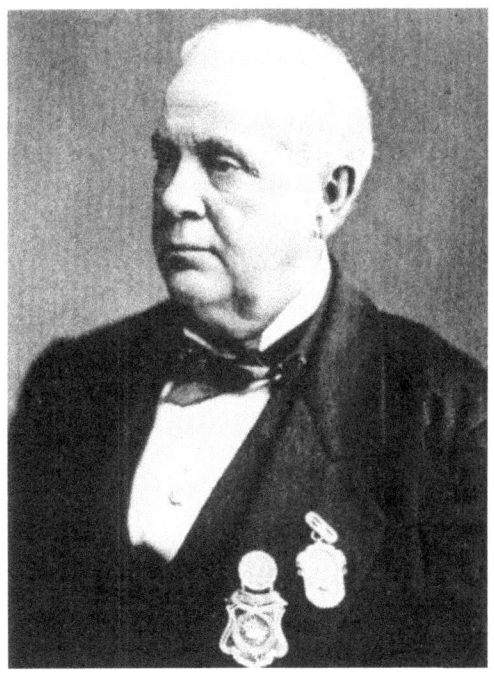

Luke Blackburn's name is inextricably linked to the distribution of yellow fever–infected clothing during the American Civil War and some sources suggest the plot to kill Northerners with biological weapons targeted victims as high as President Abraham Lincoln. Blackburn's alleged complicity notwithstanding, after returning from Canada to the United States years after the war he resumed his medical practice and later became governor of Kentucky (National Library of Medicine).

Cuba and devise means of destroying yellow fever at the source, "believing that strangling the monster in its cradle is wiser than fighting it after it has grown and begun to travel."

At the midpoint in July—as 117 deaths from yellow fever were reported from Havana—a commissioner was appointed by the National Board of Health to study the disease in that country. With permission from Spanish authorities in Cuba, the "Havana Commission" members included George Miller Sternberg, Juan Guiteras y Gener and T.S. Hardie. By July 28 Dr. Stanford E. Chaille, chairman of the commission, submitted a preliminary report describing the harbor as being built upon a thin layer of earth that covered extremely porous coral rocks "deeply saturated with the excrements of many thousands of human beings and of animals, continuously deposited throughout a long series of years. Nothing can be worse or more offensive than the privy system of Havana, associated with the evil hygienic conditions of the city." He added, "having no hesitancy," that the ballast sold and transported by ships from Havana "was eminently suited" to carry the germs of yellow fever into the United States.

After spending three months on the island the commissioners returned to Washington, noting "beyond all controversy, that yellow fever permanently dwells in Cuba ... [and] that during the period embraced between 1856 and the present time scarcely a single month has passed without deaths from yellow fever." A preliminary report issued in early December stressed that, protestations to the contrary from residents and government officials, yellow fever was prevalent, although varying greatly from place to place. While they failed to discover the cause or method of transmission, their studies confirmed that yellow fever did not affect animals in the same way it did humans and they argued there was a correlation between unsanitary conditions and yellow fever, incorrectly believing a massive public health program would significantly lower the threat of disease.[8]

Rio de Janeiro was the other hot spot during 1879, with notices from late February indicating an outbreak "of a very severe character has occurred among the shipping." The government contributed 50,000,000 milreis to alleviate distress in the northeast and asked for credit of an additional 10,000,000 milreis. By April 8, reports from New Orleans warned that the steamship *Baltimore* out of "Rio Janeiro" (the "de" was frequently omitted in the 1800s) had arrived with at least one yellow fever victim aboard. The spread of disease was clearly contained, for the official tally of yellow fever deaths in New Orleans for 1879 amounted to only nineteen.

Yellow fever in 1880 arrived early, reports from January indicating the disease had appeared in some of the West Indian islands and that outbreaks at Antigua and St. Kitts were serious. No full-scale epidemic appeared, however, as deaths in Rio, listed as 8–10 per day in February, were reduced to 7 for the week ending July 3 and 5 for the week ending July 10. The disease also appeared at Guadaloupe as the crew of the British *Jorawur* (formerly HMS *Vulcan*) came down with "a terrible outbreak of yellow fever" after putting in there for water and provisions. By the time the vessel made St. Kitts she had lost 27 out of 670 "coolie emigrants" and 12 crew. For the week ending June 22, there were 35 deaths from yellow fever at Havana, reaching 46 deaths the following week. For the week ending July 24, fifty-nine deaths were credited to yellow fever, leaving 200 active cases by the end of the month. During October, 63 yellow fever deaths were reported, the number dwindling to 5 for the week ending November 5.[9]

The news from Havana in July 1882 indicated 225 cases of yellow fever existed in that city "with a strong tendency toward becoming epidemic." Sporadic reports indicated vessels from Cuba brought the disease to the United States and by mid-month 64 ship captains were said to have died in various Cuban ports from the disease. As grim as that was, the eyes of the nation were on another country as yellow fever reports as early as January 28 indicated that in Temax, Yucatan, 1,700 cases of yellow fever had already resulted in 222 deaths. By July, the disease was considered epidemic at Matamoras, Mexico. The city was quickly quarantined and authorities at Austin promised to picket the Rio Grande with rangers if necessary to keep infected persons out of the state.

A month later yellow fever had reached Brownsville, Texas, situated near the mouth of the river across from Matamoras. The latter contained a population of about 12,000, while Brownsville had half that number. The nearest railroad point was Laredo, situated about 200 miles upriver. The distance from Laredo to San Antonio was 150 miles and Austin lay about 100 miles farther eastward. The distance from Matamoras to Galveston was so great no disease was anticipated there or at New Orleans. For those fearful that yellow fever would spread, fingers were quickly pointed at Washington, where, it was noted, "the general government has done nothing." Congress reduced appropriations to the NBA, rendering it "practically powerless," and the president declared the sum of $100,000, appropriated by him for use in an epidemic, should be distributed through the MHS, the medical bureau of the treasury. By August at least one editorialist observed, "The national board of health has come to grief through the hostility of the marine hospital service. The doctors of the m.h.s. think they know more than the doctors of the n.b.h. and they propose to run the health business of the nation. To do this they are working to smash the national board of health and the fight is a very lively one."

In mid–August Texas governor Roberts asked the treasury for help, stating 2,000 at Brownsville were unemployed due to the epidemic. Acting Secretary French replied the department would take charge of hospitals and quarantine the city but the state of Texas was responsible for citizens not in hospitals. Assistance was accepted and by mid–September 1,539 cases were reported at Brownsville with 88 deaths. Ultimately, there were 1,977 cases and 114 deaths. At Pensacola, arguments over money and authority between the city and both the NBH and the MHS and charges of dereliction of duty against naval officers abandoning their posts from fear of yellow fever made national headlines. A thorough study indicated two vessels, the *Saleta* and the *Vincenzo Accame*, introduced the disease into Pensacola, while the outbreak at the Navy Yard six miles distant likely resulted from communication with persons and articles from Pensacola and articles infected by previous epidemics. Eventually the NBH spent $6,079 combatting the disease, which affected 2,079 people and resulted in 172 deaths.[10]

In his 1883 annual report to the secretary of the treasury, Surgeon General Hamilton of the MHS recommended a national quarantine system but one that would only "effectively supplement" local efforts. He also concluded that "however desirable it might be for the government to undertake the work of general sanitation, it is evident that the limits of such a work could not be foreseen at the present time." He added, "[I]nterference by federal authority is not only unwarranted, but probably mischievous." If, however, it was deemed prudent to continue the epidemic fund he suggested inexpensive yellow fever hospitals should be established at principal gulf ports.

Proposal for U.S. Quarantine Station

Site and erection	$50,000
Warehouse	$5,000

Wharf	$10,000
South Atlantic quarantine,	
Sapeio station (Black Beard Island)	$25,000
Cape Charles (site, buildings, wharf)	$50,000
Running expenses at Ship Island	$12,000
South Atlantic	$10,000
Cape Charles	$10,000

Congress did appropriate $100,000 for the epidemic fund, but control of it remained contentious. Addressing rumors that Charleston was in danger of a yellow fever epidemic due to a refusal to enforce quarantine regulations, Hamilton visited the city. Returning to Washington, he declared there was no foundation for the rumor, stating his belief the rumor was started "in the interest of the National Board of Health which desired to obtain control of the epidemic fund."

Reports of yellow fever at Havana and Port Royal, Jamaica, made headlines in 1883. In the latter case, although quarantine of the port was severely criticized, an internal investigation by Dr. Fegan revealed that nothing had been done in recent years to improve sanitary conditions; the habits of the inhabitants "outrage[d] the laws of heath." He concluded with his belief outbreaks of yellow fever were due to "cosmic and atmospheric influences" endemic to Port Royal.

The same, in larger headlines, was said of Vera Cruz. Although Vera Cruz had once been predicted to hold great rank in Mexican commerce, "carelessness and wanton disregard of sanitary regulations" had created a breeding ground for a malignant form of yellow fever, prompting the commercial world to shun doing business there during a large portion of the year. Complicating problems in Mexico, railroads, once looked upon as a boon to economic growth, had instead become looked at as transporters of yellow fever germs. When once overland transit was equivalent to "a good and safe quarantine," travelers from Vera Cruz to any port on the Mexican Pacific coast were now capable of spreading yellow fever within the five-day incubation period between contact and infection.

In the same vein, ships passing from Panama to San Francisco often put in at Mazatlan, where yellow fever ran rampant. Notices from October 25 indicated over 5,000 had died from the epidemic, while in the Gulf of California at Guaymas, deaths were so numerous Indians were employed to bury the dead and it was believed "a number have been buried alive." Toward the end of the year an act was proposed in the Mexican congress requiring bodies of those who died of yellow fever to be cremated as "recent experiment proved yellow fever was spread by insect germs which are particularly dangerous after the death of the person attacked."[11]

A table compiled by the NBH for the years 1878 to 1883 revealed there were 115,406 cases of yellow fever with 21,797 deaths, or 18.8 percent. Of these, 73,842 were in the year 1878 with a mortality of 15,230. The following year Memphis suffered most severely, there being 2,010 cases and 587 deaths.[12]

Astral Science, Hair Ghouls, Feathers and Poetry

During the yellow fever epidemic of 1879, William Van Slooten, chemist the board of health of New Orleans, made a chemical analysis of the air from September 9 to

November 24 and found "a series of extraordinary variations in the amount of free and albuminoid ammonia to the million of cubic feet of atmosphere." The fluctuation of both, day to day and week to week, "as the wave of the epidemic rose and fell, was very striking."

If such observations were not a predictor of yellow fever, researchers looked to "Astral Science" for an answer. In 1880, "Zadkiel" wrote a paper entitled, "Perihelions Conjunctions Square and Opposition of the Four Superior Planets, Jupiter, Saturn, Uranus and Neptune, and Their Coincidence with Pestilential Periods." Historically, he deduced, in 1619 "Jupiter was in opposition to Neptune, and in perihelion" (a point in the path of a celestial body nearest the sun) and a comet appeared in 1620, both correlating to the first history of epidemic in North America. During intervals from 1618 to 1622, mortality among the Indians of New England from "bilious plague, or yellow fever," was so great that only one out of 30 survived. Interestingly, the author added that the disease "must have originated in the localities where it prevailed," as the Indians had no intercourse with the outside world. During the 18th century Zadkiel correlated yellow fever epidemics to Uranus being in perihelion.

The dire predictions did not stop Sarah Bernhardt from visiting the United States in 1880, but the arrangements were complicated "by the prevailing idea that any French artist, willing to expatriate himself or herself, ought to retire with a fortune in a twelvemonth, and also by the belief that the yellow fever devastates New York nine months of the year." It's to be hoped the artist did not require feathers for costumes or bedding, as a shipment of "yellow fever feathers" from Memphis consigned to Cincinnati was refused by the health officer there and sent on to Louisville. It was alleged the same lot had been sent out of Chattanooga a short time before that. On the subject of lucrative professions, wearing wigs had become so fashionable the "business of cutting off and selling hair" from the corpses of yellow fever victims prompted "hair ghouls" to be on the lookout for dissected bodies. They then tempted "the students or janitors to let them cut the long and flowing locks from the heads of the grave-robbed stiff." The wearer was thus subjected to "grave" danger, as it was believed the germ of infectious diseases was carried in "switches, bangs and coils."

Fortunately, one theory was "exploded" in 1882 when Professor Chaille of New Orleans debunked the southern myth that "the yield of sugar has always been highest during epidemic visitations." Calling the mischievous idea "sheer nonsense," he collected statistics proving there was no correlation between ill health and good crops or poor crops and ill health. Astrologers predicted 1883 as a "good year" for earthquake, pestilence and accident. Chaille noted "they seem to have made a hit," data from the first eight months of the year indicating "considerably more than 143,000 lives" had been lost in notable disasters. Among the most notable were the yellow fever epidemics in the South; the Poland circus fire (268); the Sunderland, England, school panic (202); the Ischia earthquake (4,500); the English fishing fleets (373); the Java earthquake (100,000); the India cholera (15,000); the Egyptian cholera (21,000) and sundry steamboat disasters, floods, mine disasters and powder explosions.[13]

Ice became a popular treatment for yellow fever in the 1800s. Unfortunately, in 1880 Dr. Carbally, associate editor of *Sanitary* magazine, warned readers that bacteria or elements of disease in water before it was frozen remained undestroyed in ice, creating the probability of contamination. A Texas professor stated that cities built of limestone kept back malarial diseases by absorbing carbolic acid arising from decomposition, and Dr.

Constantine Paul of Hospital La Riboisiere suggested inserting 36 inches of a rubber tube down the patient's throat and pouring water into the intestines as a cure. In response to the sundry remedies offered around the world, the *New Orleans Times* noted tongue-in-cheek that a German scientist claimed yellow fever germs could be destroyed by exposing them to a temperature of 70 degrees below zero, then to 800 degrees above, then being steeped in a concentrated solution of prussic acid and washed off with oil of vitriol and hung up to dry. "The chances are two to one," the writer concluded, that after this treatment the germs would "be powerless to start an epidemic."

On two equally positive notes for those in dread of death from yellow fever, the Cleveland Board of Health issued a statement that "the spread of veneral [sic] disease is alarming," affecting one in every 15 citizens. The board warned this "was more to be feared than yellow fever, cholera, and small-pox combined." Deaths by lightning in 1870 (202) disposed of more people in the United States than did yellow fever (177), gout (43), scurvy (69), hydrophobia (63), cholera (76), cancer of the mouth (105), calculus (109), Addison's disease (12), carbuncle (168), lead poisoning (31), suicide by cutting the throat (133) and suicide by drowning (110) but not as many as dyspepsia (841) and explosions (290)!

For those "fortunate" enough to be taken by yellow fever instead of the above horrors, the Knights of Honor Life Insurance Company paid $2,000 each to the beneficiaries of 191 brotherhood subscribers during the yellow fever epidemic of 1878. Claiming to have "the cheapest and safest insurance to be had," the company favorably compared their rates to another company that had the "audacity to claim that it offers 'The cheapest insurance in the world.'"

New York Mutual Life Rates

Age		Age	
25	$16.91	45	$32.27
30	19.35	50	40.10
35	22.42	55	50.92
40	26.61	60	65.99

While not offering specifics, the Knights noted its payments were gradual, "not more than once a month, unless in case of an epidemic—as the yellow fever last year—and then in so small a sum that one hardly misses it; you also have the consolation of knowing that the money you pay in goes directly to the object for which it is given, and not into the pockets of greedy insurance officials." By 1885, the Knights' rates were $9–12 per $1,000, according to the age of the member. Noting there was no greater danger to an insurance company than a yellow fever epidemic, advertisements bragged there was no danger of the "organization breaking," as the company had successfully withstood the yellow fever epidemic of 1877.

For those desiring to travel in 1881, the following table likely served as a guide of places to avoid:

Nativity of Diseases

Cholera	India
Smallpox	Known in China for 1,200 years before Christ
Plague	An Oriental disease with a distinct geographical range
Typhus fever	Ireland
Typhoid	Ireland, Galicia, Upper Silesia and Northern Italy
Military fever	Provinces of France, Germany and Italy

Scarlatina	Arabia
Epidemic dysentery	Tropics
Dengue	Southern latitudes with sharp geographical limits
Yellow fever	Distinctly traced to the Antilles
Chaoalongo	Chili
Verruga	Peru

As a word of caution, some life insurance companies had clauses in their contracts cancelling policies if tourists traveled abroad where epidemics such as cholera and yellow fever prevailed, while New Orleans was "interdicted generally" during yellow fever season.[14]

At the dawn of the "Germ Theory Era" came a short notice that seems to put a humorous period between the centuries of grouping in the dark and the leap to scientific discovery: "Southern poets are writing poetry about the yellow fever plague. Now that yellow fever has gotten into poetry, editors cannot be too careful, and this office will maintain a quarantine against poetry until the weather gets colder. The cases are only sporadic thus far, but we can't tell how soon such poetry may become epidemic."[15]

Chapter 27

Mosquitoes and Germ Theories

If we succeed in protecting ourselves against all important diseases by inoculation the world will soon become crowded. In order to keep up a respectable death rate we shall have to depend upon railway accidents; druggists' mistakes, and Fenian patriots [Irish revolutionaries]. Old age will of course kill as surely as ever, for even the boldest medical theorist has not yet ventured to suggest that old age is produced by a microbe, and that immortality can be secured by inoculation. Still, it will be very inconvenient if everybody lives to the age of three-score and ten before bidding farewell to earth. The annuity branch of the life insurance business will be entirely broken up, and ordinary life insurance will languish, since death by accident will be virtually the only kind of death against which the companies will find it worth while to insure.[1]

The last two decades of the 19th century were pivotal in the study of yellow fever, not surprisingly aided by war and financial interests. At the beginning of the 1880s the "old battle of cleanliness against mysticism" was in full force, with the latter arguing for the potential value of vaccines. They were opposed by "anti-vaccine" advocates who either held that zymotic disease was "the natural result of municipal filth," requiring severe sanitation efforts or their counterparts advocating isolation and quarantine.

On the side of "mysticism" was Louis Pasteur, who believed yellow fever—like silkworm disease, charbon (anthrax), and chicken cholera—was occasioned by microscopic parasites. If such proved to be true, he hoped the disease could be "robbed of its power by inoculation." On this basis, the French government sent Dr. Talmy to Senegal to determine the application of Pasteur's theory of specific inoculation as a preventative against yellow fever epidemics. Curiously, in the same edition of *Nature* that offered the astonishing fact that *elephantiasis* "arises from a parasite introduced by the bite of a mosquito," the "general theory" of yellow fever was that it was "simply a virulent form of malarious fever ... produced at any moment by a sudden chill."

Also from 1881 came two other declarations on yellow fever, the first from Dr. Manuel da Gama Lobo, of Rio Janeiro, physician to his majesty the emperor of Brazil, who at Vera Cruz, Mexico and Havana, Cuba, found sufficient evidence to state these localities were "fruitful sources of a poison" causing yellow fever. The toxic agent, he believed, was "derived from a species infusoria, the *spunsia Mexicana*, which belongs to the family of *bacillae*."

In 1881 Dr. Domingos Freire (frequently misspelled as "Domingo," and "Frieze" "Freise" and "Friez") of Brazil announced he had successfully treated the early stages of yellow fever with hypodermic injections of sodium salicylate. In 1883, using blood from a recently deceased yellow fever victim, Freire discovered the microscopic presence of cryptococci, considered characteristic of the disease. The organisms were in different stages of development. In order to prove these organisms propagated (were transmitted) from individual to individual, he and his assistant Sr. Menezes Doria injected a rabbit with infected blood and the animal soon succumbed. The test was repeated numerous times using rabbits and guinea pigs with like result, confirming the hypothesis. Freire also concluded yellow fever was "primarily a contagious disease but may become infectious as soon as sufficiently many focuses accumulate," adding that the disease did not reside in one organ but resided in the blood and, therefore, "in all the organs the blood traverses." He considered that his experiments established "the parasitic nature of yellow fever." Carrying his research one step further, Freire found in cemetery soil "myriads of microbes" identical with those seen in vomit, blood and urine of yellow fever victims, as well as "vibriones in rapid motion." He concluded that after passing from corpses into the earth some germs were dispersed through the atmosphere while others were carried through rain into towns, thereby provoking epidemics. In light of this, he proposed all victims of yellow fever be cremated.

The same year reports were published stating that Freire had "inoculated five persons with what he claims to be the germs of yellow fever. These germs were attenuated by successive transplantations in gelatine (in accordance with Pasteur's practice), and it is said that 'the type of yellow fever which they communicated was so mild as to cause little inconvenience.'" If further tests proved those inoculated were immune to yellow fever, the "human family ... will indeed have cause to rejoice, and to honor the doctor as a benefactor of his race."

Freire himself followed news of his discoveries carefully, writing a letter to the editor of the *Evening Telegram* on December 26, 1883. In this widely reprinted letter he informed readers that he had inoculated 173 persons of "different nationalities, ages, professions and sexes, without the least resultant inconvenience." The inoculations were accomplished by the same method as in the Jennerian vaccination and the cultures of the yellow fever microbes made in gelatine or beef tea "following the Pastorian [*sic*] method." He added that the Brazilian government, by a decree dated October 9, 1883, had authorized him to practice vaccination.

The 1884 compilation of the *Journal of the American Medical Association* offered no more than a brief notation indicating Freire had discovered a microorganism that remained indefinitely in the soil and rapidly reproduced with fatal results in rabbits and guinea pigs. American newspapers were more optimistic, noting, "The really important discovery is that a parasite peculiar to yellow fever exists; with this to work on, the hope of controlling the disease is at least somewhat increased." The *New York Times* added its own voice: "It is most singular that so important a discovery has not been more widely heralded."[2] Freire's investigation, begun in 1880, ultimately resulted in the discovery of the "micrococcus of yellow fever," called by him "Micrococcus zantogenus," from which he cultivated the fifth and sixth generations by attenuation until it became a vaccine.[3]

On June 14, 1886, a report summarizing scientific developments concerning yellow fever was presented to the Senate and House of Representatives by the American Medical Association under the author's names, J. McF. Gaston, MD, of Georgia and P.O. Hooper, MD, of Arkansas.

Requesting a committee to confirm their presentation, the authors detailed the work of Dr. Freire, beginning with the opening statement that 6,000 persons were inoculated at Rio de Janeiro during the fatal epidemic in 1885, resulting in a perfect prophylactic that was "trustworthy and safe in practice."[4]

Other research was conducted by Granizo y Ramirez of Havana; Dr. Joseph Jones of New Orleans; Dr. Girerd of Panama; Dr. Rebourgeon of France and Dr. H. de Meyrignac of Panama. In his work, Dr. Meyrignac employed the sediment of urine from yellow fever patients containing zoospores of the *Peronosperma lutea*. Few articles gained any but a casual mention, lumped under headings such as "Science and Industry," which included mentions such as the news out of Nuremberg that Dr. Barthelmess had announced the discovery of coral formations in meteorites, indicating "animal-vegetable life in other celestial bodies than our earth." After years of research, Dr. Carmona y Valle (always referred to simply as "Carmona") of Colima, Mexico, claimed in 1884 to have discovered the germ of yellow fever in a parasitic mycelium that caused black vomit. Creating a method of inoculation, the physician tried it on himself on September 29, 1881. After experiencing only slight discomfort from that test, he expanded his work. Using 300 criminals confined for murder at the fortress of San Juan de Uilon (some reports called them "volunteers"), the men were "forcibly inoculated" by hypodermic. Two or three days after vaccination the patients suffered violent headaches and all the precursory symptoms of yellow fever but after 40 hours they recovered and it was claimed they were "now impervious to the disease."

During a session of the Mexican Congress several deputies to the Secretary of the Interior requested a commission "to investigate the work of prophylactic or preventive vaccination for yellow fever." The commission rendered "a most favorable report," and Congress authorized an additional $10,000 for further follow-up. Despite strong protests of the medical faculty against the practice, "based on supposed biological principles," by 1885 the "prophylactic process of Carmona" was "being daily administered in a drug store in Colima." Satisfied with the results, the Mexican government permitted soldiers at Vera Cruz to be vaccinated, believing the process would protect a person for 4–5 years. Labeled the "Saffron John virus" by U.S. exchanges, newspapers fluffed the story by adding that soldiers might now be able to secure life insurance at a small premium, "for disease kills more than bullets."

By July, reports surfaced that three persons inoculated in Vera Cruz by the Carmona method had died. In a thoughtful editorial published by the *New York Times* of July 10, 1885, it was noted this fact did not render the work useless but certainly proved "that the methods have not yet been perfected." It being apparent that more work was needed, by the end of 1885 more than 1,250 persons were inoculated by the Carmona system. It was claimed that of the first 908 individuals inoculated, none were attacked; of the next 582, including soldiers stationed in Vera Cruz, 26 suffered symptoms. According to the records, 32 percent of soldiers not inoculated got yellow fever as opposed to only 7 percent of those who underwent inoculation. Carmona attributed the 26 failures to the fact a sufficient quantity was not injected or the original material was not properly prepared.

Dr. B.C. Nunez de Villavicencio used Carmona's methods in Panama, charging $10 per inoculation and claiming, "The microbe once injected by the syringe into the system does its work effectually within 48 hours, at which time it can be discovered by aid of the microscope in the urine of the person inoculated." It was believed the inoculation would maintain its virtue for fifteen years. In June 1886, when de Villavicencio arrived in New Orleans with a specimen of the yellow fever microbe, the board of health

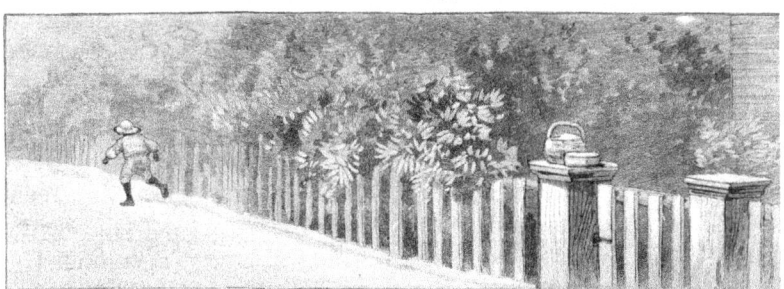
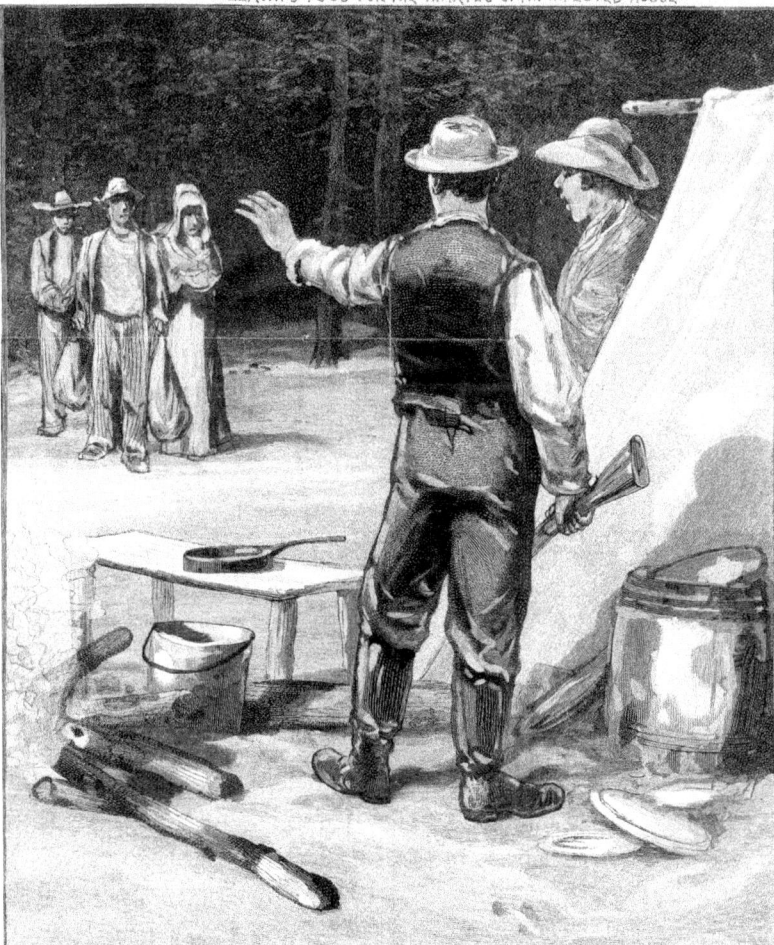

Yellow fever was a terrifying disease that seemingly struck out of nowhere, bypassing some towns and attacking others with deadly force. Those in an affected area, even one as small as a farm, were shunned by neighbors. This illustration from *Frank Leslie's Illustrated Magazine* (1888) by James Dawson, depicts a "Shotgun Quarantine" in Florida, where men warn a family to stand back while they leave them food. The upper panel shows a man fleeing after leaving a basket of food on a fence post (courtesy National Library of Medicine).

denounced the doctor and ordered his arrest. It was subsequently noted he had "disappeared."

E.H. Rogers, appointed as consul at Vera Cruz by President Garfield, became a victim of yellow fever immediately upon taking his post in July 1881. He died August 1 and his remains were immediately interred. According to the law that prevailed among all Spanish nations, victims of epidemics could not be exhumed for five years and only then upon orders from the highest authority. In 1886 the current consul attempted to have Rogers' remains returned to the United States and Congress appropriated funds for the cost of shipment. Local objections were raised when the proposal was made during the summer, as disinterment of bodies had "become surrounded with many superstitions." Therefore, it was "next to impossible" to have it done.

During the yellow fever epidemic of 1885 at Rio de Janeiro, Dr. H.M. Lane, of Carthage, Missouri, and formerly the secretary of the Southwestern Medical Society, was inoculated by Freire with one gram of the 22nd culture. The fluid was injected under the skin over the deltoid muscle at 11:00 a.m. on March 16, 1885. By 5:00 p.m. Lane developed a chill, followed by headache, nausea and the form of restlessness peculiar to the first stages of yellow fever. By 10:00 p.m. his pulse had increased and he had a temperature of 102.7 degrees. The fever gradually subsided and by 4:00 or 5:00 p.m. the following day it was entirely gone. During this 24-hour period Lane suffered an almost complete suppression of urine and his appetite did not return for two days. In exchange for this inconvenience he was able to visit victims throughout the city without suffering a full-blown attack. He subsequently gave samples of Freire's fluid to bacteriologists at Johns Hopkins and Cambridge along with the doctor's pamphlet, *Le Vaccin de la Freire Jaune*. In a letter written May 2, 1886, Dr. Freire explained his theory:

> It is very probable that by the sudden introduction into the circulation of the attenuated microbe it may have the property of attenuating in its turn the virulent microbe which exercises its destructive action over the organs; that it may have the power, so to speak, of *domesticating* this microbe by a quality similar to the crossing of breeds, which holds in certain species of animals. From the contact of the attenuated microbe with the virulent there may arise a third variety, likewise attenuated, from which comes the cessation of all morbid developments, the arrest of the disease, and the rapid cure of the patient. Should this curative and preventative effect ensure, it will be the perfection of therapeusis and prophylaxis in yellow fever.

A further statement gave details of his work: "My discovery is made. The epidemic of this year [1885] was one of the most fatal. About 4,000 persons have been victims of it. And in the mean time among the 7,000 inoculated, living in the same infected districts, and for the most part living in hovels, known to be the most dreadful foci of the disease, there are only encountered 7 or 8 [deaths] from yellow fever." Freire was "much opposed" by other physicians, the congressional report stating, "[H]is antagonists, not having discovered the paracitic theory, which is now triumphant in science, revenge themselves by abusing it and detracting him." Authors Gaston and Hopper also pleaded their case for an investigative committee by noting that opposition arose "from the antagonistic relations of the parties, on other grounds than fundamental objections to the means employed for the prevention of yellow fever in the inoculation with cultured virus. The proofs of its efficacy show the futility of all such opposition." They concluded: "The object in view ... by a simple introduction of the cultured virus on the same general principle that vaccine secures against small-pox, commends itself to the consideration of our Government, and if its claims are confirmed by further investigation, its adoption must confer incalculable benefits upon our people wherever this scourge is liable to concur."

When asked to comment on the report, Dr. T.G. Richards rejected it, denying the request for an investigative committee and adding, "I cannot discuss this subject with you at present." He was not alone in his denial. In 1885, with the backing of Dr. Joseph Holt, president of the Louisiana State Board of Health, Dr. Gaston sent an appeal to President Grover Cleveland, asking for an appropriation to investigate inoculation. Cleveland sent an unfavorable answer on July 3 and the Surgeon-General of the United States replied on September 24 stating there was no money for such a cause.[5]

The "Germ Theory"

Louis Pasteur's discovery that most infectious diseases were caused by microbial germs, a discovery popularly known as the "Germ Theory," opened the scientific door for astonishing discoveries. In 1884 the *Philadelphia Press* attempted to describe this new concept:

> There is a large class of diseases which it has been known for a long time that they all have certain characteristic peculiarities in unison. They are all apt to appear as epidemics or are endemic in certain localities. They are more or less contagious. They have a period of incubation.... Another peculiarity is that these diseases run a definite course. They are self-limited.... Then one attack of such a disease usually insures at least for a certain time, immunity against a second.
>
> All these peculiarities seemed to point to some unknown agent which needed a certain period to ripen, when at maturity it developed in the system symptoms always alike in the same disease and differing only according to the organ mainly affected and to the idiosyncrasy of the individual.
>
> These facts were known and they proved that each infectious disease was caused by a morbid agent of its own. What that agent was for more than 2,000 years no one could tell.

Through the work of Pasteur, Lister, Koch and others, microorganisms were found: "These animalculae, microbes, micro-organisms, or microzymes are known under the generic term of bacteria. According to their shape and other characteristics, they are subdivided into microcrocci, bacilli, and vibriones, the first usually appearing as diminutive cells and dots, the second as fine rods, and the last in all kinds of fantastic forms. These bacteria are exceedingly small, some of them having a length of less than three-thousandth part of an inch."[6]

In more general terms, "the germ theory of disease continues to be discussed," noted *Boy's World* (Fort Wayne, March 8, 1884, from the *Washington Chronicle*), "and great credit is given to Dr. Rudolph Koch, of Berlin, for his labor in this field of enquiry" by discovering the "bacilius of tuberculocis," while "Pasteur discovered the parasitic origin of cholera, and Dr. Declat and others have been equally successful with yellow fever." (In 1882 Declat wrote that two young ladies at Rio de Janeiro were cured of yellow fever by subcutaneous injections of phenic acid, ammonia and sulpho-phenic acid. Dr. Lacailel reported twelve others cured by similar treatment.)[7] Widening the scope of the germ theory, Dr. Cutler of Chicago announced that when serving as an Indian agent during the Civil War he experimented with inoculating beef cattle against the Texas cattle fever (Spanish fever) and also stated his belief that charbon was of parasitic origin.

The entire concept of germs would not have been possible without the microscope, and its gradual acceptance by the scientific community changed the way people looked at their world. By 1885, in an interview with a reporter from the *Indianapolis Journal*, Dr. Henry Jameson remarked that the microscope had been in use among his colleagues for about a dozen years. He added that microscopy opened up the study of the various kinds of "baccilli" that were present in, if not causative of, cholera and yellow fever. Interestingly, he added that the instrument had frequently been used "in a legal way to investigate blood-spots, and determine whether they are of human or animal origin; also in poisons, to examine their crystals." He warned, however, that lack of experience or defects in the optical instrument were sources of concern. Prices for a microscope and its furnishings ran from $150 to as high as $3,000.

When illustrations of cholera and yellow fever germs were put on display in London, one reviewer opined, "They are not what one would call pretty, being something like splashes of mud on a pane of glass. Of the two—as germs go—we would prefer the yellow fever germ, which looks quite a gentleman when compared with the little black cholera germs." On the other side of the Atlantic, at a session of the Public Health Association held at St. Louis, Dr. George Sternberg reviewed the germ theory and gave details of his own research on yellow fever conducted in Havana. It was noted, "He did not find the germ of yellow fever, and doubted if it was to be found in the blood of a person suffering from that disease."[8]

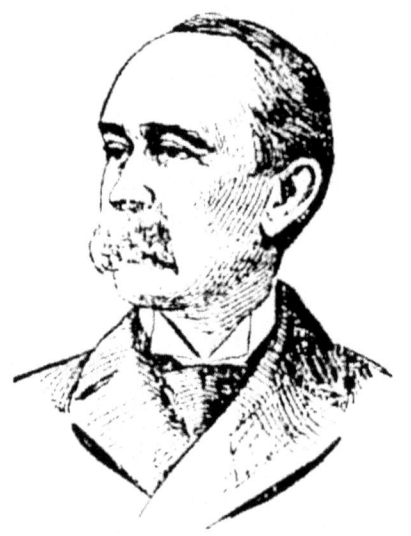

During the First Occupation of Cuba, Surgeon-General George Sternberg faced the task of ridding the island of yellow fever (*Steubenville Herald* [Ohio] *Star*, April 21, 1898).

Dr. Patrick Manson (1844–1922), a Scottish physician educated at the University of Aberdeen, spent his early career in Formosa as a medical officer to the Chinese Imperial Maritime Customs. After five years he was transferred to Amoy, on the Chinese coast, where he dedicated years to researching the filaria parasite (*Wuchereria bancrofti*), a small worm he discovered in the blood of elephantiasis victims. Using blood from his gardener, Hin Lo, who suffered from the disease, Manson discovered the worms were present only during the night and were absent in daytime. Suspecting mosquitoes as the causative agent, he dissected them, being "gratified to find that, so far from killing the Filaria, the digestive juices of the mosquito seemed to have stimulated it to fresh activity." Observing that the filaria developed no further than an embryo in human blood, he concluded the mosquito had a role in its life cycle. Expanding this theory in 1877, Manson hypothesized about the role of mosquitoes in the spread of disease and in 1878 published a paper stating that the *Culex fatigans* (*Culex quinquefasciatus*) was the intermediate host of the filarial parasite. In 1884 his work was described in American newspapers, explaining that the researcher had detected mosquitoes conveying affliction from man to man, "acting as a necessary go-between" rather than a direct carrier.

After biting an infected person, the immature worms go through a second period of development requiring four to six days. By this time the mosquito has died and the worm, which had acquired a boring apparatus, is taken into the human stomach through drinking water. Reaching the lymphatic system, it "attains full majority, and the disease elephantiasis is established." Manson's medical breakthrough stimulated the development of the mosquito-malaria theory. Under his supervision, Ronald Ross described the life cycle of the malarial parasite inside the female mosquito. He proved Manson's theory in 1898 and won the Nobel Prize for Physiology in 1902.[9]

Another leader in the quest to identify a bacterial origin of malaria was Alphonse Laveran, a French military physician born in Paris on June 18, 1845. Posted in 1878 to Algeria, where malaria was a serious problem, he studied both the clinical aspects and the anatomic pathology with an aim toward identifying the agent of the disease. Research at the time indicated a miasmic origin for malaria but Laveran sought a bacterial cause, studying the bodies of those who had died of yellow fever from both severe attacks and those suffering from chronic malaria. Paying particular attention to lesions found in the organs and in blood, he determined the one similar feature was the presence of granules of black pigment in the blood, occurring at very different frequencies depending on the case. He concluded these pigmented granules were specific to malaria and that they originated in the blood. At the hospital in Bone he identified spherical bodies, free or adherent to red blood cells, some of which were hyaline, or nearly impossible to see; others were dark, exhibiting ameboid movements and pigmented bodies in a crescent shape.

On the morning of November 6, 1880, at a military hospital in Constantine, while examining the blood of a patient who had been febrile for 15 days, Laveran saw, "on the edges of a pigmented spherical body, filiform elements which move with great vivacity, displacing the neighboring red blood cells." These were "the exflagellation of a male gametocyte, a phase in the life cycle of malaria parasites which usually occur in the stomach of the *Anopheles* mosquito." The mobility of these elements convinced Laveran the protozoan parasite was the agent causing malaria. Finding more of these agents, some adhering to the spherical bodies and others unattached, in November and again in December 1880 he sent his paper "New Parasite Found in the Blood of Several Patients Suffering from Marsh Fever" to the French Academy of Medicine.

Laveran visited Italy in 1882. His paper "Treatise on Marsh Fevers," published in 1884, cited numerous studies that indicated various algae, aquatic protozoa and bacteria found in marshland soil as the likely cause. Later, after ruling out the idea such parasites were found in the air or the soil of marshlands, he determined they were located in the bodies of mosquitoes, which were abundant in that environment. He published his hypothesis in 1884 and defended it at the International Congress of Hygiene in Budapest in 1894. His ideas were questioned by the adherents of Pasteur (except Elie Metchnikoff), who sought a bacterial cause. In 1884, while working at the Val-de-Grace School of Military Medicine, Laveran invited Pasteur to come and examine the evidence for himself. He did and was immediately convinced, but the theory was not accepted until the years 1885–1890 and not confirmed until 1899 when Ehrlich's methylene blue stains positively identified the malaria parasites. Alphonse Laveran was awarded the Nobel Prize in 1907 and donated the prize money to the Pasteur Institute for the creation of a laboratory dedicated to the study of tropical diseases.[10]

The "musquito"

Juan Carlos Finlay y Barres was born in Puerto Principe (Camaguey), Cuba, in 1833. Changing his name to Carlos Juan Finlay, he graduated from Jefferson Medical College,

Philadelphia, in 1855. Later returning to Havana, he became involved in the investigation of cholera in 1867, concluding the disease was waterborne. His theory, subsequently verified, was rejected by publishers at the time, but by 1872 his attention had been diverted to the investigation of yellow fever, and his first paper on the subject was published that year. His preliminary study, "El mosquito hipoteticamente considerado como ahent de tranmision de la fiebre amarilla," published in 1881, suggested the *Culex* mosquito be "hypothetically considered as the agent of transmission of yellow fever." The idea was not well received and only one Cuban physician, Claudio Delgado, supported the concept. In a second paper published the same year—"El mosquito"—Finlay acknowledged, "I understand but too well that nothing less than an absolutely incontrovertible demonstration will be required before the generality of my colleagues accept a theory so entirely at variance with the ideas which have until now prevailed about yellow fever."

By 1884 Dr. Finlay's name appeared frequently in American newspapers as having identified mosquitoes as the carrier and determining yellow fever was inoculable only from the third to the sixth day, while the period of incubation varied from 5 to 14 days. Symptoms from his system of inoculation included headache and pyrexia, while the injection occasionally caused "an icteric tint of the conjunctiva and in some cases albuminuria." The subsequent fever lasted 5 to 21 days. Of eleven inoculated cases, 6 were efficacious, 1 doubtful and 4 negative.

Most reports summarized Finlay's work as revealing under the microscope "spores and filaments of a particular nature on the sting of one of these insects that had just bitten a patient suffering from yellow fever, and [he] thinks that the germs may undoubtedly be introduced into a healthy individual by the bite of a mosquito." The *St. Louis Globe-Democrat*, summarizing Finlay's report in the *Annals of the Royal Academy of Sciences* (Havana), went into further detail on the mosquito theory, reporting that Finlay believed "the female alone stings and sucks blood, the male being a harmless sort of body that lives on the juice of vegetables.... The female stings, not because she likes blood particularly, but because it furnishes an amount of nourishment and heat that is necessary in order that the eggs she is about to deposit in the water may become matured": "Microscopic examination of the stinging apparatus shows that some of the blood dries, on the outside and another portion adheres to the inside, ready to be washed into the next puncture it makes along with the acid venom or saliva it injects. It is easily seen how the inoculation of a healthy person with disease germs swarming in the blood of a fever patient might occur, especially if the healthy man should be stung soon after the mosquito had been interrupted in its meal of the blood of a fever patient."

Taking mosquitos to the yellow fever hospital at Havana, Finlay allowed them to sting patients suffering from the disease. He then had them sting unacclimated men. In the first case, two days after being stung by a mosquito that had gorged itself with the blood of a patient in the fifth day of the disease the individual began to feel unwell on the ninth day "and had a well-marked attack of yellow fever, with jaundice and albuminuria, which persisted from the third to the ninth day of his illness." In three other cases results were similar except the attacks of fever were less grave. "The rest of the twenty unacclimated persons, from among whom these four were selected, showed no symptoms whatever of yellow fever during the seven weeks they were under his care and observation."

Finlay deduced that the inability of mosquitoes to reach elevated locations due to weak wings explained the long-established fact that higher elevations were a protection against the disease. He also concluded that mosquitoes hibernated during the winter and were not killed by frost. That theory explained the celebrated case of the U.S. steamship *Plymouth*, which wintered near Boston but had two cases of yellow fever as soon as it reached the warm temperatures of the Bermudas before touching in at an infected port. By December 1885 the *New York Sun* noted Finlay's research was "an important addition to the history of how zymotic diseases are spread," while in May 1886 London newspapers carried articles stressing Finlay's belief that his method "of producing artificial yellow fever will ultimately be found very valuable as a prophylactic against the natural and dangerous form of the disease."[11]

Another researcher making headlines in 1884 was Dr. L. Girerd. His early work consisted of taking blood samples of people newly arrived in Panama, reporting in all cases that none showed the malarial bacillus. Reexamination of "scores of them" after the first month, however, revealed the bacillus present in every one. He was also an early pioneer in inoculation against yellow fever. Typically this was done by removing a sample of blood from the finger of a "case of specific yellow fever" and making a culture: "The attenuated culture is used for inoculating. Natural result, a mild yellow fever, or planting corn that you may get corn, to use a homely simile. Dr. Girerd, while in that hotbed of yellow fever, Panama, inoculated himself and produced a mild yellow fever."[12]

A revelation on the preventative side, carried by numerous exchanges, stated that few Jews died of yellow fever and cholera, presumably due to "the simplicity of their diet."

Proving that yellow fever had an impact on commercial ventures, in 1884 following his summer business P.D. Armour made an additional $2,000,000 in the pork market by buying low when rumors of yellow fever were rife and selling high when the demand rose. The year 1885 proved another boom when "Phil Armour and his clique" spread the word about another possible yellow fever epidemic, depressing pork prices from $13.50/barrel to $8. Word from the Chicago market was that when Armour bought all the pork he wanted, "prices [would] be put up again without regard to cholera or anything else." The following year, when rumors of yellow fever again depressed pork prices, Armour "came to the rescue" by printing a "private" circular he scattered freely, declaring his belief that pork would soon double in value. This had its effect, as prices soared. Among conservative men, however, it remained a question as to whether Armour meant what he said "or was merely getting ready to unload on the country." Possibly the "Pork King" was also one of many wealthy men and women "annoyed" by begging letters of "unlimited extent" exacerbated after epidemics.

Pork was not the only commodity affected by reports of yellow fever. In July 1886 rumors were spread that the disease had appeared in New Orleans, creating havoc among the produce and cotton exchanges. A panic ensued, prompting one businessman to proclaim, "It is the most malicious lie that ever was written about the health of this city, and as it is bound to hurt our interests, it is very important to have it emphatically denied."[13]

The Demise of the National Board of Health

While the opening years of the 1880s were pivotal in the advancement of yellow fever discoveries, they also signaled the end of the National Board of Health, due, in part, to the absence of epidemics of infectious disease, the continuous battles between the NBH and the Marine Hospital Service, and the ongoing suspicion about the growing powers of the federal government. The original Act of 1879 set 1883 as the year the NBH would cease to exist if not reauthorized. On February 20, 1883, the appropriation for the prevention and spread of contagious diseases was granted to the Treasury Department, a clear indication the charter would not be renewed. The work of the NBH ended, but an attempt was made to reestablish the board in December 1884. This effort failed and the official demise of the NBH came on February 15, 1893, when an act of Congress granted additional powers and duties to the MHS.

In summary, the NBH fell in the crosshairs between the federal and state governments at a time when centralization of power was a hotly debated issue. Additionally, no one figure had enough authority to take control, and achieving a uniformity of opinion proved impossible. The concept itself was laudable and necessary but the temper of the times doomed it until a later date when Americans were more open to the idea of federal rules and regulations uniting the states into one cohesive nation.[14]

The Golden Rule

The attention of the nation from December 16, 1884, through May 31, 1885, was focused on the world's fair at New Orleans, or the "Exposition of the World's Progress." Acutely aware the success of the venture depended on the health of the city, local authorities worked to rid the waterfront and the city of any nuisances that might bring on an epidemic of yellow fever. Their rigid sanitation and quarantine efforts had been remarkably successful: since the horror of 1878 when 4,046 perished, fewer than twenty-five yellow fever deaths had been registered in the subsequent six years.

Quarantine was not without its economic consequences. Barring imports from Jamaica, merchants in New Orleans lost out on the sharp increase in the fruit trade as shippers were forced to reroute produce to New York and Baltimore. Increased consumption in the American markets propelled revenue from $75,000 in 1873 to $1,500,000 in 1884.

Yellow fever in New Orleans, of course, was not the only deterrent to the exposition. Advertisements for one of the major steamboat companies promoting the *Golden Rule* excursion steamer from Cincinnati to the Crescent City took pains to extol the beauty and historic significance of the water route. Passing Memphis, "that once yellow fever stricken city," the ad reassured customers, it was "now one of the cleanest, brightest, healthiest, busiest and one of the most beautiful cities on the Mississippi." For travelers skeptical of that promise, a new disinfectant on the market was "Cane Juice Clarifying" preventative. Derived from sugar cane juice that "could not be got to granulate," advertisers urged its use in hospitals, sewers and homes as being "efficacious as a preventative of cholera, yellow fever and other fevers."

As testimony to how pervasive yellow fever had become in the culture, in describing the "Pranks of Senators" a story of Arkansas senator Garland detailed his many practical jokes and noted that after his telling a tall tale the hearer often looked at him as if he were "a case of yellow fever and he was a freezing ship."

Rounding out the mid–1880s was a brief dig at the despised railroad men. One representative in particular swore, "A good many people are vowing not to spend another winter in this country; but when some of the hot days strike them next summer and they read about yellow fever in the newspapers, they will think that they don't want to go any further south." One editor flippantly responded, "'Yellow fever in the newspapers!' If any publication sends out yellow fever in his newspaper he ought to be shot."

For those far removed from the threat of contagion, however, yellow fever was regarded somewhat more facetiously. In discussing cures, *Bell's Life in London* (December 10, 1885) noted, "It would be more interesting to the British householder to know whether inoculation would afford any relief in acute cases of income-tax, election fever, and London fog."[15]

Chapter 28

Panama and Nicaragua: Two Canals, Two Views

> Two hundred years ago visionary projects were concocted for uniting the waters of the Atlantic and Pacific at Panama. Louis Napoleon theorized over it long before his coup-d'etat, or even prior to the day when he unloosed a tame eagle at Boulogne. In fact a Panama canal has been the dream of many enterprising statesmen. It is a grand work, and once completed must exert a great influence on the commerce of the world.... When the ships of all nations can in a few hours sail from the Atlantic into the placid Pacific, commerce will receive such an impetus as it has not felt since the discovery of the application of steam to navigation.[1]
>
> There is a saying that every tie of the Panama Railroad represents a tombstone for some one of those who were engaged in its construction, and it may almost as truly be said that for every yard of earth turned up on the canal there is a death in the hospitals.[2]

Visionary's dream, engineer's nightmare. Such is the history of the Panama Canal.

The need for a cut through Central America from the Atlantic to the Pacific was obvious. Prosaically, the *Indianapolis Journal,* quoted above, added, "The 'stormy cape' has been the dread of sailors since Magellan's day. Millions upon millions of property have been lost in the effort to turn it. Vessels, cargoes and crews without number have gone down within sight of the inhospitable shores where Darwin saw what he thought the lowest type of humanity, naked Indians living on the blubber of rotting whales. To this is added the diseases of the tropics and the lower Atlantic, dreaded by sailors always."

When German scientist Alexander von Humboldt renewed interest in a canal, the Spanish government in 1819 authorized the creation of a company to construct it. After numerous surveys were made, three viable routes were identified: that across Panama (then a part of Colombia), another through Nicaragua and a less attractive option across the Isthmus of Tehuantepec in Mexico. Beyond surveys, nothing substantial was done until the completion of the Suez Canal in 1869 prompted the French to readdress the idea of a canal across Central America. In 1876 the investment company La Societe internationale du Canal interoceanique was developed to carry out operations and in 1878 the company gained permission from Colombia to begin construction.

Unfortunately, those involved in this first serious attempt grossly underestimated the complexities of the mission. In May 1879 a congress was held at Paris under the leadership of Ferdinand de Lesseps, who had gained renown on the Suez Canal project. Although the mountains of Central America reached a low point at Panama, they still rose 361 feet above sea level at the lowest crossing point. De Lesseps believed this terrain could be excavated and a sea-level canal constructed. Early estimates placed the cost at $214,000,000, although, apparently to attract investors, this was unrealistically lowered to $120,000,000, with a six year completion date. The additional problem of the need to rechannel the Chagres River, which crossed the proposed site, was left unresolved.

Other intangibles also went ignored. The first was the application of the Monroe Doctrine and how the United States would view the intervention of a foreign power assuming control of a strategic passageway.

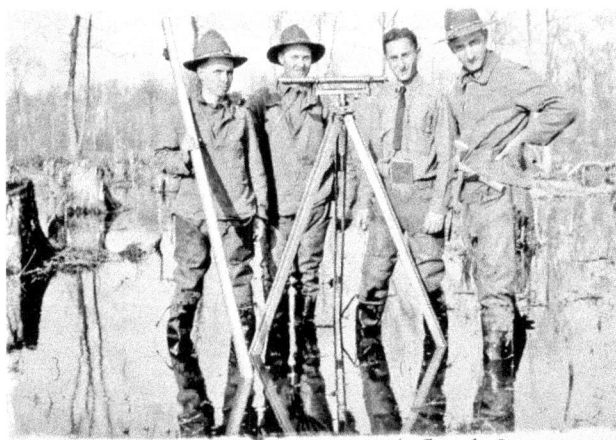

These engineers, replete with survey equipment, were involved in a swamp drainage project at New Market Street Swamp (probably Panama) around 1910 (courtesy National Library of Medicine).

The second rested on whether a merging of two oceans would affect "the equipoise of the earth" by pouring furious tide waters of one ocean into another. One scientist argued that as the Atlantic Ocean was "full of seeds of contagious diseases," with seaweed "supposed to be full of germs of yellow fever," there was great risk of contaminating the Pacific Ocean. All, or any, of these might trigger "an artificial cataclysm."

Nevertheless, the official start of the project was on January 1, 1881. The expression "plagued with problems" was apt, as excavating the canal proved far more complex than that of the Suez Canal. Worse, the problem of yellow fever proved virtually insurmountable. By August, more than fifty laborers per day were dying; subdirector Etinene died on the 25th, followed by the bridge chief Borbier on the 28th; other influential officers among the deceased included Des Songes, Dusseau and Zeimbraske. The situation along De Lessep's canal line was described as "discouraging and gloomy. The whole of the location of the canal stretches along an endless morass, and is inhabited by alligators and poisonous serpents." Malarial fever had already left "a mass of human skeletons" bleaching in the tropical sun. The same month, reports indicated there were only "200 colored men and 60 Europeans at work on the ditch. One half of the number are either lying sick or are being passed over to the silent majority. Frequently laborers are found dead in the woods. Medicine and doctors are scarce."

A dispatch dated August 24 stated it was "a positive fact that two-thirds of the yellow fever patients in the hospital here are taken out dead. No attention is paid to them in the last stages, they being removed to the dead-house and there left without even a drink of water, and this by Sisters of Charity." Additionally, food proved insufficient and wages were only $17 per month, with wet, nonwork days deducted. "Many devices are employed to make it difficult for laborers to get away from Panama, while ships carry men there from almost all parts of the free world." However, when word spread about poor treatment "and almost certain death," speculation ran rampant that "De Lessep's canal [wa]s a failure."

Official announcements were considerably brighter. By early October, the manager of the canal company, Armand Reclus, was in New York, stating that work on the canal was "advancing rapidly," with 1,200 men employed. Expectations were that by December there would be 8,000 workers. He indicated that to date the sum of $250,000 had been spent on the works, and drafts were in the hands of bankers for half a million more from shareholders in Europe. Brazenly, he denied there had been "an epidemic of yellow fever on the Isthmus."[3]

Chief Engineer Jules Dingler arrived in Panama with a party of 32 on October 29, 1883. Within a week Count de Cuerno died and he was soon followed by Mr. Zimmerman. Within a year, eleven of the group had died of yellow fever (also called malarial and Chagres fever), including his daughter, son, canal chiefs, a priest and staff officers. After his wife succumbed on January 2, 1885, he became so distraught he attempted to shoot himself. One American described the situation as critical, noting that unless the victims had money or influence they were dumped into pits and covered with quick-lime.

By 1884 matters had deteriorated considerably. Lack of progress, escalating costs and the horrific death toll of workers from yellow fever led many to question the advisability of the Panama site, and calls were renewed for work to begin on a canal in Nicaragua, where the terrain was felt to be easier to work and yellow fever was not a problem. There was also a growing interest in having either the United States or the British government assume control of the project from the French. The only positive news came from Dr. L. Girerd, the French physician. Bringing his three-year experiments to a close, he and Didier, both connected to the canal company, announced Girerd had successfully inoculated himself and was ready to perform the operation with attenuated yellow fever germs on workers. This was good news, for reports indicated 600 out of 7,000 canal workers were sick in bed. Most of the workers at this point were Jamaicans and the summer death rate was calculated at 110 per 1,000. "Yellow fever kills the whites," the report added, "malaria the natives and negroes. Many an able-bodied, well-built negro is cut off in from twenty-four to thirty-six hours after his seizure. Many are placed in the ambulance cars of the canal company and die en route."[4] Complicating matters was the political situation, summed up by one American newspaper:

> The situation down in that land of volcanoes, yellow fever and creoles is briefly stated as follows: There are five little Republics in Central America, whose entire population is but little more than that of the State of Iowa. These five, Guatemala, Nicaragua, Honduras, San Salvador and Costa Rica, have been worrying along for the past few years as independent States. The President of Guatemala, Gen. Barrios, seems to have been a man of Napoleonic tastes, and five-story ambition, each story of which he kindly dedicated to the services of these miniature Republics. After having been practically a Dictator at home, he proposed to unite the five States into a confederation, with himself at the head, as President, in name, Dictator, in fact.... Nicaragua promptly declined the offered compliment.... So far the United States has little interest and no concern with the trouble at the Isthmus.

No one was really certain, however, what the implications were, and many feared that European complications in the region might involve the United States in a Central American war. Equally significant was the consideration that France had designs on making Panama a French protectorate. Political savants felt this act would please the Panamanians, who desired to separate themselves from the United States of Colombia but again opened the question of a foreign power controlling a strategic military and economic canal.

On January 3, 1885, Surgeon General John B. Hamilton received a warning from an official at Panama: "All information as to deaths occurring here is studiously concealed. You can readily see that if it were known abroad that the mortality on this isthmus is alarmingly great, it would probably check the flow of laborers, contractors, tourists, and others in this direction, to the detriment of the Canal Company, steamship lines, hotel keepers, merchants, and all who gather gain from the people that flock hither.... In the new cemetery opened in this city during July last, there are already more than one thousand graves.... I have no doubt that 3,400 persons were buried in Panama in 1884. The death rate at Colon and along the line has been very heavy." Based on this information, Hamilton ordered extreme caution at ports receiving vessels from Panama and Colon.

Reports on the revolution continued to fill U.S. newspapers throughout the spring and summer of 1885. Admiral James Jouett, aboard the flagship *Tennessee*, was sent to Carthagena (Cartagena) with a number of commissioners for the purpose of securing a peaceful settlement with the revolutionists. He failed in that, and his report indicated yellow fever was liable to become epidemic and had struck a number of his marines. The disease also prevailed aboard several ships at Colon and was prevalent in the harbor and cities of Aspinwall (the American name for Colon) and Panama. Complicating matters, naval officers of the Panama expedition announced the people of Panama were "anxious that the United States should make its temporary possession of Panama permanent."

In light of these developments, Captain Bedford Pim, RN, an 1861 advocate of the Nicaraguan canal plan, reiterated his beliefs that a sea-level Panama canal was "preposterous," adding that among those working in Panama yellow fever was "raging in its deadliest form; men are taken down and are dead in a week. They are dying off by the wholesale."[5]

In an interview given in September 1885, W.J. Crosby, a contractor providing lightering services in Panama remarked, "The history of [the Panama] canal will be a record of fraud almost unparalleled in the annals of any nation. Already it has cost the sum of $120,000,000. The projectors have in addition a debt of $30,000,000 and now they estimate that to compass its completion $500,000,000 additional will be needed. What have they accomplished? Nothing more than the transportation to the objective point of an unlimited amount of machinery, which is useless."

The company erected a great number of houses along the line, as well as an immense office that "seemed at once a hospital and an asylum for broken-down relics of French nobility. Each window of the office had a small balcony, and each balcony its lolling Frenchman. When one got tired and went within to either pore over the pages of a French novel of questionable moral purity or the Paris papers another Frenchman took his place."[6]

After spending the years 1880–1885 as a practicing physician in Panama, Dr. Wolford Nelson returned to New York in 1886 and gave an interview to the *World*, stressing the filthiness of the canal sites. In March he stated there had been 33 deaths in the city of Panama and 15 in Colon. Nelson published a book, *Five Years at Panama,* in 1890, stressing "that the Isthmus of Panama is a disease-producing and disease distributing center.... Such a condition is a disgrace to our Civilization and a constant menace to all countries doing business with, or by way of, the Isthmus of Panama." In a November 1887 letter, Nelson declared yellow fever was a "blood disease, pure and simple." Remarking that germs could not propagate in fluid even slightly acidulated, his specific included the administration of phosphoric acid, vapor baths and sulphate of soda. He also stressed adherence to the theories of Drs. Freire, Findlay, Delgado and Girerd.

A.P. Smith, another eyewitness, reported to the *Boston Globe* the death rate in Panama was "enormous, particularly among the colored laborers from Jamaica.... Among the whites I should estimate that not above ten per cent survive many years." When asked to describe the workers, Smith stated, "Most of them are blacks, who receive $2 per day, equivalent to something like $1.60 in our money. This means affluence to these men, and all higher grades of labor are paid proportionately. But the money is the only possible inducement, and the wages must necessarily be high to attract men to a region which will in all probability prove fatal to them if they remain there long. So the men and women who come are the very lowest and vilest. Convicts and outlaws and prostitutes make up a large part of the sojourners there, and murder and arson are common. Police regulations are a farce, and justice is almost impossible to obtain." He added:

> There is little compassion shown to the sick and unfortunate, if the unhappy victim of disease happens to have an empty purse. There is a special police established to look for and take care of dead bodies, and the "police coffins" have been made to do service for hundreds of victims, for as soon as one corpse has been placed in the coffin, it is conveyed to the notorious Monkey Hill burying ground, is there thrown into the ditch, and the coffin brought back to do service for another unfortunate.
>
> A special train is run from Aspinwall [Colon] to Monkey Hill every day to carry out the dead. There they are miserably buried, and so imperfectly and hurriedly is the work done that bones may frequently be seen protruding from the ground and bleaching in the sun.

Smith added that there were so many bodies piled up in the brush they were simply burned. Notwithstanding, reports continued to circulate that the high number of deaths from yellow fever were "not true," and that the exchange was "still high, although the Canal company draws every month for upward of $400,000 on France, England and the United States. Their drafts are taken up immediately by merchants and those who can not procure them consider themselves most unfortunate." Augmenting the positive, in August 1886 the *New York Times* published a report stating, "Panama is healthier now than it has been for a long time, and of the much dreaded yellow fever there has not been a single case in 40 days." The article added, "The Government has called to New-York, Jamaica, and Guayaquil for a supply of vaccine matter, and on its receipt there will be a general resort to vaccination here." As much as those involved continued to spin positive press, men kept dying. In early 1887 one thousand Negro workers were brought from Liberia. Between April 1 and December 20 of the same year, 389 had died, a death rate of 53 percent. Those left alive in the spring of 1888 were returned to Africa.[7]

Matters could not continue in this way and in 1889 work on the canal came to an inglorious close. Called "the shameful collapse of a mighty work, perhaps the greatest engineering feat ever undertaken in the history of the world" in a scathing expose done for the *New York World,* the article summarized the eight-year colossal enterprise as having cost 20,000 lives and two hundred million dollars, two-thirds of which was "stolen in the most shameless manner." Other accounts reported the death toll reached as high as 35,000–40,000, including 141 doctors. Within the year Colon had "assumed the sorrowful and gloomy aspect of a necropolis."

Speculators were eager to move on. By May 1889 attention turned to Nicaragua. The warlike conflict in Central America clouded that situation, however, with many prominent people and their organs calling for the president of the United States to step in and negotiate a settlement.[8]

The World Outside Central America

A correspondent of the *South Side* (VA) *Democrat* in September 1885 wrote, "For one who has never witnessed a city suffering from a pestilence I can convey no adequate idea of the weary desolations of Portsmouth. It looks like a fallen city of the Arabian Nights in which everything was suddenly petrified and frozen into silence and death. Closed stores, perfectly deserted streets, window shutters everywhere fastened, and nothing to relieve the frightful and unnatural blankness of the scene but hearses and coffins and corpses!" He reported yellow fever seizing citizens at a rate of 50 per day, nothing that in a population of 2,500 "death stares us all in the face," leaving no civil government and no trade in anything but drugs. Panic among the remaining whites was "tremendous," and reports from Norfolk indicated a daily mortality of 70. A month later, as the epidemic subsided, the Howard Association Hospital at Norfolk reported its staff treated 275 patients of whom 191 were white and 84 colored. Of those who died, 100 were white and 7 colored.

The following year, residents of San Antonio gleefully reported that as warring Indians would never come that far eastward into their state, the threatened war with Canada was far to the north (U.S. citizens were fearful six imperial British warships were on their way to Halifax to enforce fishery rights) and they had no "sewer committee" to stir up cholera and yellow fever they were lucky indeed.

In June 1886 unlucky residents of Key West were warned by the board of health to leave the area immediately, as 13 cases of yellow fever had been reported. This started an exodus to New York and New Orleans, those being the only routes not quarantined. By the end of the month 46 cases had been confirmed, and 19 deaths. New York might not have been the safest destination, however, as the "unfortunate" city, which had just "been rid of her boodle aldermen," faced reports of a "dire plague" of yellow fever due to the "carelessness" and "ignorance" of her quarantine officers who permitted a "full fledged" case to be admitted to a city hospital. New Orleans might not have been any better, as "A War Among the Doctors" was raging between Dr. Holt, president of the Louisiana Board of Health, and Dr. Godfrey of the United States Marine Hospital Service over the true diagnosis of two persons at Biloxi suffering—or not—from yellow fever in that city. The question appears to have been resolved by locals who adopted a "shotgun quarantine" against Biloxi, where the number of yellow fever cases was variously estimated from 40 to 285 and fatalities from 5 to 30.

In any case, Geronimo, "like other epidemics," was apt to break out and attack a western community when least expected. By "untiring perseverance," he "rose step by step," until, it was claimed, the Indian leader was "more fatal than the yellow fever." On the sanitation front, warnings were issued to dairymen to clean up their barns: "It is now known that all decaying and fermenting matter develops millions and millions of bacteria and other microscopic forms of animal and vegetable life; that the air is loaded with these, and they are taken into the lungs of animals and men who inhale it. In hot weather these microbes are very active and destructive. Yellow fever rages only in hot weather, when these low forms of life are most active."

Although total numbers were small compared to previous epidemics, yellow fever in Florida dominated the medical news for the rest of the decade. By September 4, 1888, for example, total cases at Jacksonville were 245 with 86 fatalities. In the South, exiling refugees became a standard practice, culminating in Chattanooga's reward of $25 to anyone who reported a refugee entering the city. Pecuniary losses in 1888 from yellow fever, and more specifically from the fear of contagion, cost Americans $25,000,000, with a wildly exaggerated mortality set at 25,000. The disease continued to ravage other parts of the world as well. In Rio de Janeiro from January to late March 1889 the mortality from yellow fever was placed at 1,500, with the death rate from all causes placed at 2,000 a month in a city of 300,000.⁹

As with most tragedies, Yellow Jack found its way into folklore. One ballad, written by Herbert E. Clarke in the *Youth's Companion* and memorialized in the *Pall Mall Gazette* of London, recounted the true story of a ship that sailed into an English port seemingly without a crew. An angry delegation from town went to investigate. The balland read, in part:

> Not a soul to meet them, and they stared aghast;
>   Empty was the deck—no helmsman at the wheel—
> Only one dead sailor, lying huddled by the mast,
>   Grinned as if defying their pistols and their steel.
>
> Down the hatch they stumbled—back they rushed amazed—
>   For the crew and Captain were lying dead below;
> Helter shelter o'er the bulwark to their boat again.
>   And back to shore in terror, hard as they could row.
>
> Quickly as they landed rumor went before,
>   Pier, parade and terrace emptied as they came;
> For the King of Terrors was steering for that shore,
>   And they recognized his colors now and knew his name.
>
> Now the town has dwindled, now the fort is mute;
>   But men still remember, and ballad-mongers sing,
> How they challenged Death—grim Death—himself for a salute,
>   And how Yellow Jack avenged the insult to his king.¹⁰

Medical Congresses and Lack of "Satisfactory Evidence"

Members of the doctor's congress convened in Washington in September 1887 were presented with a paper by Dr. Domingos Freire entitled "Vaccination with the Attenuated Culture of the Microbe Under the Microscope." Agreeing that Freire's research "afford[ed] a reasonable assurance of its protective influence in Rio de Janeiro," they recommended a "co-operative investigation" with "adequate appropriations by the governments represented in this congress." In explaining his technique Freire noted the following:

> The two methods of cultivation are those of Pasteur and Koch, but the latter is preferable, and the microbe is colored with analine [aniline] red or violet, to render it more visible in the medium which it is to inhabit. As it multiplies it forms a compact and crowded colony, which ever grows denser and denser without apparent inconvenience to itself. The animalculas that thus develop do not lose the natural characteristics of their ancestors by reason of their artificial surroundings. They remain the same until they are transmitted to the blood of some animal, and then to another and another. This is an important part of the process. The malignancy of the microbe is attenuated by it. The beasts chosen for these experiments were usually guinea pigs and rabbits. The microbes usually killed them in a very few days, the average time being not more than a week. They were taken with the yellow fever. The autopsy showed the same symptoms which distinguish the disease in man.
> After each murder the microbes commit in this way they are less vigorous than before. When they have thus become sufficiently enfeebled the paste or gelatine containing the microbes is prepared by proper dilution to be injected in the arm of the patient who is menaced by the fever.

By 1887 the *New York Ledger* reported that "the Freire system of inoculation against yellow fever certainly seems efficacious," the uninoculated in Rio de Janeiro being ten times greater than those treated by Freire's method.

In the fall of 1887 the French government sent Dr. Paul Gibier to study yellow fever at Havana. Reaching that city in November he conducted numerous experiments but was unable to find the microorganism reported by Freire. He did discover "a creature somewhat resembling the comma bacillus of cholera that was present in the bodies of yellow fever victims." This led him to the conclusion that the microbes developed in the intestines and the disease was, therefore, a local one. He added that they were killed by acidity and disappeared during the process of decomposition, and that fact eliminated the fear of cemeteries and the danger from bodies of yellow fever victims. The following year the Southern Medical Society meeting at St. Louis announced the belief that yellow fever was not contagious "in the ordinary sense," and that quarantine should only be applied to personal effects rather than people.

The picture became more muddled early in 1888 when Dr. George M. Sternberg submitted to the president a "voluminous report" on his investigations in Brazil and Mexico. He stated, "There is no satisfactory evidence that the method of inoculation by Dr. Domingos Freire has any prophylactic value. The claims of Dr. Carmona y Valle, of Mexico, to have discovered the specific cause of yellow fever have likewise no scientific basis, and he has failed to demonstrate the protective value of his proposed method of prophylactics." Sternberg repeated his findings in September 1888 at the International Medical Congress in Washington, announcing that he could find no microorganisms in the blood and tissue of yellow fever patients and pronouncing Freire's theory "utterly fallacious." Ultimately, the congress seemed to favor the theory of microorganisms entering via the mouth and invading the intestines. That being the case, the cure was deemed to be through the internal administration of some form of powerful acid.

Adding to the confusion, in 1888 Thomas A. Edison announced he had "discovered a remedy for the extermination or effectual check of the yellow fever." Without having access to yellow fever germs and drawing his conclusions from "analogy," Edison stated his belief that yellow fever germs were "either of two things—animal organization or fungus growth.... I believe that the fever microbe is parasitic, as it travels slowly along the ground." His disinfectant included gasoline, exhigoline and a 10 percent solution of caustic soda.

For those interested in what yellow fever germs looked like, the *Herald of Health* published an article describing them as having "the appearance of three joints of sugar cane." The theory proposed was that these microbes "eat up one's blood so fast as to take it away from him in a very short time. Some men can stand the letting of more blood better than others, and consequently some men recover from the yellow fever."[11]

On October 13, 1889, the annual report of Supervising Surgeon General Hamilton of the Marine Hospital Service was issued. Covering the fiscal year than ended June 30, much of the 400-plus pages concerned yellow fever. Included were regulations on how officers were to deal with the disease in Florida, as well as articles such as "The Diagnosis on Yellow Fever," by surgeon John Guiteras, and "Treatment of Yellow Fever," by Dr. C. Faget. Surgeon W.H.H. Hutton, commander of Camp Perry, Florida (the first camp of "detention and observation" known in the history of epidemics), described the establishment and measures taken to prevent the spread of the disease, while Dr. John P. Wall wrote, "The Yellow Fever in Tampa, Plant City, Manitee and Palmetto," arguing that smugglers introduced the disease into Tampa in 1887. Investigations done at the Bacteriological Laboratory, New York, under the supervision of surgeon Kinyon were included, as well as a "voluminous" paper by Sternberg arguing against inoculations done in Mexico and Brazil.

In a move perhaps more applicable to the general reader, in the summer of 1889 Dr. Robert H. Lamborn offered a prize to anyone offering original investigation into the methods of destroying mosquitoes. Compiling the essays and publishing them in August 1890, the winner was Mrs. C.B. Aaron, who discussed the migration of mosquitoes, arguing against the popular belief they were brought to the seaside by land breezes, based on the idea the insects were capable of long sustained flight. Her research revealed they were able to fly only short distances and then only during lulls in the wind. Another suggestion promoted the idea of an "artificial remedy" pouring coal oil into swamps to coat the surface of the water and prevent mosquito eggs from hatching.[12]

"Miniature vampires"

With politics in Central America and Cuba taking center stage in the minds of many Americans, the presence of yellow fever in these areas of contention complicated both situations. On August 20, 1885, a mild panic arose in New York when a stowaway on the bark *John Gibson,* late from Havana, came down with the disease and charges were flung at quarantine and sanitary officials who allowed the vessel to come into harbor. The panic quickly spread to Philadelphia when two sailors from the ship made their way to that city, reportedly with symptoms of yellow fever.

On the subject of New Yorkers and the odd quirks of Americana, in 1885 the *New York World* reported that a "queer phase of yellow fever" had broken out in the city. "Since the new and cheap cab company started their sun-

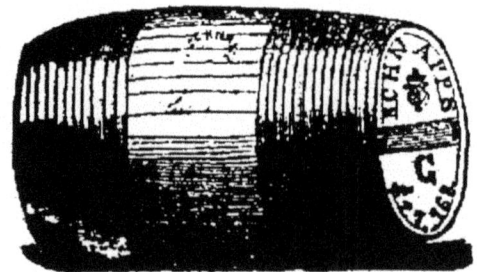

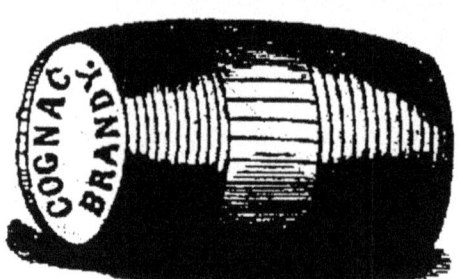

Depending on one's point of view, spirituous liquors were either the best or the worst thing in the world. Alcohol either served as a strengthener and a preventer of malicious fevers or it weakened the body and made it susceptible to disease. Clearly agents for the "Celebrated Wormwood Cordial" promoted the former idea (*Milwaukee Sentinel,* July 2, 1879).

shiny vehicles all the old cab and hack proprietors" gave their sombre carriages a bright yellow covering. The reporter deduced the "epidemic" was either a reminiscence of the street corner "yellers" who ran after the omnibuses and surface road cars or resulted from a superstition stemming from a story told by Artemus Ward about a cemetery operator in Africa who catered to the locals' penchant for bright colors by painting the front gates red. His cemetery was soon filled and he returned to New England a wealthy man. At all events, the writer concluded, "proprietors and the public believe just now in yellow cabs and will have no other."

Fortunately the reaction of those citizens was less drastic than those taken by authorities at Barbados when several seamen aboard the German bark *Mozart* arrived at Carlise Bay about January 1, 1891. Following the custom of affording no medical treatment to those stricken with yellow fever, the ship was quarantined and no physician was allowed aboard. Three men died but the captain was not permitted to send them ashore for burial, forcing him to dump the bodies overboard. Later that month the Royal Mail Steamer *Esk* brought in a sick passenger named Christlausen. He and three of the crew who had fallen ill were transferred to a quarantine lighter, where they were left to fend for themselves. The passenger died after two days and the health officer pushed his body overboard where it floated for three days before finally sinking.

For those who did not believe in inoculation as a preventive against the "miniature vampires" and their yellow fever germs, *Blackwood's* magazine ran an article in 1885, widely reprinted in newspapers across the country, asserting that "to keep well saturated with alcohol is a safeguard against yellow fever." Another method of "prevention" involved international mails. In 1888 recipients were informed that if they received letters with rows of small round holes punched in the envelope it indicated the missives originated from districts where yellow fever raged.

On the humorous side, a number of lighthearted tidbits are worth mentioning. From 1885 it was noted that Atlanta had not yet been visited with the roller skating epidemic, but the city was subject to visitations of yellow fever, "which is almost as bad." From the *Merchant Traveller* came this sentiment: "Yellow fever is epidemic in Mexico, small-pox in Canada and prohibition in Ohio. We need frost badly." A "Philosopher" in Pennsylvania noted that "base ball fever has struck the town worse than small pox or yellow fever, and will stick closer than a brother." The Census Bureau announced that the average American's life span was 66.27 years but statistics indicated that for those living in the "malarial and yellow fever swamps of Mississippi" life was prolonged to an average of 77.57 years. The article concluded: "Truly the ways of Providence are inscrutable in making life shortest where it is enjoyable and longest where it is unendurable." According to the *St. Paul Herald*, "some scientific person ... discovered that 'Cryptococcuszanthogeniacus' causes yellow fever. It will also produce lock-jaw if you try to pronounce the word with undue haste." Finally, from 1886 came this deduction: "At the present rate of alleged discoveries or remedies by inoculation the child of the future will look like a tattooed South Sea Islander, or a work[-]out pin cushion. He is already destined to be punctured for smallpox, hydrophobia, yellow fever, cholera, consumption and scarlet fever."[13]

CHAPTER 29

Cuba and the "Patriotic Disease"

Havana (Cuba) papers state, that the yellow fever prevails in many parts of the island, and has excited considerable alarm. Many have died who have been inoculated by the celebrated Dr. Humboldt. On this subject of inoculation the [press] is publishing from day to day a volumious and exciting controversy, to which we have but briefly alluded. So far as we have read it, we have only arrived at this conclusion, that in Cuba, as elsewhere, "doctors disagree"[1]

Although Spain was the imperialistic power controlling Cuba, "ownership" of the island had been a contentious affair. The Ten Years' War (1868–1878) and the Little War (1879–1880) fought between Spain and Cuban revolutionists made clear to the world that matters would only escalate until a final resolution was reached. Yellow fever would prove one deciding factor in the island's fate. In 1886 it was observed of the disease, "In Cuba they call this the patriotic disease, as it attacks only foreigners." However, three years later Spanish authorities would proclaim, "We have 200,000 troops on the island, perfectly acclimated, and any Americans who are landed there will die like flies." But by 1891 reports from officers of the Ward Line Steamship *Seguranca* touching in at the island avowed that 7,000 Spanish soldiers were hospitalized with the fever and mortality was very high.[2]

In the United States, the new administration of President Benjamin Harrison was just coming into power in 1889. James G. Blaine, who would become Harrison's secretary of state, was immediately forthcoming on his views on Cuba. In February 1889 word spread throughout the press that he intended to "acquire" Cuba, first because "Cuba is the hotbed of yellow fever, and he believed if it was the property of the United States we would discover some means of stamping out the curse, and thereby benefit the gulf and south Atlantic states." Owning Cuba would also put a stop to "smugglers and coasters … the very best means possible of spreading the germs of yellow fever," who constantly landed at Pensacola from Cuba and other infected islands.

Logically, it followed in many people's mind, "if Cuba were annexed[,] to annex also Santo Domingo and the whole island of Haiti." Blaine's project was in the "peaceful way of purchase" following the precedents set with the Louisiana and Alaska acquisitions and would "probably fuse—by an almost magical process—with the revived notions of negro colonization." Not everyone agreed. Calling Blaine's policies "jingoistic," the *New York World* among others noted "the 'Uncrowned King' would have to seize Hayti, and Mexico and Central America might be deemed essential to the full success of his sanitary crusade. Then Samoa and Canada would have to be captured in order to kill the germs of discontent in those localities."[3]

Nor was there any consensus among physicians about yellow fever. This same year Dr. George M. Sternberg returned from Cuba after a six-month stay. In preparing his report to President Harrison he "confirmed his previous conclusions as to the absence of a specific microbe organism" and failed to confirm "the germ which Dr. [Freire] of Brazil, has claimed to be the cause of the disease." For this reason, he continued, "I have given my attention entirely to the bacilli of the alimentary canal. As none of the lower animals are subject to yellow fever, and inoculations will therefore be impossible, it will be extremely difficult to arrive at a positive demonstration."[4]

Preventive Inoculators

Sternberg was not convinced, but the March 20, 1891, issue of *Science* carried an article on the work of Drs. Finlay and Claudio Delgado (other sources cite Finlay and Anderson). The practice of inoculating persons newly arrived in Cuba against yellow fever was performed "by means of mosquitoes which have been caused to contaminate themselves by stinging a yellow fever patient." Over the past ten years, the physicians offered 52 cases of "preventive inoculations" that had been fully followed up. Of these, 12 experienced between the 4th and 26th day after inoculation a mild attack of yellow fever; 12 experienced no symptoms of yellow fever during the next three years; 24 experienced no symptoms within 25 days but contracted a mild attack before the end of three years; 3 had no symptoms within 25 days but contracted well-marked yellow fever within three years; and one patient died of the disease.

Finlay and Delgado also offered the case of 65 monks who arrived from Spain and Italy and lived under similar conditions. Of these, 33 were inoculated and 32 were not. Only two of those inoculated contracted the fever but neither died, while 11 of the uninoculated suffered severely from the fever and five died. Even better results were claimed from a "Camara Polar" (polar chamber) where the cold was said to cure all sufferers. Based on the theory that cold killed fever germs, a Cuban physician named Garcia practiced a similar method by placing patients in a freezer box.

In 1897 world headlines announced that Dr. Guiseppe Sanarelli (the name was routinely misspelled in American newspapers), an Italian bacteriologist working on the island of Flores, in Montevideo, announced the discovery of "the strangest of all microbes that are known," claiming to have discovered the bacillus of yellow fever, which he named *B. icteroides,* or icteroid. He concluded the microbe did not reside in the intestinal tube, "and that its toxin, instead of being absorbed by the intestinal walls, is elaborated in the interior of the organs and in the blood." He believed the disease was conveyed principally by the atmosphere, noting the bacillus favored damp or moldy places, accounting for its development and vitality aboard ships and wetlands.

Following Sanarelli's research, the following year Dr. Alvah H. Doty, health officer of the port of New York, produced a stronger serum than that developed by Sanarelli that he hoped would be a remedy and serve as a preventative for the disease. Dr. Sternberg, surgeon general of the army, conducted his own research on icteroid, initially concluding it to be the same as his "Bacillus X," an organism his team had extracted from approximately 50 percent of the yellow fever victims they had studied. Preliminary results indicated icteroid and Bacillus X were identical. But after receiving a sample of Sanarelli's culture from Professor Roux of Paris the team determined the former's bacillus was "nothing more or less than the common hog-cholera bacillus," while Bacillus X was identified as belonging to the group of colon bacilli. Ironically, Sanarelli was awarded large pecuniary prizes and honors as the discoverer of the causative agent of yellow fever, while American papers ran this notice: "It is solemnly announced from Washington that Surgeon General Steinberg [sic] lays claim to being the discoverer of the yellow fever germ."[5]

Costs Continue to Accumulate

After years of guerrilla-like fighting, on February 24, 1895, the last of three Cuban revolutions against Spain began. Interest in the outcome affected the United States, as it had considerable financial concerns in the sugar, tobacco and mining operations. The question of whether the United States should annex Cuba resounded throughout the newspapers and public forums, while reports of victories, whether true or not, were claimed by Spanish and revolutionary forces. By May 16, the typical sentiment was expressed by the *Boston Globe*: "The Cubans have not to fear yellow fever, that scourge of Cuba which will prove one of the greatest generals of the war. It is because yellow fever

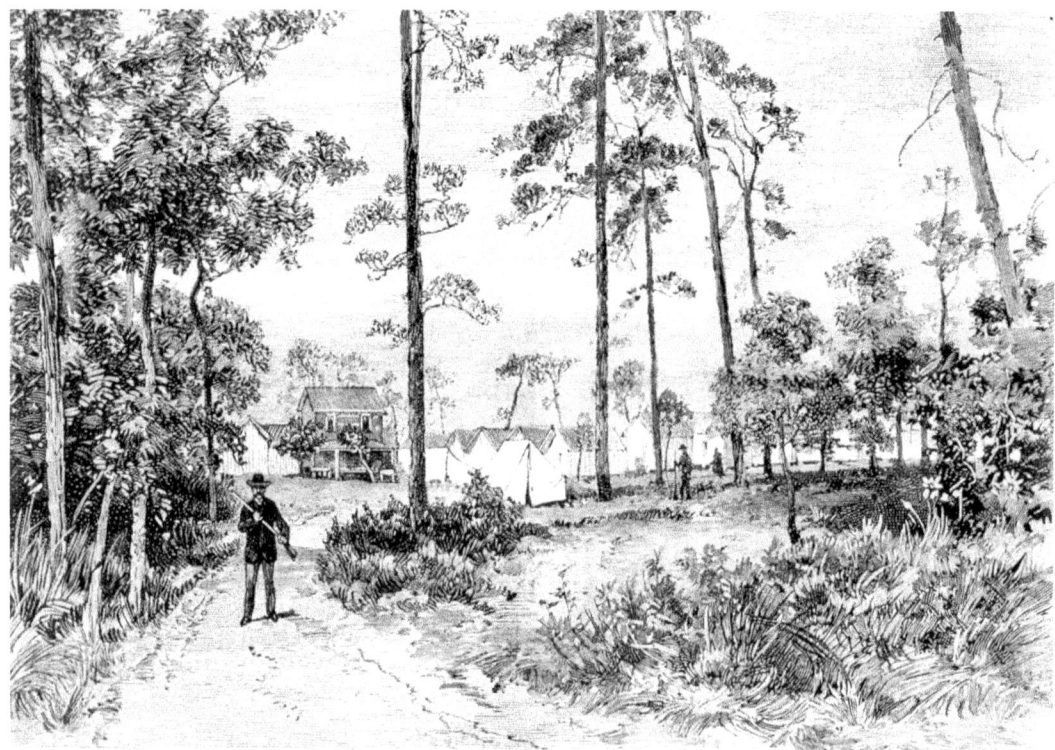

One reason for annexing Cuba was the claim that once the United States had control of the island, sanitary officers could rid the country of the yellow fever mosquito. The argument was based on the fact smugglers between Cuba and the mainland were notorious for introducing the disease into Florida. Sand Hill Hospital, in Jacksonville, was one facility used during the yellow fever epidemic of 1888 (originally published in *Harper's Weekly,* Vol. 32, p. 728, September 29, 1888) (courtesy National Library of Medicine).

is expected about June 1 that this date has been chosen by the Cubans for a decisive onslaught on the Spaniards."

Yellow fever appeared as promised. During June, 400 cases were reported throughout the Spanish army. By July the Reuter's Agency reported the outbreak of an epidemic; thereafter, 76 deaths occurred in Santiago de Cuba, 26 of who were Spanish soldiers. The tragedy was not all one-sided. By December, as the disease continued "without abatement," reports indicated rebels suffered as much as the Spanish with "enormous" fatalities. In February 1896, Dr. L.A. Hines, who served as a physician in the Cuban army, noted that the Spanish hospital at Havana had nearly 100 patients. According to his testimony, "None ever get well. Shortly after a victim gets it he begins to curl up like a withered leaf, and as soon as his head and feet touch, he dies."

The same month reports stated that over 60 percent of horses and mules imported into Cuba died of the yellow fever within a year. Consequently, those animals withstanding two summers on the island were worth between $400 and $700 each.

Horror stories notwithstanding, in February 1896 the United States Senate resolved to "maintain a strict neutrality between the contending powers, according to each all the rights of belligerents in the ports and territory of the United States." The minority report, offered by Senator Cameron, requested the president to "interpose his friendly offices with the Spanish government for the recognition of the independence of Cuba."[6] That same month, the minister of war in Madrid offered the following statistics:

Cost of the Spanish War to Spain

Soldiers at Cuba when war broke out	13,000
Soldiers sent as of March 10, 1896 [sic]	118,000
Cost of the insurrection to Feb. 29, 1896	10,000,000 pounds sterling
Estimated cost for 1896	15,000,000 pounds sterling
Cost of 1 soldier per year	100 pounds sterling
Killed in battle	286
Dead from wounds	119
Mortality in 1895 from yellow fever	3,190
Dead from all other diseases	282

The report concluded by offering the grim assessment that field General Valeriano Weyler stated he could not crush the insurrection "within two years at the least."[7]

Matters did not improve during 1896. Limes, considered beneficial to yellow fever victims, were prohibited from being brought to the cities, as Spanish authorities feared the fruit would aid the civilian population. By July, 4,500 Spanish troops were hospitalized at Santiago de Cuba and it was estimated 40 percent of all cases were fatal, while the hospitals at Havana held nearly 6,000 patients. Not surprisingly, physicians and nurses were "utterly incapable of coping with the disease," and as of August the epidemic was considered "the worst ever known." Unrest in Spain over these continued losses and the bankrupt state of affairs in that country led one American observer to opine, "A panic of anger and humiliation is imminent and a declaration of war against our country is the only remedy apparent." Perhaps more ominous was an article in the *San Antonio Light* (July 24, 1896) that began as follows: "The mosquito has few friends and none are so poor as to be his apologist. *Since the scientists have turned upon him their roantengon rays it is affirmed that these little pests are swift and wide disseminators of yellow fever and malarial fevers of all kinds* [italics added]." Although "roentgen" (named after Wilhelm Röntgen, who on November 8, 1895, produced wavelengths that became more familiarly

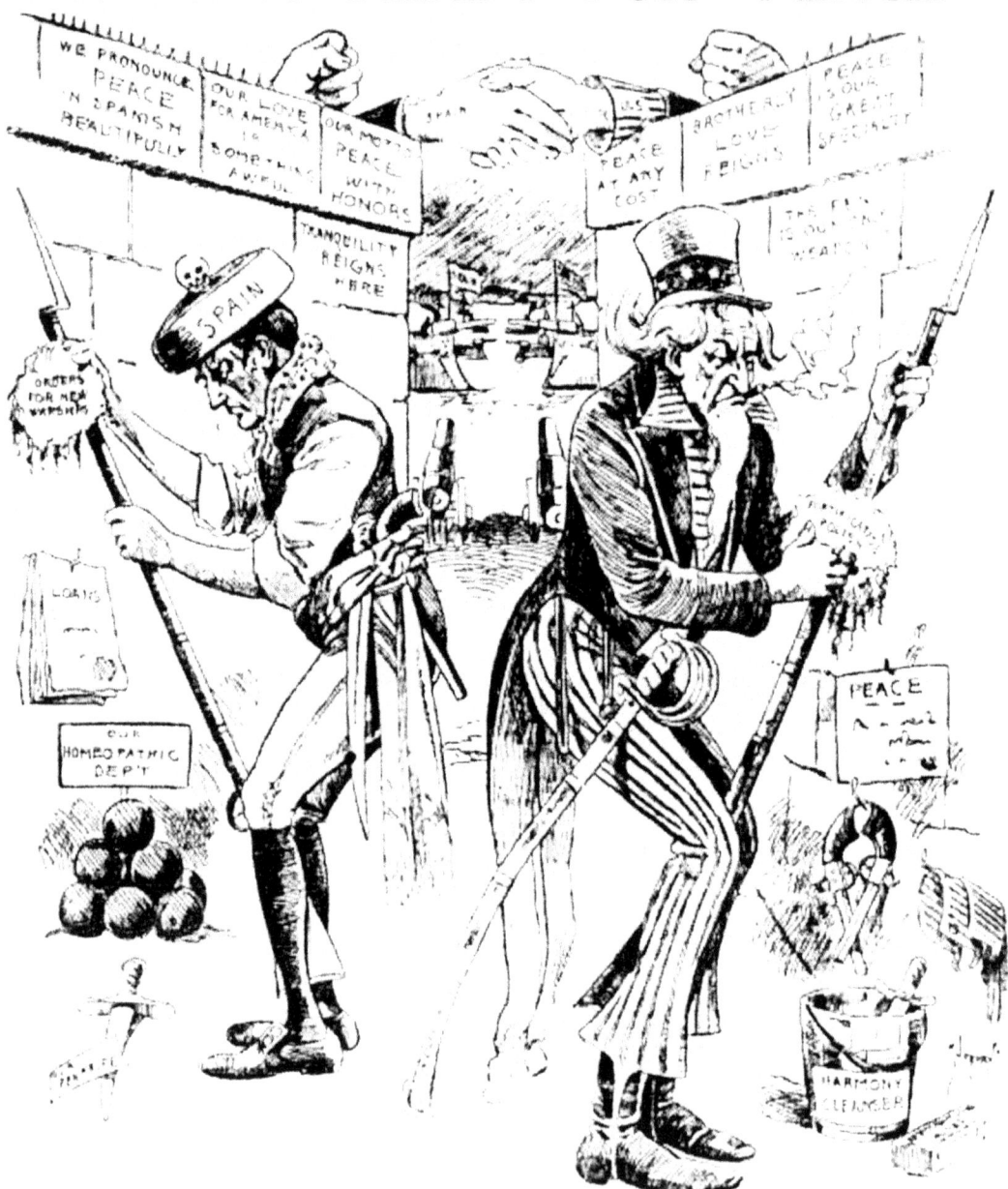

By showing the word "Peace" in quotes, this political cartoon conveys a mixed message: two grim enemies standing with their backs to one another. Uncle Sam rubs his rifle with "fortification polish," under the declaration, "Brotherly Love Reigns" (*Boston Post*, March 6, 1898).

known as X-rays) was misspelled, this paragraph aptly demonstrates the fear of science and the dissemination of false knowledge commingled with statements of truth. Along more creative lines, it marked an early beginning of the science fiction genre that dealt with technology run wild, mad scientists and mutant creatures.[8]

Official Spanish figures placed the annual death rate among their forces at 74 percent for 1896, or nearly 15,000 per year, while estimating a 51.9 per thousand mortality from yellow fever. No account of deaths among civilians from yellow jack was given but news reaching the United States described the numbers as "frightful" and phrases such as "dying like sheep" were common.

By January 1897, newspapers were alerting war-crazed Americans that in order to hide the disastrous direction of the war Spanish authorities were altering statistics to indicate soldiers died from yellow fever rather than wounds. The numbers hardly needed to be "softened." In May, reports indicated six Spanish generals, 65 colonels, lieutenant-colonels and majors, almost 600 subaltern officers and 2,000 soldiers had perished from war-related causes. Ten thousand more died from "various maladies" and 13,400 succumbed to yellow fever, while 22,000 were returned to Spain with disabilities. The report by Dr. W.F. Brunner, sanitary inspector of the United States Marine Hospital, gave the official statistics.

Deaths from Disease in the Spanish Army in Cuba During 1897

Deaths from yellow fever	6,034
Deaths from enteric fever	2,500
Enteritis and dysentery	12,000
Malarial fevers	7,000
All other diseases	5,000
Deaths from all diseases	32,534

These numbers did not include deaths among certain troops sent back to Spain. It was estimated 10 percent of those 30,000 "were destined to an early and positive death."

Spurred by the "yellow journalism" of Joseph Pulitzer of the *New York World* and William Randolph Hearst of the *New York Journal,* many Americans demanded that the United States enter the war. These were countered by headline news from officials at the White House indicating the president was concerned over the "Dread of Exposing Soldiers to the Deadly Climate." Reports also stated that the administration had confidence in the eventual evacuation of Spanish forces without U.S. intervention. Less stressed but equally potent was the fear that France or Germany would come to the aid of Spain should the United States involve itself in a colonial struggle.

England was another nation that had the power to alter the course of events. Through the early months of 1897 its most powerful journals had taken the side of Spain, defending the terror tactics used by the Spanish commander, Captain-General Valeriano "The Butcher" Weyler, in suppressing Cuban rebels. By August, however, the *Chronicle,* among other leading London papers, began criticizing the inhuman torture of citizens and dissidents. Not insensitive to this changing tide, Senor Canovas, head of the Madrid government, decided to replace the ineffective and controversial commander.[9]

The Second War for Independence took a heavy toll on Cuba and her mother country. In 1895 the export of sugar to the United States amounted to over $80,000,000, while imports were a mere $12,000,000, garnering a substantial profit. By 1898, however, the trade had nearly ceased. Spain was spending $300,000 per day to carry on the hostilities and of the 200,000 soldiers sent to Cuba it was reported that half were dead and 60,000 were hospitalized. Although General Blanco brought new leadership after Weyler's departure, matters did not improve.

In January 1898 Spanish loyalists rioted in Havana. The United States consul general cabled Washington he feared for the lives of American citizens in the city and at the end of the month the battleship USS *Maine* was dispatched to Havana. On February 15 the vessel exploded and sank, killing 258 crew members. Spurred by Hearst's newspaper battle cry, "Remember the *Maine*, to hell with Spain!" war became all but inevitable.

Investigations into the *Maine* disaster centered on the question of why the vessel had been tied to a buoy in the harbor rather than set at anchor. Two weeks after the disaster the Navy Department explained that if a ship cast her anchor in Havana waters, when hoisting it the mud adhering to it would be so fouled by yellow fever germs the ship would be required to go into quarantine upon arrival at any Florida port.

National guard units around the country prepared for war. Major Edward J.T. Marsh, surgeon of the 71st New York, provided "excellent advice" to his men by telling them to drink and bathe in nothing but boiled water. Professor Edwin Klek of Rush Medical College went further, stating troops "may be rendered immune from yellow fever simply by cooling the food thoroughly and boiling the water." Surgeon-General Sternberg dampened expectations by remarking, "We know of no preventative measures by which an army of unacclimated troops could be protected from yellow fever if they should be stationed in an infected locality during the months from May to the end of October." The only prevention measure was to remove the men to a noninfected area. He added that the native population had an immunity "which probably results from the fact that the people have suffered a mild attack of the disease during childhood."

The *New York World* (April 24, 1898) had a better answer. To belay fears of the "Senseless Yellow-Fever Scare," the newspaper offered four facts:

(1) Even at its worst, yellow fever does not attack one man in five

(2) Morality of those attacked does not exceed 17 per cent, or 3.4 per cent of the whole number exposed. This does not compare to the battle mortality of Fredericksburg, Cold Harbor, Antietam or Gettysburg

(3) There is never any yellow fever outside the cities in Cuba until July and US troops would be encamped outside those cities

(4) Even in the rainy season sanitation is a pretty effectual check upon yellow fever and our military commanders will "fight dirt as vigorously and successfully as they fight the Spaniards."

The article concluded, "ACTION is the word!" Or, as rephrased by the *San Antonio Light* (April 26, 1898), "The American with his purer blood and better morals and greater knowledge of hygiene and better food and medicine will not be anything like as subject to yellow fever as the Spaniards." The *St. Louis Post-Dispatch* added, "The lessons taught by General Butler in New Orleans in 1862 may be applied in Cuba in 1898. Yellow fever is no match for energy and common sense." Another authority, Dr. William C. Gorgas, chief of the Medical Department at the United States Army building in New York, added, "I do not think [American soldiers] would run any greater risk than our soldiers ran during the civil war." But he added, "I do not underestimate the risk. In the civil war disease killed twice as many men as were killed by bullets."[10]

Not everyone believed yellow fever was so easily conquered. As early as February

29. Cuba and the "Patriotic Disease"

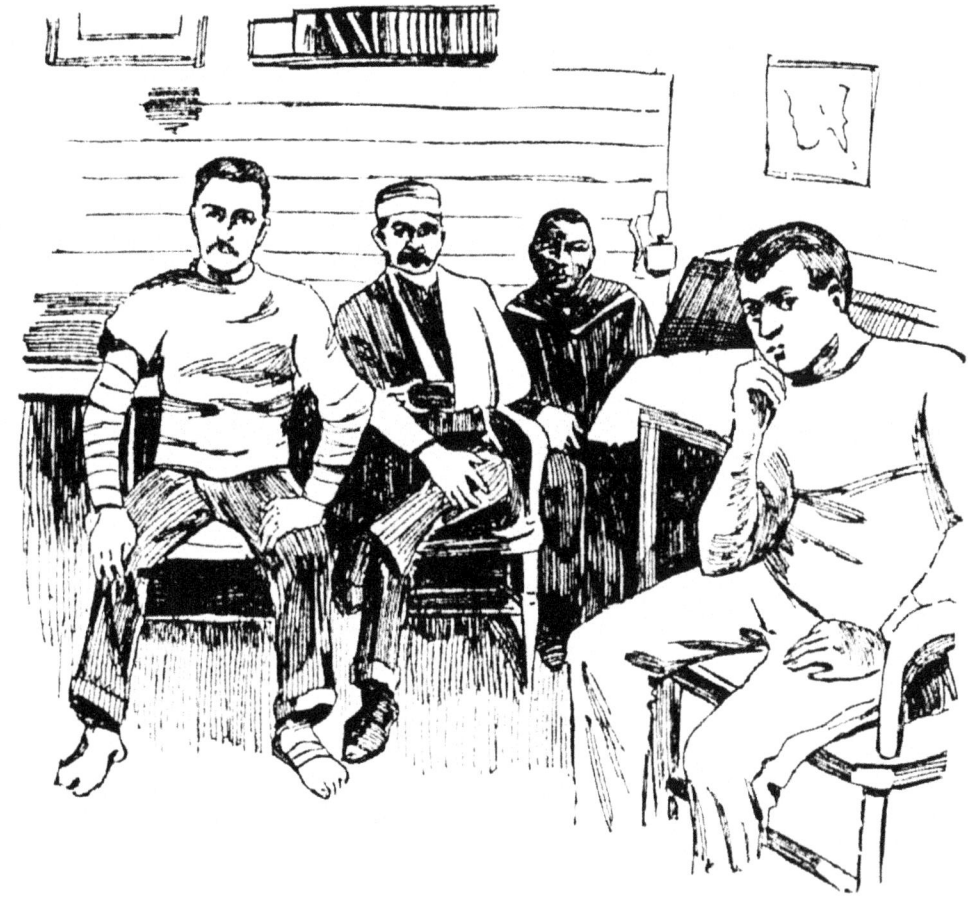

SURVIVORS OF THE MAINE ABOARD THE STEAMER BACHE.

Not even the survivors of the *Maine* disaster were spared the quarantine regulations. Sketched by an artist several days after their removal from the fever-infested military hospital at Havana to the coast survey vessel, the passengers were to be transported to the Dry Tortugas and remain in quarantine until it was certain they did not have yellow fever (*Boston Globe*, March 9, 1898).

1898 "a gallant ex–Confederate officer," Colonel Mallory of Rome, Georgia, floated the idea of recruiting "the floating negro population into troops" and landing them in Cuba, on the supposition they could "stand the torrid climate better than white men and the pestilences that sweep the marshes of that island will not hurt them." In exchange for their service, Mallory proposed to give the black soldiers the old post–Civil War carrot of 40 acres of land and a mule.

Two months later the idea of raising "fever-immune regiments" began to gather steam. Secretary of War Alger came out strongly in favor of an amendment to the existing volunteer law permitting the recruitment of at least half a dozen special regiments of yellow fever immunes for service in Cuba. Senator Caffrey promised to raise 20,000 such volunteers in New Orleans alone. This idea was seconded by General A.F. Moralis, veteran campaigner in the West Indies, who called for troops from the Gulf region to be the first sent to Cuba. Those going, it was noted, were to receive $13 per month, or "just 50 cents more than a councilman's salary, which is earned (?) at two sittings of half an hour each." On the assumption "the colored soldiers [were] not susceptible to diseases ... prevalent in a climate like that of Cuba" and were "naturally acclimated" to yellow fever, five regiments of such "immunes" were added to the five white "immune" regiments recruited for military service.

The Spanish-American War

On April 25, 1898, Congress declared war on Spain. By May 2 the Senate had passed a bill for the enlistment of a volunteer brigade of engineers and 10,000 men in the South who were immune to yellow fever to be added to the 125,000 volunteers called for by the president. Soldiers were not the only ones preparing for war: profiteers were already anticipating their share. Under the category "Life Imitates Art," an article in the *Westville* (IN) *Indicator* (May 5, 1898) described a new venture by the Klondike and Cuba Ice-Towing and Anti–Yellow Fever Company. The idea was to tow icebergs to "such countries in the southern seas as are

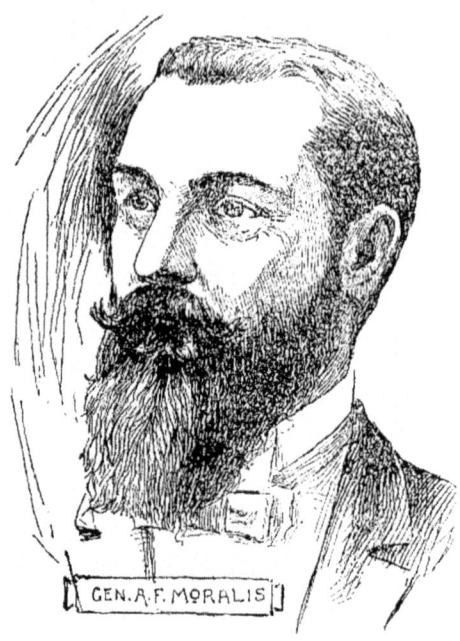

A revolutionist in San Domingo, General A.F. Morales offered his opinion to New York reporters that April was "the worst time of the year for the United States to engage in war with Spain.... [W]ith the season of rain comes yellow fever, and with yellow fever death" (*New York World*, April 10, 1898).

in need of refrigeration or cooling applications, ice water, ice cream, cracked ice for fever patients, etc." The value of the icebergs was based on three assumptions: ice would cure yellow fever; when the bergs melted they would yield large quantities of gold; and the ice could be towed without serious diminishment of size and value. The scheme was credited to a man from Denver who added, "Our profits will be established as we appear down there with a few icebergs to begin on. They will pay us at the rate of $1,000 per patient, in cases of speedy cure. That will generate $419,000 per iceberg, if all goes well." Apparently that gentleman had never read Ambrose Bierce's "The Failure of Hope and Wandel" (originally published as "Cool Correspondence" in the London publication *Fun* in September 1874. It described an eerily similar (and disastrous) scheme. As if the Klondike Company needed worse news, an article in the *Boston Globe* on June 16, 1898, noted that there had been splendid success "in making liquid air by the barrel," suggesting there was more refrigeration in a thimbleful of liquid air than in an ice cart, having the potential to "wipe out a whole ice monopoly."[11]

Tracing the history of the disease, the concept that yellow fever was originally spread by the importation of Africans resurfaced: "Yellow fever is the heritage of the era of slavery. Had we never imported Africans we might never have known what yellow fever was.

HEALTH BANDS and HEALTH FLANNEL
(Dr. DURAND'S Patented).

All who value their health and would prolong their lives should wear this remarkable Flannel, curative of organic and nervous affections, and preservative against cholera, small-pox, yellow fever, and all epidemics.

Bands for chest and stomach from 7s. 6d. each. Flannel, from 5s. per yard.

Catalogues free.

Sole agents, Messrs. MARTIN, 27, Coleman-street, E.C.

The use of flannel was highly promoted in the 18th and 19th centuries to ward off deadly diseases. If worn as protective clothing it might actually have had some positive effect in preventing mosquitoes from biting exposed arms, but that rationale was unknown. Instead, the properties of flannel were promoted as almost mystical rather than common sense (*Anglo-American Times*, London, September 16, 1871).

The virus of yellow fever comes originally ... from the discharge of the sick negro and from the scourings of slave ships [that discharged bilge water into ports]." Falling back on old science, many continued to believe the disease arose "from noxious exhalations or miasmata, and flourishe[d] in stagnant water or under a hot sun." Excerpts from the government commission's voluminous report more bluntly stated, "Cuba has become the greatest nursery and camping ground of one of man's most ruthless destroyers. Itself most afflicted, it annually disseminates to other lands, as from a central hell, disease and death."

Everyone felt free to offer an opinion on how to counter the effects of disease. Dr. Cyrus Edson of New York suggested that every man ought to wear a "cummerbund," a "light flannel band placed around the abdomen to keep it warm." Authorities in Indiana ordered their troops to shave so yellow fever germs would not root in their whiskers. In some circles tobacco was considered a preventative, as was putting refined sulphur in the boots or taking sulphume (liquid sulphur) internally. Those using feather pillows on their beds were warned by the L.E. Patterson Feather-Cleaning Company to have them cleaned, as such pillows were "the recipients of the waste matter from your system!" and would bring on yellow fever. The Swanson Rheumatic Cure Company, makers of "5 Drops" medicine, urged that quinine be supplanted by their remedy, noting, "It's a wonder. Try it [for the cure of] rheumatism, neuralgia, catarrh, asthma, hay-fever, yellow fever and other kindred ills." The use of alcohol was believed to predispose a man to yellow fever by "by destroying the power of resistance and enfeebling all the powers of life," while a remedy of one-half ounce Peruvian bark, 20 grains salt of wormwood, and 20 grains snake root mixed together was sure to cure all ills. Slightly more palatable was the statement by physicians that a daily dose of tomatoes would make a person immune from yellow fever. So great was the belief in this that the government placed large orders with canning factories, and agents were paying 11 cents a can, 1 cent more than the retail price.

On that subject, one paragraph perhaps sums it up best:

> On the matter of specific for the diseases that are liable to inflict our soldiers the number is legion. All the quack preparations in existence are offered the government, from patent corn exterminators to magic salves that will draw out all hidden knots on a wooden leg. It is passing strange, but nevertheless pitiable, that even medicine is now having a "yellow" streak in it. Yellow pills are offered the government which, it is claimed, will cure yellow fever. Then there are pink pills for pale-faced soldiers, brown pills for the negroes, and green pills for those who are afflicted with jaundice. The inventors of these don't take into account color-blind people, it would seem.

An equal number of suggestions for preserving heath were offered, all similar to this one:

Keeping Well in Cuba
(from Colonel Pedro Cardo, an Insurgent Veteran)

(1) Keep the body clean
(2) Change underclothing as often as possible
(3) Keep in the shade
(4) Don't eat sun-warmed fruit; let it cool
(5) Only drink boiled water with a few drops of brandy added
(6) Don't sleep on the ground
(7) Don't sleep without covering
(8) Rest in the middle of the day and march in the morning
(9) Have medicine to keep the bowels clear
(10) Don't think you have yellow fever every time you get a headache[12]

Immediately after war was declared, a naval fleet under Admiral William T. Sampson blockaded Cuban ports, the ultimate objective being the capture of Santiago de Cuba. Between the 22nd and 24th of June soldiers commanded by General William R. Shafter were landed at Daiquiri and Siboney, east of Santiago. To achieve their goal, soldiers had to pass through Spanish defenses concentrated in the San Juan hills and the town of El Caney. Guantanamo Bay, with its excellent harbor, was chosen as protection from summer hurricanes and was attacked on June 6, followed by the Battle of Santiago de Cuba on July 3, resulting in the destruction of the Spanish Caribbean Squadron. Ground battles took place at Las Guasimas on June 24 and El Caney and San Juan Hill on July 1, after which the United States forces began a siege. The city finally surrendered on July 16 and Spain sued for peace the following day. The Treaty of Paris, which recognized Cuban independence, was signed on December 10, 1898.

War news, particularly that of yellow fever among the troops, gripped those back home. In early May, when word was received that the disease had broken out among some of the prize crew that captured the *Argonauta*, a quarantine was quickly established at Key West, Florida. This brought up the question of what to do with the "White Elephant," those Spanish prisoners captured in Cuba. The suggestion they be sent to the States until released home brought immediate protest from those fearing the importation of yellow fever.

The numbers of those stricken with the disease also made headline news, although they fluctuated greatly. To control both the disease and the rumors, strict quarantines were established by military commanders in Cuba, resulting in "considerable inconvenience to the newspaper dispatch boats." On July 11 Lieutenant Colonel Pope, chief surgeon in Shafter's army, released word that 14 cases of yellow fever had been diagnosed in the field hospital at Santiago. By July 15 "only" 23 new cases were reported. By July 17, a dispatch advised the number of fever cases at Santiago "did not exceed 300. This lowered the estimate by one half and was a source of satisfaction to the authorities. Alden, acting surgeon general says the disease is much less serious than would appear at first glance." Simultaneously, Clara Barton reported that "immunes are not needed as nurses, all the fever patients are doing well."

> **YELLOW-JACK IN THE ARMY.**
>
> **The Dread Disease Breaks Out Among Our Troops.**
>
> Startling Information Contained in Offcial Dispatches Received at Washington--Hospitals and Quarantine Camps to be Established at Once--Immunne Doctors and Nurses Ordered to the Front--Gen. Toral Still Seeking Terms for Surrender--Indications That Most of the Spanish Troops Have Slipped Out of the Beleagured City--No Engagement Since Monday.

It was a fact of public record that disease killed more Spanish soldiers than Cuban bullets. In order to mitigate that happening to United States soldiers, a call went out for "immunes," or men who had survived an earlier attack of yellow fever, to join the ranks for service in Cuba. Unfortunately, there were not enough of them or those thought to be immune were not, and by mid-July headlines such as this were filling newspaper mastheads (*Massillon* [Ohio] *Item*, July 13, 1898).

Writing from the yellow fever camp near Siboney on July 26, Thomas W. Steep informed those back home: "The yellow fever camp is spread out on hills swept by the ocean breezes. The medicine given is in the tablet form and the treatment simple. The doctors are Americanized Cuban experts. A number of Red Cross ladies have bravely ventured into camp. The general convalescence indicates that yellow fever will not marginally affect the garrison now here."

On the same date, a reporter from the *New York World* writing from Siboney indicated that city had been burned to the ground in an effort to stop the spread of yellow fever. "Still," Steep added, "the fever is increasing, and cases of it are reported at Firmeza, El Caney and Santiago, which are from five to 12 miles away." However, Dr. John Guiteras, a leading expert in yellow fever, stated the fever was of a very mild form and praised the colored troops for their work in "burning buildings and doing other sanitary work."

H.L. Beach of the Associated Press claimed yellow fever was first introduced into the ranks of the American army when army ambulances were used to carry infected Cuban refugees fleeing Santiago. Worse, he complained commissary wagons going to Siboney with food returned full of infected refugees. Quoting Dr. Ducker of Chicago he stated, "No yellow fever appeared in the army before the lines were opened to these people from Santiago."[13]

On July 30 the War Department released the following message from General Shafter: "Sanitary conditions for July 28: Total sick, 1,278; total fever cases, 3,400; new cases of fever, 696; cases of fever restored to duty, 590; death, private Michael McGoldrick, First Infantry, cause, athenia following malarial fever."[14]

By August 4 the Associated Press supplied newspapers with the information that

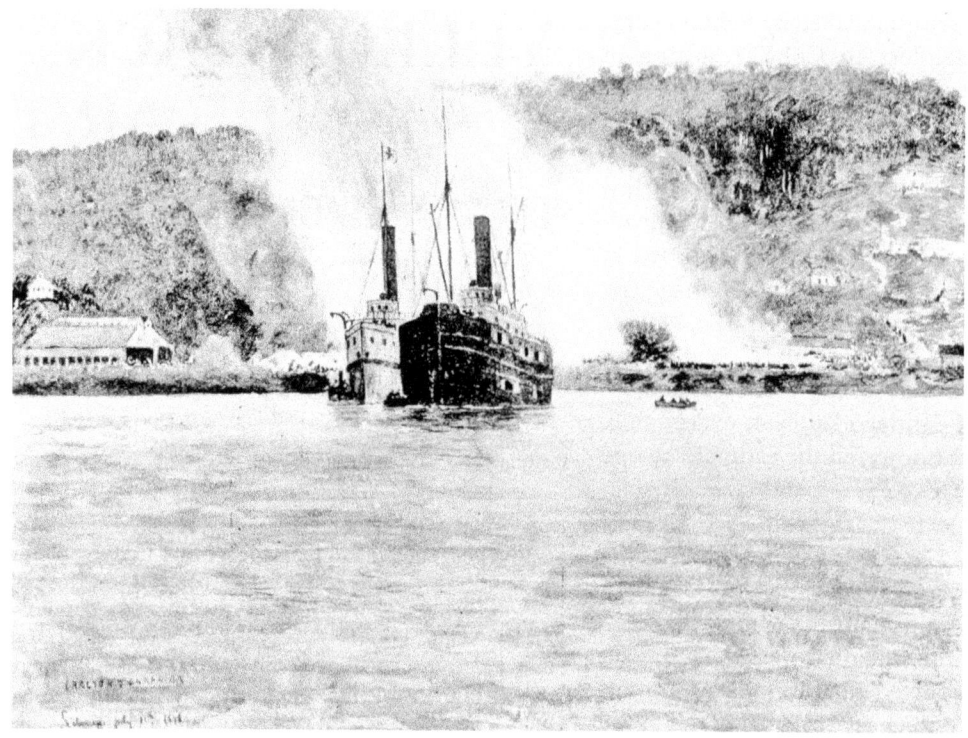

In an effort to control the spread of yellow fever in Cuba, United States officers burned the city of Siboney. This image (published in *Harper's Weekly*, V. 2, p. 761), depicts the start of the blaze July 11, as viewed from the water. The hospital ship *Relief* is in the foreground (courtesy National Library of Medicine).

"after Col. Roosevelt had taken the initiative in demanding that the army be sent north," other officers united in a round-robin address to General Shafter requesting that the army "be moved at once, or perish," due to the destructive power of yellow fever. The government responded by notifying General Shafter that in response to returning troops all West Indian ports under United States control and all medical officers of the Marine Hospital Service were to be detailed for duty to carry out requirements of the quarantine law of 1893. Furthermore, Secretary Alger ordered that troops from Santiago arriving at Montauk Point be inspected by quarantine officers and the yellow flag raised; those found sick were to be isolated, with no visitors permitted.

For those waiting transport, life was hard. In a letter to his brother, Lou Foeltzer wrote in a letter dated July 30:

> Most of our men are sick with fever. One man of our company died yesterday. The sickness comes on in a few minutes. I was appointed head mogul of the burial detail. I have to bury all the dead and it keeps me busy. Eight today that died of yellow fever. We dig a hole three feet deep, roll the corpse in a blanket, put their name in it, also my name and address, so if their bodies should ever be taken up they will have to come and get me so as to find the spot. I handled all the noted men, such as Hamilton Fish, Jr. and Captain O'Neil of the Rough Riders. We shipped their bodies to the United States.

By mid–August the naval base at Key West, including hospital personnel, was transferred to Norfolk, but those suffering from yellow fever remained behind. Left without proper facilities or physicians, the marines were placed in an old cigar factory. While newspaper headlines lambasted the authorities over the deplorable conditions, the *Chicago Tribune* published statistics from the war, listing 350 officers and men killed in battle or dead of wounds and between 1,200 and 2,000 volunteers and regulars dead of disease.

Deaths from Disease in the Spanish-American War

Typhoid fever	515
Yellow fever	84
Dysentery	68
Meningitis	47
Malaria	81
Pneumonia	61
General fever	106
Miscellaneous	327

Deaths According to State

Regular army	200
Massachusetts	130
Illinois	100
Michigan	91
New York	85

Not incidentally, in an article published in the *American Journal of Medicine* (September 1898), Lieutenant Colonel Nicholas Senn, U.S. Volunteers, chief of the operating staff in the field, noted that while the national guard surgeon "more than [held] his own," he decried that many seeking commissions did not possess adequate preliminary education, "a reflection upon the system of medical education which continues to prevail in the country." He added, "Many militia Surgeons are illiterate, because no proof of competency has been demanded, except the presentation of a diploma, no matter from what institution." In light of this, the *Temple* (TX) *Tribune* supplied the following:

THE DIAGNOSIS

You have yellow fever if you die.

If lots of people take it from you, it is yellow fever, otherwise it is typhoid.

If you have yellow fever and get well it is "suspicious," but if you had vomited it would have been yellow fever.

You can tell yellow fever principally by the big death rate.

Fright causes over 50 percent of deaths in yellow fever.

If you have dengue in Temple, it is dengue, but if you have the same thing in New Orleans it is yellow fever.

Black vomit is a sure sign of yellow fever, but you can have it with dengue or black jaundice.

If you have yellow fever once you are an "immune," but you can keep on having it.

A full-blood negro is immune, although lots of black people die with yellow fever.

Some experts can tell a yellow fever case as soon as they see it, but they pronounce a case as "suspicious" until several days elapse and if he gets well it is most probably something else.

Yellow fever always has a "history," and contact or exposure with another case is a pre-requisite; it is often sporadic.

The above facts regarding yellow fever were gathered by the *Tribune* from reading expert testimony within the past year, noted the *Galveston News*: "There are a great many more 'sure signs,' and the quarantine goes merrily on."[15]

Chapter 30

After War: Science and Sanitation

> *11:50 p.m. Dec. 31st 1900—Only ten minutes of the old Century remain, lovie, dear. Here I have been sitting reading that most wonderful book—LaRoche on Yellow fever—written in 1853—Forty-seven years later it has been permitted to me & my assistants to lift the impenetrable veil that has surrounded the causation of this dreadful pest of humanity and to put it on a rational & scientific basis—I thank God that this has been accomplished during the latter days of the old century—May its cure be wrought out in the early days of the new century!*—Walter Reed letter to his wife[1]

After the Spanish surrender, arrangements were made for the transport of the Spanish Army to Spain. United States ships were then sent to Santiago, where they collected eighteen thousand U.S. soldiers and removed them from Cuba. The soldiers were then "detained" at Montauk Point, New York. Fully half were reported to be "very sick or in a feeble condition." Of these, over 5,000 were received in the general hospital, while "as many more sick" were cared for in the camps. On September 11, 1898, acting Secretary of War Melklejohn announced the object of the camp had been accomplished, "undoubtedly preventing an epidemic of yellow fever throughout the country."

Fifty thousand soldiers remained in Cuba as part of the First Occupation (1898–1902). As they were responsible for the overall supervision, Governor General Leonard Wood (a former army surgeon) and Surgeon General George Miller Sternberg were to rid the island nation of yellow fever. Sternberg, a bacteriologist, believed at the time the disease "could fairly easily be controlled" by following the rules of proper hygiene. To assist them, Major William Crawford Gorgas and his sanitation officers were assigned to clean the island.

Within two months, news from Santiago was all positive. The town was divided into five sections, each under the control of a medical man, and sewers, streets, houses and dispensaries were cleaned. Five hundred cubic yards of refuse were burned daily, disinfectants were distributed and heavy fines were imposed for uncleanliness or failure to report unhealthful conditions and deaths. The death rate rapidly decreased from an average of 70 per day to 20 per day. On September 9 Wood wrote to Secretary Alger that expenses for the upkeep of Santiago amounted to between $4,500 and $5,000, of which $1,600 had gone for sanitary work and engineering and the balance for hospital work and police. Although warned by the yellow fever expert Dr. Guiteras that an epidemic was "absolutely unavoidable," Wood was of the opinion there was a great chance of escaping an outbreak. His prediction proved to be correct, and for a short period it was believed yellow fever had been permanently arrested.

This was good news, for Dr. Z.R Molina, the surgeon in change of the military hospital at Veracruz for 30 years, delivered his paper, "Yellow Fever, a Self Limited Disease," at the medical congress held in Kansas City, stating that yellow fever was "an incurable disease, and there was no eipecial [specific; special] treatment for it." On the lighter side of the equation came the story of the "1600 Outcast Goats." According to the *New York Sun*, an enterprising Texan bought 1,600 goats and had them shipped via New Orleans to Havana, where he anticipated selling them at a huge profit. There being no known tariff on such animals, Governor General Blanco set the duty so high it would have meant a heavy loss to the owner. After a wait aboard in the harbor of several days the goats were returned to New Orleans. Their stay at Havana made them suspect as carriers of yellow fever, however, and authorities refused them entrance until they had been disinfected. No one knew how to disinfect a goat and no southern state would accept them for the same reason, so they were landed at the quarantine station and ordered to remain there until ice was seen, which was about Christmastime.

Dr. Alvah P. Doty made headlines in June 1899 when he claimed success in identifying and curing yellow fever. Beginning in the spring of 1897 and continuing for 18 months he experimented with horses and guinea pigs with an eye toward confirming Sanarelli's identification of the yellow fever germ and verifying his curative serum. On July 6 the transport *McClellan* from Santiago brought in two people suffering from yellow fever: Miss Clendenin and Oscar F. Lackey. Isolating the two of them on Swinburne Island, Doty found Lackey to be in "very bad shape" and administered his serum to him three times. Over the course of two weeks Lackey's progress was tracked by the newspapers and on July 24 Doty declared him cured and discharged him. While making no claims as to the discovery or cure, Doty considered the case a rousing success of Sanarelli's claims and hoped to have it further tested in Havana.

Yellow fever remained controlled in the United States, but was still enough of a threat that in an advertisement for a land sale in Hamilton County, Illinois, a major selling point was there qas "no southern yellow fever and negroes."[2]

The Yellow Fever Commission

By mid–July 1899 yellow fever struck again in Cuba, dashing the hopes and expectations of Sternberg and Wood, who had anticipated, due to their sanitation efforts, a summer as healthful as 1898. The resurgence caused them to reevaluate the situation and they assembled a yellow fever commission to be led by Major Walter Reed, with assistants Jesse Lazear, James Carroll and Aristides Agramonte.

Walter Reed (1851–1902) graduated from the University of Virginia in 1869 and earned a commission in the United States Army Medical Corps in 1875. He attended bacteriology courses at Johns Hopkins and in 1893 he was appointed professor of Clinical and Sanitary Microscopy at the Army Medical School in Washington. In 1898 he, Victor Vaughn and E.O. Shakespeare served on a typhoid board to examine military camps in Cuba. At the time of his appointment, Reed was an advocate of the fomites theory, meaning that yellow fever was spread by direct contact with an infected person or by infected objects such as clothing.

Jesse W. Lazear (1866–1900) was educated at Washington and Jefferson College, Pennsylvania, completed undergraduate work at Johns Hopkins and studied at the University of Edinburgh before taking his medical degree from the College of Physicians and Surgeons in New York. After working in Berlin and at the Pasteur Institute in Paris he became head of clinical laboratories at Johns Hopkins. In 1898 he developed a method of using thyonin to stain malarial parasites and in January 1900 he applied for and accepted a temporary assignment in the Medical Corps.

James Carroll (1854–1907) was an English-born Canadian and earned his medical degree in 1891 at the University of Maryland. He did postgraduate work at Johns Hopkins and in 1895 he was assigned to the Army Medical Museum, where he worked on bacteriology. In 1899 he was involved with Walter Reed, studying Sanarelli's *bacillus icteroides*

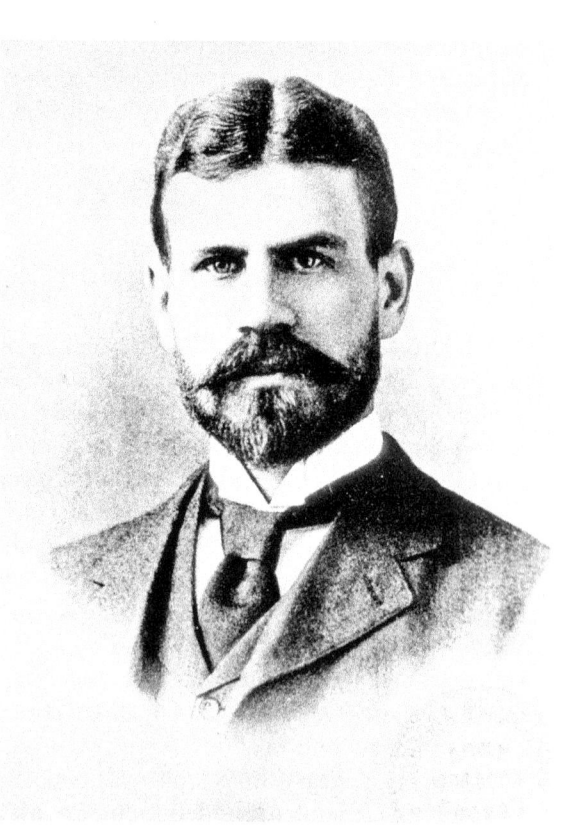

Top: This illustration of a young Dr. Walter Reed was placed on the cover of the *Health Heroes* pamphlet that described the advances Reed and his associates made in Cuba concerning the transmission of yellow fever. The pamphlet was published by the Metropolitan Life Insurance Company in 1926, and the countenance on the cover presumably was meant to convey American youth and ingenuity. The opening paragraph describes Reed as a "master detective" who was "helped by brave American soldiers who offered their lives in the conquest of this disease" (author's collection, pamphlet written by Grace T. Hallock and C.E. Turner). *Bottom:* Jesse Lazear, MD, was an original member of Walter Reed's Yellow Fever Commission to Cuba after the Spanish-American War. He was either bitten accidentally, or allowed himself to be bitten by a suspected yellow fever-carrying mosquito in an ongoing attempt to prove the precise species responsible for spreading the disease and the period of incubation required between the time a mosquito fed upon an infected person to the time it was capable of infecting a disease-free individual. Tragically, Dr. Lazear died from yellow fever, one of many heroes who sacrificed themselves in the cause of science (courtesy National Library of Medicine).

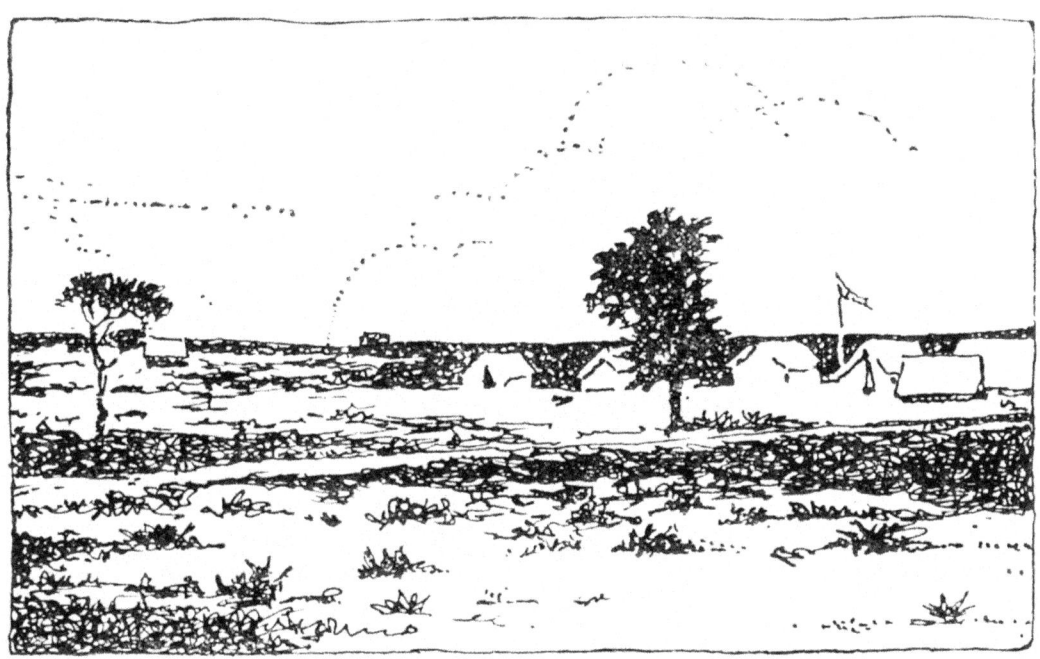

Camp Lazear, a second research site in Cuba, was named after Jesse Lazear (author's collection, from *Health Heroes*, 1926).

and ultimately helping to disprove the theory. In 1900 Sternberg promoted him to acting assistant surgeon in the Medical Corps and appointed him second-in-command of the Yellow Fever Commission.

Aristides Agramonte (1868–1938) was born in Cuba but was raised in the United States after his father was killed in the First Cuban War for Independence. He earned his medical degree from the College of Physicians and Surgeons and worked as a bacteriologist for the New York Health Department until 1898, when he was appointed acting assistant surgeon in the army. As Agramonte was immune to yellow fever from early exposure, Sternberg sent him to Cuba to study it in Shafter's forces. In conjunction with Carroll and Reed, Agramonte helped discredit Sanarelli's claims, but when Drs. Wasdin and Geddings issued a report in 1899 confirming Sanarelli's findings, Agramonte returned to Cuba. During the outbreaks that year he verified his previous findings that *icteroides* was not present in all yellow fever victims.[3]

Two areas of interest were immediately apparent to the investigators who met at Columbia Barracks, Quemados, Cuba, on June 25, 1900: the mosquito theory and the presence of microorganisms in the intestinal canal of yellow fever victims. The researchers decided to follow the mosquito theory because of its similarity to malaria, already proven to be conveyed by mosquitoes through the work of Ronald Ross and Patrick Manson in 1897.

Similarity of Yellow Fever to Malaria

(1) Yellow fever resembled malaria, already identified as being conveyed by mosquitos
(2) Both diseases were airborne
(3) Both were contracted primarily at night

(4) Both jumped from house to house in an unknown manner
(5) Both were non-contagious
(6) Both prevailed in the season when mosquitoes were numerous
(7) Infections ceased with a sharp frost
(8) The interval of time between the first case and a second in an infected dwelling suggested an intermediate host in the conveyance of the disease
(9) Soldiers leaving Columbia Barracks, near Havana, after sundown were the only persons who contracted yellow fever and after recovering, did not infect others

The last similarity seemed to indicate the cause of the disease was not present on the body, the clothing or the dejecta. This idea was supported by Henry Rose Carter, who had studied the disease during outbreaks of yellow fever while a quarantine officer with the Marine Hospital Service. He determined that, regardless of exposure to infected persons or clothing, two weeks elapsed between the first and subsequent outbreaks. During an outbreak in Orwood and Taylor, Mississippi, in 1898, he confirmed that a period of 9–14 days elapsed between the first and second cases, which he termed an "extrinsic incubation period" before the disease was transmitted, suggesting an intermediate host.

The members of the board visited Dr. Finlay, whose work with mosquitoes and yellow fever was far advanced. Working with Sternberg and the Yellow Fever Commission of 1879, Finlay had concluded the disease was spread from an infected person's blood vessels to another by the *Aedes aegypti* mosquito, but he had never been able to prove it. He supplied the new team with these dried mosquito eggs for the purpose of hatching them for the study. Lazear was placed in charge of the mosquitoes, Carroll worked on the cultures and Reed returned to the United States.

Due to the fact it was believed no animal was susceptible to yellow fever, human subjects were required. The physicians agreed to subject themselves to the experiments and a number of attempts were made to infect nine American volunteers, including Lazear, with mosquitoes that had been incubated and infected over the period of August 11–25, 1900, but these attempts were unsuccessful. Finally, Carroll was bitten by a mosquito that had been infected by a victim twelve days earlier. Four days later, on August 29, Carroll came down with a fever and the following day was removed to the isolation camp. On the day Carroll came down with fever, Lazear applied the same mosquito, along with three others, to a soldier ("X.Y.," identified as Private William Dean of the 7th Cavalry) who was taken sick on the fifth day with a mild attack. The incubation periods proved to be the missing link in Finlay's experiments. James Carroll wrote of the tragic event that followed:

> Scarcely more than a week later, Dr. Lazear was applying mosquitoes, as usual, late in the afternoon, to patients in the yellow fever hospital, known as Las Animas, and while thus engaged a mosquito alighted upon his hand. He allowed it to take its fill, and concluded it was one of the common culex mosquitoes which were present in the hospital in large numbers. So little importance did he attach to the incident that he made no note of it, and related the circumstance to me when he was first taken sick, five days afterward. A week from that date he died, having been delirious and affected with black vomit for several days. Thus ended the first set of experiments, with the death of our esteemed and unfortunate colleague.

Before dying, Lazear stated the bite had been accidental but speculation persists that he had allowed himself to be bitten, denying the fact in order that his life insurance policy be paid to his family. Results of the team's preliminary findings were presented at the annual meeting of the American Public Health Association held in Indianapolis on

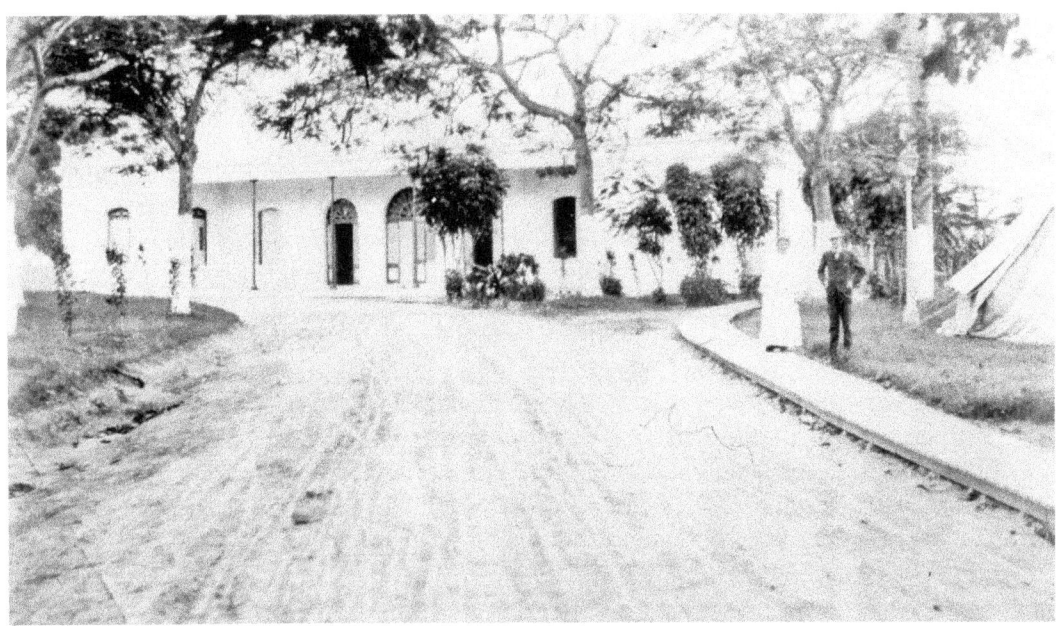

One can only guess at the conflicting hope and misery hidden behind the walls of this yellow fever ward, Las Animas, Cuba (courtesy National Library of Medicine).

October 23, 1900.[4] On October 27 the *New York Times* published a summary of the board's work to be released in summary form by the *Philadelphia Medical Journal*. Declaring the mosquito to be "the 'intermediate host' for the parasite of yellow fever," they concluded "it is highly probable that the disease is only propagated through the bite of this insect." The death of Dr. Lazear was also described in clinical detail.

> Dr. Lazear was bitten on August 16, 1900, by a mosquito, (Culex fasciatus,) which ten days previously had been contaminated by biting a very mild case of yellow fever, (fifth day.) No appreciable disturbance of health followed this inoculation.
> On Sept. 13, 1900 (forenoon,) Dr. Lazear, while on a visit to Las Animas Hospital, and while collecting blood from yellow fever patients for study, was bitten by a Culex mosquito (variety undetermined.) As Dr. Lazear had been previously bitten by a contaminated insect without after-effects, he deliberately allowed this particular mosquito, which had settled on the back of his hand, to remain until it had satisfied its hunger.
> On the evening of Sept. 18, five days after the bite, Dr. Lazear complained of feeling "out of sorts," and had a chill at 8 p.m. On Sept. 19, 12 o'clock noon, his temperature was 102.4 degrees, pulse 112; his eyes were injected (sic) and his face suffused; at 3 p.m. temperature was 103.4 degrees, pulse 104; 6 p.m. temperature was 103.8 degrees and pulse 106. Jaundice appeared on the third day. The subsequent history of this case was one of progressive and fatal yellow fever, the death of our much-lamented colleague having occurred on the evening of Sept. 25, 1900.

The report concluded: "Since we here, for the first time, record a case in which a typical attack of yellow fever has followed the bite of an infected mosquito, within the usual period of incubation of the disease, in which other sources of infection can be excluded, we feel confident that the publication of these observations must excite renewed interest in the mosquito theory of the propagation of yellow fever, as first proposed by Finlay."[5]

Camp Lazear and Informed Consent

Walter Reed returned to Cuba in November 1900 and obtained over $10,000 from Governor General Wood to begin phase two of the yellow fever experiments for the purpose of confirming what they had already established and to disprove the fomite theory. Camp Lazear was established a mile from Columbia Barracks and consisted of seven large hospital tents, separated by a wide interval and pitched in an arc. The plan was to "establish the fact that cases [of yellow fever] could be produced at will by the application of infected mosquitoes."

Several Spanish immigrants participated in the experiments but the majority of volunteers came from Lieutenant Albert E. Truby's Hospital Detachment at Camp Columbia. For their participation they were given a $100 gold piece. Because of the potential for great bodily harm, the team devised what later became the standard for human participation: the "informed consent," outlining the risks and potential benefits of the study. This consent made note of the fact there was a great likelihood of contracting the disease naturally and argued it was better to do so under controlled conditions, but it stated the

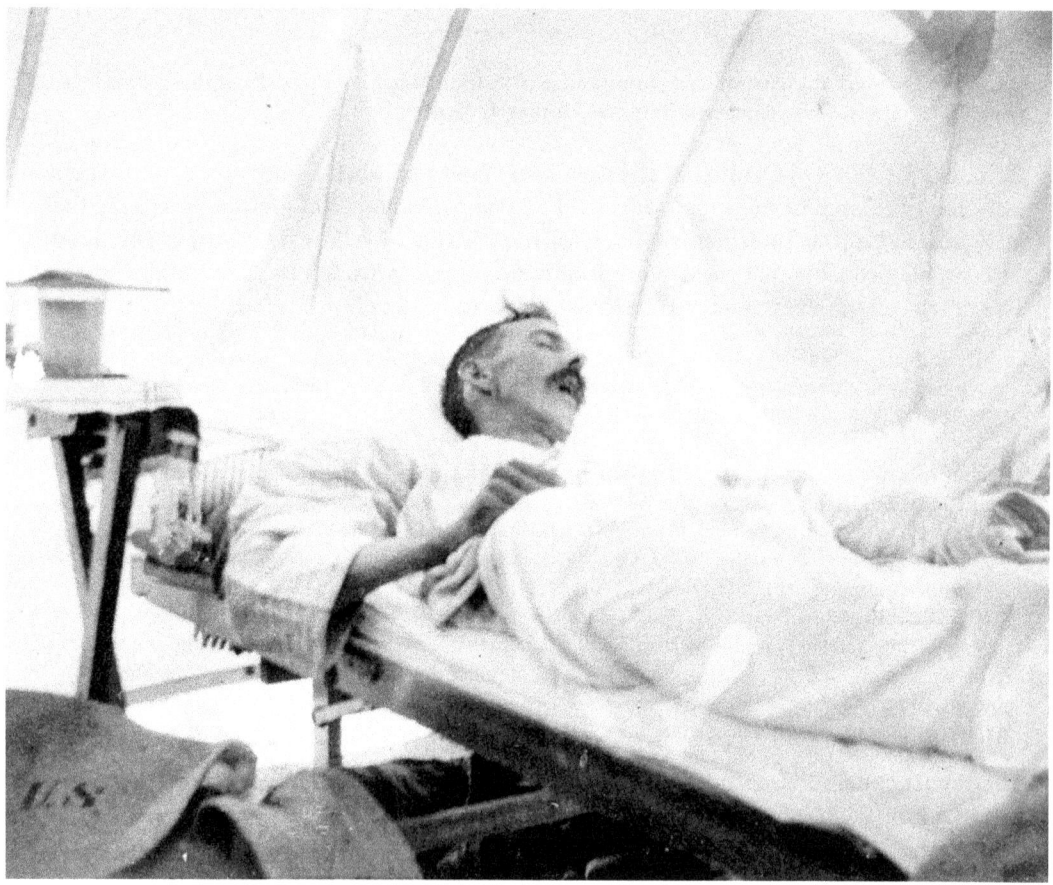

If anything puts a face to the horrors of yellow fever, this unidentified man in a yellow fever hospital at Siboney, Cuba, July 1898, expresses the pain, suffering, isolation, dread and mystery of the disease (courtesy National Library of Medicine).

possibility the volunteers might die during the experiment. This novel and humane approach garnered for members of the commission an acknowledgment of being the first to advocate and implement informed consent. Ralph E. Gregg of the hospital corps put it in laymen's terms: "We have an experimental station where the doctors are studying yellow fever. If any soldier wants to earn $200 all he has to do is to volunteer to be experimented upon. If he gets yellow fever and recovers he gets $200 cash and a three-months' furlough. If he does not recover under the experimental treatment he gets a pine box and a final resting place in the soldiers' cemetery at Quemados."

To prove or disprove the fomite theory a secured area was heated to 90 degrees and kept warm and dark, simulating the hold of a ship in the tropics. It was filled with bedclothes and garments taken from yellow fever victims and handled by two non-immune Americans volunteers, one of them a physician. Neither was affected with yellow fever. After repeated tries, four of these volunteers were subsequently infected by mosquitoes or blood infusions and contracted the disease, effectively disproving the fomite theory.

The technique of infecting a volunteer was to let loose fifteen contaminated mosquitoes in a secured apartment similar to the one used in the fomite study. The nonimmune subject was to lie for 30 minutes with arms and legs exposed; the experiment was then repeated later for 20 minutes, during which time the subject would be bitten as many times as possible. John R. Kissinger (Liberty Mills, Wabash County, Indiana) was the first volunteer at Camp Lazear. Coming from Truby's corps, he developed a very severe case of yellow fever on December 8, 1900. He recovered ten days later and at the end of the month he agreed to allow doctors to transfuse blood from a yellow fever patient into his veins as a means of testing his immunity. The operation was successful and he was given a gold watch in recognition of his courage. Unfortunately he suffered permanent damage and was given a discharge the following year. In 1910 Congress awarded him a $100 a month pension for his service.

John J. Moran volunteered and was bitten six days after Kissinger but did not develop yellow fever. He was subsequently confined in the "Infected Mosquito Building," where he was repeatedly bitten. On December 25 he fell ill with yellow fever. Further experiments were tried by directly injecting four volunteers (including Kissinger) by subcutaneous injection with small quantities of blood drawn in the first and second days of the disease. This demonstrated the presence of the infectious agent in the blood, although the researchers did not discover anything by microscopic examination that could be identified in all persons with yellow fever. In all, ten cases of yellow fever were brought on "at will." In no instance was a mosquito found to be capable of infecting in a shorter time than twelve days after biting the patient, and one patient was infected with two mosquitoes kept as long as 57 days.

The work progressed until the end of February 1901, when confirmatory experiments were assumed by Dr. John Guiteras of Havana. Dr. Carroll returned to Havana in August 1901. After obtaining some of Guiteras's mosquitoes he infected two Spanish nonimmune subjects. Drawing blood from one, he separated the serum and passed it through a filter that "was shown to be capable of holding back the ordinary bacteria. Injection of the filtered serum into two Americans infected them with yellow fever." This explained that bodies smaller than ordinary bacteria (viruses) were responsible for producing yellow fever.

Results Produced by the Army Board

(1) *Bacillus icteroides* had no relation to yellow fever

(2) Yellow fever was transmitted by the mosquito of the genus Stegomyia and all attempts to bring on the disease by fomites resulted in failure

(3) Yellow fever could be produced experimentally by the injection of blood drawn in the first and second days of the disease but this had no bearing upon the transmission or prevention of the disease in its epidemic form

(4) The germ of yellow fever was sufficiently minute to pass through a bacteria-proof filter

Safely Assumed Assumptions

(1) Disinfection in the prophylaxis against yellow fever is effective only when it takes the form of fumigation and destroys mosquitoes

(2) Yellow fever patients could be the source from which other cases spring only when they have been bitten by the proper mosquitoes. In the yellow fever zone, all acute febrile cases should be kept rigidly behind mosquito screens

(3) Hospitals treating yellow fever cases should be built on high ground away from open standing water and secured by close-meshed wire screens.

(4) Petroleum should be poured over standing water

(5) Water should not be allowed to stand uncovered in houses. *Stegomyia fasciata*, the yellow fever mosquito, is a house-dwelling and house-breeding insect that breed in even small amounts of open water so all vessels, large and small, should be covered

(6) After the removal of a patient the room should be fumigated with insect powder, tobacco or sulphur to destroy mosquitoes

(7) So long as an infected patient is rigidly protected against mosquitoes, he may be safely transported through a city

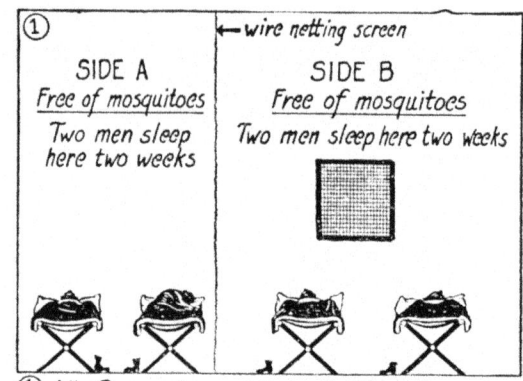

① All four men remain well. Therefore the building is not infected with yellow fever

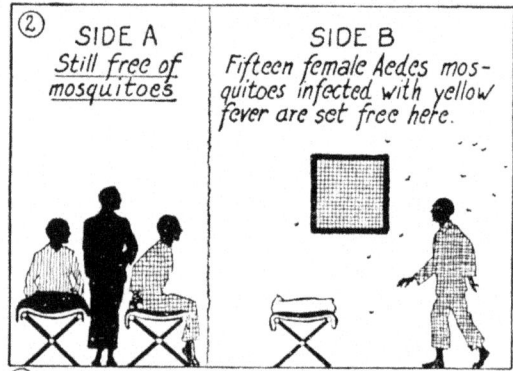

② J. Moran enters side B, is bitten and has yellow fever in four days. The men in side A remain well. Therefore the presence of contaminated mosquitoes infected side B.

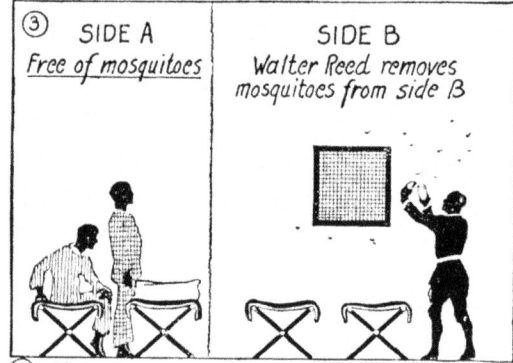

③ Men sleep on both sides of wire netting as before without taking yellow fever. Therefore side B has been disinfected by removing mosquitoes

This line drawing illustrates one of the techniques used by the scientists in Cuba to prove yellow fever was transmitted by mosquitoes rather than by fomites. The second soldier to volunteer to be exposed in the mosquito room was John Moran. He contracted the disease and recovered. The first volunteer, John R. Kissinger, also contracted yellow fever but suffered a lifelong disability and was eventually granted a pension from the government (author's collection, from *Health Heroes*, 1926).

(8) The belief in the supposed contagiousness of yellow fever arose because it was not then known mosquitoes transmitted the disease

(9) An infected house is one that contains infected mosquitoes. In the absence of this insect no amount of filth, heat or moisture is capable of generating the disease

(10) Vessels from infected ports should be compelled to anchor at least a fourth of a mile from shore unless in winter, to prevent mosquitoes reaching the city

(11) As the yellow fever mosquito does not generally bite between 9 a.m. and 3 p.m. it is practically safe for non-immunes to visit infected localities during these hours

(12) Before the lapse of many years yellow fever will become extinct. The length of time will depend on the cooperation of many countries

(13) Another epidemic of yellow fever should never occur in the United States[6]

In February 1901 at the Pan American Medical Congress in Havana, an end to quarantine regulations against vessels which had been exposed to yellow fever was suggested. It was also hoped that an international treaty could be drafted for removing the sources and suppressing the causes of yellow fever in the American hemisphere. This would prove easier said than done, however, as not everyone accepted the results of the Reed Commission. Great attention was paid to Drs. Herbert E. Dunham and Myers, of the Liverpool School of Tropical Medicine, who claimed to have proven yellow fever was a bacterial disease, while Dr. Sanarelli refused to believe his *icterodes* were not the actual cause. Nor were they alone. Assistant Surgeon S.H. Hodgson, of the Marine Hospital Service, claimed that the cimex, or bedbug, was "more than liable" to transmit yellow fever than "the buzzing mosquito." He added that the bean of the cedron, with its antibiotic properties, made into a tincture and administered hypodermically, was a specific (remedy) for the disease.[7]

On August 14, 1901, the War Department announced it had issued an order convening a board of medical officers at Havana to examine the claims of Dr. Caldas of Brazil and Dr. Angel Bellinzaghi that they had perfected a method of preventing the contraction of yellow fever and also developed a cure for the disease. Headed by Major Harvard (chief surgeon of the Department of Cuba), the committee comprised Drs. Gorgas, Finlay, Guiteras and Agramonte, who were to supply the mosquitoes used in the controlled experiments. The eight mosquitoes were to be separated into two divisions: two persons inoculated with the serum were to be bitten by two mosquitoes each, while the other four mosquitoes were to bite two nonimmune subjects. The test did not go well, as two of the volunteers died. The third victim, Miss Clara Maass, from New Jersey, a contract nurse with the U.S. Army working in Cuba, died August 24. On August 27 American newspapers carried the story of the "Girl Martyr," noting her death was "particularly pathetic, as she had served long, had been bitten by infected mosquitoes many times, and volunteered with perfect serenity, yet the result was death." "Devotion to her calling and a desire to immediately help her mother by offering herself—for a paltry sum—as a subject for a scientific experiment made a martyr of Clara Maass."

By August 29 Major Harvard announced the Caldas serum to be useless and stated the commission "has definitely severed connection with the Brazilian expert and will not supervise any further experiments conducted by him." Major Gorgas, chief sanitary officer, quickly denied any connection "with the recent experiments conducted by the Yellow Fever Commission nor with those conducted by the officials sent by the War Department to investigate the origin and propagation of yellow fever, although it did supply the Carroll commission with mosquitoes." He added that the Sanitation Department "stands ready to immunize any one who desires to undergo the treatment.... The

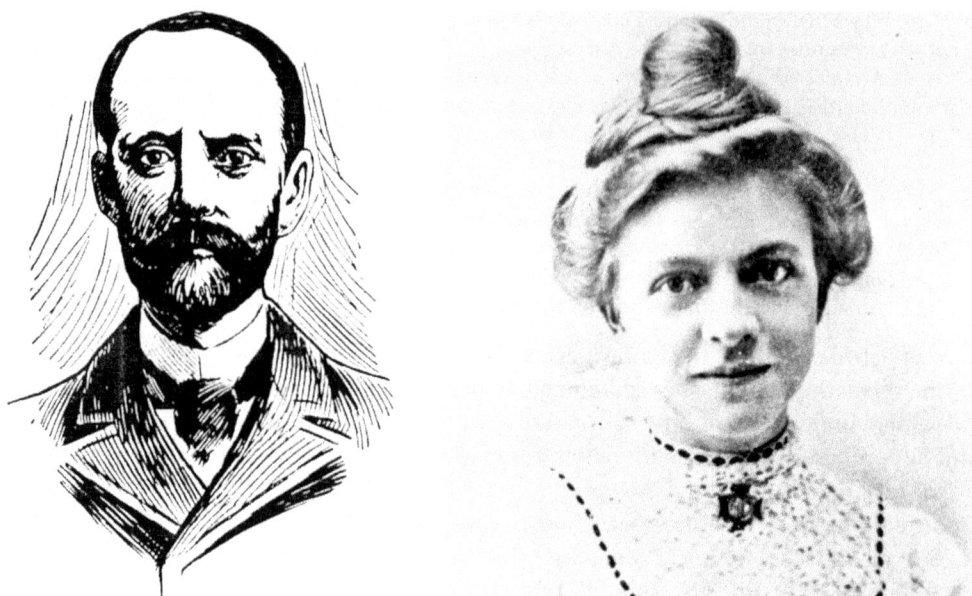

Left: Dr. Caldas was one of several scientists proclaiming he had developed a serum to prevent yellow fever. It was ultimately declared "useless," but in a larger sense it required a great many minds to add small pieces to the larger puzzle (*Upland* [Indiana] *Monitor*, September 5, 1901). *Right:* The most recognized woman in the fight against yellow fever, Clara Louise Maass was a nurse who volunteered for a yellow fever research study in Cuba. Tragically, after contracting the disease she died. Her death caused an outcry in the United States and brought an end to this human-based study (courtesy National Library of Medicine).

person who submits to mosquito infection, however, stands a better chance of recovery than one who contracts the disease accidentally, as the former has care from the beginning."

Inveighing angrily against the authorities in Havana and claiming "the theory that mosquitoes are the only transmitting medium of yellow fever is a scientific brag," Caldas took a ship to the United States, where, ironically, he was detained at Hoffman Island, New York, when he was unable to prove his immunity from yellow fever. Ordered home by his government, he stated his intention to continue his work at Rio de Janeiro.

Ultimately, with the efforts of General Wood and the Sanitary Office to clean the cities and the streets of Havana and to drain areas of open water, Dr. Gorgas declared "for the first time since 1762 Havana has been free from yellow fever in October, while malaria has decreased more than one-half," adding that Mr. Le Prince, who had charge of the anti-mosquito work, estimated that mosquitoes decreased 90 percent.

Prefatory to the last day of American occupation of Cuba, on May 19, 1902, General Wood cleaned out his office, issuing the announcement appointing Dr. Carlos Findlay as chief health officer of the island. With an eye to the future, one newspaper declared, "Probably General Wood is to have charge of the isthmian canal work in order that he may accomplish the first stage by telling the yellow fever to vanish from the isthmus."[8]

Chapter 31

Into the 20th Century

In speaking of yellow fever, the Express states that it carries the stamp "Fumigated" across its head, not that it believes such precaution to be necessary, but because the "public" has not yet accepted the scientific claim of scientists that yellow fever is inoculated by the mosquito bite.[1]

If mosquitoes really were the vectors carrying yellow fever, what did the germ look like? That was the question foremost in the minds of scientists as the world marched into a new century. In 1902 Surgeon General Walter Wyman of the Marine Hospital Service appointed Drs. Parker and Pothier and Professor Beyer to try to identify the animal parasite at a research facility in Vera Cruz. They began their experiments by raising mosquito larvae under controlled conditions. A few days after leaving the pupal stage the insects were given their first meal biting a yellow fever victim. The mosquitoes were subsequently sacrificed from three to fifteen days after infection, hardened and cut into cross-sections one sixteen-hundredths of an inch in thickness and then examined under a compound microscope by J.C. Smith.

Smith identified rod-shaped sporozoites, or "germs" (subsequently named "myxococcidium stegomyiae") and tracked their progress through the digestion cycle of the mosquito, where they eventually reached the proboscis. From that the commission deduced the yellow fever germ was passed to a nonimmune subject via a bite through the female's salivary secretions.

Report of the Yellow Fever Commission, 1903

(1) In the blood of a yellow fever patient which constituted the first meal of a mosquito they identified the yellow fever parasite in its first stage

(2) The cycle in the mosquito was similar to the plasmodium malariae of malarial fever

(3) The time required for the complete development of the parasite into the sporozoites was 12 days, corresponding to the timeline developed by the Reed Havana study

In summing up the report for the *New Orleans Picayune*, Smith concluded with the following: "As a result of the light which has been thrown on the etiology of yellow fever there should no longer be any dread of that disease, as, knowing its cause and the method of its propagation, our health guardians should be able to throttle it on its first appearance." Unfortunately, there was an outbreak of yellow fever in 1905 in New Orleans, where the board of health estimated 437 deaths from the disease. This, however, was the last substantial appearance of the disease in the United States.[2]

The debate was hardly conclusive to the scientific mind or the general population although inroads were made. Based in part on the yellow fever research conducted at the laboratory of the Public Health and Marine Hospital Service on the grounds of the old naval observatory at Washington overlooking the Potomac, Congress passed an act in 1902 regulating the sale of "vaccine virus and antitoxine serum," requiring all interstate dealers to obtain a license from the secretary of the treasury. Before issuing the license, the secretary's office was obliged to see that the products were "up to the standard."

In 1903 Dr. Ludvig Hektoen announced that hydrophobia, smallpox and yellow fever were neither toxic nor inherently poison but were infectious transmittable diseases caused by "minute living organisms capable of proliferation, bacteria so small that they work their way through the best made filters of the laboratories, and so minute that they cannot be detected by the strongest microscope in existence." By 1905, Surgeon General Wyman backtracked from the report of Drs. Pothier and Watson of New Orleans by announcing "the notion that Pothier and Watson have found the origin of yellow fever itself is wrong. What they have discovered is certain phenomena which will be of the utmost value in diagnosing yellow fever cases." He added that Drs. Rosenau and Goldberg of New Orleans were investigating the same subject, marking the third in a series of "earnest efforts on the part of the Public Health and Marine Hospital Service ... to break through the clouds of mystery that have so long enveloped yellow fever."

Two years later, in 1907, headlines read, "Texas Doctor Finally Succeeds in Identifying Dreaded Microbe," announcing the "lucky discoverer" to be Dr. A.E. Thayer of the University of Texas. Thayer claimed the yellow fever germs "were blue" and varied in size from "a point, barely distinguishable under the most powerful microscope, to a mass almost filling up a red blood cell."[3]

If these were new names to the study of yellow fever, old ones continued to make the news. The most shocking was the death of Dr. Walter Reed. Only 51 years of age, he succumbed to a ruptured appendix on November 22, 1902. By August 1903 a memorial association was incorporated in Washington to collect $25,000 in order to erect a monument commemorating Major Reed "in recognition of his important discovery of the transmission of yellow fever by mosquitoes." By December 1906 only $17,000 had been raised, prompting President Roosevelt to ask Congress for funding to further the aims of the association. The following year, it was hoped some of the money raised could be used to "make up for the part cut from his widow's pension by Congress when it was proposed to give her his monthly pay."

Dr. Lazear's widow was eventually given a pension of $17 a month with $2 additional for each child until they reached the age of 16 years, while a bill was entered in Congress by Senator Dick in January 1907 to raise the rank of the ailing, 52-year-old Dr. Carroll from first lieutenant to major. When this special act was passed, President Roosevelt immediately signed it. Carroll died soon afterward, on September 16, 1907. In March 1908 pension bills for the widows of Lazear and Carroll were put before Congress, seeking to provide them a $125 monthly stipend.

Finally, in January 1909, a relief bill for John R. Kissinger was put before Congress, asking that he receive the same pension as the widows of Lazear and Carroll (reported to be $100 a month). It was stated the first volunteer of the Cuban yellow fever experiments suffered from myelitis and as a result was an invalid and required a wheelchair when outside. On May 24, 1910, the House Committee on Military Affairs finally voted Kissinger a pension of $72 a month, denying the Senate request to pay him $125 on the grounds $72 was all that was allowed a private soldier for total disability.[4]

Mosquito Netting, "the Doctors who make no cures," Chimpanzees and Biological Warfare

Questioning the exact path from mosquito to yellow fever proved to be problematic for many Americans. Questions arose and continued to linger: "Why is it that years elapse from one epidemic to another?"; "How is it that some cities along a direct route are spared and others depopulated?" For true believers, accepting the theory occasionally made for good fun. "Mosquito parties" sprang up in which the "umbrella cage," or a full-length netting affixed to an umbrella, became the rage. Designed with various colors to compliment a lady's outfit or a gentleman's suit, guests could sit outside during periods when the insect was particularly annoying and be safe from both itchy bites and yellow fever. Carrying that idea one step further, it was noted, "If you are an adult, baldheaded and have learned to swear, you can keep flies off yourself. If you are a woman you can fan away the mosquito. But what about the baby? ... Cover the baby with netting. A mosquito marked babe in this scientific age should be a cruel anarchronism [sic]."

Dr. Leland O. Howard, chief of the Bureau of Entomology, Department of Agriculture, led the anti-mosquito campaign in the United States, working to drain the Potomac marshes to protect citizens in South Washington. (In 1892 Howard had advanced the idea of placing oil or kerosene on open water to discourage mosquitoes from laying eggs, as well as serving to destroy larvae already in the water, since they needed air to survive. This technique, using "any common oil," was used as early as the yellow fever epidemic in Philadelphia in 1793.) Baltimore authorities took active steps to locate and eradicate mosquito breeding places. The same was true in New Orleans, where squads of special workers poured oil over marshes, stagnant pools and cisterns. In addition, houseboats were converted into "fruit steamers" and placed at the mouth of the Mississippi to rush perishable goods into the city without the costly delays of strict quarantine. Even the railroads got into the act. In 1907 the Texas state health officer notified the general managers of the various railroads in the state to extinguish the "stegomyia" mosquito in an effort to control outbreaks of yellow fever. "I hope that 'shot gun quarantines' are a thing of the past," he said, "but this ounce of prevention is, I think, well worth the effort on your part."

In Mexico, wider precautions were taken when the board of health distributed thousands of small bowls containing a mixture of sulphur and saltpeter to rid homes of insects or to be suspended by wires and lowered down wells to destroy mosquitoes.

While nations were questioning and revising their quarantine practices, the search for a cure remained elusive. A special report made in 1907 noted, "So far no cure for yellow fever has been perfected. During the course of an attack medicines are of little avail and nature must be left to battle with the invading organisms almost unaided." Immunizing serums "did not come up to expectations," and the suggestion that "blood from patients who have conquered the disease and are convalescent be injected into the veins of healthy persons to immunize them ... has not proved practically successful."

The positive news was that universities were beginning to make special provisions for training scientists to work toward stamping out disease "rather than to curing it after it has attacked mankind." George Washington University was singled out as a leading example, having George M. Sternberg serve as professor of preventative medicine. Advocating that an ounce of prevention served better than a pound of cure, Sternberg announced that in the 16th century the average life was a mere 20 years, while in 1907 that estimate had doubled and in the previous 25 years the number had been lengthened by another 6 years. "So," one newspaper concluded, "the doctor who never makes a cure will be one of the most useful members of the community, devoting his life to research work and to service on boards of health and similar bodies."[5]

Two other items of note occurred in the first decade of the 20th century. In 1906 the expedition of the School of Tropical Medicine, which had been in Brazil for nearly two years researching yellow fever, announced that it had been proven chimpanzees could be infected with the disease by the bite of a mosquito. "The discovery," one report announced, "is considered of the highest importance." Work on establishing the first convincing evidence that animals other than human beings were susceptible to yellow fever was established by H. Wolferstan Thomas. On October 23, 1906, fifty-seven *stegomyia fasciata* mosquitoes raised in the laboratory were allowed to feed on two cases of yellow fever of the virulent and fatal type. On November 13 the 21st day after feeding, the 29 surviving mosquitoes were allowed to feed on a chimpanzee. The animal subsequently developed a mild case of yellow fever. In 1907 the Liverpool School of Tropical Medical further announced that Rupert Boyce, dispatched to Brazil to study yellow fever, had successfully applied his antidote to monkeys. He subsequently received a request from President Roosevelt to lay his theory before the United States government. Boyce's two texts, *Mosquito v. Man* and *Yellow Fever and Its Prevention*, stressed the importance of sanitation and explained how mosquitoes survived in ships and thus introducing the disease the distant countries across oceans.[6]

Far more disturbing was the idea of using bacilli in war. In July 1903 a rumor was publicized by the *London Daily News* that revolutionary leaders in Turkey had obtained a quantity of plague bacilli from India and were threatening to infect Constantinople, Salonica and possibly Berlin if world powers did not intervene on their behalf with the Turkish government. Noting that in the American Civil War Confederate sympathizers attempted to infect Northern cities with yellow fever, the author questioned what would happen if similar maniacs attempted to destroy their enemies with such deadly "weapons." With that in mind, "among the curious exhibits at the World's Fair [St. Louis, 1904] will be several hundred mosquitoes and larvae which have recently been brought from Havana." The purpose was to prove how yellow fever was transmitted, but it prompted one journalist to write, "The mere idea suggests what a dangerous factor in war the power thus to introduce yellow fever into an army would be.... Turning loose the yellow fever mosquito impregnated with the fatal germs in either of the two armies in Manchuria would be a more terrible engine of destruction than any now in use."[7]

Cuban Relations Strained

In 1903 Dr. William C. Gorgas proudly announced the United States had spent $100,000 driving yellow fever out of Havana but two years later, complaints about the sanitary conditions in that city culminated in a marine quarantine applied at all ports between Baltimore and Galveston. Dr. Finlay, chief of health and sanitation, acknowledged yellow fever was epidemic in Havana but expressed hope the situation was under control. Major Jefferson Randolph Kean, chief sanitary officer in Cuba, who had convinced Governor General Leonard Wood to enforce the Yellow Fever Commission's findings and base efforts on mosquito eradication rather than the disinfection of homes and goods, seconded that hope by stating December 1, 1906, as the time frame for wiping out the *Aedes aegypti* mosquito's breeding places that had become reestablished. Among the methods used was the importation from the United States of citronella, "one of the few things on earth that seem to cause the mosquito to hesitate."

In August 1907 reports that the disease had broken out among the Hospital Corps at Cienfuegos prompted Dr. Agramonte to investigate the situation. He found conditions in the city favorable to a rapid spread of the disease due to an inadequate water supply and inefficient sanitation. In response, Governor Magoon issued a decree creating a national department of sanitation, consisting of one chief and a national board of five members. Matters were complicated in 1908 over the quarantine maintained against Cuba, prompting Governor Magoon to visit President Roosevelt and express his displeasure.

United States forces permanently withdrew from Cuba on March 31, 1909, when the garrison flag at Camp Columbia was replaced by that of the Cuban republic and home rule was restored. Less than three months later, however, newspaper headlines lamented the fact Cuba's "last gift" to the United States was the fresh importation of yellow fever to St. Petersburg.[8]

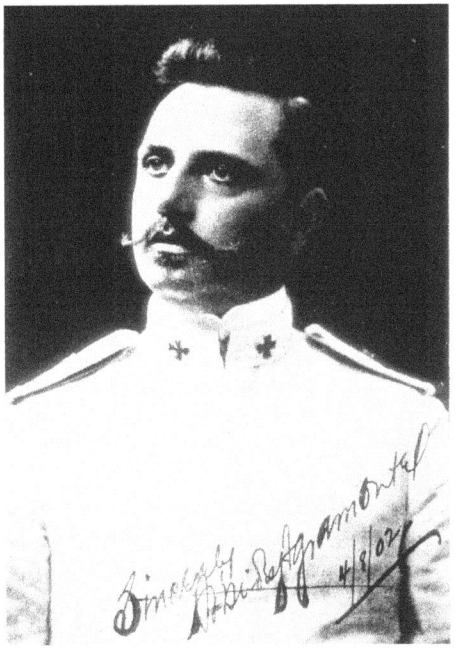

Aristides Agramonte was a member of the Yellow Fever Commission established in Cuba after the Spanish-American War. He and his fellow scientists were instrumental in confirming the discovery that mosquitoes were the actual vector in transmitting the disease (courtesy National Library of Medicine).

CHAPTER 32

Panama!

One complaint is that the doctors in charge of the sanitation of the canal zone have no funds to properly disinfect houses in which the disease occurs. Because of the red-tape methods of the Canal Commission it is said that when the necessary funds and materials are received, the family or tenants of the house are generally dead.[1]

Theodore Roosevelt became president in 1901 after the assassination of William McKinley. One of his earliest goals was to establish a United States–controlled canal across Central America. At the time, there was a great push to abandon the work done in Panama and proceed with a Nicaragua canal, which had already been approved by the Walker Commission. The debate came to a head in 1902 when the Senate Commission on Inter-oceanic Canals debated the idea. Alfred Noble, a civil engineer and a member of the Isthmian Canal Commission was brought before the Senate to testify. He advised that it would be necessary to have absolute control of the cities of Panama and Colon in order to control sanitation. When pressed, Noble conceded conditions in Panama favored the development of yellow fever and admitted the disease did not exist in Nicaragua. He testified that the price of $40,000,000 asked by the Panama company for its property was fair and reasonable. "Taking the whole proposition, do you consider the Panama proposition better than the Nicaragua proposal?" asked Senator Hanna. "I think it is," Noble responded. The Panama plan was successfully championed by George S. Morrison and on June 28, 1902, $40 million was authorized by the Spooner Act. Roosevelt opened negotiations with the Colombians to obtain the necessary rights and in early 1903 the Hay-Herran Treaty was signed by both nations, although the Colombian government failed to ratify it.

This renewed interest in Panama stirred memories of the French disaster and the prevalence of disease. By October, newspapers published notices that Captain Porter of the United States ship *Ranger* stated conditions on the isthmus were "unsatisfactory and that yellow fever and dysentery prevails among the Colombian troops stationed there." Bold headlines dated November 13 warned, "TERRIBLE EPIDEMIC of Yellow Fever Breaks Out Among United States Marines Stationed on Isthmus of Panama." Although the U.S. Navy was "reticent" about releasing details of Admiral Casey's report, Acting Secretary Samuel Darling admitted the marine force would probably be concentrated in Colon "and active steps taken to prevent any spread of the epidemic."

By April 1903 the newly formed Society for the Study of Tropical Diseases in Philadelphia addressed a concern about the canal construction voiced by many scientists both at home and abroad: "Thousands of laborers … will be employed. They can export yellow fever and they can import plague. In fact, they might be the means of introducing yellow fever into regions of the globe where it has never prevailed within the historic period. The canal will not only be a new route for commerce, but it will also be a new route for disease. Pestilence always follows on the heels of trade." Original predictions were that it would require fourteen years to complete the canal and that the unskilled labor would come principally from Jamaica: "The workmen must necessarily be negroes, as white men cannot stand the climate. The negroes of Jamaica and other British West India colonies are fairly good workers and are immune from yellow fever. It is estimated that about 30,000 will be required."

The political situation deteriorated between Panama and Colombia and with some behind-the-scenes manipulation by Roosevelt, Panamanians declared their independence on November 3, 1903. The Hay-Bunau-Varilla Treaty between Panama and the United States was signed on November 18, 1903, and by January 1904 a seven-member Isthmian Canal Commission was established. The same month, headlines declared, "Medical Eyes Turned on Isthmian Canal Strip," an article in which Assistant Surgeon Charles G. Smith was quoted as saying sanitary conditions at Colon were very poor": "There is no system of sewage. Garbage, slops, old clothes and excreta are thrown on the streets and into back yards.... Every condition exists for creating an epidemic of smallpox." Other physicians stated that many victims of yellow fever had actually succumbed to "pernicious malaria."

The United States assumed control of the Canal Zone on February 23, 1904, and on June 30 the Sanitary Department was formed, with Colonel William Gorgas, by then the surgeon general of the Atlantic Division of the Army, as its head. Gorgas spent the summer there but returned to New York in late August. Summing up his early work, he stated, "We have established quarantine stations at both ends, at Panama and Colon, and every vessel arriving at either port is now regularly examined just as at this port [New York]. This was our first step." After describing several cases of bubonic plague brought into Colon from Peru, he continued:

> Yellow fever and its carriers are now receiving attention, and we have the disease so well in hand that within two years it will be practically unknown. We have ordered all people to kill the mosquitoes found in the houses, and a band of mosquito killers that we have organized looks after the work on the outside. All through the zone swamps are to be found in which are the mosquitoes that cause the fever. We have learned by scientific investigation that it is the larvae that are infected, and the only way to prevent yellow fever is to fill in the ponds and swamps. The mosquitoes there are bad, but they do not compare in numbers with those in New Jersey.
>
> We have also learned by investigation that a yellow fever bearing mosquito never moves more than 100 yards. Knowing this we think it would be foolish to try to fill in all of the swamps at this time. When the canal is finally completed, I think we will have one of the most healthy places in the world.[2]

THE SEVEN TENETS OF MOSQUITO CONTROL IN PANAMA

(1) Drainage: All pools within 200 yards of villages and 100 yards of houses. Subsoil drainage was preferred, followed by concrete ditches.

(2) Brush and grass cuttings: Foliage was trimmed to fewer than one foot within 200 yards of villages and 100 yards of homes on the rationale that mosquitoes would not cross open spaces greater than 100 yards

(3) Oiling: When drainage was impossible, oil was poured along the edges of swamps and ponds

(4) Larvicding: Joseph Augustin LePrince developed an insecticide of carbolic acid, resin and caustic soda that was liberally spread

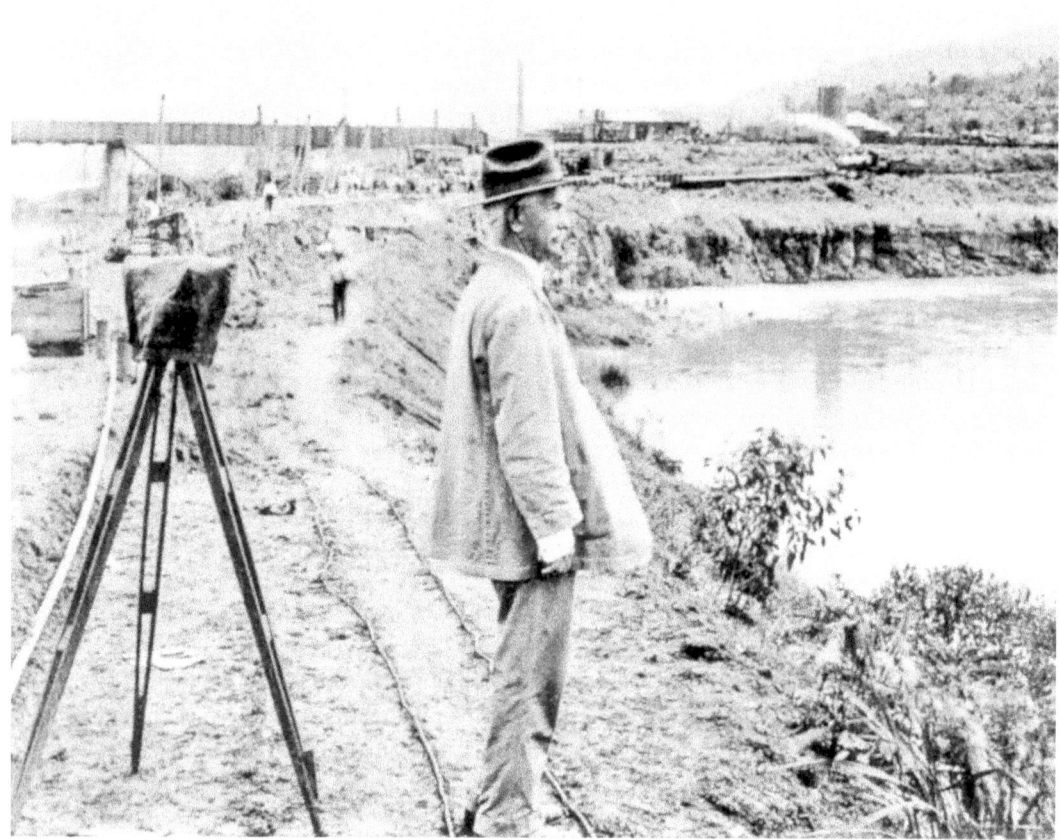

William C. Gorgas, whose father, Josiah Gorgas, was a general in the Confederate army, became renowned in a far different field. After attending the University of the South and studying at Bellevue Hospital Medical College, he was appointed to the United States Medical Corps in June 1880. Surviving an attack of yellow fever at Fort Brown, Texas, he became immune to the disease, making him a logical candidate for service in Cuba after the Spanish-American War. Appointed chief sanitary officer in Havana, his dogged determination to rid the city of yellow fever mosquitoes proved so successful he was re-posted to Panama where he ordered and oversaw the drainage of swamps, mass fumigations and the mass distribution of netting (author's collection).

(5) Prophylactic quinine: This treatment was given to workers along the construction line at 21 dispensaries and dispensers were available at all hotel and mess tables. On average, half the work force received a dose daily

(6) Screening: All government buildings and quarters were secured with netting

(7) Killing adult mosquitoes: Collectors were hired to collect mosquitoes from houses during the daytime. Those captured in tents were examined by Dr. Samuel T. Darling, Chief of the Board of Health Laboratory. The cost of adult mosquito killing was $3.50/per capita/per year for the entire population of the strip (Panama).[3]

After spending three months in Panama, John F. Wallace, chief engineer of the Panama Canal, returned to the United States for a brief visit. Well satisfied with conditions as he saw them, he declared the idea that yellow fever was still prevalent in the isthmus was "erroneous": "It, as well as the malarial fevers common to tropical countries, is being eradicated." He went on to explain the mosquito theory, adding that the system of drainage then being put into effect was gradually getting rid of the insects. His statement proved somewhat premature. A report from Governor Davis of the Canal Zone, dated January 17, 1905 (at Ancon), to Rear Admiral Walker, chairman of the Isthmian Canal Commission, stated only three deaths from yellow fever had occurred since the United States took charge, and that a systematic fumigation of the entire city of Panama was underway. The report also noted Chief Sanitary Officer Gorgas "confidently believed that all mosquitoes capable of transmitting yellow fever will be destroyed within a month." Yellow fever was subsequently found aboard the cruiser *Boston,* but Minister Barrett, at Panama, assured the State Department there was "not a single case of the disease among the employees on the canal."

The notices continued to worsen. By January 22, newspapers reported unofficial advices from the zone indicating yellow fever cases were increasing and speculating on the probability of an epidemic. Blame for the outbreak was "placed on the Canal Commission by those who know

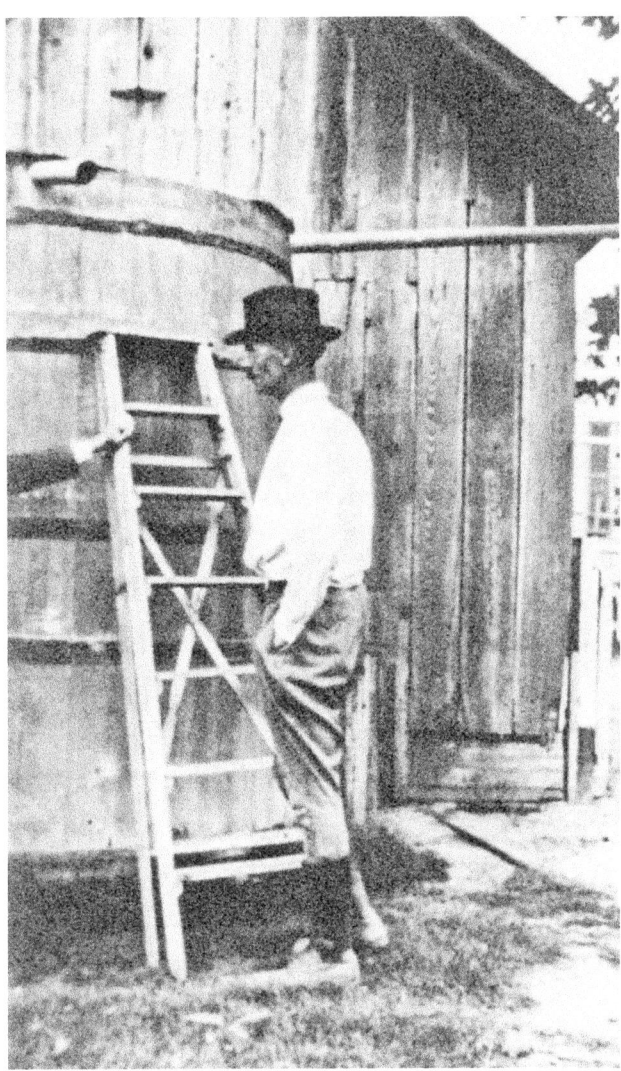

Senior Sanitation Engineer J.A. LePrince, wearing a field uniform, inspects a large rain barrel for signs of mosquito infestation, Robstown and Corpus Christi, Texas (courtesy National Library of Medicine).

the methods used by the commission in dealing with the doctors and sanitary experts.... In addition to the lack of proper sanitary arrangements, the commission refused to make appropriations sufficient properly to protect canal workers from the mosquitoes."

Gorgas returned to Panama on June 5, 1905, aboard the SS *Allianca.* Accompanying him were Dr. Henry R. Carter, Dr. John Ross, Major James Turtle, two additional physicians, a sanitary engineer and a head nurse. Realizing there was a great deal more work to be done, Gorgas requested more workmen from the commission. The request was denied. He then cabled his superiors in Washington but was chastised for the expense and advised to make all future requests by mail. What was more frustrating, the governor of the zone, George Davis, ignored the scientific revelations discovered in Cuba and was quoted as saying, "A dollar spent on sanitation is like throwing it into the Bay."

John Wallace, chief engineer, resigned and was replaced by John Frank Stevens, who arrived in the zone on July 26, 1905. He was credited with shoring up the infrastructure, helping to improve sanitation in Panama and Colon and recruiting workers for the project. Watching from a distance in 1906, those in the United States read headlines such as "Waiting for the Dirt to Fly at Panama" and "Uncle Sam's Big Ditch." A reporter from the *New York Times* wrote, "[T]he efforts of Col. Gorgas and the Sanitary Department to eradicate it completely from the Isthmus have been absolutely necessary and worthy of all praise. While I am not sanguine as to believe that there will never be another case on the zone, it is evident that the danger from this cause is slight, and that if the present careful supervision is continued a serious epidemic is improbable."

With sanitary matters under control, Theodore Roosevelt became the first sitting president to travel outside the United States when he visited Panama in November 1906. Extreme precautions were taken to ensure that neither he nor his wife was exposed to yellow fever. Although there had been no recently reported cases of the disease, the party

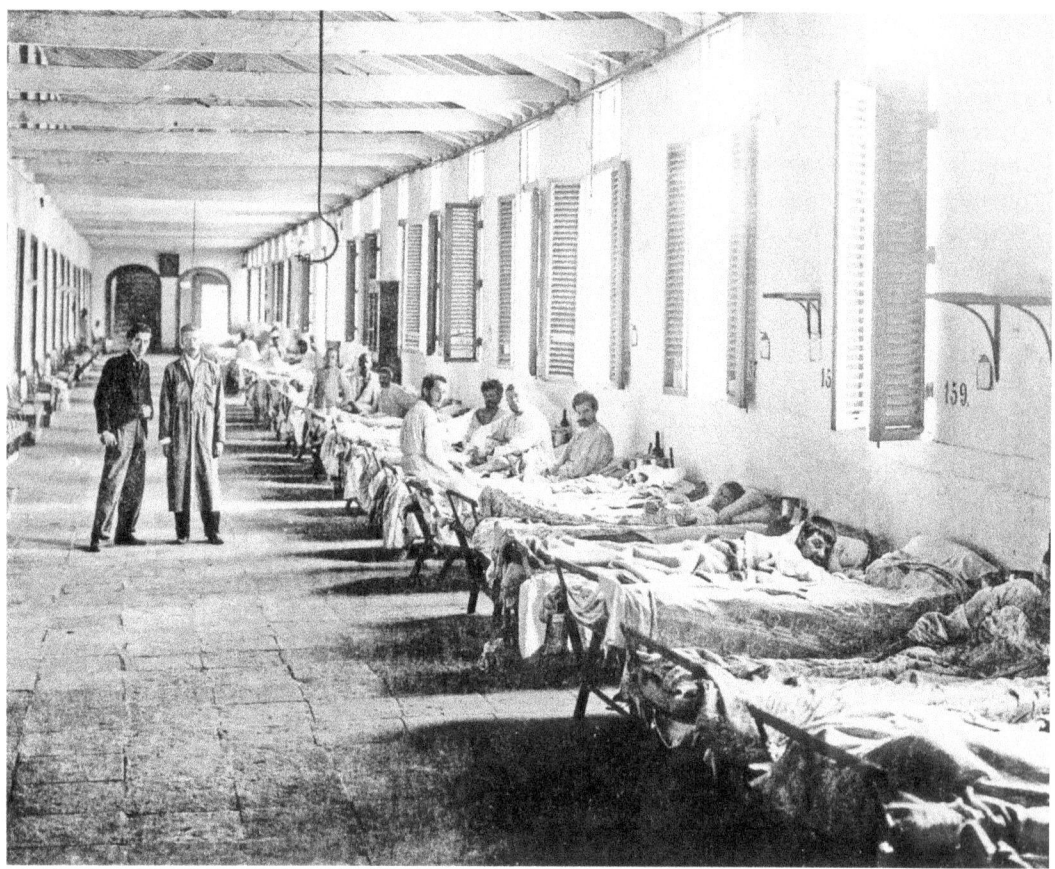

Yellow fever was, and continues to be, a deadly disease flourishing in tropical climates where the *Aedes albopictus* mosquito thrives. Hundreds of preventatives and "cures" were tried, but mortality was staggeringly high. Despite the advances in medicine, sick wards such as the one depicted here continued to be known as death houses (Library of Congress).

headquarters at the Hotel Tivoli was completely enclosed in mosquito netting. But, "if by ill luck the President is bitten by one of the insects carrying the fever germ the physicians at hand will immediately employ heroic measures to eradicate all trace of the infection. However, the proverbial Roosevelt luck and the President's splendid physique are counted upon to constitute the best preventatives."

It was likely that Dr. Gorgas was not one to hold that last sentence to heart, but he had become a hero to the American people. On December 31, 1906, under the heading "Won Victory at Panama," an article in the *Goshen* (IN) *Times* announced that the greatest achievement in Panama was the eradication of yellow fever: "It was not an easy task, but still one about which clings a romance of successful endeavor. Fully 4,000 men were employed in this campaign for freedom from a dread disease, and they had behind them an appropriation of $2,000,000. Science and money, working together, have proved an all-powerful combination." The story might have added that through Gorgas's dedication and determination he was able to achieve success over the doubts of Admiral Walker, Governor Davis and those on the Isthmian Canal Commission who had doubted from the start that mosquitoes were the vector through which yellow fever was spread or that sanitation efforts were the tool through which they could be combatted.

In June 1907, at the graduation exercises of Cornell University Medical College, Gorgas offered his own opinion: "I am inclined to think that the advances made in recent years in tropical sanitation will have a much wider and more far reaching effect than freeing Havana from yellow fever or enabling us to build the Panama Canal. I think that sanitation can now show that any population coming into the tropics can protect itself against disease by measures that are both simple and inexpensive." Gorgas called the February 1908 health report on Panama the most favorable the health department had been able to make. Such success at Panama "may do more than furnish a great new trade route to the world and remain a monumental engineering work. It has already aroused the wonder of South America at the possibilities of sanitation and is apt to be quite as much use in that direction as it will be to the trade of the world." (Sanitation efforts also made possible the work of August Busck, a "government bug hunter" who secured the larvae of 83 species of "skeeter" in Panama, of which 30 species were new to science.)

In July 1908 William Gorgas was recognized by his profession when he was elected to the presidency of the American Medical Association and in August a special commission composed of James Bronson Reynolds, Samuel B. Donnelly and Henry Beach Needham reported to President Roosevelt that "the terrible scourge of yellow fever, against which the French struggled in vain, the filthy and pest breeding state of the principal Panamanian towns, the rough labor camps and pioneer hardships of the first two eras have been eliminated through the brilliant and persistent activities of the department of sanitation, the department of municipal engineering and the building department. Today we find yellow fever driven from the Isthmus, the deadly Stegomyia mosquito thus rendered innocuous, malaria and pneumonia greatly reduced and a high average of health established."

On January 7, 1914, the *Alexandre La Valley* became the first vessel to make a complete circuit of the Panama Canal under its own power. On April 1 the Isthmian Canal Commission ended operation. William Gorgas redirected his efforts to fight pneumonia in the South African gold mines and later became surgeon general of the Army. The price for the Panama Canal under the occupation of the United States was stiff: the total cost amounted to approximately $10,000,000. More than 75,000 men and women worked

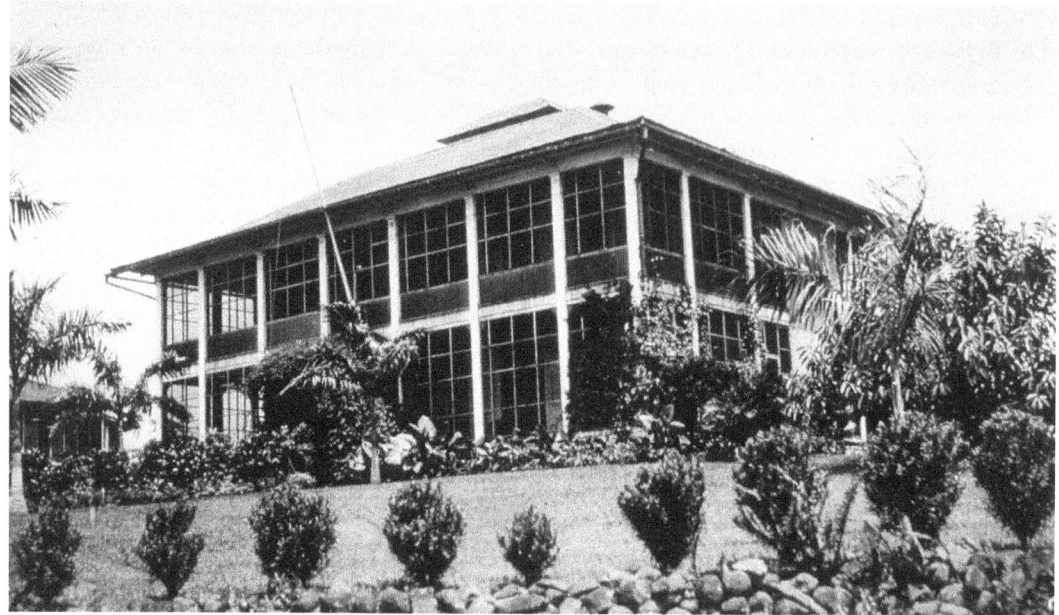

This building is most likely the headquarters of the Mosquito Control Unit in Panama, circa 1910 (courtesy National Library of Medicine).

on the project and, according to hospital records, 5,609 workers died from a combination of disease and accidents.[4]

As a sad yet somehow fitting footnote to the Panama Canal, on August 20, 1915, Dr. Charles Finlay died from what was described as "senile debility." In recognition of his work on yellow fever, the Cuban government took charge of his funeral and the body lay in state for several days. One of numerous United States obituaries stated, "Thirty years ago, Dr. Finlay made tentative and practically conclusive demonstration of the cause [of yellow fever]. He 'took it' himself; he showed how it worked in the cases under his supervision. And today, in the triumph of sanitation of the Panama Canal region there is to be seen the result of the application, in effective form, of the discovery of this physician and investigator of conditions existing in our tropical possessions."[5]

The canal was a technical marvel, sanitation miracle and economic asset, and on September 7, 1977, President Jimmy Carter made a bold political move by signing the Torrijos-Carter Treaty, starting the process that would rightfully return control of the canal to Panama. In both a poetic and scientific sense, "Book One" of a two-part series on yellow fever came to a close on December 31, 1999, when the final turnover of the Panama Canal to the Panama people took place. Humanity had marched from the gloom and fear of mystery and superstition through the illumination of international cooperation and discovery into a new era where a mighty foe had been identified, confronted and controlled. But what remained in 1914 was to actually *see* the yellow fever virus, cure those who suffered from the disease and ultimately wipe this insensate enemy off the books of human misery.

Despite the optimism of the late 18th and the early 19th centuries, the figurative "Book Two," although filled with advances and optimism, contains dire threats for the future. Although yellow fever remains "controlled," that measure of comfort pertains to

North Americans. The disease lives on in Central and South America, where the very real danger of global warming threatens to expand its influence. Of potentially greater concern is the possibility that terrorists may use yellow fever as a biological warfare weapon of mass destruction. For today and for all the tomorrows one can predict, yellow fever remains without the final *finis*.

Chapter 33

"America to Slay the World's Disease Germs"[1]

> *Take a newspaper of a decade or so ago and read about the terrible scourge of yellow fever. Note how all of the clothing of the infected persons was burned, how the gutters and sewers were flushed with disinfectants, how even buildings were burned because of the fact that deaths had occurred in them from the terrible "black vomit." Then note how it always disappeared upon the approach of frost. And all these precautions being taken were useless. It was a little thing that spread the disease. The yellow fever mosquito, almost too insignificant an insect to be cared for. But in an epidemic of yellow fever today [1909] the first thing is to destroy the mosquito, and when that is done the fever is gone.*[2]

"The complete eradication of epidemic disease from the world is entirely possible by eliminating conditions which favor them, according to Major General William C. Gorgas, whose work in cleaning up the Panama Canal zone gives authority to his words," proclaimed the *Ogden Standard* on August 14, 1915. As news spread around the country that Gorgas had been engaged by the Rockefeller foundation to undertake a campaign to stamp out yellow fever wherever it existed, Americans rejoiced. As the Rockefeller Foundation, under the auspices of its mission statement "to promote the well-being of mankind throughout the world," had already been praised for its work on the global effort to eradicate hookworm, its treatment of war-related problems in Belgium, Serbia, Poland, Germany and China, as well as its efforts to stamp out typhus fever, this added task seemed no less impossible.

In explaining its newest quest, the Rockefeller Foundation announced, "The opening of the Panama Canal has wrought radical changes in trade relations. Countries and ports between which there has been little or no exchange are to be brought into close relation. Pest holes of infection that have been relatively harmless are going to be on or near the world's highway of commerce and travel." Gorgas wasted no time. As chairman for the Yellow Fever Commission constituted by the International Health Board of the Rockefeller Foundation, his initial itinerary included Caracas, Venezuela, and then Colon, Panama. After crossing the isthmus, he was to sail down the west coast of South America making a number of stops, especially at Guayaquil, Ecuador, one of the chief points where the fever prevailed. Leaving in June 1916, the commission returned to New York in September.

Gorgas's report, released in December 1916, stated that the commission found yellow fever at Guayaquil, the chief port of Ecuador, a town of 50,000 people. He noted the governments of Ecuador and Brazil had consented to have American physicians work to stamp out the disease. Noting that the mosquito could retain the poison from a yellow fever patient for 55 days, he optimistically added, "When it is known finally that for two months' time there has been no patient from whom it is possible for the mosquito to get a supply of poison, all danger of the spread of the disease or of its springing anew is passed, and dreaded Yellow Jack finally will be put into his grave."[3] The news continued to be positive. Dr. Juan Guiteras, Cuban director of sanitation who had worked with Gorgas for the Rockefeller Foundation, stated in February 1917, "Yellow fever is ended within the world. I only found one center of infection of this disease at Guayaquil, Ecuador. Brazil is cleaned of it, or practically so. Its existence in Venezuela, Colombia, Porto [sic] Rico or Trinidad could not be proved."

In June 1918, however, an epidemic was reported at Guatemala and Drs. Joseph H. White and M.E. Conner were sent to the scene. In November there were 75 cases and in December the number rose to 87. But after they organized an "energetic campaign" the numbers were reduced to 72 in January 1919, to 42 in February, to 13 in March, and to 2 in April and May. Mindful that more research needed to be done, in July 1918 Gorgas gave Guiteras full authority under the International Health Board of the Rockefeller Foundation to seek out further seedbeds and eradicate the disease. The foundation's proposed expenditures for 1918 in relation to hookworms, malaria and yellow fever were placed at $1,076,000. Unfortunately, the full work of the Yellow Fever Commission was delayed due to World War I. By November 25, 1918, George E. Vincent, president of the Rockefeller Foundation, announced that the cessation of active warfare in Europe made it possible to resume work on yellow fever, and late in the year a corps of 123 men were put to work destroying stegomyia mosquitoes in Guayaquil. Gorgas himself arrived at Guayaquil in mid–September 1919 and by October, on his return through Panama, he announced only a few isolated cases were left and he expected the disease to "burn itself out" for lack of nonimmune persons. Two months later, while the world celebrated Gorgas's announcement that there was no more yellow fever in the world, "practical science" was heralded as being the savior of mankind.

In its December 1919 report, the Rockefeller Foundation also announced Dr. Hideyo Noguchi, a Japanese-born scientist who had previously received worldwide acclaim for discovering the syphilis spirochete in the brains of those already demented by the disease, had isolated, during work in Guayaquil, "an organism (spirochete) which he named *Leptospira icteroides*," claiming it to be the specific organism of yellow fever. (This name was chosen to distinguish his discovery from *Leptospira icterohemorrhagiae*, the cause of Weil's disease, thought to be identical or closely related to yellow fever.)

Following World War I, Dr. Henry Hanson was asked by the Peruvian authorities to "study sanitary conditions in [the] Province of Lima and the Rimac Valley, with special reference to malaria." Hanson, then with the Army Medical Corps in Panama, accepted and went to Peru in the fall of 1919. While there, Noguchi briefly visited the town of Paita (which Hanson subsequently burned to destroy the rat-infested buildings, thus preventing an outbreak of bubonic plague) to test his Pfeiffer serum meant to cure yellow fever. Hanson described the procedure: "To do this they took blood from a group of people who had had yellow fever within the last few months. The blood of such people is lytic to the bacterium or agent responsible for the disease; which means that when a culture of the organism and blood from such a recovered case is mixed, it causes the etiologic organism to disintegrate, a phenomenon known as bacteriolysis." Noguchi added *L. icteroides* to blood from the recovered victims and observed the destruction of *L. icteroides*. Although further experimentation was needed, there was a "strong feeling" he

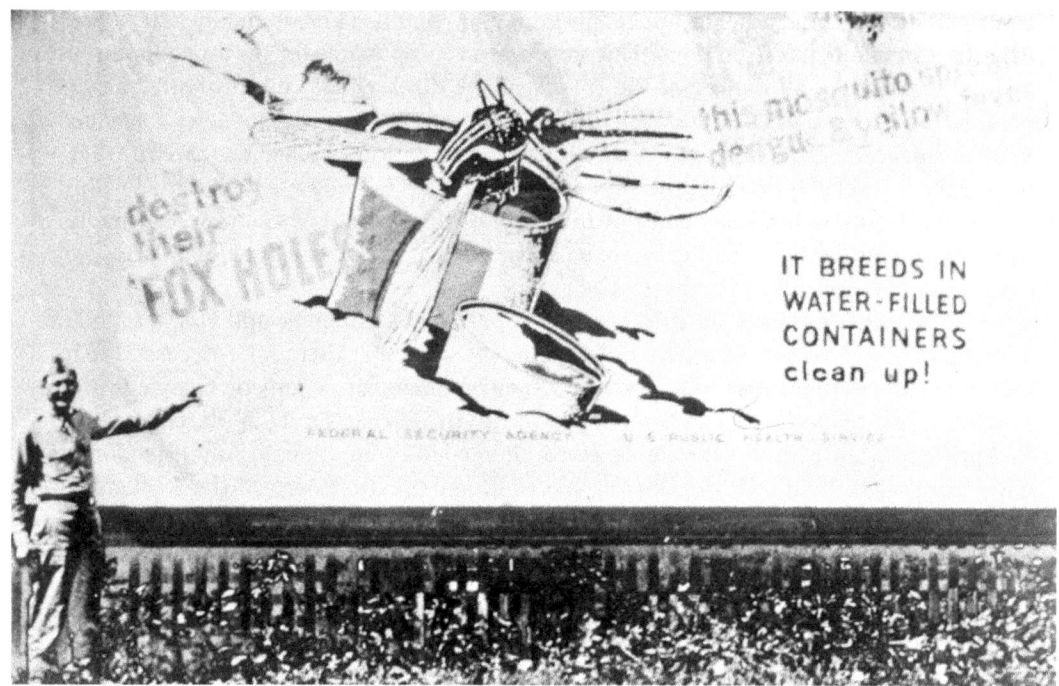

Using a war theme, this billboard goes to the heart of the matter: Destroy mosquitoes carrying yellow fever and dengue in their "fox holes" (courtesy National Library of Medicine).

had "caught" the organism of yellow fever and that "the total disappearance of this dread malady from the earth is predicted for the near future." By December 4, 1919, headlines proclaimed yellow fever was "the first of the great diseases to suffer extirpation."

The claim that yellow fever was caused by a bacterium was directly opposed to the work of the Walter Reed Commission. In 1902 James Carroll announced that the agent that caused yellow fever could pass through a bacteria-proof filter, therefore determining it was smaller than a bacterium. Notwithstanding the contradiction, Dr. Gorgas coauthored a paper in 1920 declaring, "The brilliant work of Noguchi in discovering the organism causing yellow fever already is having some effect on the control of the disease." That point was stressed at the American Association for the Advancement of Science conference held in St. Louis in January 1920. A month later, Noguchi set up an extensive laboratory in the Yucatan for the purpose of studying the origin, prevention and cure of yellow fever, for which he was made an honorary member of the Mexican Academy of Medicine. The Rockefeller Foundation announced in May that Noguchi's serum had cured a member of the Mexican Ministry and had thereby "opened the way for work in Mexico by the foundation."[4]

While this good news from Mexico was being celebrated, a deadly attack of "yellow jaundice" was discovered on the Gold Coast Colony of western Africa known as the "White Man's Grave." Preliminary reports in March 1920 left it uncertain whether this disease was a form of yellow fever or not, prompting the foundation to send Gorgas to investigate. He noted that the disease was "believed to be a heritage from the days of the slave traffic" and "thought to have been introduced by the slave traders carrying the infected mosquitoes over from the West Indies."

Ironically, when Dr. George Vincent announced the trip, he added, "Dr. Gorgas would probably live to see the final chapter in the fight against yellow fever written." Sadly, Gorgas suffered a stroke on the trip and was transported to London. On June 8, during a visit to Milbank Hospital, King George bestowed upon him the insignia of Knight Commander of the Order of St. Michael and St. George in recognition of his service to the British Empire and "making possible the construction of the great canal." Reports to the contrary, William Gorgas did not recover and died in the early morning of July 3, 1820.[5]

The Yellow Fever Vaccine

On December 10, 1920, the *New York Times* promoted the Noguchi serum by advising travelers to South and Central America to get his vaccine, noting "the efficacy of the vaccine seems to be thoroughly established." This vaccine and antiserum, both manufactured by the Rockefeller Foundation, became immediately popular and was used extensively in the United States, Latin America and French African colonies.

During the next five years Noguchi published successful results on 7,964 vaccinations but investigators were unable to duplicate his findings. Suspicions grew about his "sloppy statistics," the easy filterability of the causative agent (bacteria) and the inability to infect laboratory animals. But it was not until 1926 that Max Theiler and Andrew Watson Sellards demonstrated the *L. icteroides* was serologically identical with *L. icterhemorrhagica*. That fact proved Noguchi had been incorrect and the Rockefeller Foundation discontinued use of the vaccine. The Rockefeller foundation established the second West African Yellow Fever Commission in 1925 with four goals: "to learn the characteristics and epidemiology of yellow fever in West Africa and its relationship to the fever in the Western Hemisphere; to attempt the isolation of the organism that causes the disease; to discover the method of transmission; and to identify those areas in which the disease is continually present."

Dr. Henry Beeuwkes, a Johns Hopkins–trained bacteriologist and a retired United States Army colonel whose background was in fighting typhoid and cholera in Russia, was placed in charge. He was assisted by Adrian Stokes, a London-based professor of pathology. They established headquarters and a laboratory in Yaba, near the capital city of Lagos, Nigeria. On seven and a half acres the study group built an office, lab, animal house, two dorms and a staff house. The headquarters provided a central locale that would be used as a "field program with a rotating staff" among the Nigerian population of "approximately 99,000 Africans and 1,000 British."

After two years of work, in June 1927, a 28-year-old African named Asibi (from the Gold Coast, now Ghana), who was suffering from a relatively mild case of yellow fever, had blood drawn by Dr. Alexander F. Mahaffy. Asibi's blood was injected into two different species of monkey and two guinea pigs. The *Macacus rhesus* monkey (imported from India) proved susceptible, establishing, for the first time the transfer of this infection into a suitable (animal) laboratory host. Significantly, the commission proved that the "agent of yellow fever passed through a Berkefeld filter," confirming James Carroll's work that the agent was smaller than a bacteria.

Tragically, death seemed to haunt the commission. Three months after their initial success, Adrian Stokes contracted yellow fever and died on September 19, 1927. The same year, Dr. Noguchi arrived in November, hoping to confirm his *leptospira* theory, which Stokes had already disproved. This caught the attention of the newspapers, which noted that the bacteriologist from the Rockefeller Foundation had gone to Nigeria "to introduce the vaccine and serum he has perfected. The treatment was successfully used by the French last summer in treating yellow fever in Senegal."

Noguchi's techniques were described as "haphazard" and "careless," and his "secretive" behavior added to the tension of those conducting extremely dangerous work. Disaster struck again when Noguchi contracted yellow fever and died May 21, 1928. In one obituary it was written, "Before he died he had made a serum from his own blood that was successful in immunizing animals and men." The newspaper concluded that he added his name "to the list of those who have died for the cause of science and to improve the condition of the human race." The investigator, William Young, who performed Noguchi's autopsy, also contracted the disease and died.[6]

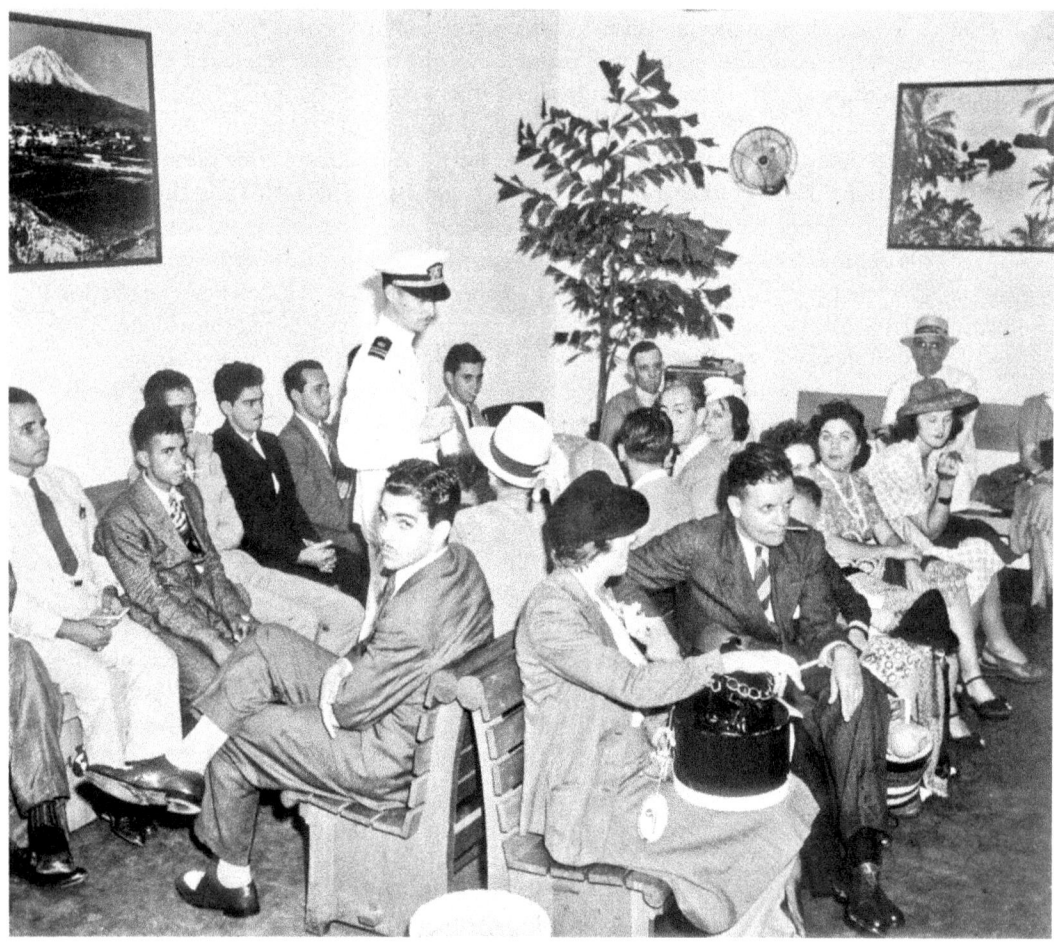

In an effort to control the importation of yellow fever sufferers into the United States, overseas passengers were checked for symptoms of the disease by registering their temperatures, one of the first and easiest-to-identify symptoms. In this photograph, many of the quarantined passengers from Latin America have thermometers in their mouths. Checking them is a Public Health Service officer wearing his summer whites (courtesy National Library of Medicine).

In April 1931, delegates from 14 Latin American nations met at the Second Pan-American Health Conference to discuss recommendations on yellow fever and aerial transmission of the disease. In a letter greeting the delegates, President Herbert Hoover noted that their work would "have a profound effect throughout the world." In tracing the progress of this and other conferences, Hoover added that many pestilences in the American republics have been "robbed of the power for harm." The consensus of attendees was that aerial (airplane) transportation of infectious diseases posed the greatest threat to the Western Hemisphere, while Dr. Frederick Russell of the Rockefeller Foundation added this gloomy observation: "There is no vaccine for yellow fever and all attempts to make one have failed." He added, "As a new generation grows up, it will have no immunity. Twenty years may pass without an outbreak and then a country may have a frightening epidemic."

Despite, or because of, Russell's warning, work progressed at a literal fever pitch. Traveling to Dakar, Senegal, Andrew Sellards learned of the success of the West African Commission in transferring the yellow fever germ to rhesus monkeys. Teaming with Constant Mathis, director of the local Pasteur Institute, and Jean Laigret, the sanitation expert, the team handled the yellow fever outbreak there. Laigret took a sample of blood from a youth named Francois Mayali and transfused it into a rhesus monkey, succeeding in bringing on an acute case of yellow fever. This virus was subsequently referred to as the "French strain," while the other notable virus was referred to as the "Asibi strain," identified by the Rockefeller team.

Further work by Sellards' group revealed that the virus survived freezing, allowing it to be transported in liver tissue rather than in monkeys. The next breakthrough came when Max Theiler succeeded in inoculating mice intracerebrally, finding the virus grew well: "More important, with multiple passages, while there was an increase in neurotropism, there was diminished hepatic damage and systemic illness ('viscerotropism') when given back to rhesus monkeys." This became the first attenuated strain. Theiler contracted yellow fever while working on the process but fortunately survived.

The International Health Division (IHD) of the Rockefeller Foundation, under the directorship of Simon Flexner, appointed Wilbur Sawyer as head of a new laboratory and Theiler left Harvard to join the team. He was well aware of the danger (the 1931 report from the IHD indicated 32 cases of acquired yellow fever in eight laboratories and 5 deaths) and knew the need to protect laboratory and field workers was acute. "Because of concern over inducing an encephalitis, the [Rockefeller] virus was combined with immune human serum obtained from recovered laboratory staff." Dr. Bruce Wilson of the IHD was the first person given the vaccine/serum. He suffered no ill effects and it was then tried on others. Serum obtained from these subjects was then given to mice (a technique developed by Theiler and called the "mouse protection test") and it protected them against infection. This serum became the standard used by the Rockefeller Foundation.

Following a similar path, Laigret and Sellards went to the Pasteur Institute in Tunis, where they experimented with their mouse brain vaccine. Preparing a vaccine from mouse brain cultures using the French strain but without the human serum, they created an attenuated virus. They began with a three-dose regimen using virus dried for varying periods but found systemic and neurologic reactions. The next method was to "coat the virus particles with oil or egg yolk and freeze-dry the mixture, creating a fine powder of coated virus particles" that could be reconstituted in saline and given as a single dose.

This was important, as it could be administered by the scarification method (as oppose to injection), allowing it to be administered as a combined smallpox–yellow fever vaccine. The attenuated but neurotropic French strain, passed more than 100 times in mouse brains, was put out for trial.

On October 1, 1934, the discovery of a vaccine against yellow fever was announced to the French Academy of Science by Professor Charles Nicolle, director of the Pasteur Institute at Tunis. Experiments carried on by Dr. Jean L'Aigret of the Tunis Pasteur Institute had been extended into the French-African possessions, where 5,000 vaccinations had already been so successfully completed the governor general made them obligatory. The report from three physicians declared, "[O]ne of the most terrible curses of tropical regions for the white man has been vanquished."

At this point there were two vaccines being offered. The Rockefeller vaccine was used in the Western Hemisphere and England, while the Pasteur Institute one-dose combined vaccine was used in France and its African colonies. Ultimately, the "French strain" was linked to "a high incidence of encephalitic reactions in children," which "led to its use in children under 10 years being stopped in 1961." Its manufacture was ultimately discontinued.[7]

The 17D Strain

In May 1932 Dr. W.A. Sawyer of the Rockefeller Foundation announced researchers had discovered an antitoxin against yellow fever: "The serum, made from a strain of virus developed in mice together with some immune serum from persons who have recovered from the malady, constitutes the new vaccine, and in at least six cases it has proved effective.... The discovery that yellow fever could be introduced into mice provided the means of reproducing a mild form of the disease and what appears a successful immunization.... The development of an anti-toxin may make yellow fever as much of an anachronism as smallpox."

The same year, attempting to eliminate concerns over neurologic reactions, Theiler and Eugene Haagen "succeeded in cultivating yellow fever virus in both mouse and chicken embryo tissue. But extensive passages of both the Asibi and the French strains failed to affect their neurotropic tendency, so a strategy of dissecting out the nervous tissue from the chick embryos was adopted." At the 100th subculture of the Asibi strain in nervous tissue-deprived embryo, Hugh Smith observed the virus had passed the acid test: failing to kill mice when injected intracerebrally. The team subsequently discovered the attenuation was the result of a chance mutation that proved to be safe and immunizing. This breakthrough, used without the protective immune serum, was called 17D. According to the Rockefeller foundation, 17D was developed in three stages.

Development of the 17D Vaccine

(1) Small-scale vaccination with a "living virus, derived from a strain first transferred from man to monkey and thence to mice, was employed with immune human serum. This prevented disease in the lab and the field but was not feasible for large-scale use.

(2) Vaccination with a "virus strain cultivated in tissue culture" which required the use of immune serum to reduce its virulence.

(3) 17D, a "modified virus strain of exceedingly low virulence which could be used without any immune serum whatever."

Also in May 1932, Dr. Bolivar J. Lloyd, medical director of the United States Public Health Service, made a startling announcement before the American Medical Association in New Orleans. He advocated the use of condemned criminals for experimentation of the yellow fever vaccine. If the criminals should survive the experiment, he favored their pardon, contending that "in view of the relative immunity of criminals and gangsters both in and out of court, the releasing of a few more would not matter very much." He went on to volunteer himself for testing but qualified the offer by saying he would participate only if he could obtain sufficient life insurance to protect his family "in case of any untoward result."

Other unwelcome news the Public Health Service was the threat of commercial air travel between the United States and Central and South America. Not unlike the dilemma officials encountered when steamers replaced sailing vessels, lowering the time it took infected passengers to reach distant shores, airplanes virtually eliminated the wait period, so that a passenger leaving an infected locale might feel well on departure but could arrive in the U.S. only to develop the disease days later. The other scenario involved the mosquito as a stowaway on airlines.

In 1936 the basis of insect spray at the time was pyrethrum, found in kerosene. Considered harmless to humans, low concentrations were effective against *Aedes aegypti*. The disadvantage was that the insecticide was highly flammable, making it inappropriate for airplanes. Consequently, Drs. C.L. Williams and W.C. Dreesen developed a noninflammable carbon tetrachloride as a substitute. When this proved irritating to human respiratory systems, a mixture of both was developed. The fear that mosquitoes might still be present in the wings and fuselage and escape once the plane landed suggested the old and disruptive idea of quarantine. In order to avoid that whenever possible, once the insecticide was sprayed the plane was vacuumed. If more than one mosquito was found on ten planes of any one airline, the company was issued a warning by the Public Health Service to do a better job of mosquito killing. If mosquitoes were persistently discovered, passengers and cargo would be held for "search and destruction"—presumably of the insects. Keeping infected passengers out of the country proved to be a harder task. To avoid catastrophe, the United States, Great Britain and nearly two dozen other countries signed the International Sanitary Convention Act, agreeing to keep persons from yellow fever areas under surveillance before they boarded a plane and for long enough after to determine whether or not they had yellow fever.

In 1937 Hugh Smith took 17D to Brazil for a large-scale trial. Because animals had been found to be susceptible to yellow fever, thus eliminating the possibility of eradication, the only hope of preventing wide-scale epidemics was in containing small outbreaks. To do this required an immune population and that could be achieved by vaccination. The newly developed technique of culturing virus in embryonated eggs and freeze-drying them was used.

On March 22, 1938, the Rockefeller Foundation announced the development of this new yellow fever vaccine. The report disclosed that scientists had found "yellow jack was running rampant in South American jungles. The startling fact appeared that the jungle fever needed no mosquitoes to spread its ravages. This was a new fact in medicine, and was accepted as an immediate world menace." The report confirmed that 40,000 persons in South America had already been vaccinated within the past year. That number soon reached 59,000 individuals who were vaccinated with 17D without severe complications. By June 1939 the total reached 1.3 million people, again without problems. Smith took his field operation to Colombia and conducted another successful program.

The cycle, however, was not yet complete. Beginning in 1937 delayed cases of jaundice were detected in England and Brazil. The small amount of human serum, used as a protein source to provide stabilization during filtration, was suspected as the cause. The use of this serum was abandoned in Brazil and the matter appeared to be resolved. This was followed, in July 1941, by 119 cases of encephalitis identified in Brazil, all of which were traced to one lot of vaccine. It was concluded that an unfavorable mutation had occurred during the manufacture of these subcultures. Consequently, researchers developed the concept of the "seed lot" system whereby "master seeds" were created from parent strains and kept frozen for future use, thus eliminating extra subcultures. At the 1944 International Sanitary Convention for Aerial Navigation, the 17D vaccine was approved, followed by the French vaccine administered by scarification.

Dr. Max Theiler became the first (and to date, only) "yellow fever" scientist to win the Nobel Prize, which he received in 1951 for the development of 17D. The Rockefeller Foundation's work on yellow fever ultimately lasted almost forty years, with 75 staff members involved in the various projects. The foundation spent over $14 million and lost six researchers in the process, including William A. Young, Paul A. Lewis and A. Maurice Wakeman.[8]

The Threat of Biological Warfare

The danger from biological warfare grew with the development of microbiology that began with Louis Pasteur and Rudolph Koch, "because it allowed agents to be chosen and designed on a rational basis." In 1874 in Brussels and again in 1899 in The Hague, two international declarations were created prohibiting the use of poisoned weapons. However, these were little more than gentlemen's agreements, containing no way for countries to ascertain whether or not the rules were being adhered to. Of note, the only dissenting vote was the United States representative, Naval Captain Alfred Mahan, who protested "it is illogical and not demonstrably humane to be tender about asphyxiating men with gas, when all were prepared to admit that it was allowable to blow the bottom out of an ironclad at midnight, throwing four or five hundred men into the sea, to be choked by water, with scarcely the remotest chance of escape."

Threat became reality in World War I when the German army developed both chemical and biological weapons. The first chemical attack came on April 22, 1915, when chlorine gas was used against French and Algerian troops at the Belgium city of Ypres. Haze from the German trenches, first blue-white, then yellow-green, blew over the terrain to a height of six feet, settling over "every depression in the landscape." French soldiers emerged from the cloud, "running wildly, and in confusion" and ultimately blinded and choked from the poison. All who breathed the gas were killed within a matter of minutes. A month later the Germans released 264 tons of chlorine gas along a 12-kilometer line southeast of Warsaw. Before the war ended, more than 200 chemical attacks were documented, producing an estimated 1.3 million casualties. The Germans also used biological weapons, particularly anthrax and glanders, although on a limited and relatively ineffective manner.

Although having refused to sign The Hague agreement, the United States had no chemical warfare experts and after entering the World War I military experts acknowledged it would take "several months" before troops could be issued defensive gas masks and gear. At war's end, peace treaties prohibited the importation or manufacture of poisonous or other gases. In 1925 the Geneva Protocol stated, in part, "Whereas the use in war of asphyxiating, poisonous or other gases, and all analogous liquids, materials or devices, has been justly condemned by the general opinion of the civilized world [the signees agree to prohibit] such use, accept this prohibition, agree to extend this prohibition to the use of bacteriological methods of warfare and agree to be bound as between themselves according to the terms of this declaration." The concept was high-minded but did not prove a defense against reality. After the bombing of Pearl Harbor, the United States feared Japan, which it had reason to believe had covertly researched yellow fever as a means of warfare, would launch a biological attack on its shores. Suspected targets were California, the Midwest and the South, as well as overseas areas where there was likely to be ground combat.[9]

Dr. Karl F. Meyer, University of California bacteriologist and member of the United States Public Health Services' National Advisory Committee, disclosed on December 6, 1940, that half of the growing army was being prepared for service in tropical regions by inoculation against yellow fever, without mentioning the only yellow fever vaccine available was not licensed for civilian use in the United States. The country, he continued, was bolstering its health defenses by establishing a laboratory at Hamilton, Montana, which would produce vaccines against typhus and yellow fever on a huge scale. To aid the effort to stem epidemics in Europe, the United States was rushing 1,000,000 doses of influenza vaccine to England and in excess of 1,500,000 doses of yellow fever vaccine to military centers. At that time, Meyer continued, most of the influenza vaccine came from the Rockefeller Institute. The lab at Hamilton was expected to turn out between 500,000 and one million doses a year for treatment of that and yellow fever. Later that month, Americans were told "national defense means that in 1941 attention will be devoted to the health of youth, military and industrial [persons]. Mass production of yellow fever vaccine, for instance, means likely security against exposure to yellow fever areas as defense zones move south."

Following an order from Secretary of War Henry L. Stimson, the War Department prepared to immunize "the whole American Army against yellow fever." (Soldiers who refused to be vaccinated were subject to court-martial, a rule that was initiated during World War I.) Stimson added it would "be the first large-scale vaccination against the tropical disease ever attempted by a military force." Vaccination for soldiers stationed in Panama, Puerto Rico and Caribbean bases began around February 15, 1941. Soon to follow were troops stationed in the Western Hemisphere and all other troops prior to their departure for such regions. Large quantities of the vaccine were made by the U.S. Public Health Service and other medical laboratories in cooperation with the Rockefeller Foundation's International Health Division laboratories, where the vaccine was first developed.

Figures released by the Rockefeller Foundation indicated that during 1941, a total of 959,300 doses were provided for the army; 960,000 for the navy; 3,000 for the Public Health Service; 12,000 for the Virgin Islands; 152,000 for West Africa; 158,000 for South Africa; 1,662,380 for East Africa; 222,000 for India; 100,000 for Brazil and 28,000 for Singapore, a total of 4,260,680 doses, all at no charge. By April 10, 1942, seven million doses had been distributed. This vaccine, still created with serum used as a stabilizer, employed a strain in use in Colombia, as more than 600,000 doses had been given without serious complications.

Biological warfare was also on the minds on many Americans. In an editorial published by the *Port Arthur* (TX) *News* on August 10, 1941, Frank Thone wrote, "There is one army Adolf Hitler's panzers cannot whip. It won't be encircled, cut-off, blitzkrieged. Stuka dive-bombers, giant howitzers and flame-throwers don't dent its armor. It is the army of disease, and when it strikes even the well-oiled Nazi war machine must retreat." After discussing natural diseases, Thone mentioned the threat from yellow fever, noting, "Yellow fever is more likely to become dangerous to our troops if we have to send an army to protect South America, where it still lurks in the jungle." He then expended the idea of disease to a much more ominous threat:

> The specter of bacterial warfare inevitably rears its ghastly head whenever war-pestilences are mentioned.... The idea fascinates but so far no attempt has been made by either side. Fear of reprisals may be one restraining factor, just as it has apparently retarded gas attacks on civilian populations.... Probably, though, the real reason why bacteriological warfare isn't attempted is that it is too difficult to control. Wind shifts sometimes made cloud gas attacks more dangerous to one's own side than to the enemy during World War I. Similarly, the uncontrolled migration of germs could easily backfire against the nation who turned them loose. Until someone discovers or invents a one-way germ, bacterial warfare will remain a two-edged sword, highly hazardous to use.

On July 24, 1942, Stimson held a press conference to announce that 28,585 cases of jaundice had developed among army men between January 1 and July 4, apparently from the yellow fever vaccine. He revealed there had been 62 deaths, a ratio of 1:461 cases. The peak was reached during the week ending June 20, when 2,997 hospital cases were reported, compared with 2,575 cases for the week ending July 4. Of the cases in the six-month period, 24,057 occurred at home and 4,523 abroad. Stimson explained there "appeared to be a long period of incubation before jaundice developed." Thus, considerable time elapsed between the time of the first inoculation and the source of the malady became evident. The change in the serum, which Surgeon General James C. MaGee thought would "eliminate the whole trouble," had been made some time before, "but cases of jaundice continued to develop from the old inoculations." Otherwise, the health of the army was "excellent."

In editorials of July 27 and 30, the *Chicago Tribune* expressed outrage that twenty times as many soldiers had fallen victim to the vaccine as had been wounded to that point in combat and called for an investigation. In response, on July 28 the *Journal of the American Medical Association* came out in defense of the War Department, stating the vaccination of American soldiers to protect them from yellow fever "was warranted." The article added, "The occurrence of 62 deaths and some 28,000 cases of jaundice associated with the vaccination of millions of men is far less serious than would be an epidemic of virulent yellow fever among soldiers sent to the tropical areas in which our army is now engaging the enemy." The editorial added that Stimson "did not state what proportion of those injected failed to develop jaundice. Actually between 2,000,000 and 2,500,000 men have been inoculated." The *Tribune* soon had company. On August 6, 1942, the *Frederick* (MD) *News Post* published an editorial entitled, "Army Jaundice: Disturbing Rumors about an epidemic," in which it stated the following:

> Assurance by the Surgeon General of the Army that the vaccine has been modified to eliminate the trouble is timely, but it will hardly satisfy the people, especially the families of victims of the disease. The American Medical Association did not help matters by defending the Army's health record with

the statement that "its sickness and death rate today are, even with the temporary invalidism associated with the vaccination, far less than those of similar age groups in civilian life."

Since soldiers are picked men, must be in good health to enter the Army, and are under constant medical supervision, their health should be far better than that of "similar age groups in civilian life."

Secretary Stimson's frank confession of the fault is commendable, but Congress should make a complete investigation and report to the people. The Army Medical Corps should welcome a Congressional inquiry and report.

On August 1, 1942, the *El Paso Herald Post* published what amounted to a group admission, stating that "newspapers of the nation have known about the outbreak for some time but withheld the information at the request of Army authorities pending results of the scientific investigation which started when the first cases occurred." In a remarkably thorough description of the process, the article continued: "Contrary to rumors circulating for some weeks, no case of yellow fever has occurred in any of the troops. The sickness was catarrhal jaundice.... Jaundice occurred only in men vaccinated with certain batches of yellow fever vaccine. The vaccine was made from chick embryo pulp which had been suspended in normal human blood serum.... The human blood serum was used because it keeps the vaccine active longer when it is stored before use. The unidentified germ of catarrhal jaundice may have gotten into certain batches of vaccine from this serum." The newspaper gave the date of this change as April 15.

Details obtained by researchers indicated that in March 1942, one hundred cases of jaundice and hepatitis were discovered in army training camps in California soon after yellow fever immunization. They determined that the diluent for the vaccine contained human serum that had not been heat treated. The "albumin was contaminated with a previously unrecognized virus that caused hepatitis [B]." This discovery "helped reveal the differences between hepatitis A (then called "infectious hepatitis") and the newly recognized hepatitis B virus ("serum hepatitis"). The decision to use human serum had been made on the basis that the link between serum and jaundice "was not fully established and there was too little experience using vaccine without serum stabilization to recommend it on so large a scale. The high demand for vaccine required a weekly supply of eight to 10 liters of pooled serum, and procurement of serum was the limiting factor in production." Serum had been collected from medical people at the Johns Hopkins School of Public Health, some of whom, later studies concluded, had prior histories of jaundice. In 1985 a follow-up study interviewed and sero-screened 597 army veterans from 1942. The researchers concluded that hepatitis B caused the outbreak and that approximately 330,000 persons may have been infected.

Immediate action was taken to address the problem. The first and most obvious task was to eliminate serum in the vaccine and the second was to restrict vaccination to those personnel who were to be sent into high-risk areas. Thereafter, the problem was resolved.[10]

Researching Biological Weapons of Mass Destruction

When it became known that Germany had developed quick-kill nerve gases such as tabun and sarin, the United States quickly turned its attention from the suspected but unsubstantiated threat of yellow fever as a biological weapon toward the more immediate danger of nerve gas. President Franklin Roosevelt warned of massive retaliation against German cities if chemical or biological warfare was used against the United States or its troops, and ultimately Germany did not use its massive chemical arsenal. Japan, however, was less intimidated. As early as 1930, the Japanese scientist Shiro Ishii had started biological research at the Tokyo Army Medical School. In 1939 the Japanese attempted legally, and then illegally, to obtain the yellow fever virus from the Rockefeller Institute in New York. Ishii became head of Japan's biological weapons program during World War II, which at its height employed more than 5,000 people and killed as many as 600 prisoners a year during human testing at one center in a single year. Japan tested at least 25 different disease-causing agents, poisoned 1,000 Chinese water wells to study cholera and typhus outbreaks and dropped plague-infested fleas over Chinese cities, in rice fields and along roads.

In the fall of 1941 Secretary of War Stimson requested the National Academy of Sciences (NSA) to investigate the idea of biological weapons for use by the United States. The NSA formed the War Bureau of Consultants, which issued a report in 1942 recommending "the research and development of an offensive biological weapons program." In November that same year President Roosevelt officially approved a U.S. biological weapons program, ordering Stimson to organize the War Research Service (WRS). In the spring of 1943 the U.S. Army Biological Warfare Laboratories were established at Camp (later Fort) Detrick in Maryland. The facility was completed in November and three other facilities—a biological agent production plant at Vigo County near Terre Haute, Indiana; a field-testing site on Horn Island in Mississippi; and another field-testing site near Granite Peak, Utah.

Little was known by the American people about the government's biological warfare (BW) programs. In May 1947 a 40,000-word explanation of BW, published in the *Journal of Immunology* and written in 1942, was released. It contained "all the basic facts, excepting only secret work of World War II." Along with the statement by George Merck (president of the drug company that bore his name and who led efforts to develop poison gases at Camp Detrick) that "the only real defense against bacteriological warfare is peace," the diseases listed as having war possibilities included "rabit [*sic*] fever" (a pneumonia type transmitted by air), the great plague, and melioidosis, a disease that resembled glanders: "Also, anthrax, yellow fever to be transmitted not by mosquitoes, but possibly directly through the air, undulant fever, parrot fever, the tick-borne typhus-like disease, botulinus poisoning ... and maybe malaria." In November 1947 another report surfaced, noting that the army had plans "to protect the civilian population from the two newest and deadliest forms of warfare, atomic and germ attack." Among the diseases capable of being spread by airplane or from guided missiles were anthrax, undulant fever and yellow fever.

Biological weapons are relatively inexpensive to make and use. Two rules for selecting a BW is that it must be highly infective and possess high potency. Due to the fact most BWs are slow to develop, they are less useful for the battlefield and fall under the category of "strategic" or "terrorist" weapons. The process involved is relatively simple and inexpensive: obtain a sample of the microorganisms to be used (the seed culture), cultivate and concentrate the cultures and then add a stabilizer. Yellow fever is among the viruses NATO considers a viable BW.

Yellow fever falls into the category of viral hemorrhagic fevers, under the category of Flaviviridae, a virus that also includes dengue, Kyasanur Forest and Omsk hemorrhagic fevers. Mortality from Flaviviridae ranges from 0.2 percent to 50 percent. Of all the flaviviruses, yellow fever is primarily hepatotrophic. Black vomit caused by hematemesis is common, and victims usually develop clinical jaundice and die from hepatorenal syndrome. Although there are better and more efficient BW choices, yellow fever remains a viable threat because virtually no one outside tropical regions is vaccinated against it, and treatment is primarily supportive, as opposed to medical science possessing a definitive cure.

Biological programs in the United States from 1943 through the end of World War II cost $400 million, while the budget for 1966 alone stood at $38 million. Research and testing in the U.S. continued throughout the Cold War. By the time President Richard Nixon ended the program on November 25, 1969, the U.S and Russia had combined "to produce enough biological weapons to kill everyone on Earth." Nixon's administration "became the world's leading anti-biological weapons voice" and called for an international treaty on the subject. In 1972 the Biological Weapons Convention (BWC) banned the development, stockpile, transfer and use of BWs worldwide. This was the first comprehensive disarmament treaty having as its primary purpose the destruction of existing stockpiles of BWs and the prevention of their proliferation. The 144 signees renounced the right to either use or retaliate in kind against any country using BW. The United States belatedly signed the Geneva Protocol in 1975.

When the U.S. ended its biological weapons program in 1969 it had mass-produced, battle-ready weapons in the form of anthrax, tularemia, Q-fever, VEE and botulism. In addition, staphylococcal enterotoxin B, smallpox, EEE and WEE, AHF, Hantavirus, BHF, Lassa fever, glanders, melioidosis, plague, yellow fever, psittacosis, typhus, dengue fever, Rift Valley fever, CHIK V, late blight of potato, rinderpest, Newcastle disease, bird flu and the toxin ricin had been investigated as weapons.

Is this the end of the threat of biological weapons of mass destruction? It would be naive to think so. Following the Cold War, member countries realized that to strengthen the BWC a process of verification needed to be implemented. After taking office in 2001, President George W. Bush reversed support of these negotiations, destroying any opportunity to institute a legally binding compliance. Furthermore, critics of United States policy claim that the country's interpretation of biological warfare has changed, in that the U.S. now claims Article 1 of the BWC does not apply to nonlethal biological agents. In the Biological Weapons Anti-terrorism Act of 1989, the law defined a biologic agent as follows: "any micro-organism, virus, infectious substance, or biological product that may be engineered as a result of biotechnology, or any naturally occurring or bioengineered component of any such microorganism, virus, infectious substance, or biological product, capable of causing death, disease, or other biological malfunction in a human, an animal, a plant, or another living organism; deterioration of food, water, equipment, supplies, or material of any kind." As of 2009, the Federation of American Scientists considers that United States work on nonlethal agents exceeds limitations set forth in the BWC.

Guidelines have been established for the detection of BW agents.

CRITERIA FOR DETECTING A BIOLOGICAL ATTACK

(1) Disease or strain not endemic
(2) Unusual antibiotic resistance
(3) Atypical clinical presentation or classic presentation of a BW agent
(4) Case distribution geographically inconsistent
(5) Inconsistent elements such as mortality and morbidity rates

INDICATIONS OF A POSSIBLE BIOLOGICAL ATTACK

(1) Disease entity unusual or one that does not occur naturally in a given area
(2) Multiple disease entities in the same patient indicating mixed agents
(3) Large number of civilian and military causalities from the same area
(4) Data suggesting a massive point-source outbreak
(5) Apparent aerosol route of infection
(6) High morbidity and mortality relative to the numbers at risk
(7) Illness limited to a localized geographic area
(8) Low attack rate among persons who work in areas of filtered air or closed ventilation systems
(9) Sentinel dead animals of multiple species
(10) Absence of a compelling natural vector in the area of outbreak

According to a State Department report, more than ten countries are believed to have ongoing BW programs: Russia, Israel, China, Iran, Libya, Syria and North Korea. The only established and FDA-licensed, virus-specific vaccine against any of the VHF viruses is the 17D live-attenuated yellow fever vaccine. It is mandatory for those traveling through endemic areas of South America and Africa.[11]

Chapter 34

Taking Steps Against a Deadly Enemy

Rio De Janeiro: Brazil Links dengue-like virus to birth defects in babies: **November 30, 2015:** *The dengue-like Zika virus has been linked for the first time to cases of babies being born with small heads, or microcephaly, Brazil's government said. It is said scientists studying a surge of such cases in northeastern Brazil found the presence of the virus in the blood of a baby born with birth defects in Ceara state. The girl died.... So far in* **2015** *the ministry has reported 739 cases of babies born with microcephaly in nine states that have been hit hard by Zika infections, while last year the same region had only 45. The same mosquito that carries the dengue virus,* **Aedes aegypti,** *is also responsible for spreading Zika, a disease that until now was known as a mild version of dengue with symptoms such as fever, rash and joint pain. Before Brazil, outbreaks of Zika have occurred in Africa, Southeast Asia and the Pacific Islands. The virus is not found in the United States, but cases of Zika have been reported in returning travelers, according to the CDC.*[1]

In 1943 the United Nations Relief and Rehabilitation Administration (UNRRA) was created to assist nations in post–World War II Europe. Among its functions was to assist in public health matters. One of its prime directives was the oversight of international quarantine. This effort was guided by the regulations established by the International Sanitary Conventions of 1944, which included yellow fever control measures. Among them were rules on quarantining travelers from endemic areas who might have been exposed to the disease that became the precursor of formal yellow fever vaccination requirements. To administer the 1944 rules, it was necessary to create a map of endemic yellow fever areas. The UNRRA assumed this task and created the first official map. As World War II came to an end the World Health Organization (WHO) was organized and quickly formed a Yellow Fever Panel. In 1949 this group modified the yellow fever map and issued its first report, recommending that "measures be applied permanently against arrivals from endemic areas."

WHO authorities drafted the International Sanitary Regulations (ISR) to replace older regulations and these were adopted by the World Health Assembly in 1951. These rules required vaccination against yellow fever by "any person leaving an infected local area on an international voyage and proceeding to a yellow fever receptive area." This was the first "regulatory language that overtly mandated yellow fever vaccination requirements for country entry. The IRS were modified and renamed the International Health Regulations (HR) in 1969. Most recently these were completely revised in 2005 and most clearly demand "vaccination against yellow fever may be required of any traveler leaving an area where the Organization has determined that a risk of yellow fever transmission is present."

In the United States, yellow fever vaccine is given only at designated yellow fever vaccination centers. Those being vaccinated are given an International Certificate of Vaccination. The certificate becomes valid 10 days after vaccination and is valid for ten years.[2]

The Pan American Sanitary Organization and the 17D Vaccine

The Pan American Sanitary Organization was given the responsibility of investigating outbreaks of jungle yellow fever through laboratory testing of dead monkeys from Panama southward to Colombia. An outbreak was first discovered in Panama in 1948. It was learned these individuals had been infected in the forests east of the Panama Canal on the South American side. The infection was determined to be a forest strain spread by mosquitoes that had bitten infected monkeys. Subsequently, the disease was found on both coasts of Costa Rica and southern Nicaragua and Honduras in 1952 and 1953. An emergency vaccination campaign in Nigeria using the French scarification method was employed. But neurologic reactions were evident and for the first time vaccine virus was recovered from affected brain tissue. A similar result was found in cases in Costa Rica and the Congo.

The disease was believed to have died out by September 1954. The final outbreak was in the vicinity of San Pedro Sula, where the river valley had been cleared of forests for the cultivation of bananas. However, by November and December 1955 rumors of dead monkeys from the Puerto Barrios area of Guatemala reached scientists. The reports were confirmed, prompting Dr. Fred L. Soper, director of the Pan American Sanitary Organization, to warn that jungle yellow fever had resumed its northward march, coming "fairly close to the borders of British Honduras and Mexico."

In 1962 a potentially disastrous discovery was made when avian leukosis virus was detected in a seed lot of 17D vaccine in England and shortly after that in the United States: "These viruses, the cause of avian leukosis, displayed oncogenic activity in animals. They were widespread in the fowl population and the eggs used for virus culture.... The challenge was to eliminate the avian virus while keeping additional passages of vaccine virus to a minimum." The British solved the problem by incubating the vaccine with antibody against avian virus and in the United States by ultra-filtration.

Since 1982 the 17D vaccine, presumed clear of all contamination, is manufactured from a small number of seed lots. Two substrains, 17DD and 17D-204, were originally obtained from passage numbers 195 and 204, respectively, at the Rockefeller Foundation. These strains share 99.9 per cent homology. The 17DD vaccine is manufactured in Brazil and used there and in many other South American countries. The 17D-204 vaccine is manufactured and used outside of Brazil, including the United States. Studies indicate the immune responses of both do not differ and thus persons vaccinated with either of these two strains are considered protected against yellow fever. Following yellow fever vaccination the recipient often develops a low-level viremia with the vaccine virus. The viremia usually occurs within 3–7 days and persists for 1–3 days, abating as yellow fever antibodies (YFV IgM) are developed. The level of viremia is high enough to be transmitted through transfusion. A study of 1,440 healthy adults found that males and Caucasians had higher LNI levels when compared with females, blacks and Hispanics. Age did not appear to affect immunologic response. Historically, "the 17D vaccine has been considered to be one of the safest and most effective live viruses ever developed."

In 1985 the complete genome of the virus was published. Further development of the vaccine has been along technical lines, such as greater stabilization to allow for a greater shelf life.[3] The United States Public Health Services' Centers for Disease Control (CDC) declared "war" on the "city slicker mosquito" in 1964, pledging $100 million to eradicate the fearsome yellow fever carrier. This five-year campaign was to be carried out in nine southeastern states, Puerto Rico and the Virgin Islands and was acknowledged to be of "international political significance bearing on the maintenance of friendly relations with Latin America." Explaining the threat, scientists informed the public that yellow fever might recur in the U.S. due to the possibility of unsuspecting yellow fever victims traveling from Central and South America, which still harbored the virus in jungle areas, and the continued presence of the yellow fever mosquito in the U.S., which "constitutes a greater immediate threat to 14 countries in Latin America which have eradicated the mosquito after long campaigns."[4]

Present Impact of Yellow Fever

Yellow fever remains a major health problem today as it is endemic in tropical regions of South America and Africa, where nearly 90 percent of yellow fever cases and deaths occur. In 2009 WHO announced the "Yellow Fever Initiative," targeting nearly 12 million people at risk in Benin, Liberia and Sierra Leone. Supported by WHO, UNICEF, national Red Crosses and Red Crescent Societies, *Medecins sans Frontieres* and other partners, it was hoped "high vaccination coverage [would] prevent outbreaks of yellow fever, a disease that is very difficult to diagnosis in the early stages of infection," according to Dr. William Perea, coordinator of the WHO Epidemic Readiness and Intervention unit. He hoped the vaccination campaign would be carried out throughout all high-risk African countries by 2015.

Vaccination against yellow fever early in life is also a critical goal, Dr. Jean-Marie Okow-Bele, director of the Department of Immunization, Vaccines and Biologicals at WHO, stressed: "Thirty-seven countries in Africa and the Americas have introduced yellow fever vaccine in their routine childhood immunization schedule, up from 12 countries a decade ago." That said, if further funding was not forthcoming, yellow fever, which is "reappearing in countries that have not reported cases in many years," will add to the deadly toll of tragically lost lives.

During the 1990s it was widely publicized that 200,000 persons yearly contracted yellow fever, causing an estimated 30,000 deaths. During the October 2011 Quantitative Immunization and Vaccine Related Research (QUIVER) meeting, it was decided to initiate new modeling techniques to measure the yellow fever disease burden in Africa, work that began in 2012. It did not paint an encouraging picture.

According to this study, it was estimated that yellow fever infected between 840,000 and 1.7 million people in Africa *each year,* resulting in approximately 84,000–170,000 cases and 29,000–60,000 deaths. These numbers are staggeringly higher than previously given and mark the potential for massive tragedy. Even before this study was completed WHO warned, "Recent increases in the density and distribution of the urban mosquito vector, Aedes aegypti, as well as the rise in air travel increase the risk of introduction and spread of yellow fever to North and Central America, the Caribbean, the Middle East, Asia, Australia, and Oceania." As difficult as it is to believe, WHO further stated, "The pathogenesis and pathophysiology of the disease are poorly understood and have not been the subject of modern clinical research." Even more distressing is another statement issued by WHO: "Since the 1980s, epidemics of yellow fever in Africa have affected predominately children under the age of fifteen years. The failure to control yellow fever arises from a misapplication of public health strategies and insufficient political commitment by governments in yellow fever endemic areas, especially in Africa, to control the disease."

Where to go from here? More money and more commitment for control of yellow fever are needed, obviously. WHO recommends that every at-risk country have at least one national laboratory where basic yellow fever tests can be conducted, and it stresses that even one laboratory-confirmed case in an unvaccinated population should be considered an outbreak. Medical teams must then assess and respond to the outbreak with emergency measures and long-term immunization plans.

On an even wider scale is the effect global warming has, and will continue to exert, on the international spread of infectious diseases. Responding to a slight increase in temperatures, the insect population will find a greater range in which to thrive, making it probable that the northern latitudes, as far up as Canada could find the yellow fever mosquito an unwelcome arrival. In 1999 WHO released a warning that not only North America but also Britain and the rest of Europe, where the average temperature has risen by nearly 1 degree centigrade, will see an increase in humidity and rainfall, two prime ingredients in the propagation of *Aedes aegypti*. As James Dickerson wrote in his book, *Yellow Fever*, "Perhaps the best method of determining the effect of global warming on yellow fever is to examine the effect that warmer temperatures are having on related mosquito-borne diseases such as dengue, malaria, West Nile fever, and encephalitis. If they show signs of increased incidence, then it is only a matter of time before the yellow fever virus makes its reappearance."[5]

We must acknowledge that yellow fever and its family of viruses are a legitimate concern. They aren't just relics of a bygone age, synonymous with the 19th century and the Panama Canal. Yellow fever, dengue, Ebola and viruses yet to be discovered pose a real threat to life on earth, as evidenced by the lead paragraph in this chapter. Not until nations fully cooperate and dedicate themselves to peace, research, education and application can the world we live in be truly safe.

Glossary

Definitions are from the Lexicon Medicum; or, Medical Dictionary *(1842) and the* Dispensatory of the United States *(1845) unless otherwise indicated.*

Addison's disease A rare illness marked by gradual and progressive failure of the adrenal glands and insufficient production of steroid hormones.[1]

Alkaline salts Alkalines neutralize acids; the principal alkalines in use are carbonates and sub-carbonates of soda and potassa, the sub-carbonate of ammonia, lime-water, chalk, magnesia and its carbonate.

Ammonia (Muriate of) An alkaline used for neutralizing acidity.

Anodyne Something that relieves pain; a soothing agent.

Antimetic A medicine used to suppress nausea and vomiting.

Antimonials A composition containing antimony.

Antimony A brittle, brilliant metal of a silver-white color when pure but bluish-white as it occurs in commerce. First described by Basil Valentine in the 15th century. It was imported into the U.S. from France, Trieste and occasionally Cadiz; that from France was the most esteemed. Preparations containing antimony were stated to be alternative, diaphoretic, purgative or emetic, according to the dose in which it was given. It was frequently used in fevers for its diaphoretic effect in a dose of 3–8 grains every 3–4 hours, given in the form of a powder or pill. In larger doses it was purgative or emetic.

Antiphlogistic A term applied to those medicines, plans of diet and other circumstances which tend to oppose inflammation, or which, in other words, weaken the system by diminishing the activity of the vital power.

Antiphlogiston regimen Cooling drinks, cool air, cool baths and soft diet, intended to remove all inflammatory stimulus, or inquiline humors, from the body.

Antiscorbutic Medicines which cure scurvy; those considered superior were lemons, limes and molasses.

Antiseptic medicines Those medicines which possess a power of preventing animal substances from passing into a state of putrefaction and of obviating putrefaction when already begun. Such medicines fell into four orders:

Tonic antiseptics: such as cinchona and cusparia, which are suited for every condition of the body and are preferable to other antiseptics for those with relaxed habits.

Refrigerating antiseptics: As acids which are principally adapted for the young, vigorous and plethoric.

Stimulating antiseptics: As wine and alcohol, best adapted for the old and debilitated.

Antispasmodic antiseptics: as camphor and asafoetida, which are to be selected for irritable and hysterical habits.

Apozem   A decoction.

Aquafortis   A weak and impure nitric acid.

Arbovirus   Any of a large group of viruses that multiply in both vertebrates and anthropods such as mosquitoes and ticks. Arboviruses cause diseases such as yellow fever and viral encephalitis.

Aromatic   A term applied to a spicy scent and an agreeable pungent taste such as cinnamon bark and cardamons.

Aromatopola   A druggist; a vender of drugs and spices.

Arrowroot   (Maranta) Early uses consisted of a warm stomachic bitter and generally ordered in bitter infusions but seldom employed by the mid–1800s. After this time it was believed to contain "a greater proportion of nourishment than any other yet known," superior to saga or tapioca. It was made into a jelly and fed to debilitated frames.

Arteriotomy   Cupping.

Athenia   Referring to malaria; a layman's term.

Bark   (Peruvian) See Quinine.

Bleeding   (Blood-letting) This term includes every artificial discharge of blood taken with an aim to cure or prevent disease. Blood-letting was categorized as either general or topical. The former included *arteriotomy* and *venaesection,* while the latter included the application of leeches, cupping-glasses and scarification.

Blisters   (*Vesicatorium;* Epispasticum) Used to increase and strengthen the pulse. A topical application which, when put to the skin, raises the cuticle in the form of a vesicle, filled with a serous fluid (blister).

Bomb-ketch   A ketch was a fore-and-aft rigged vessel; the term bomb-ketch indicated a strongly-built ketch having mortars mounted for use in naval bombardments.

"Broken bone fever"   (also known as "break-bone fever" or "breakbone fever") Benjamin Rush was the first to use "broken bone fever" in 1789 in a report on the 1780 epidemic at Philadelphia. Although these names fell out of use in the 1830s (replaced by Dengue fever) they remained in the popular vernacular. In 1866 broken bone fever was considered one of the most common diseases in Texas and along the Rio Grande. Symptoms included aching from head to toe, making it impossible to find a position of comfort. The duration of the disease was considered "co-equal with that of the yellow fever, of which it is a modified type." Frost put an end to epidemics. When it broke out with violence, this was considered a blessing in that yellow fever never encroached "to much extent upon the region which it may chance to be infecting."[2]

Bulam fever   (Bulam, from the coast of Bulam, in Africa) Yellow fever.

Calculus   Small, sand-like concentrations (gravel, stone) that pass from the kidneys through the ureters.

Calomel   (Hydrargyri Chloridum Mite; mild chloride of mercury) Composed of mercury, sulphuric acid, chloride of sodium and distilled water, reduced by boiling. Calomel united the general properties of the mercurials as a purgative and anthelmintic. It was the most valuable of the mercurial preparations, "and in extent of employment is inferior to few articles of the Materia Medica." It was peculiarly useful in the commencement of bilious fevers, in hepatitis, jaundice, bilious and painters' colic, dysentery, especially that of tropical climates and all other affections attended with congestion of the portal system, or torpidity of the hepatic vessels. In very large doses it is supposed to act as a sedative and with this view, has been given in yellow and malignant bilious fevers. A common dose is 1–2 scruples, repeated ever one half to one hour, or less frequently. In yellow fever, from 20 grains to a drachm have been given but this is justifiable only in cases of extreme urgency. (It was not generally recognized until late in the 19th century that mercury was actually a poison, although early medical literature often offered antidotes to mercury given in excess.)

Calumba (Colombo or colomba root) The root has an aromatic smell, with a pungent and bitter taste. The powder, added to brandy and water, made a pleasant infusion. As a corrector of putrid bile, it was used to treat yellow fever.

Camara polar (Camera; polar chamber) A sanitarium reduced by means of ice to a temperature nearly 40° below the average of the outdoor atmosphere. Popular in the 1880–1890s to cure yellow fever patients.

Camphor Commercial camphor was derived from the *Camphora officinarum* of Nees or *Laurus Camphora* of Linnaeus, an evergreen tree native to the most eastern parts of Asia. Camphor was brought to the United States in the crude state primarily from Canton. It was believed to allay nervous irritations, quiets restlessness and produced a general placidity of feeling. By its moderately stimulating powers, its diaphoretic tendency and its influence over the nervous system it was admirably adapted to the treatment of all diseases of a typhoid character.

Cape stone The topmost stone of a building, associated with Masonic history; the "Cape stone of medical research," thus indicating the highest degree of authority.

Carbolic acid Widely used in the 1800s as a disinfectant against yellow fever but discredited in the late 1870s as failing to prevent the formation or spread of bacteria.

Carbuncle *Anthrax*. A hard and circumscribed inflammatory tubercle like a boil, forming on the cheek, back or neck, and in a few days becoming highly gangrenous. It discharges a highly foetid sanies from under the black core and destroys the surrounding tissue. It was thought to arise from a peculiar miasma and was most common in warm climates and often attended the plague.

Castor emulsion Made with 6 or 8 almonds and one castor nut, stripped of its pellicle and boiled in a pint of water.[3]

Castor oil The oil of the seeds of the *Ricinus communis*. A mild cathartic speedy in its action, usually operating with little gripping or uneasiness.

Catarrh See Influenza.

Chagres fever Named for the river in Panama that cut across the Isthmus where the canal was being dug. It was used interchangeably with yellow fever, described as being "insidious and often fatal years after the victim has left the region."[4]

Chalk Carbonate of lime, found in the South of England and North of France. Prepared chalk was used in the preparation of the alkaline bicarbonates.

Chalybeate A term given to any medicine into which iron enters; a mineral water containing iron.

Chalybeate system Drinking and bathing in iron-rich waters; very popular in the 17th and 18th centuries. The regimen, or "cure," was taken to strengthen digestion and rid the body of impurities.

Chaoalongo A fever specific to Chile.

Charbon Anthrax; a bacterial infection of animals.

Cinchona (Quinine) The bark of a species of Cinchona from the western coast of South America; Peruvian bark. It came into use in the middle of the 17 century; also known as *Jesuits' powder*. It was used to cure intermittent diseases and as a remedy in fever and ague.

Cinnamon water Used as a warm cordial to the stomach, carminative, astringent, chiefly used as an adjuvant to less pleasant medicines, or used with chalk and astringents to stop diarrhea.

Citronella An essential oil obtained from the leaves and stems of the *Cymbopogon* (lemongrass), used in perfumes and as a plant-based insect repellant.

Clyster An enema.

Colluvies A collection of pus or, more generally, of rubbish or odds and ends.

Copperas Sulphate of iron, a disinfectant used for promoting the purity of sinks and drains.

Cordial Medicines which possess warm and stimulating properties given to raise the spirits.

Costive Affected with or causing constipation.

Cream of tartar The popular name of the pulverized super-tartrate of potassa; a cathartic, diuretic and refrigerant. In large doses it produces large, watery stools. It is advantageously used in some febrile affections.

Creosote A volatile oil derived from the distillation of wood, discovered in 1830 by Dr. Reichenbach. It was considered an irritant, narcotic, styptic, antiseptic, and moderately escharotic. Externally, it was used as an ointment for treating wounds and ulcers; it was administered internally for the treatment of diabetes mellitus, epilepsy, hysteria, neuralgia, chronic catarrh and haemoptysis. More commonly, it was use for nausea, vomiting and seasickness. When given in overdose, it acts as a poison.

Croaker A person who spread gruesome details about diseases.

Cupping Topical bleeding. Performed with a scarificator and a cupping glass, the air within the glass rarefied by the flame of a little lamp containing spirit of wine and a thick wick, blood is removed by the suction created. A common medical practice in the 1700s.

Cusparia One of many names for Angustura bark, changed to *Galipea officinalis* sometime before 1845. Its operation is that of a stimulating tonic and in large doses it evacuates the stomach and bowels. However, certain physicians employed it extensively in the treatment of malignant bilious intermittent fevers.

Delirium ferox The mental disturbance noted in the early stages of acute fevers.

Dengue fever (See also Broken bone fever) The term "dengue fever" came into general use after 1828. Dengue is an infectious tropical disease; symptoms include fever, headache, muscle and joint pains, and a characteristic skin rash similar to measles. It is transmitted by several species of mosquito within the genus *Aedes*, principally *A. aegypti*.

Diathesis Any particular state of the body; thus, in inflammatory fever, there is an inflammatory diathesis, and, during putrid fever, a putrid diathesis.

Distemper A vague medical term of the 1600s used to describe any disease not otherwise named, or of an unknown name; a malady

Dysentery (Dysenteria; contagious pyrexia) Symptoms include frequent gripping stools, tenemus, stools chiefly mucus, sometimes mixed with blood. In the 1800s it was described as occurring chiefly in the summer, occasioned by the use of unwholesome and putrid food and by noxious exhalations and vapors.

Effluvia Miasma.

Emetic That which is capable of exciting vomiting.

Empiric Based on observation; subject to verification by observation or experiment. An empiric physician of the 18th and 19th centuries was one who practiced by treating symptoms rather than basing a diagnosis on the classification of disease (nosology), its nature and cause.[5]

Ether (eather; sulphuric aether) A volatile liquor obtained by distillation from a mixture of alcohol and a concentrated acid; when taken internally, the properties are antispasmodic, cordial and serve as a stimulant. Applied externally, it was used for pain relief in toothache and headache.

Extravasation   A term applied by surgeons to fluids that are out of their proper vessels or receptacles. Thus, when blood is effused on the surface, it is said to be an extravasation. Also applied to urine and bile.

Fixed air   Carbonic gas. Carbonic acid gas was considered to be much denser than common air, occupying the lower parts of such mines or caverns as contain materials which afford it by decomposition. Miners called it "choke-damp."

Flux   Another word for dysentery.

Gamboge   (*Stalagmitis*) A concrete vegetable juice from a tree grown in the East Indies, chiefly used as a drastic purge.

Glanders   A contagious infection caused by *pseudomonas mallei* in horses, donkeys and mules. It is communicable to humans but no cases have occurred in the Western Hemisphere since 1938. Sulfadiazine is the recommended therapy.[6]

Glauber's salt   Sodae sulphas. A sulphate of soda, found native in Bohemia. Created from the salt remaining from the distillation of muriatic acid. It possessed cathartic and diuretic qualities.

Glyster   (Glister) Alternate spellings of clyster: enema.

Hartshorn   (Cornu cervi) The horns of several species of stag. When boiled, they impart to the water a nutritious jelly. The chief use of the horns is for calcination (oxidation).

Heat   High body temperature; fever.

Humors   (Humours; British spelling).

Hypochonders   The spaces in the abdomen that are under the cartilages of the spurious ribs on each side of the epigastrium. A hypochondriac is a person of low spirits.

Icterical (Icterus)   A genus of disease characterized by yellowness of the skin and eyes; white faces and urine of a high color.

Inflammable air   Hydrogen gas.

Inflammatory fever   A fever characterized by heat, pain and redness; characterized as acute or chronic, local or general, simple or complicated with other diseases.

Influenza   So named because it was supposed to be produced by a peculiar influence of the stars. Cross-referenced under "Catarrhus," or "catarrh," symptoms included increased secretion of mucus with fever, attended with sneezing, cough, thirst, lassitude and want of appetite. In epidemic catarrh (*Catarrhus a contagio*), more active evacuations through expectorants, cathartics and diaphoretics are required, as well as cupping or through the use of blisters. These should not be carried too far as the disease is apt to assume typhoid characteristics. The chief danger seemed to be through suffocation.

Infusion   A process that consists of pouring water on a substance and allowing it to stand (soak) a certain time. The resulting mixture is then taken by mouth or inserted into the body by various means.

Infusum rosa   (Rosa dog rose, wild briar; heptree) Produces a smooth, oval, red, sweet fruit with citric and malic acids. The petals are used as a laxative but they are chiefly employed in infusion, as "an elegant vehicle for tonic and astringent medicines."

Inst.   Instant. When used in 19 century letters and newspapers, the abbreviation was used to refer to a date within the current month.

Ipecacacuanha   Derived from various emetic roots of South American origin; administered as an emetic in the form of powder suspended in water.

Iron, tincture of   (Ferrum) Acetate of Potassa, two parts; Sulphate of Iron, one part; rectified spirit 26 parts. It was considered an "agreeable chalybeate," meaning any medicine into which iron enters.

Jalap (Jalapa) First recognized by Dr. John Redman Coxe, of Philadelphia, who received a plant from Mexico in 1827; a description was first published by Mr. Nuttall in the *American Journal of Medical Sciences* in January 1830. Jalap is an active cathartic, operating briskly and sometimes painfully on the bowels and producing copious, watery stools. The dose is from 10 grains; the dose of calomel and jalap is 10 grains of each. (1854).

Juleps (cooling) Usually a mixture of fruit juices, occasionally mixed with alcohol used as a restorative.

Kibbee fever cot A bed which is filled with meshes and contains beneath an India rubber receptacle to hold water. Designed by Dr. Kibbee for ice water treatments of yellow fever victims (1870s).

Manna Obtained from several different species of manna tree. Used medically as a gentle laxative, it is usually prepared with senna, rhubarb, magnesia, and the neutral salts, the taste of which it conceals.

Mercury, preparations of The metal is found pure. Its most abundant form is the bisulphuret, or native cinnabar. In combination it acts as a peculiar and universal stimulant. The 1845 *Dispensatory of the United States* noted, "Indeed, there is no fact better established in medicine, than that of the influence of the mercurial preparations over the hepatic system; and whether the liver be torpid and obstructed as in jaundice, or pouring out a redundancy of morbid bile as in melaena, its judicious use seems equally efficacious in unloading the viscus, and restoring its secretion to a healthy state."

Miasma Poisoned air, arising from decaying matter and swamps.

Musk (Moschus) The musk animal, a ruminating animal resembling the antelope. An unctuous substance is contained in excretory follicles about the navel of the male animal. This substance is prescribed as a powerful antispasmodic; in cholera it frequently stops vomiting; combined with ammonia it is used to arrest the progress of gangrene.

Night soil Human feces.

Nitre (*Nitrate of Potassa*) Saltpetre. Nitre is considered a refrigerant, diuretic, and diaphoretic much used in inflammatory diseases. It was a powerful antiseptic, producing urine and sweat, lessens the heat of the body and the frequency of the pulse. It is frequently given in active hemorrhages, particularly haemoptysis.

Nosology The doctrine of the names of diseases. The most quoted authority on nosology was William Cullen, who published, *Synopsis and Nosology* (Hartford, 1792, abridged from *Genera Morborum* in *Synopsis Nosologiae Methodicae,* 1769; *Synopsis and Nosology* (2nd edition, Hartford, 1793; *Synopsis of Methodical Nosology* (Philadelphia, 1793).

"On the grunt" An expression used in the mid–19th century to mean someone who complains, especially about their own illnesses.

Opium Thebaic tonic.

Oxymel A preparation that combines honey and vinegar. It was used in expectorant medicines and to impart flavor to drinks in febrile complaints.

Palliative measures Treatment designed to relieve or ease painful conditions without attempting to cure.

Paludal A plant, animal or soil living or existing in a marshy habitat.

Pearlash Pearl ash or salts of tartar Potassium carbonate; a white salt which forms a strong alkaline solution in water. First identified in 1742 by Antonio Campanella. Derived from wood ashes and used as a cheap chemical levener in bread and cakes in place of yeast. Combined with an acid such as sour milk, a chemical reaction is created with carbon dioxide as a by-product. It was most commonly used between 1780–1840, after which it was replaced by Saleratus, chemically similar to baking soda.[7]

Pepper grass Lepidium virginicum; a member of the mustard family. The leaves are nutritious and generally detoxifying and have been used in vitamin C deficiency, diabetes and to expel intestinal worms. The herb is also diuretic and of benefit in easing rheumatic pain.[8]

Petechia Hemorrhagic spots on the skin that appear in many patients with febrile illnesses.[9]

Pfeiffer reaction (Syndrome) A rare autosomal-dominant disorder marked by early closure of the cranial sutures that may lead to mental retardation.[10]

Pleurisy Inflammation of the pleura (membranous sacs) that enclose the lungs and line the chest) usually with fever, painful breathing and coughing.

Pneumatic medicine (early 1800s) "Pneumatic": "of or belonging to air or gas." The science of studying diseases caused by miasmata or bad vitiated air and the practice of curing diseases by the admission of pure, vital air.

Potassa, chlorate of Substance made by passing an excess of chlorine through a solution of either caustic hydrate or carbonate of potassa. It is used as a refrigerant and a diuretic.

Pratique License granted to a ship to proceed into port after compliance with health regulations or quarantine.

Precordia (Praecordia: British spelling) The area on the anterior surface of the body overlying the heart and lower part of the thorax.

Quicksilver See Mercury. A term used especially in reference to that element, employed in thermometers.

Quinine (also referred to as "bark"; *Cinchonina*) Typically Peruvian bark used to treat fever. Considered the most valuable remedy in continual fevers connected with debility in such diseases as typhus, confluent smallpox, dyspepsia, rickets and dropsy; the powder was given orally or as an enema or as a nasal spray (see "bitters"). Quinine was highly effective in treating malarial infections but was worthless for the treatment of yellow fever.

Ratanhia (*Krameria*) A genus in the Krameriaceae family. The biological action is caused by the astringent rhataniatannic acid, similar to tannic acid. Rhatany is a gentle tonic and powerful astringent, used in chronic diarrhea, passive hemorrhages and bowel complaints. It became in general use in 1816 and by 1845 was extensively employed around the world. It was also used in tooth powders, as a gargle and as a local application to spongy gums. Most *Krameria* are native to tropical regions.[11]

Rhubarb Used as a purgative.

Rochelle salt A combination of carbonate of soda, bilartrate of potassa (cream of tartar) and water. It is a mild, cooling purgative, well suited to delicate and irritable stomachs, being among the least unpalatable of the neutral salts. It is an ingredient in the effervescing aperient called Seidlitz powders.

Saffron (Crocus) A perennial plant native of Greece and Asia Minor. Originally believed to moderately excite the different functions, exhilarate the spirits, relieve pain and produce sleep. In large doses it gives rise to headache, intoxication and can prove fatal. By 1845 its chief use was to impart color and flavor to tinctures.

Saline draughts Typically composed of salt of wormwood, lemon juice and cinnamon water.

Sanies A thin, greenish discharge; or a thick and bloody pus.

Scarification A superficial incision made with a lancet, or a chirurgical instrument called a scarificator, for the purpose of taking away blood, or letting out fluid, or, in the case of vaccination, administering a small amount of serum.

Scarificator An instrument used by physicians and cuppers. It is made in the form of a box with twelve or more lancets fitted on the same plane. When "cocked" and fired, they are depressed together and driven equally into the skin.

Scarlatina Scarlet fever. Symptoms include facial swelling and scarlet eruptions on the skin in patches, fever, chills, anxiety, shivering and thirst.

Scarlatina anginosa (Angina Scarlatina) Scarlet fever with ulcerated sore throat; approaches very near the malignant form. The patient is seized with coldness and shivering, great languor, debility, fever, nausea and vomiting of bilious matter, soreness of the throat, inflammation and ulceration of the tonsils.

Serpentaria Virginian snake root; first used as a of extraordinary power in counteracting the poisonous effects of bites of serpents; it possesses tonic and antiseptic virtues, and is generally administered as a powerful stimulant and diaphoretic in some fevers.

Slow fever A low-grade fever.

Snakeroot See Serpentaria.

Spiritus mindereri Spirit of Mindererus. A solution of acetate of ammonia; a powerful diaphoretic used in febrile and inflammatory diseases.

Spruce (Essence of Spruce; Spirit of Spruce) Turpentine. Prepared from the young branches by boiling them in water and evaporating the decoction, it is a thick liquid, having the color and consistency of molasses, with a bitterish, acidulous, astringent taste. It is used in the preparation of spruce beer and much used in long sea voyages as a preventive of scurvy.

Spruce beer The formula calls for half a pint of essence of spruce, pimento bruised, ginger bruised, hops, each four ounces, water three gallons. Boil 5–10 minutes, then strain, add 11 gallons of warm water and a pint of yeast and 6 pints of molasses. Mix and allow to ferment 24 hours.

Sudor Sweat or perspiration.

Sudorific Diaphoretic.

Sulfate of quinia See Quinine and Cinchona.

Tabardillo (Spanish) Spotted fever.

Tabes dorsalis A late-stage form of syphilis.

Tamarinds (*Tamarindus indica*) Employed as a laxative and for abating thirst or heat in various inflammatory complaints and for correcting putrid disorders, especially of a bilious kind in which cathartic, antiseptic and refrigerant qualities are useful.

Tertian A recurring fever, usually used to indicate recurrence every second or third day.

Thebaic tonic Opium, a stimulant narcotic. Taken by a healthy person in a moderate dose, it increases the force, fullness, and frequency of the pulse, augments the temperature of the skin, invigorates the muscular system, quickens the senses, animates the spirits, and gives new energy to the intellectual faculties. It excites the brain to intoxication or delirium. In a short time this excitation subsides, leaving a calmness and a delightful placidity of mind. The individual, insensible to painful impressions, forgets all sources of care and anxiety and is subject to pleasing fancies. Unless the dose is frequently repeated and the powers of nature worn out by over-excitement, no injurious consequences ultimately result. In 1845 it was more frequently prescribed than perhaps any other article in the materia medica. It was used as a stimulant, for pain relief, as a sleeping aid, an antispasmodic, for allaying general and local irritations, suppressing morbid discharges and to produce perspiration. In combination with ipecacuanha it served as a powerful diaphoretic and was extensively employed for this purpose. Opium was generally given in pill form or in tincture. The medium dose in ordinary diseases was 1 grain.

Thebaica (*A Thebaide regione,* from the country about the ancient city of Thebes in Egypt, where the plant flourished) Egyptian poppy.

Tonics Medicines which increase the tone of the muscular fibre, such as vegetable bitters; also stimulants and astringents.

Turpentine, oil of Used in frictions.

Typhus icterodes Typhus with symptoms of jaundice.

Ultimo (ult) When used in 19th century newspapers, the abbreviation was used to refer to a date from the previous month.

"Unity of fevers" A prevailing belief in the 1700s and through half of the 1800s meaning that all fevers stemmed from a common source. Therefore, all fevers could be treated with the same remedies.

Vapors A fainting spell.

Venaesection (Venesection) Surgical opening on a vein for withdrawal of blood (phlebotomy).

Verruga Peruvian virus associated with warts.

Vesicatories See Blisters.

Vinum croceum A mixture of wine, typically with oil, saffron and myrrh.

Viremia The presence of viruses in the blood.

Virginiana, rad. serpent (Aristolochia Serpentaria) Virginian snakeroot. First used to counter the poisonous bite of snakes but soon disregarded for this purpose. It possessed tonic and antiseptic virtues and was generally administered as a powerful stimulant and diaphoretic; used in some fevers where those properties were required.

Vis vitae The natural power of the animal machine in preserving life.

Vital air Pure air; uncontaminated air.

"Walking case" (of yellow fever) A patient who refuses to go to bed and keeps on his feet until he drops dead of yellow fever.

Water cure (Ice water cure) Developed by Dr. Choppin to treat yellow fever victims in the 1870s. The patient was stripped naked and ice water sprinkled over him to reduce fever and lower the pulse.

Whey The fluid part of milk that remains after the curd has been separated.

Wormwood (*Artemisia absinthium, common and mountain*) A plant native to Britain, used in intermittent fevers.

"Yellow disease" The southern name for a noncontagious malarial disease peculiar to local swamps. It was thought to be caused by the heat of the sun decaying vegetative matter and creating sickly exhalations that contaminated the atmosphere. It was often used as an alternate theory to explain yellow fever outbreaks. The significance of misdiagnosis stemmed from the fact that during the 19 century true yellow fever was believed to be contagious and of foreign origin, requiring strict quarantine, whereas "yellow disease" became epidemic from purely local causes and raged as long as the cause existed or there was material upon which it could feed.

Yellow fever names Yellowjacket, yellow jack, jack, yellow plague, Yellow Rainer, Bronzed John, dock fever, ship fever, stranger's fever, American plague, plague, bilious fever, *febris continua, mal de Siam,* "Great Sickness," "pestilential distemper," *La Fievre Matelotte* (French), summer complaint, autumnal disease, remittent disease (also used to describe malaria), Philadelphia fever, "Barbados distemper," Palatine fever (so-called because it appeared German immigrants suffered heavily from it); tropical continued, or proper yellow fever; highest grade of bilious fever; fever of Bolama; black vomit; *vomito*; Saffron-hued Angel of Death (Mississippi, 1871).

Yellow fever, transmission of Sylvatic (jungle); Intermediate (savannah) and Urban (city).

Chapter Notes

Preface

1. *New-York Times,* November 16, 1821.
2. *Anti-Jacobian Review and Magazine* (London), February 1, 1807.
3. *Oshkosh Daily Northwestern,* December 7, 1878.
4. *Ames* (IA) *Intelligencer,* August 6, 1885.

Chapter 1

1. *London Gentleman's Magazine,* December 1, 1754.
2. "Colonial Diseases," http://mayflowerfamilies.com.
3. *Newark* (OH) *Advocate,* July 16; *Syracuse* (NY) *Herald,* July 19, 1885; *Lawrence* (KS) *Gazette,* April 21, 1892; Richard Ligon, "A True and Exact History of the Island of Barbadoes," 1657; *McKean County* (PA) *Miner,* October 3, 1878; Rupert Boyce, "Discussion of Yellow Fever," February 1, 1911.
4. R. McGrew, and M. McGrew, *Encyclopedia of Medical History* (London: Macmillan, 1985), 357.
5. W.C. Gorges, "Recent Experiences of the United States Army with Regard to Sanitation of Yellow Fever in the Tropics," February 2, 1903 (extracted from Sheldon Watts' *Yellow Fever Immunities in West Africa and the Americas in the Age of Slavery and Beyond: A Reappraisal,* 2001.
6. R. Padmanabhan, "Molecular targets for flavivirus drug discovery"; D. Fontenille, "First evidence of natural vertical transmission of yellow fever virus in Aedes aegypti, its epidemic vector; "Yellow Fever," http://en.wikipedia.org/wiki/Yellow_Fever; J.M. Powell, *Bring Out Your Dead: The Great Plague of Yellow Fever in Philadelphia in 1793* (Philadelphia: University of Pennsylvania Press, 1949, reprinted 1993).
7. Molly Crosby, *The American Plague* (New York: Berkley Books, 2006), 9, 11.
8. "Yellow Fever," http://www.who.int/mediacentre/factsheets/fs100/en/index.html.
9. A.D. Barrett, and S. Higgs, "Yellow Fever: a disease that has yet to be conquered," *Annual Review of Entomology.* 52: 209–230.
10. "Yellow Fever," http://www.ncbi.nlm.nih.gov/pubmedhealth/PMH0002341/.
11. Ibid; "Yellow fever," http://www.who.int/mediacentre/factsheets/fs100/en/imdex.html.
12. Hooper, Robert, *Lexicon Medicum; or Medical Dictionary* (New York: Harper, 1842), 353.
13. Ibid., 170, 365.
14. "Yellow fever," http://who.int.mediacentre/news/release/2013/yellow_fever20130517/en/.

Chapter 2

1. *London Evening-Post,* April 14–17, 1739.
2. John B. Blake, "Yellow Fever in Eighteenth Century America," *Bull NY Acd Med* 44, no. 6, June 1968.
3. Ibid.; Claude Edwin Heaton, "Yellow Fever in New York City," *Bull Med Library Assoc.* 34, no. 2, April 1946.
4. Samuel Choppin, "History of the Importation of Yellow Fever into the United States, from 1693 to 1878."
5. Ibid.
6. Ibid.
7. Ibid; Heaton, *Yellow Fever in New York City.*
8. Choppin, "History of the Importation."
9. "King George's War"; "King George's War: The Third of the French and Indian Wars."
10. Choppin, "History of the Importation."
11. *London Evening-Post,* May 17–19, 1739 (spelling modernized).
12. *Dublin Daily Post and General Advertiser,* May 26, 1740 (spelling modernized).
13. *London Daily Post,* February 10, 1743.
14. David Hosack, John W. Francis, editors, "Account of the Yellow Fever which prevailed in Virginia in the years 1737, 1741 and 1742, in a Letter to the late Cadwallader Colden, Esq. of New-York, from the late John Mitchell, M.D., F.R.S. of Virginia," 181–215.
15. *London Daily Advertiser,* October 15, 1742.
16. *London Evening-Post,* December 31, 1745.
17. Hooper, *Lexicon,* 135–136.
18. Ibid., 355.
19. Blake, "Yellow Fever in Eighteenth Century America."
20. *Whitehall Evening-Post; or, London Intelligencer,* August 17–19, 1749; *British Spy; or, Universal London Weekly Journal,* December 17, 1757.
21. Blake, "Yellow Fever in Eighteenth Century America."
22. J.M. Powell, *Bring Out Your Dead: The Great*

Plague of Yellow Fever in Philadelphia in 1793 (Philadelphia: University of Pennsylvania Press, 1949, reprinted 1993), 14–15.
  23. Hooper, *Lexicon*, 207.
  24. Powell, *Bring Out Your Dead*, 14–15.
  25. *Dunlap's American Daily Advertiser* (Philadelphia), August 28, 1793.
  26. *European Magazine* (London), September 1, 1794.
  27. *Monthly Review* (London), October 1, 1765.
  28. *Gentleman's Magazine* (London), December 1, 1768.
  29. *London General Advertiser*, October 22, 1751; *London Gazetteer and New Daily Advertiser*, October 26, 1765.
  30. *London General Advertiser*, June 19, 1750.
  31. *Whitehall Evening-Post*, June 28–July 1, 1755.
  32. *London General Advertiser*, May 30, 1750.
  33. Hooper, *Lexicon*, 76; George B. Wood, and Franklin Bache, *The Dispensatory of the United States* (Philadelphia: Grigg & Elliot, 1845), 853.
  34. *London Gazette*, November 19–23, 1754, May 3–6, 1755; *Whitehall Evening-Post*, December 19–21, 1754, June 28–July 1, 1755; *London Public Advertiser*, June 3, 1756.
  35. *Read's* (London) *Weekly Journal, Or, British Gazetteer*, September 30, 1758; *Gazetteer and London Daily Advertiser*, March 10, 1759.
  36. Wood and Basche, *The Dispensatory*, 522.
  37. *A New Review* (London), November 1, 1785.
  38. *Gazetteer and London Daily Advertiser*, May 16; *Grand Magazine of Magazines; or, Universal Register* (London), July 1, 1759.
  39. *London Monthly Review*, October 1, 1765.
  40. *Gentleman's Magazine*, February 1, 1765.
  41. *London Gazetteer and New Daily Advertiser*, February 22, 1766.
  42. *Monthly Review*, May 1, 1799.

Chapter 3

  1. John S. Fulton, "Quarantine: The Delirium Ferox of American Sanitation," *Pub Health Pap Rep* 31, no.1, 1905.
  2. S.L. Kotar and J.E. Gessler, *Cholera: A Worldwide History* (Jefferson, N.C.: McFarland, 2014) 269–270.
  3. *Gentleman's Magazine*, December 1, 1754.
  4. *Monthly Review*, October 1, 1765.
  5. *Gentleman's Magazine*, December 1, 1768; *London Evening-Post*, September 18–20, 1766; *Lloyd's Evening Post*, August 15–17 (a continuation of Dr. Lind's "Observations on the Diseases Which a Strangers in North America").
  6. S.L. Kotar and J.E. Gessler, *Smallpox: A History* (Jefferson, N.C.: McFarland, 2013), 40–43.
  7. Richard L. Blanco, "Medicine in the Continental Army, 1775–1781," *Bull NY Acd Med* 57, no. 8, 1981.
  8. Gilbert Blane, *Observations on the Diseases Incident to Seamen* (London: Murray, 1785), 389–407; *A New Review* (London), November 1, 1785.
  9. Blanco, "Medicine in the Continental Army."
  10. Peter McCandless, "Revolutionary Fever: Disease and War in the Lower South, 1776–1783," 2007 (unless otherwise cited, references in this chapter were extracted from this study).
  11. Blanco, "Medicine in the Continental Army."
  12. S.L. Kotar and J.E. Gessler, *The Steamboat Era: A History of Fulton's Folly on American Rivers, 1807–1860* (Jefferson, NC: McFarland, 2009), 244.
  13. Blanco, "Medicine in the Continental Army."

Chapter 4

  1. Clemency Chase Coggins, "Medical Articles in Eighteenth Century American Magazines," quoting Hippocrates as published by the Middlesex Medical Society, *Massachusetts Magazine*, February 1789.
  2. John Hunter, *Observations on the Diseases of the Army in Jamaica; and on the Best Means of Preserving the Health of Europeans in that Climate*, 88–91.
  3. *Monthly Review*, March 1, 1789.
  4. *London Times*, November 9, 1790.
  5. Philip Beaver, *African Memoranda: Relative to an Attempt to Establish a British Settlement on the Island of Bulama, on the Western Coast of Africa, in the Year of 1792* (Westport, CT: Negro Universities Press, 1970) ; George Brooks, "Bolama as a Prospective Site for American Colonization in the 1820's and 1830's," 1973.
  6. Blake, "Yellow Fever in Eighteenth Century America."
  7. "A Revolution in Haiti," http://schlor.library.miami.edu/slaves/san_domingo_revolution/revolution.html; "The Slave Rebellion of 1791," http://www.latinamericanstudies.org/haiti/slave-rebellion.htm.
  8. *Philadelphia Federal Gazette*, July 11, 1793.
  9. Powell, *Bring Out Your Dead*, 1–3.
  10. Ibid., xviii.
  11. S.L. Kotar and J.E. Gessler, *The Rise of the American Circus, 1716–1899* (Jefferson, NC: McFarland, 2011), 50–52.
  12. *London Times*, December 10, 1793.
  13. William Currie, *A Description of the Malignant Infectious Fever Prevailing at Present in Philadelphia; with an Account of the Means to Prevent Infection, and the Remedies and Method of Treatment, Which Have Been Found Most Successful* (Philadelphia: Thomas Dobson, 1793).
  14. *Free-Mason's Magazine*, November 1, 1793.
  15. *Public Advertiser; or, Political and Literary Diary* (London), January 16, 1794. This letter was widely published in England.
  16. Powell, *Bring Out Your Dead*, 12–18.
  17. Ibid., 21–22.
  18. *Dunlap's American Daily Advertiser*, August 28, 1793.
  19. *Philadelphia, Federal Gazette*, August 24, 1793.
  20. Ibid., August 29, 1793.
  21. Powell, *Bring Out Your Dead*, 36–42.
  22. *Pennsylvania Journal*, August 28, 1793.
  23. *Federal Gazette*, August 28, 1793.
  24. *Free-Mason's Magazine*, January 1, 1794.
  25. Powell, *Bring Out Your Dead*, 56.
  26. *Philadelphia Independent Gazetteer*, August 31, 1793.

27. *Federal Gazette,* August 31, 1793.
28. *Dunlap's American,* September 4, 12, 1793; Powell, *Bring Out Your Dead,* 61–62.
29. Kotar and Gessler, *Ballooning: A History 1782–1900* (Jefferson, NC: McFarland, 2011), 59.
30. *Federal Gazette,* August 21, 24, 28, October 9, 1793.
31. Powell, *Bring Out Your Dead,* 59–63.

Chapter 5

1. *Free-Mason's Magazine,* January 1, 1794.
2. "Cock Lane Ghost," www.localmythsandlegends.com.
3. Powell, *Bring Out Your Dead,* 72–73.
4. Ibid., 66–67.
5. *Free-Mason's Magazine,* January 1, 1794.
6. Powell, *Bring Out Your Dead,* 65.
7. *General Advertiser,* September 11, 1793.
8. *Federal Gazette,* September 13, 1793.
9. "Thomas Young." Gilder Lehrman Institute of American History: http://gilderlehrman.org.history-by-era-war-for-independence/timeline-terms/thomas-young; "Dr. Thomas Young, Early American Deist." http://www.christiandeistfellowship.com/dryoung.html.
10. Powell, *Bring Out Your Dead,* 78–80.
11. "Four Thieves Vinegar," http://en.wikipedia.org/wiki/Four-Thieves_Vinegar.
12. Kotar and Gessler, *Cholera,* 19–20.
13. Powell, *Bring Out Your Dead,* 88–89.
14. *London Star,* November 7, 1793.
15. *London Evening Mail,* November 6–8, 1793.
16. Absalom Jones and Richard Allen, *A Narrative of the Proceedings of the Black People During the Late Awful Calamity in Philadelphia, in the Year 1793* (Philadelphia: William W. Woodward, 1794).
17. Ibid.
18. *London Evening Mail,* November 6–8, 1793.
19. *Dunlap's American Daily Advertiser,* September 14; *Federal Gazette,* September 14, 1793.
20. *London Evening Mail,* November 6–8, 1793.
21. *London Star,* November 7, 1793.
22. Ibid.
23. Heaton, "Yellow Fever in New York City."
24. *Federal Gazette,* September 30, 1793.
25. Ibid., September 11; *General Advertiser,* September 13, 1793.
26. *Federal Gazette,* September 16, 1793.
27. Ibid., September 12, 1793
28. *Dunlap's American,* September 14, 1793, from the *Federal Gazette.*
29. *Federal Gazette,* September 13, 1793.
30. Ibid., September 23, 1793.

Chapter 6

1. *Free-Mason's Magazine,* November 1, 1793.
2. *London Star,* November 7, 1793, letter written in New York dated September 26.
3. Powell, *Bring Out Your Dead,* 118–119; Donald Venes, editor, *Taber's Cyclopedic Medical Dictionary,* ed. 20 (Philadelphia: F.A. Davis, 2005), 1989.
4. Powell, *Bring Out Your Dead,* 124–125.
5. Thomas C. Danisi, *Uncovering the Truth About Meriwether Lewis* (New York: Prometheus Books, 2012).
6. *Federal Gazette,* September 11, 1793.
7. Ibid., September 17, 1793.
8. *Free-Mason's Magazine,* January 1, 1794, letter dated November 18, 1793.
9. *London Morning Post,* November 29, 1793.
10. *General Advertiser,* September 25; *Independent Gazetteer,* September 28, 1793.
11. *Federal Gazette,* September 27, 1793.
12. *Free-Mason's Magazine,* November 1, 1793, January 1, 1794.
13. Powell, *Bring Out Your Dead,* 153–158.
14. *Federal Gazette,* September 27, 1793.
15. Powell, *Bring Out Your Dead,* 163–164.
16. *Free-Mason's Magazine,* January 1, 1794.
17. *London Morning Chronicle,* December 26, 1793.
18. *St. James Chronicle; or, London British Evening-Post,* December 24, 1793.
19. *European Magazine* (London), September 1, 1794.
20. *Pennsylvania Star and Banner,* April 26, 1850.

Chapter 7

1. *Scots Magazine,* May 1, 1798.
2. *London Times,* September 22, 1794.
3. *Edinburgh Advertiser,* August 29–September 2, 1794; *Star,* May 19, 1797.
4. *London Times,* September 8, 1794.
5. *Lloyd's Evening-Post,* July 3–6; *London Morning Post and Fashionable World,* July 7, 1795.
6. *Star,* September 6, 1796.
7. *Lloyd's Evening-Post,* October 21–24, 1796.
8. *St. James Chronicle,* February 21–23, 1797.
9. *Star,* May 19, 1797.
10. *Daily Advertiser,* October 12; *Edinburgh Advertiser,* November 11–15, 1796; *Monthly Review,* August 1; *Monthly Magazine,* February 1; *London Times,* December 15, 1797; *Morning Post and Gazetteer,* March 10, 1798.
11. *Morning Chronicle,* March 5, 1795; *London Times,* October 1, 1796; *London True Briton,* February 9, 1797; *London Observer,* December 23, 1798.
12. *London Monthly Mirror,* October 1, 1797.
13. Reprinted in *Bell's Weekly Messenger,* May 6; *Evening Mail,* April 30–May 2, 1798.
14. *London Monthly Magazine,* Supplemental Number, July 20, 1799.
15. *Monthly Review; or, Literary Journal,* September to December, 1799, inclusive.
16. *Monthly Review,* November 1, 1799.
17. *London Observer,* February 3, 1799
18. *London Times,* December 24, 1794.
19. *Edinburgh Advertiser,* November 4–7, 1794.
20. Heaton, "Yellow Fever in New York City."
21. *London Scientific Magazine, and Freemasons' Repository,* November 1, 1797; letter dated August 28, 1797.
22. *Monthly Review,* April 1, 1798.
23. *London Times,* October 23, 1795.

24. *London Times,* December 3, 1795, January 23, 1796.
25. *St. James's Chronicle,* November 5, 1795.
26. John Duffy, "Yellow Fever in the Continental United States During the Nineteenth Century," *Bull NY Med* 44, no. 6, June 1968.
27. Heaton, "Yellow Fever in New York City."

Chapter 8

1. *Greenleaf's New York Journal,* September 4, 1798.
2. Ibid., September 1, 1798.
3. Heaton, "Yellow Fever in New York City."
4. *New York Spectator,* September 19, 1798.
5. Heaton, "Yellow Fever in New York City."
6. *Spectator,* September 19, 1798.
7. Heaton, "Yellow Fever in New York City."
8. *New York Commercial Advertiser,* February 12, 1799.
9. "Hamilton and Burr together for the last Time," http://todayshistorylesson.worldpress.com/2010/22hamilton-and-burr-together-for-the-last-time; "Aaron Burr takes everyone to the bank," http://todayshistorylesson.worldpress.com/tag/manhattan-company; "The Manhattan Company," http://en.wikipedia.org/wiki/The_Manhattan_Company).
10. Edward K. Spann, *The New Metropolis: New York City, 1840–1857* (1981), 117.
11. Choppin, "History of the Importation."
12. *London Times,* October 19, 1798.
13. *London Evening Mail,* September 19–21, November 2–5; *New York Daily Advertiser,* September 17; *New York Spector,* September 22; *New York Commercial Advertiser,* September 25; *London Weekly Register,* November 14, 1798, January 2, 1799; *London Observer,* December 2, 30, 1798; *Morning Post and Gazetteer,* November 1, 29; *London Times,* December 29; *Gentleman's Magazine,* December 1, 1798; *Annual Register on a View of the History, Politics, and Literature of the Year 1798* (London), January 1, 1799.
14. *Evening Mail,* August 9–12, 1799.
15. *Philadelphia Gazette,* April 16, 1799.
16. Ibid., April 11, 1799.
17. Ibid., April 16, 1799.
18. *Philadelphia Universal Gazette,* July 18, 1799.
19. *Philadelphia Gazette,* July 24; *Claypoole's American Daily Advertiser,* August 2, 1799.
20. *London Observer,* October 13, 1799.
21. *New York Weekly Museum,* July 13, 1799.
22. *Philadelphia Gazette,* July 10, 1799.
23. *Lloyd's Evening-Post,* October 16–18, October 21–23; *Star,* November 27, 1799.
24. *New York Commercial Advertiser,* July 30, 1799.
25. George B. Shattuck, ed., *Boston Medical and Surgical Journal* 3 (July–December 1844).
26. *New York Daily Advertiser,* September 4, 1799.
27. *New-York Gazette,* September 5, 1799.
28. *New York Commercial Advertiser,* September 6, 1799.
29. "Elisha Perkins." http://archive.org/details/2566065R.nih.gov; "Elisha Perkins," http://en.wikipedia.org/wiki/Elisha_Perkins.
30. *Philadelphia Gazette,* August 27, 1798.
31. *London Monthly Review,* August 1, 1799.
32. *London Anti-Jacobin Review and Magazine,* July 1, 1799; *London Monthly Review,* April 1, 1798.
33. *London Monthly Review,* August 1, 1799.
34. Kotar and Gessler, *Cholera,* 19–20; *London Monthly Magazine,* September 1; *Philosophical Magazine* (London), July 1, 1799.

Chapter 9

1. *New York Spectator,* September 19, 1798, reprinted from the *New York True American.*
2. *Star,* April 7, 1800.
3. *London Albion and Evening Advertiser,* August 25, 1800; *London Courier and Evening Gazette,* October 29, 1801.
4. *London Times,* October 30, 1801.
5. *Courier and Evening Gazette,* February 20, 1804.
6. *London Times,* July 30, 1804.
7. *London Courier,* December 12, 1807.
8. Ibid., December 12, 1807.
9. Ibid., July 25, 1807.
10. *European Magazine,* February 1, 1803; *British Press,* October 24, 1804; *Bell's Weekly Messenger,* July 27, 1806.
11. *Monthly Mirror* (London), October 1, 1800.
12. *Monthly Magazine,* October 1, 1805.
13. *London Times,* August 30, 1802.
14. *Dublin Journal,* May 10, 1803.
15. Ibid., March 7, 1805.
16. *London Times,* November 8, 1803.
17. *Edinburgh Weekly Journal,* January 4, 1804.
18. Ibid., December 21, 1803, January 4, 1804.
19. *Bell's Weekly Messenger,* January 22, 1804.
20. *Monthly Mirror,* November 1, 1806.
21. *Bell's Weekly Messenger,* January 1, 1805.
22. Ibid.; *Courier,* February 23, 1805.
23. Unless otherwise cited, all data in this subchapter is from James Fellowes, *Reports of Pestilential Disorder of Andalusia Which Appeared at Cadiz in the Years 1800, 1804, 1810 and 1813* (London: Printed by A. Strahan for Longman, Hurst, Rees, Orme, and Brown, 1815), see also Edward Nathaniel Bancroft, "An Essay of the disease yellow fever, with observations concerning Febrile Contagion," 1811.
24. *Lloyd's Evening-Post,* November 7–10, 1800.
25. *Dublin Journal,* November 25, 1800.
26. *Annual Register* (London), January 1, 1802.
27. *Edinburgh Advertiser,* October 5–8, 1802; *Adams (PA) Centinel,* August 18, 1802.
28. *Adams Centinel,* October 19; *London Times,* November 21, 1803.
29. *Gentleman's Magazine and Historical Chronicle,* January–June 1810.
30. *Pennsylvania Sprig of Liberty,* July 20; *London Times,* November 9, 1804.
31. *Yellow Fever,* Louisiana Office of Public Health, Annual Report, 1934, dhh.louisiana.gov.
32. J. Hardie, *Account of the Malignant Fever Lately Prevalent in the City of New York,* 100–107, cited in Heaton, "Yellow Fever in New York City."

33. *Dublin Journal,* October 19, 1805; *European Magazine,* February 1, 1806.
34. Heaton, "Yellow Fever in New York City."
35. *Morning Post,* September 3, 1806; *London Day,* September 26; *Dublin Journal,* January 14, November 25, 1809; *British Press,* October 23, 1810; *London Times,* December 21, 1810.
36. *Davenport* (IA) *Gazette,* April 10, 1851; "Thorburn, Grant," http://en.wikisource.org/wiki/Thorburn_Grant_(DNB00).

Chapter 10

1. *Pennsylvania Adams Sentinel,* January 21, 1801.
2. *Annual Register,* January 1; *Monthly Magazine,* January 1; *Monthly Mirror,* September 1, 1800; *Repertory of Arts and Manufactures* (London), January 1; Supplementary Number to the *Monthly Magazine* (London), July 1, 1801; *London British Critic,* November 1, 1802.
3. *Monthly Magazine,* July 1, 1803.
4. *Monthly Review,* October 1, 1803.
5. *Philosophical Magazine* (London), January 1, 1803.
6. *New Annual Register and General Repository of History, Politics and Literature* (London), November 1, 1804.
7. *Monthly Magazine,* January 1, July 1, December 1, 1805; *New Annual Register* (London), January 1, 1805; *Gentleman's Magazine and Historical Chronicle,* January 1, 1806.
8. Kotar and Gessler, *Cholera,* 36–37; *Monthly Magazine,* October 1; *British Press,* August 16, 1805.
9. *Monthly Magazine,* January 1, 1805; *Monthly Review,* July 1; *Pennsylvania Centinel,* July 9, 1806.
10. *Anti-Jacobin Review and Magazine,* February 1, 1807; *British Critic,* April 1, 1809.
11. *Monthly Magazine,* July 1, 1808.
12. *Gentleman's Magazine,* August 1, 1809.
13. *Anti-Jacobin,* October; *Monthly Review,* October 1, 1809.
14. *Monthly Review,* July 1, 1814.

Chapter 11

1. *London New Times,* August 6, 1824.
2. *New Annual Register,* January 1, 1811.
3. *New Times,* August 29, 1818; *Pennsylvania Sentinel,* September 4, 1811.
4. *London Times,* October 8, 1811.
5. Anthony Willich, Florian Madinger and James Mease, *The Domestic Encyclopedia; or, A Dictionary of Facts and Useful Knowledge,* 1804 (Philadelphia: William Young Birch and Abraham Small, 1804), 92–94.
6. *Scots Magazine and Edinburgh Literary Miscellany,* January 1, 1812; *Antigallican Monitor and Anti-Corsican Chronicle* (London), September 22, 1811.
7. *London Times,* September 27, 1811.
8. *London Courier,* September 26, 1811.
9. *London Times,* February 21; *Evans and Ruffy's Farmer's Journal* (London), February 24, 1812.
10. *Courier,* October 5; *London Times,* November 16, 1812.
11. *Monthly Magazine,* January 1, 1814.
12. *Courier,* October 8, December 21; *Evans and Ruffy's Farmers' Journal,* October 11; *Drakard's Paper: A London Weekly Journal,* October 17; *Dublin Journal,* October 21, 1813.
13. *London Times,* September 19, 1814; Supplementary Number to the 38th volume of the *Monthly Magazine,* January 30, 1815.
14. *Monthly Magazine,* December 1, 1816.
15. *New Annual Register,* January 1, 1819.
16. *British Press,* August 25, September 16; *London Times,* September 15, 16, 22, October 4; *London Philanthropic Gazette,* September 29, 1819.
17. *Surrey, Southwark, Middlesex, Sussex Gazette,* October 9; *British Press,* October 11, December 16; *London British Statesman,* October 18; *London New Times,* October 23; *London Times,* October 27; *London Correspondent,* November 1; *Evans and Duffy's,* November 22, 1819; *London Times,* January 1, 1820.

Chapter 12

1. *London Courier,* November 6, 1819.
2. *Evans and Ruffy's,* January 19; *Courier,* February 12, 1811; *London Times,* December 9, 1811, February 6, 1812.
3. *British Press,* June 17, 1811; *Edinburgh Advertiser,* June 26, 1812.
4. *Bell's Weekly Messenger,* October 6; *Dublin Journal,* October 8; *London Times,* November 29, 1816.
5. *Courier,* January 6; *Champion: A London Weekly Journal,* January 12, 1817; *Monthly Magazine,* January 1; *Edinburgh Advertiser,* August 28; *British Press,* September 16; *New York Times,* December 14, 1818.
6. *New Times,* September 23; *Edinburgh Advertiser,* December 18, 1818.
7. *British Press,* October 25, 1819.
8. *Edinburgh Advertiser,* January 28; *London British Freeholder,* April 15, 1820.
9. *London Times,* September 7; *Pennsylvania Republican Compiler,* October 20, 1819.
10. *Baldwin's Weekly Journal* (London), January 4; *London Times,* July 29, October 24, December 16, 1817; *Courier,* November 5, 1818; *Cumberland* (MD) *Daily Times,* March 31, 1885.
11. *Dublin Journal,* July 17; *London Times,* November 6, 1817.
12. *Republican Compiler,* September 8, 1819.
13. *Yellow Fever,* Louisiana Office of Public Health, Infectious Disease Epidemiology Section, Annual Report, 1934, dhh.louisiana.gov.
14. Ibid., "Yellow Fever Deaths in New Orleans," Louisiana Dicision, New Orleans Public Library, http://nutrias.org/facts/feverdeaths.htm.
15. *British Press,* August 7, September 21, October 5, November 10; *Republican Compiler,* September 8; *London New Times,* October 5; *London Courier,* October 21, 1819.
16. Heaton, "Yellow Fever in New York City."
17. *London Times,* November 3, 1819.
18. Molly Crosby, *The American Plague,* p. 13.
19. *Washington* (D.C.) *Daily National Intelligencer,* November 4, 1826.

20. *Edinburgh Advertiser,* October 19, November 9; *London New Times,* November 5, 1819.
21. *London Courier,* November 6, 1819.
22. *New Times,* December 28, 1819, from the *London Hull Advertiser.*
23. *Evans and Ruffy's,* November 22, 1819.
24. *London Times,* July 10; *New Times,* December 9, 1819.
25. *Monthly Magazine,* April 1, 1816.
26. *Monthly Review,* February 1, 1818.
27. Ibid., May 1, 1818.
28. *London Times,* October 28, 1819.
29. *Courier,* October 8, 1821.

Chapter 13

1. *Evans and Ruffy's,* November 9, 1829.
2. *Baldwin's London Weekly Journal,* September 22; *London Courier,* September 25; *London Times,* October 2; *New Times,* October 2, 1821.
3. *Courier,* October 8, 15; *Dublin Journal,* October 5; *New Times,* October 5, 19; *London Observer of the Times,* November 12, 1821.
4. *New Times,* November 16, 22; *London Times,* December 24, 1821.
5. *New Times,* November 19, 1821.
6. *London Philanthropic Gazette,* November 21; *Courier,* November 21, 1821.
7. *New Times,* December 8, 1821.
8. *Edinburgh Advertiser,* September 19; *London Times,* October 1; *London Atlas,* November 2, 1821.
9. *Atlas,* December 28, 1828.
10. *New Times,* November 16, 1821.
11. *Sandusky (OH) Clarion,* July 31; *Maryland Torch Light, Public Advertiser,* October 15; *British Press,* November 22; *New Times,* December 26, 1822.
12. *Edinburgh Advertiser,* October 16, 1823; *Republican Compiler,* October 13, 1824, December 7, 1825; *Courier,* October 20, 1824; *Logansport (IN) Telegraph,* December 2, 1827; *Washington (D.C.) National Intelligencer,* September 3, 1829.
13. "Yellow Fever Deaths in New Orleans," http://nutrias.org/facts/feverdeaths.htm, from George Augustin, *History of Yellow Fever* (New Orleans: Searcy & Pfaff, 1909).
14. "Yellow Fever," Louisiana Office of Public Health, 1934.
15. *British Press,* April 23, 1825.
16. *New Times,* July 27, 1820, September 27, 1821; *London Times,* October 2; *Edinburgh Advertiser,* November 2, 1821.
17. *Sandusky Clarion,* August 28; *Torch Light, Public Advertiser,* September 3; *London Times,* September 24; *Republican Compiler,* September 18, November 6; *British Press,* October 2, 30, 1822.
18. *Torch Light, Public Advertiser,* June 17; *New Times,* July 30, 1823.
19. *Republican Compiler,* September 13, 1820; *New Times,* October 2, 1821; *Torch Light, Public Advertiser,* October 15, 1822.
20. *Courier,* October 20; *New Times,* October 21; *Torch Light,* November 30; *Republican Compiler,* December 8, 1824.

21. *Adams Sentinel* (PA), July 5, 1826; *London Morning Journal,* October 9; *Logansport Telegraph,* November 23, 1829.
22. *London Times,* January 22, 1824.
23. *British Press,* September 30; *London Times,* December 29, 1825; *Edinburgh Advertiser,* May 17, 1825; *National Intelligencer,* November 4, 1826, November 13, 1827.
24. *National Intelligencer,* September 19, 1829.
25. Ibid., November 30, 1826.
26. *New Times,* October 12, 1821.
27. *Philosophical Magazine* 39, no. 167 (1812).
28. *National Intelligencer,* May 8, 1832.
29. *New Times,* June 18, 1825.
30. *Sandusky Clarion,* May 12, 1827; *Quarterly Journal of Science, Literature and Art* 23 (January–June 1827).
31. *National Intelligencer,* June 28, 1831.

Chapter 14

1. *London Courier,* July 23, 1831.
2. "Yellow Fever," Louisiana Office of Public Health, 1934.
3. *National Intelligencer,* October 7, 1830, October 16, November 7, 1832; *Adams Sentinel,* October 9; *Frederick (MD) Herald,* October 20; *Washington (D.C.) Globe,* November 14, 1832.
4. *Republican Compiler,* November 27; *Hagerstown (MD) Mail,* December 1, 1832; *London Patriot,* January 2, 1833.
5. *Patriot,* October 16; *London True Sun,* October 7, 14; *Washington (D.C.) Globe,* September 26; *Republican Compiler,* October 15, 1833.
6. *National Intelligencer,* October 22; *Alton (IL) Telegraph,* August 17, 1836.
7. *Bangor (ME) Daily Whig, Courier,* September 21; *Logansport Herald,* November 9, 30; *National Intelligencer,* September 28, October 9; *Globe* (D.C.), November 1, 1837.
8. *National Intelligencer,* October 12; *Courier,* July 14, 1838.
9. *Washington Globe,* August 29, 1839.
10. *Globe,* June 26, 28, August 10, 19, 22, 28, 29, September 9; *National Intelligencer,* August 19; *Hagerstown (MD) Mail,* September 13, 1839.
11. *Globe,* September 17, October 22, 28; *National Intelligencer,* September 19, December 18; *Bangor (ME) Whig,* September 20; *Courier,* November 7, 1839.
12. Augustin, *History of Yellow Fever.*
13. *National Intelligencer,* November 7, 1832; October 22, November 14, 1838; *Globe,* September 21; *Courier,* October 15, November 6; *Calhoun County (MI) Patriot,* November 2; *Adams Sentinel,* November 12, 1838.
14. *Globe,* September 25, November 2; *National Intelligencer,* November 6, 21; *Hagerstown Mail,* November 8; *Courier,* December 3, 1839.
15. *Globe,* June 26, September 9, 30; *National Intelligencer,* September 2, 19, 21, 26; *Mail,* August 30, 1839.
16. *National Intelligencer,* August 4; *People's Press* (Pennsylvania), August 28, 1835; *Globe,* July 15, 1839; *Cleave's Penny Gazette of Variety* (London), March 24, 1838.

17. *Sandusky Clarion,* January 2, 1830; *Globe,* July 6, October 4; *National Intelligencer,* July 6, 11, 1833; *Daily Evening News* (Indiana), September 19, 1835; *London True Sun,* November 30, 1836.
18. *True Sun,* August 11, 1835; *Republican Compiler,* August 8, 1837; *Globe,* August 31, 1838.
19. *National Intelligencer,* September 7; *Courier,* August 5, 1837; *Patriot,* June 18, 1838.
20. *London Colonial Gazette,* December 1, 1838; *Adams Sentinel,* February 11; *London Age,* September 22, 1839.
21. *Morning Chronicle,* July 8, 1853.
22. William Stevens, *Observations on the Healthy and Diseased Properties of the Blood* (London; John Murray, 1832), preface.
23. *National Intelligencer,* September 15, 1831, June 19, 1832; *London Times,* September 18, 1832; *Cleave's Penny Gazette,* December 28, 1839; *Republican Compiler,* June 28, 1836; *Colonial Gazette,* May 18, 1839, March 22, 1843.
24. *Colonial Gazette,* January 26, 1839; *Globe,* March 28, 1833, June 6, 1834; *Carlton Chronicle* (London), August 6, 1836.
25. *Globe,* August 10, 1837.

Chapter 15

1. *Weekly Wisconsin,* November 15, 1848.
2. *Hagerstown Mail,* September 3, 10; *Globe,* September 14, 1841.
3. *Globe,* September 17; *Mail,* September 24; *Bangor Whig,* November 4, 5; *Southport* (WI) *American,* November 11, 1841; *Southport* (WI) *Telegraph,* January 18, 1842.
4. *Indiana Palladium,* October 7; *Globe,* October 11, 19, 1834.
5. *Adams Sentinel,* November 27, 1843.
6. *Burlington* (IA) *Hawk-Eye,* November 30, 1843.
7. *Bangor Whig,* October 10, 1843.
8. *Bell's Messenger* (London), July 14; *London Atlas,* November 2, 1844; *Palladium,* October 4, 1845, October 24, 1846.
9. *Alton* (IL) *Telegraph, Democratic Review,* August 13; *Palladium,* August 14; *Hawk-Eye,* August 19; *Adams Sentinel,* August 23, September 6; *Independent American and General Advertiser* (Wisconsin), August 27; *Daily Sentinel and Gazette* (Wisconsin), September 1, 1847.
10. *Adams Sentinel,* September 13, 1847.
11. *Weekly Wisconsin,* September 22; *Green Bay* (WI) *Advocate,* September 23; *Adams Sentinel,* September 27, 1847.
12. Reprinted in *Weekly Wisconsin,* September 29, 1847.
13. Reprinted in *Hillsdale* (MI) *Whig Standard,* October 5, 1847.
14. Reprinted in *Fort Wayne* (IN) *Times, People's Press,* October 14, 1847.
15. Reprinted in *Sandusky Clarion,* November 16, 1847.
16. *Davenport* (IA) *Gazette,* October 19; *Wisconsin Tribune,* November 24, 1848; *Democratic Pharos* (Iowa), July 4; *Zanesville* (OH) *Courier,* September 4, 1849; *Sanduskian,* April 16, 1850.

17. Augustin, *History of Yellow Fever.*
18. *Wisconsin Democrat,* September 18, 1847.
19. *Globe,* November 5, 1842, September 18, 22, October 28, 1843; *Albany* (NY) *Log Cabin,* August 14, 1841; *Civilian and Galveston Gazette* (Texas), July 20; *Guernsey* (OH) *Jeffersonian,* September 27, 1844.
20. *Globe,* August 31; *Tioga* (PA) *Eagle,* September 6, 1843.
21. *Hawk-Eye,* September 7; *Weekly Wisconsin,* September 13; *Sandusky* (OH) *Clarion,* September 11; *Defiance* (OH) *Democrat,* September 14, 1848.
22. *Southport Telegraph,* December 17, 1844, August 18, 1847; *Newport* (RI) *Daily News,* June 2, 8; *Palladium,* June 13, August 29; *Logansport Telegraph,* June 13, 1846; *Weekly Wisconsin,* June 9; *Fond du Lac* (WI) *Whig,* July 14, 1847; *Potosi* (WI) *Republican,* June 1, 1848.
23. *Log Cabin,* November 6; *Globe,* December 11, 1841; *London Argus,* January 22, 1842; *London Daily News,* February 13; *London Nonconformist,* May 30, 1849.
24. Reginald Horsman, *Josiah Nott of Mobile* (Baton Rouge: Louisiana State University Press, 1987), 141–143.
25. *National Intelligencer,* March 4, October 5, 1840; *American Freeman* (Wisconsin), January 5; *Davenport* (IA) *Gazette,* October 21, 1847; Horsman, *Josiah Nott,* 141–142.
26. *Bell's Life in London and Sporting Chronicle,* October 15, 1848; *London Nautical Standard,* June 9, 1849.
27. Horsman, *Josiah Nott,* 144–148.
28. Wood and Basche, *The Dispensatory,* 281–282.
29. Ibid., 157–158.
30. *Marshall* (MI) *Statesman,* February 25, 1845; *Indiana Democrat,* March 27, 1846; *Star and Banner* (Pennsylvania), June 18, 1847.

Chapter 16

1. *Janesville* (WI) *Gazette,* August 20, 1853.
2. *Davenport* (IA) *Gazette,* April 10, 1851; "Thorburn, Grant," http://en.wikisource.org/wiki/Thorburn_Grant_(DNB00).
3. *Weekly Wisconsin,* October 16, 1850, October 13, 1852; *New-York Daily Times,* October 28, December 1, 1851, September 10, 15, 20, 21, 30, October 13, 16, 1852; *Daily Zanesville* (OH) *Courier,* November 27; *Danville* (IN) *Advertiser,* November 27, 1852.
4. *New Albany* (IN) *Daily Tribune,* July 30; *Zanesville Courier,* July 30; *Democratic Banner* (IA), August 5; *Daily Free Democrat* (Wisconsin), August 6; *Alton Telegraph,* August 11; *New-York Times,* August 11; *Racine* (WI) *Advocate,* August 11, 1853.
5. *New-York Times,* March 3, 1854.
6. *Adams Sentinel,* August 15; *London Morning Chronicle,* August 18; *New Albany Tribune,* August 16; *New-York Times,* August 19; *Weekly Wisconsin,* August 31, October 5, 1853.
7. *Republican Compiler,* August 22, 1853.
8. *Star and Banner,* August 26; *Adams Sentinel,* August 29; *Logansport* (IN) *Journal,* September 3; *Weekly Wisconsin,* August 31, September 21; *New Albany Tribune,* September 12; *New-York Times,* August 17, 1853.

9. *Democratic Pharos,* September 7, 1853.
10. *New-York Times,* September 5, 1853.
11. Ibid., September 5; *Weekly Wisconsin,* September 8; *Democratic Banner* (Iowa), September 16; *Alton Weekly Courier,* September 23, 1853.
12. *New Albany Tribune,* October 24, 1853.
13. *New-York Times,* September 13, 17; *Defiance Democrat,* October 29; *Weekly Wisconsin,* October 26, 1853; *New Albany Tribune,* January 16, 1854.
14. Horsman, *Josiah Nott,* 151, 160–167.
15. *Weekly Wisconsin,* October 5; *Star and Banner,* September 9; *Morning Advocate* (Wisconsin), October 14; *New-York Times,* August 4, 1854.
16. *New Albany Tribune,* July 15, September 1; *Janesville Gazette,* September 6; *Herald* (Wisconsin), September 13; *Globe,* October 2, 9; *Kenosha* (WI) *Telegraph,* October 19; *Weekly Wisconsin,* November 5; *Alton Courier,* November 23, 1854; Augustin, *History of Yellow Fever.*
17. *Sheboygan Lake* (WI) *Journal,* September 20; *Jackson County* (IN) *Democrat,* September 26; *Globe,* October 2, 1854.
18. *Weekly Wisconsin,* June 7; *Alton Courier,* August 3; *La Crosse* (WI) *Independent Republican,* September 20, 1854.
19. *New-York Times,* September 2, 14, 15, 19, 27, 28; *Grant County* (WI) *Herald,* September 11; *Lorain County* (OH) *Argus,* September 20; *Sheboygan Lake Journal,* September 20; *Oshkosh Courier,* September 23; *Janesville Gazette,* September 30; *Warrick Democrat,* October 3; *Free Democrat* (Wisconsin), October 4; *Globe,* October 2, 9; *Weekly Wisconsin,* November 1, 1854; *Atlanta Constitution,* September 30, 1876.
20. *Weekly Wisconsin,* November 15; *New-York Times,* April 11, September 14, 1854.

Chapter 17

1. *New-York Times,* August 25, 1855.
2. *Evansville* (IA) *Daily Enquirer,* May 2; *Newport News,* May 24; *Milwaukee Daily News,* August 6, 1855.
3. *Galveston News,* August 14; *New-York Times,* August 16, 1855.
4. *Wisconsin Patriot,* July 17; *New-York Times,* July 18, 30, August 3, 21; *Warrick Democrat,* September 11; *Democratic Pharos* (Indiana), October 24, 1855.
5. *Baraboo* (WI) *Republic,* September 15, 1855.
6. *Warrick Democrat,* October 16, 1855.
7. *Democratic Pharos,* October 24; *Hawk-Eye, Telegraph,* October 22; *Galveston News,* November 6; *Warrick Democrat,* October 16, 1855.
8. *Monroe* (WI) *Sentinel,* July 8, 1857.
9. *Kenosha* (WI) *Times,* December 22, 1859.
10. *Hawk-Eye, Telegraph,* July 27; *Patriot* (WI), July 30; *New-York Times,* July 31, August 6, 11, 15, 18, 21, 25; *Milwaukee News,* July 31; *Delaware State Reporter,* August 21, 1855.
11. *New-York Times,* August 24, 1855.
12. Ibid., August 25, 1855.
13. Ibid.
14. Horsman, *Josiah Nott,* 166–167.
15. *New-York Times,* August 31, 1855.
16. *Hornellsville* (NY) *Tribune,* September 20, 1855 from the *National Intelligencer.*
17. *New-York Times,* August 27, 1855; Vera Brodsky Lawrence, *Strong on Music: The New York Music Scene in the Days of George Templeton Strong,* vol. 1 (Chicago: University of Chicago Press, 1995), 647.
18. *New-York Times,* September 6, 22; *Waupaca* (WI) *Spirit,* October 8, 1855.
19. *Free Democrat* (Wisconsin), October 15; *New-York Times,* September 11, 1855.
20. *New-York Times,* September 22, 1855.
21. Ibid., September 24; *Fort Wayne Times,* September 24, 1855.
22. *Weekly Wisconsin,* September 26, 1855.
23. *New-York Times,* August 14, September 18–20, 1855.
24. Ibid., September 18–20, 1855.
25. *New Albany Tribune,* August 15; *Weekly Wisconsin,* August 20, September 3, 10, 1856, January 14, 1857; *London Daily News,* August 25; *Milwaukee American,* August 30, September 1, 5; *New-York News,* September 3, 6, 1856.

Chapter 18

1. *Civilian and Gazette* (Texas), April 28, 1857.
2. *London Chronicle and Register,* July 4, 1857.
3. *New York Herald,* April 26, 1857.
4. Ibid., May 20, 22, June 2, 6; *New-York Times,* June 5, September 7, 1857.
5. *New York Herald,* May 12; *New-York Times,* June 10, 15, 1857.
6. *New York Herald,* April 17, June 23; *New Albany Tribune,* July 23, 1858.
7. *New-York Times,* August 5, 1858.
8. Ibid., September 6–9, 1858. For a thorough discussion of the Staten Island arson, see Kotar and Gessler, *Smallpox: A History,* 126–133.
9. *Milwaukee News,* September 9; *Janesville Gazette,* September 11; *New-York Times,* September 16–18, 21, 27, 29, 1858.
10. *New-York Times,* April 29, 30, May 20, June 2, 1859.
11. *New-York Times,* June 16, 24, 25, 29, 30, August 2, 11, 1859.

Chapter 19

1. *New-York Times,* "The Yellow Fever of New Orleans," March 3, 1854.
2. *Davenport* (IA) *Gazette,* May 18; *Weekly Gazette and Free Press* (Wisconsin), May 22; *New-York Times,* June 19, 1858.
3. *Washington* (IN) *Telegraph,* July 15; *Berkshire County* (MA) *Eagle,* July 16, November 5; *Adams Sentinel,* August 2, September 13, 20; *Warrick Democrat,* August 10; *New Albany Tribune,* August 14, September 20; *Civilian and Gazette,* August 17, October 12; *New-York Times,* August 23, September 21; *Evansville* (IN) *Enquirer,* September 4, October 9; *Monroe* (WI) *Sentinel,* October 27; *Warren* (IN) *Republican,* November 4; *Mount Carmel* (IL) *Register,* October 29; *Seymour* (IN) *Times,* November 18; *Milwaukee Sentinel,* December 8, 1858.

4. *Wabash* (IN) *Express,* February 18; *Wautoma* (WI) *Journal,* June 15; *Racine Journal,* July 2; *New Albany Tribune,* July 14; *New-York Times,* August 6, 1859.
5. Augustin, *History of Yellow Fever.*
6. *Davenport Gazette,* June 24; *Richland County* (WI) *Observer,* September 14; *Washington* (IN) *Telegraph,* September 9; *Adams Sentinel,* September 20; *New-York Times,* September 28; *Wabash* (IN) *Express,* October 20, 1858.
7. *Milwaukee Sentinel,* July 27; *New-York Times,* June 21, August 4, 1859.
8. *Daily News* (London), August 28, 1861.
9. *Wisconsin Free Democrat,* March 13; *London Church, State Gazette,* April 5; *Logansport Journal,* May 18; *Weekly Wisconsin,* May 22, November 6; *London Patriot,* May 23, June 13, 1850.
10. *Bell's New Weekly Messenger* (London), March 9; *London Patriot,* March 10, 1851.
11. *Adams Sentinel,* June 9; *Patriot,* September 4, 1851; *London Morning Chronicle,* October 18, 1852; *Weekly Wisconsin,* May 12, 1852, February 16, 1853; *London Weekly Paper and the Organ of the Middle Classes,* June 19, 1852; *Evening London Star,* May 25, 1857; *London Evening Herald,* July 6; *Evening Star,* September 17, 1858.
12. *Nonconformist,* October 8; *Lloyd's Weekly Newspaper* (London), October 12, 1856.
13. *Morning Chronicle,* September 25; *British Standard,* October 9; *London Watchman and Wesleyan Advertiser,* October 28; *Evening Herald,* December 5; *London Christian Cabinet,* December 11; *British Banner,* December 31, 1857; *Decatur* (IN) *Eagle,* January 8; *New-York Times,* January 25; *London Illustrated Times,* March 20, 1858.
14. *London Weekly Paper,* July 24, September 4; *Morning Chronicle,* September 23, October 1, November 4; *Weekly News and Chronicle,* December 11; *Nautical Standard,* December 18; *Tallis's London Weekly Paper,* December 25, 1852; *London Daily News,* January 11, 19, 20; *Nonconformist,* January 12, 1853.
15. *Nautical Standard,* February 12, 1853.
16. *Tallis's London Weekly Paper,* October 29, 1853; *Morning Chronicle,* January 16, 1855.
17. *Weekly Chronicle and Register,* August 22, 1857.
18. *Defiance* (OH) *Democrat,* August 27, 1853; *Janesville Gazette,* July 15, 1854; *New-York Times,* June 30, 1855; *Newport News,* February 4, 1858.
19. *Lloyd's Newspaper,* July 21, 1850; *Nonconformist,* February 28, 1855.
20. *Morning Chronicle,* March 25; *New-York Times,* May 31, October 1; *Kenosha Democrat,* August 26, 1853; *Weekly News and Chronicle,* March 11; *Weekly Wisconsin,* May 24, 1854; *Civilian and Gazette,* July 28, 1857; *Wabash* (IN) *Express,* September 21, 1858.
21. Charles Neidhard, *On the Efficacy of Crotalus Horridus in Yellow Fever: Also in Malignant, Bilious, and Remittent Fevers* (New York: William Raddle, 1860), 61–69; *Free Democrat* (Wisconsin), February 8; *Manchester Guardian,* March 7; *White River* (NJ) *Standard,* March 29; *New-York Times,* July 19, 1855.
22. *London Mail,* February 10; *Nonconformist,* February 25; *Atlas,* February 7, 1857; *New Albany Tribune,* November 10, 1858.
23. *Janesville Gazette,* November 26, 1853; *Zanesville Courier,* May 11, 1854; *New Albany Tribune,* February 24; *Galveston News,* January 19; *Weekly Argus and Democrat* (Wisconsin), September 16, 1856; *Democratic Expounder* (Michigan), July 2; *Adams Sentinel,* August 24, 1857; *Hawk-Eye,* October 26, 1858; *New-York Times,* May 11; *Atlas,* July 11, 1859; "The History Dish: Pearlash, The First Chemical Leavening," www.fourpoundsofflour.com.
24. *Atlas,* January 24; *Patriot,* January 22; *London Daily News,* April 13, 1852.
25. *Atlas,* January 24, 1852.
26. *Weekly Wisconsin,* December 27, 1854; *New-York Times,* June 6, 1854, January 29, 1855. The settlement given to the owners of the *George Law,* as written in the article, was $2. Presumably, the actual amount was $200, as that, added to the other awards, equaled $1,000.

Chapter 20

1. *New Albany* (IN) *Register,* August 2, 1860 from the *New Orleans Bee.*
2. *New-York Times,* June 7, 18 (italics in original); *World,* July 20, August 27, 1860.
3. *New Albany Register,* May 21, December 6, 1860.
4. *Seymour* (IN) *Times,* April 18; *Fort Atkinson* (WI) *Standard,* May 2; *New Albany Ledger,* July 10; *Wisconsin State Journal,* June 10, 1861.
5. Augustin, *History of Yellow Fever.*
6. *White River* (IN) *Gazette,* June 26; *Guardian,* July 30; *Evening Star,* August 20, 1862; *New-York Times,* January 16, 1862, November 10, 1863; *New Albany Ledger* (Indiana), October 8, 29, 1862, January 16, 1863, November 10, 1864; *Dawson's Daily Times and Union* (Indiana), November 13; *Weekly Standard* (North Carolina), September 17, 24, October 1, 8, 15; *London Daily News,* November 6; *Crown Point* (IN) *Register,* December 4, 1862; *Home League* (Wisconsin), August 8, 1863; *Dubuque* (IA) *Herald,* July 2; *Dubuque Democratic Herald,* October 7; *Janesville Gazette,* November 1, 1864; *Colonies and India* (London), December 29, 1882; *Cedar Rapids Evening Gazette,* May 16, 1885; Edward McClachlin, "Prison Life," *Stevens Point* (WI) *Journal,* March 14, 1885; Robert E. Denney, *Civil War Medicine: Care, Comfort of the Wounded* (New York: Sterling, 1994), 131, 147.
7. *Hawk-Eye,* June 1; *New Albany Daily Register,* May 6, 29; *New-York Times,* April 26, May 11; *Wisconsin State Journal,* May 17; *Madison* (IN) *Weekly Courier,* May 17; *Janesville Gazette,* May 25, 1865.
8. *Davenport Gazette,* May 30; *Milwaukee News,* May 25, June 6; *Syracuse Courier and Union,* May 31; *Wisconsin State Journal,* June 23; *Fort Wayne Gazette,* October 17, 1865.
9. Edward Steers, Jr., *Blood on the Moon* (Lexington: University Press of Kentucky, 2001), 54.
10. *West Eau Claire Argus,* January 18; *Dubuque Herald,* June 21; *Indianapolis Journal,* April 29; *Flake's Semi-Weekly Galveston Bulletin,* September 28, 1867; "Luke P. Blackburn," http://en.wikipedia.org/wiki/Luke_P._Blackburn.
11. *Burlington* (IA) *Hawk-Eye,* April 23; *Lemars* (IA)

Semi-Weekly Sentinel, May 1; *Monticello* (OH) *Express*, July 2, 1885.
  12. *Galveston News*, June 16, July 3, 1866.
  13. Ibid., July 5; *New Albany Commercial*, October 1; *Hawk-Eye*, October 13; *Indianapolis Journal*, October 18, 1866.
  14. *North-West* (Illinois), September 13, 1866.

Chapter 21

  1. *Indianapolis Journal*, October 4, 1867.
  2. Ibid., July 8, August 17; *Galveston News*, August 4, 13, September 8; *New-York Times*, August 25; *Hawk-Eye*, August 27; *Milwaukee News*, September 1; *Thomasville* (GA) *Southern Enterprise*, September 17, 1867.
  3. *Flake's Bulletin*, September 28, October 23, November 20; *Milwaukee News*, October 5; *Galveston News*, October 18, 1867.
  4. *Indianapolis Journal*, August 26; *Flake's Bulletin*, August 15; September 28, October 17, 1867.
  5. *Flake's Bulletin*, September 21; *Indianapolis Journal*, September 25; *Dubuque Herald*, November 9, 1867.
  6. *Indianapolis Journal*, August 6, 23, September 10, October 12; *Weekly Arkansas Gazette*, August 10, September 24; *New Albany Commercial*, August 14; *Milwaukee News*, August 31, September 22; *Galveston News*, September 3; *New Castle* (IN) *Courier*, September 26, 1867.
  7. *Indianapolis Journal*, October 16, 31; *Fort Wayne Gazette*, November 1; *Dubuque Herald*, November 7; *Arkansas Gazette*, October 22; *Davenport Gazette*, October 25, 1867; *Flake's Bulletin*, June 6, 1868; Augustin, *History of Yellow Fever*.
  8. *Galveston News*, September 12; *Benton* (IN) *Tribune*, December 15, 1868.
  9. *New York Herald*, June 24, 28, October 8, 1869.
  10. Augustin, *History of Yellow Fever*; *Coshocton Age*, October 15, 1869; Venes, *Tabers*, 42.

Chapter 22

  1. *Gettysburg* (PA) *Star and Sentinel*, December 1, 1885.
  2. *Civilian and Gazette*. March 27, 1860; *London Express*, March 19; *Gleaner* (Jamaica), March 8, 1867.
  3. *New-York Times*, May 29, 1862, August 26, 1867, November 22, 1869; *Appleton* (WI) *Motor*, July 24, 1862; *Lloyd's Weekly* (London), October 27, 1867; *New Albany Ledger*, May 18, 1869.
  4. *New-York Times*, January 5, 1862, April 12, July 6, 1868; *Indiana Journal*, February 27; *Aurora* (IN) *Commercial*, March 9; *Bangor Whig and Courier*, April 12; *Indianapolis Journal*, June 12, July 16, 1868; May 22, 1869; *London Express*, December 2, 1867; *London Daily News*, June 6, 7; *Flake's Bulletin*, June 17; *New Albany Ledger*, June 18; *London Morning Post*, August 12, 1868; *Stratford Times, Bow, Bromley News and South Sussex Gazette*, July 17, 1869.
  5. *New York World*, November 24, 1860.
  6. *New Albany Ledger*, December 5, 1860; *London Magnet*, May 27; *London Patriot*, December 11, 1862; *London and China Telegraph*, May 27; *London Standard*, May 30; *London Daily News*, May 31 (italics added), August 8; *Nonconformist*, June 19, 1867.
  7. *London Express*, April 6; *Guardian*, April 12; *Daily News*, April 15; *Warren* (IN) *Republic*, May 18, 1865.
  8. *Patriot*, October 5, 1865; *Daily News*, October 6, 1865, December 3, 1866; *London Watchman and Wesleyan Advertiser*, February 7; *Guardian*, December 19; *London Standard*, November 13, 1866.
  9. *Daily News*, October 29, 1862, January 2, 1868; *London Evening Herald*, January 7, 1862; *Standard*, December 4, 1863; *Edinburgh Courant*, June 19; *London Express*, April 24, 1867.
  10. *London Morning Chronicle*, December 26, 1860.
  11. *London Australian Mail*, June 12, 1866.
  12. *Galveston News*, August 17, 1867; *New-York Times*, March 12, 1866; *Grand Traverse* (MI) *Herald*, June 10, 1869; *Indianapolis Journal*, October 5, 1867, from the *New York Sun*.
  13. *Galveston News*, August 7, 11, 22, 1867; *London Evening Herald*, June 20, 1864; *New Albany Ledger*, January 16, 1869; *Flake's Bulletin*, January 12, 1868.
  14. Wood and Basche, *The Dispensatory*, 696–697.
  15. *Gleaner*, July 10, 17, 24, August 1, 3, 24, September 24, October 10, 17, November 29, December 30; *Galveston News*, September 18, 1867.
  16. *Indianapolis Journal*, October 11; *Flake's Bulletin*, November 2, 1867; *Guardian*, September 2, 1868.

Chapter 23

  1. *Fort Wayne Daily Democrat*, October 28, 1870.
  2. *Rockingham* (VA) *Register*, April 21; *Flake's Bulletin*, September 15, 18, October 23, 1870; Augustin, *History of Yellow Fever*; *Fort Wayne Sentinel*, February 15, 1871, places the total number of deaths from yellow fever at 587.
  3. *New-York Times*, August 17; *New York Herald*, September 12, 14, November 18, 1870.
  4. *Wayne* (IN) *Citizen*, August 30; *Galveston News*, September 11, 1870.
  5. *New York Herald*, July 16, 1870.
  6. *Flake's Bulletin*, September 30, 1870.
  7. Ibid., November 1, 1870.
  8. *Janesville Gazette*, January 3, 1872.
  9. *Flake's Bulletin*, January 18; *Galveston News*, March 3, December 7; *London Sun, Central Press*, August 17; *Evening Journal* (Indianapolis), December 16, 1871.
  10. *Flake's Bulletin*, November 9, 1871.
  11. *Tioga County* (PA) *Agitator*, August 20; *New Albany Standard*, August 25; *Hawk-Eye*, August 26; *Fort Wayne Sentinel*, August 26; *New-York Times*, August 27; *Fort Wayne Gazette*, August 28, November 13; *New York Herald*, August 29; *Atlanta Constitution*, August 30, September 20; *Indianapolis Journal*, September 2; *New Harmony* (IN) *Register*, October 14, 1871.
  12. *Indiana Democrat*, January 11, 1872.
  13. *New York Herald*, February 23, 1872.
  14. *Flake's Bulletin*, June 14; *Galveston News*, June 12, 1872.
  15. *New York World*, August 13, 14, 16, 17, 19–21, 23, 25, 27, 31; *New York Herald*, August 15–19, 23; *New York Times*, August 18, 1872.

16. *Titusville* (PA) *Herald*, November 8; *Galveston Tri-Weekly Civilian*, November 29, 1872.
17. *Galveston News*, May 7, 1873.
18. Ibid., June 7; *World*, June 8, 1873.
19. *Sullivan* (IN) *Democrat*, September 3; *Dubuque Herald*, September 7; *New York Evening Gazette*, September 16; *Boston Globe*, September 12, 16, 18, 24, October 23; *Salt Lake Tribune*, September 13, October 14; *Fort Wayne Gazette*, September 15, 30; *Galveston News*, September 16, November 5, 17; *Jackson* (IA) *Sentinel*, September 18; *World*, September 20, 30, October 5, 17, November 13; *Corydon* (IN) *Democrat*, October 6; *New Castle* (IN) *Courier*, October 10; *Greencastle* (IN) *Press*, October 15; *New Harmony* (IN) *Register*, October 18; *Sioux County* (IN) *Herald*, October 24; *Hawk-Eye*, November 5; *Herald and Torch Light* (Maryland), October 29; *Carroll County* (GA) *Times*, November 7; *Greenville* (PA) *Advance*, December 4, 1873.
20. *World*, March 15, 1875.
21. *Titusville Herald*, October 3, 1870; *Greenville* (PA) *Argus*, August 16, October 4; *Brownstown* (IN) *Banner*, August 31; *Orrville* (OH) *Crescent*, November 7; *Sullivan County* (IN) *Union*, November 22, 1871; *Farmer and Mechanic* (Indiana), January 7; *Galveston News*, August 21, 1874; *Perry* (IA) *Chief*, June 12, 1875.
22. *Decatur Republican*, January 1, 1874.
23. *Freeport* (IL) *Journal*, from the *Lions* (Iowa), December 24, 1873.
24. *Galveston News*, January 17, April 10, September 9; *World*, September 12, 1874.
25. *Semi-Weekly Wisconsin*, April 3; *Fort Wayne Sentinel*, April 13, 1875.

Chapter 24

1. *Indianapolis Journal*, October 12, 1876, from the *Philadelphia Press*, October 3, 1876.
2. *Athens* (OH) *Messenger*, November 9, 1876.
3. Ibid.; *Indianapolis Journal*, October 12, 1876.
4. *Galveston News*, December 9, 1876.
5. "Historical Yellow Fever Epidemics," www.WHO.int/csr/disease/yellowfev/en.
6. *Atlanta Constitution*, September 8, 9, 11, 15, 1876.
7. *Herald, Torch Light* (Maryland), October 4; *Waterloo* (IA) *Courier*, October 4; *Camden* (ME) *Herald*, November 18; *Georgia Constitution*, October 5, November 1; *Thomasville* (GA) *Southern Enterprise*, September 6, December 6; *Carroll County* (GA) *Times*, November 17, 1876.
8. *Galveston News*, August 5, 1876.
9. *London Echo*, January 10, September 21; *New York Herald*, March 9; *Dubuque Herald*, April 10; *London Anglo-American Times*, January 29, 1870.
10. *London Standard*, September 22, 30, October 10, 19; *London Daily News*, September 23; *New York Herald*, September 24; *Echo*, November 9, December 10, 1870.
11. *London Daily News*, June 10; *Indianapolis Journal*, June 24; *London Standard*, June 28; *London Sun, Central Press*, June 28; *Alton* (IL) *Telegraph*, December 1, 1871.
12. *Cannelton* (IN) *Register*, October 14, 1871; *World*, September 11, 1873; *Fitchburg* (MA) *Sentinel*, August 10; *World*, January 18, 1875; *Galveston News*, July 2, 1876; *Free Press* (Wisconsin), May 13; *Decatur Republican*, May 20, 1875; *Boston Globe*, September 25; *Indianapolis Journal*, November 1; *People* (Indiana), November 25, 1876; *Reports of Cases Argued and Defended in the Supreme Court of Louisiana*, vol. 27 (New Orleans: Republican Office, 1876), 715–719.
13. *Lebanon* (IN) *Patriot*, March 3; *Galveston News*, September 16, 1870; *London Week's News*, February 3, 1872.
14. *Fort Wayne Sentinel*, March 17; *Dearborn* (IN) *Independent*, April 15, 1875; *Cambridge* (OH) *Jeffersonian*, January 13; *Goshen* (IN) *Times*, October 19, 1876.
15. *London Central Press*, February 1, 1871; *World*, February 9; *Galveston News*, August 20, 1875; *Reno Gazette*, December 14, 1876.

Chapter 25

1. *Dubuque* (IA) *Herald*, August 30 (title quote); *Delphi* (IN) *Times*, December 27, 1878.
2. *Petersburg* (VA) *Index-Appeal*, September 10; *Republican Journal* (Kansas), September 11; *Boston Globe*, September 27, October 13; *Rockingham* (VA) *Register*, October 4; *Evening News* (Indiana), October 26; *Butte* (MT) *Miner*, November 27, 1877.
3. *Wisconsin State Journal*, July 30; *Galveston News*, July 30; *Logansport Journal*, August 3, 10; *Algona* (IA) *Republican*, August 7, 1878.
4. *Constitution*, August 3, 13; *Logansport Weekly Journal*, August 10; *Logansport Daily Journal*, August 20; *Hawk-Eye*, August 10; *Galveston News*, July 30, August 10, 11, 21, 25; *Indiana State Sentinel*, August 21; *Fort Wayne Gazette*, August 26; *Chester* (PA) *Times*, August 28; *Dubuque Herald*, August 30; *Petersburg* (VA) *Index-Appeal*, September 10; *Salt Lake Tribune*, September 15; *Alton Telegraph*, November 28, 1878.
5. *Constitution*, August 7, 1878.
6. *Iola* (KS) *Register*, September 7, 1878.
7. *Galveston News*, August 22, September 1; *National* (IN) *Democrat*, August 22; *World*, August 28, October 29; *Freeport* (PA) *Bulletin*, August 28; *Hawk-Eye*, August 30; *Fort Wayne Sentinel*, August 30; *Derrick* (PA) September 9; *Decatur Republican*, September 14; *Greenville* (PA) *Advance Argus*, November 21; *Indianapolis Journal*, December 8, 1878; *Wyoming Post Herald*, April 18, 1885.
8. *British Mail*, June 1, 1877; *Boston Globe*, February 16; *Hawk-Eye*, March 6; *Gleaner* (Jamaica), April 13; *London Daily News*, April 18; *Wellsboro* (PA) *Agitator*, June 11, 1878.
9. *Boston Globe*, February 23; *Galveston News*, March 2, 1878.
10. *World*, October 22; *Salt Lake Tribune*, November 17; *Davenport Gazette*, November 21; *Monticello Express*, November 21; *London American Register*, December 14; *Atchison* (KS) *Globe*, December 13; *Connersville* (IN) *Examiner*, November 28; *Constitution*, December 15, 31; *Indianapolis Journal*, December 21, 1878.
11. *Petersburg* (VA) *Index-Appeal*, November 28; *New Brunswick* (NJ) *Times*, November 16, December 19; *Journal* (Indiana), December 1, 1878.

12. *Gleaner,* May 19, 1877; *Salt Lake Tribune,* August 30; *Titusville* (PA) *Herald,* August 30; *Petersburg Index-Appeal,* August 30, September 28; *Chester Times,* September 10; *Mountain Democrat* (California), November 23, December 28; *Indiana State Sentinel,* October 2; *Hawk-Eye,* March 12, 21; *Independent Goshen* (Indiana), April 13; *Logansport* (IN) *Journal,* February 12, September 18, December 11; *Ukiah* (CA) *City Press,* September 6; *Greencastle* (IN)*Press,* September 11; *Waterloo* (IA) *Courier,* February 27; *New Brunswick* (NJ) *Times,* September 6; *Freeport* (IL) *Bulletin,* September 10; *Wisconsin State Journal,* November 25; *North Manchester* (IN) *Journal,* November 21; *Indianapolis Journal,* November 30; *World,* November 25; *National Democrat* (Indiana), December 26; *Lebanon* (PA) *News,* October 28; *Manitoba* (Canada) *Free Press,* September 9, 1878.

Chapter 26

1. *Indiana* (PA) *Democrat,* February 6, 1879.
2. *Port Jervis* (NY) *Gazette,* May 31; *Milwaukee News,* January 10, 12; *Gleaner,* January 13; *Indianapolis Journal,* January 18, March 27; *Davenport* (IA) *Gazette,* January 31; *Constitution,* January 31; *World,* February 26, 1879.
3. Michael M. Jerrold, "The National Board of Health: 1879–1883," http://www.ncbi.nlm.gov/pmc/articles/PMC3001811/.
4. Bob Kobres, "A Nickle Pickle: The Problem of Building High-Tech from a Meteorite Wreck," http://abob.libs.uga.edu/bobk/nica.html; *Freeport Bulletin,* January 14; *Athens* (OH) *Messenger,* January 30—italics added; *Cedar Rapids* (IA) *Times,* January 30; *Galveston News,* April 5, 6, June 10; *Constitution,* April 9; *Dearborn* (IN) *Independent,* April 17; *Hawk-Eye,* April 20; *Rushville* (IN) *Republican,* May 29; *Iola* (KS) *Register,* June 6; *Independent* (IN), July 19; *Alton Telegraph,* September 11, 1879; *Index-Appeal,* August 6, 1881.
5. *New York Times,* February 3; *Galveston News,* April 14, July 1, 21; *Brownstown* (IN) *Banner,* July 8; *Titusville Herald,* August 5; *Boston Globe,* September 13; *Chester Times,* October 13; *Marshall Statesman,* November 18, 1880; *Decatur Republican,* September 16, 1881.
6. *Logansport Journal,* February 1; *Constitution,* February 12; *Hawk-Eye,* February 1; *Lowell* (MA) *Sun,* February 15; *Milwaukee News,* March 21; *Atchison* (KS) *Globe,* April 25; *Ukiah City Press,* May 2; *Indianapolis* (IN) *People,* May 17; *Connersville* (IN) *Examiner,* May 29; *Elkhart* (IN) *Democrat,* September 25; *Fort Wayne Sentinel,* July 10; *Alton Telegraph,* August 1; *Harrisonburg* (VA) *Rockingham Register,* August 6, October 30; *Ledger-Standard* (Indiana), November 27; *London Magnet,* November 24; *Janesville Gazette,* September 1; *Iowa State Register,* September 10, 1879; *Reno Gazette,* March 12; *Galveston News,* April 7; *Miami County* (IN) *Sentinel,* April 22; *London American Register,* August 14, 1880; *Dixon* (IL) *Telegraph,* October 6, 1884; *Lima* (OH) *Democratic Times,* July 20; *Marshfield* (WI) *Times,* August 28, 1885.
7. *Oshkosh* (WI) *Northwestern,* September 3; *Greensburg* (IN) *Standard,* October 3, 1879.

8. *World,* January 21; *Kennebec* (ME) *Journal,* July 16; *Galveston News,* August 6; *Chariton* (IA) *Patriot,* October 27; *Janesville Gazette,* December 9, 1879; "The Havana Commission and Finlay's Theory," http://exhibits.hsl.virginia.edu/yellowfever/yellow-fever-research-end-19th-century/.
9. *Salt Lake Tribune,* March 1; *Ledger-Standard,* April 13, 1879; *London Colonies and India,* January 10; *Manitoba Free Press,* February 21; *Chester Times,* August 6, November 12; *London Daily News,* November 8, 1880.
10. *Sullivan* (IN) *Democrat,* February 1; *Dearborn* (IN) *Independent,* July 6; *Iowa Liberal,* August 2; *Fort Wayne Gazette,* July 30; *Constitution,* August 16; *Colorado Springs Gazette,* August 20; *Indiana* (PA) *Progress,* September 21; *New Albany Ledger,* August 15; *Constitution,* October 3; *Ligonier* (IN) *Ledger,* November 16, 1882; R.B.S. Hargis, "The Pensacola Yellow Fever Epidemic of 1882," Pub Health Pap 1883:9: ncbi:nlm;nih.gov/pmc/articles/PMC2272478/pdf/publichealthpap00020–031.pdf.
11. *Illinois Courier,* April 18; *Logansport Pharos,* May 3; *Gleaner,* July 12; *Galveston News,* August 9, September 21; *Helena* (MT) *Independent,* September 23; *Miami* (OH) *Helmet,* September 27; *Westville* (IN) *Indicator,* November 1; *Boston Globe,* November 16; *London American Settler,* December 8, 1883.
12. *Ripley County* (IN) *Journal,* May 29, 1884.
13. *Chester Times,* April 14; *Dearborn Independent,* April 15; *Boston Globe,* August 3; *Logansport Journal,* August 11, 1880; *New Albany* (IN) *Public Press,* March 1, 1882; *Aurora* (IN) *Spectator,* October 18, 1883.
14. *Star* (Indiana), March 1; *Indianapolis Journal,* May 18; *Western Mirror* (Indiana), December 11, 1897; *Dubuque Herald,* February 14; *Indianapolis Sentinel,* February 20; *Indiana Democrat,* April 15, 1881; *Logansport Journal,* July 30; *Decatur Democrat,* September 23, 1881; *Newark* (OH) *Advocate,* December 18, 1882; *Goshen Times,* September 25, 1884; *Carroll* (GA) *Free Press,* March 20, 1885.
15. *Iowa State Reporter,* November 19, 1879 from the *Norristown Herald.*

Chapter 27

1. *New-York Times,* November 7, 1883.
2. *London Echo,* February 3, September 23; *Colonies and India,* October 8, October 22; *Malvern* (IA) *Republic Leader,* May 3; *San Antonio Light,* August 2; *Boston Globe,* August 2; *Anglo-American Times,* August 3; *Galveston News,* November 10; *Hagerstown* (IN) *Exponent,* November 28, 1883; *Galveston News,* February 27; *New-York Times,* December 22, 1884.
3. "Yellow Fever," JAMA, vol. 29 (Chicago: AMA Press, 1884), 849.
4. N.S. Davis, ed., "Yellow Fever," *Journal of the American Medical Association* (Chicago: Review, 1884), 569.
5. *Galveston News,* February 23; *New-York Star,* reprinted in the *Syracuse Herald,* July 19, 1885; *Gleaner,* February 13, March 22, 1886; *Syracuse* (NY) *Standard,* June 22, 1886; Congressional Serial Set. United States Printing Office, 1886, pp. 1–8; Samuel Maxwell, "E.H.

Rogers," University of Nebraska–Lincoln, http://digitalcommons.unl.edu/cgi/viewcontent.cgi?article=1017&context=ncbhisttrans.

6. Reprinted in *Piqua* (OH) *Call,* October 9, 1884.

7. *Indepencia Medica: Therapeutic Gazette,* February 1882, reprinted in the *Edinburgh Medical Journal* 27, no. 2 (January–July 1882).

8. *Fort Wayne Journal,* February 14, 1885; *London American Register* (Middlesex), October 4; *Biddeford* (ME) *Journal,* October 18, 1884.

9. *Cedar Rapids Gazette,* August 28, 1884; "Patrick Manson," http://en.wikipedia.org/wiki/Patrick_Manson.

10. "Laveran and the Discovery of the Malaria Parasite," http://www.cdc.gov/maleria/about/history/laveran/html.

11. *London Evening Gazette,* August 28; *Monroe's Iron-Clad Age* (Indiana), February 2, 1884; *Iowa State Register,* December 24, 1885; *Waterloo* (IA) *Courier,* May 19, 1886; "Carlos Juan Finlay," http://yellowfever.lib.virginia.edu/reed/finlay.html; "Carlos Finlay," http://en.wikipedia.org/wiki/Carlos_Finlay.

12. *Wellsville* (NY) *Reporter,* August 19, 1884; Wolfred Nelson, "Yellow Fever," *JAMA,* vol. 13 (Chicago: Printed at the Office of the Association, 1889), 301; J. McFadden Gaston, "Present State of Inoculation Against Yellow Fever," *JAMA,* vol. 29, (Chicago: AMA Press), 849.

13. *Rochester* (IN) *Republican,* September 29, 1881; *Goshen News,* September 19; *Boston Post,* September 23; *Dixon* (IL) *Telegraph,* October 6, 1884; *Rushville* (IN) *Republican,* March 5; *Galveston News,* July 11; *Madison* (IN) *Herald,* July 21, 1885; *Galveston News,* September 7, 1886.

14. Jerrold M. Michael, "National Board of Health: 1879–1883."

15. *Gleaner,* January 1, February 5; *Eau Claire* (WI) *News,* from the *Philadelphia Times,* February 7; *Rockport* (IN) *Democrat,* February 7; *Ames* (IA) *Intelligencer,* February 21, 1885; Augustin, *History of Yellow Fever.*

Chapter 28

1. *Indianapolis Journal,* December 17, 1880.

2. *Williamsport* (IN) *Warren Republican,* November 27, 1884.

3. *Indianapolis Journal,* December 17, 1880; *Fort Wayne Gazette,* August 12, 31; *Weekly Wisconsin,* September 7; *Kennebec* (ME) *Journal,* October 8, 1881.

4. *London Mid-Surrey Times,* March 1; *Constitution,* June 28; *New-York Times,* July 23, December 24; *Hawk-Eye,* October 26; *Williamsport* (IN) *Warren Republican,* November 27; *Newport* (RI) *Mercury,* November 29, 1884; *East Liverpool* (OH) *Saturday Review,* February 14, 1885.

5. *Titusville Herald,* January 9; *Olean* (NY) *Democrat,* February 3; *Gleaner,* February 11; *Waterloo* (IA) *Courier,* March 18; *Humeston* (IA) *New Era,* March 19; *New-York Times,* May 24; *Yates County* (NY) *Chronicle,* May 27; *Decatur Republican,* May 28; *Lamars* (IA) *Sentinel,* June 8, 1885.

6. *Davenport* (IA) *Gazette,* September 4, 1885.

7. *Gleaner,* May 24; *Madison* (IN) *Herald,* June 24; *Galveston News,* June 27; *New-York Times,* August 2; *Titusville Herald,* August 7, 1886; *Gleaner,* August 29, 1889; *Marshfield* (WI) *Times,* November 28, 1890.

8. *World,* May 19, 21, 25; *Fitchburg* (MA) *Sentinel,* May 21; *Logansport* (IN) *Journal,* August 2, 1889; *Centralia* (WI) *Enterprise and Tribune,* February 15, 1890.

9. *Madison* (IN) *Dollar Weekly Courier,* September 12, October 17, 1885; *San Antonio Express,* June 5; *Coshocton* (OH) *Semi-Weekly Age,* June 7, July 1; *Frederick* (MD) *Age,* September 7; *Bloomington* (IL) *Leader,* September 8; *Eufaula* (OK) *Indian Journal,* June 17; *Spirit Lake Beacon* (IA), July 2; *Hutchinson* (KS) *News,* September 7; *Van Wert* (OH) *Bulletin,* May 21; *Postville* (IA) *Review,* October 23; *Atlantic* (IA) *Telegraph,* September 5; *London St. James Gazette,* September 25, 1888; *Lebanon News,* March 20; *New Philadelphia* (OH) *Times,* March 28, 1889.

10. *Decatur Republican,* April 8, 1887.

11. *Lawrence* (KS) *Journal World,* September 7, November 13; *Dunkirk* (NY) *Observer,* November 17, 1887; *Galveston Tribune,* May 5; *Portland Oregonian,* September 29; *Eau Claire Free Press,* September 27; *Bloomington* (IL) *Ledger,* September 27; *Syracuse Standard,* September 28, 1888; *Manitowoc Lake Shore* (WI) *Times,* March 12, 1889; "Paul Gibier," http://en.wikipedia.org/wiki/Paul_Gibier.

12. *Syracuse Herald,* August 17; *Boston Globe,* August 17; *Massillon* (OH) *Independent,* October 18, 1889.

13. *Fort Wayne Gazette,* April 5; *Ames* (IA) *Intelligencer,* May 23; *Titusville Herald,* May 23; *Ligonier* (IN) *Ledger,* May 28; *Huntingdon* (PA) *Journal,* June 5; *Janesville Gazette,* August 8, 20; *Biddeford Journal,* August 22; *Republic City* (KS), September 18; *Warren* (PA) *Mirror,* October 4; *Lebanon News,* December 10, 1885; *Logansport* (IN) *Critic,* January 10, 1886; *Logansport Pharos Tribune,* September 14, 1888; *Middletown* (NY) *Press,* February 7; *Gleaner,* March 7, 1891.

Chapter 29

1. *Madison* (IN) *Dollar Weekly Courier,* June 13, 1885.

2. *Salt Lake Tribune,* April 11, 1886; *New-York Times,* April 16, 1889, August 8, 1891.

3. *Constitution,* February 9; *World,* February 9; *Newark* (OH) *Advocate,* February 14; *Galveston News,* February 15; *San Antonio Light,* August 16, 1889.

4. *Galveston News,* September 26; *Syracuse Standard,* December 22, 1889.

5. *Kingston Gleaner,* July 2, August 3; *London Man of the World,* August 4; *Alton* (IL) *Telegraph,* September 9, 1897; *Ackley* (IA) *World,* August 17; *Monmouth* (IL) *Gazette,* September 2, 1898; James Carroll, "Yellow Fever: A Popular Lecture," pp. 195–215; U.S. Congressional Serial Set, 1911, pp. 195–215.

6. *Piqua* (OH) *Miami Helmet,* April 9; *Gleaner,* November 17; *Salem* (OH) *News,* September 28; *Oshkosh Northwestern,* July 10, 1891; *Indiana County* (PA) *Gazette,* November 9; *Colonies and India,* December 24, 1892; *Thomasville* (GA) *Times Enterprise,* July 13; *London Standard* (Middlesex), July 13; *Marion* (OH) *Star,* July 18; *Boston Globe,* December 2, 1895; *Mil-*

waukee Weekly Wisconsin, February 15, 19; Hawk-Eye, February 28, 1896.

7. London Standard, February 29; World, March 22, 1896.

8. NY World, June 26; Austin Herald, July 13; Fort Wayne News, July 14; Monmouth (IL) Gazette, August 6; Waterloo (IA) Courier, September 8; San Antonio Light, July 24, 1896.

9. Brownsville (TX) Herald, January 11; Salt Lake (UT) Tribune, May 9, September 19; Bloomington (IL) Pantagraph, July 2; Newark (OH) Advocate, July 3; Logansport (IN) Pharos-Tribune, July 15; Elkhart (IN) Truth, May 26; Bloomington (IL) Leader, August 12, 1897; NY World, May 22, 1898.

10. London American Register, January 22; Burlington (IA) Gazette, March 2; Bryan (TX) Eagle, April 17; Monmouth (IL) Gazette, April 18; Steubenville (OH) Herald Star, April 21; New York World, May 22; Monmouth (IL) Republican Atlas, June 3, 1898.

11. New York World, February 3, April 10; Boston Globe, April 28; Columbus (IN) Times, May 1: question mark in original; Boston Post, May 3; Bloomington (IL) Leader, July 18, 1898.

12. Lowell (MA) Sun, May 9; Racine (WI) Journal, May 12; NY World, May 25, July 3; Boston Globe, May 20; San Antonio Light, May 26; Bryan (TX) Eagle May 8; Cynthiana (IN) Argus, June 4; Perry (IA) Chief, June 16; Renwick (IA) Times, June 23; Church Weekly (London), July 1; Corona (CA) Courier, July 2; Newark (OH) Advocate, June 3, 1898.

13. NY World, May 8; Centralia (IL) Sentinel, July 7; Boston Globe, July 13, 15, 28, 30; Fort Wayne (IN) Sentinel, July 13; Middletown (NY) Argus, July 18; San Antonio Light, July 19; Indianapolis Sun, July 27, 1898.

14. Reno Gazette and Stockman, August 4, 1898; Van der Eijk, "An Episode of Malaria in the Ancient World," from Medicine and Healing in the Ancient Mediterranean, 115.

15. Lowell (MA) Sun, August 4; Salt Lake Tribune, August 12; Hutchinson (KS) News, August 13; New-York Times, August 19, September 2; Atlantic (IA) Telegraph, September 2; Galveston News, September 2, 1898.

Chapter 30

1. Crosby, The American Plague, 219–220.

2. NY World, September 3, 12; East Liverpool (OH) News Review, September 28; Salt Lake City Desert News, October 1, 1898; Boston Globe, October 30, 1898, June 21, July 7, 8, 26; El Paso Herald, October 10, 1899; Bloomington (IL) Pantagraph, May 25, 1900.

3. "The Walter Reed Yellow Fever Commission in Cuba," http://exhibits.hsl.virginia.edu/yellowfever/commission/.

4. "Mosquitoes: Finding the Yellow Fever Vector through Experiments in Cuba," http://exhibits.hsl.virginia.edu/yellowfever/mosquitoes: James Carroll: Lecture.

5. NY Times, October 27, 1900.

6. Indianapolis Sun, February 27; Logansport (IN) Journal, April 9, 1901; James Carroll, "The U.S. Army Commission Experiments," http://exhibits.hsl.virginia.edu/yellowfever/mosquitoes; "Mosquitoes: Finding the Yellow Fever Vector through Experiments in Cuba"; "Case 5 Roots of Informed Consent," http://highschoolbioethics.georgetown.edu/units/cases/unit3_5.html.

7. Des Moines (IA) News, February 15; Loogootee Martin County (IN) Tribune, April 19; Galveston News, April 21; Goshen (IN) Democrat, August 20, 1901.

8. NY Times, August 15, 25, 30, September 6; Janesville (WI) Gazette, August 20; Boston Globe, September 3; London St. James Gazette, December 12, 1901; Boston Globe, May 20; Bluefield (WV) Telegraph, July 23, 1902; Journal of Tropical Medicine 4 (January–December 16, 1901), 403–404; George Sternberg, "The Transmission of Yellow Fever by Mosquitoes," Popular Science Monthly (July 1901); Roger S. Tracy, "Yellow Fever," Popular Science Monthly 13 (October 1878).

Chapter 31

1. Lockhart (TX) Post, November 19, 1903.

2. NY Times, August 9, 1903; "Yellow Fever Deaths in New Orleans," http://nutrias.org/facts/feverdeaths/htm.

3. Covina (CA) Argus, October 3, 1903; Kokomo (IN) Tribune, August 24, 1904; Washington Post, October 3, 1905, March 19, 1907.

4. Elyria (OH) Chronicle, May 16, 1903; Boston Post, August 6, 1904; Hammond Lake County (IN) Times, December 6, 1906; NY Times, February 1; London Standard, April 5; Bessemer (MI) Herald, May 25, 1907; Decatur (IN) Democrat, March 16, 1908; Albion (IN) New Era, January 27, 1909; Indianapolis Sun, May 24, 1910.

5. Lowell (MA) Sun, August 13; Lockhart Post, November 19, 1903; Cedar Rapids Gazette, February 2; Moberly (MO) Monitor, June 21, 1904; Boston Globe, July 29, 1905; Washington Post, March 26, 1905, July 8, 1906; San Antonio Light, May 26; Salt Lake Tribune, September 15; Syracuse Herald, October 13, 1907; David McCullough, "Mosquitoes, Malaria, and the Panama Canal," http://ralphmag.org/panama.html.

6. Washington Journal, November 24, 1906; "Yellow Fever," British Medical Journal, 1, no. 1 (January 5, 1907), 138; Ferdinand (IN) News, February 15, 1907; London Standard, November 1, 1909, May 1, 1911; NY Times, May 28, 1910.

7. Brandon (Manitoba) Sun, July 30, 1903; Frederick (MD) News, May 9, 1904.

8. NY World, December 17, 1903; Brownsville (TX) Herald, November 17, 1905; Racine (WI) Journal, October 29; Kingston Gleaner, November 28; New North (Wisconsin), October 25, 1906; NY Times, August 13; Goodland (IN) Herald, August 31, 1907; Washington Post, August 24, 1908; Brownstown (IN) Banner, April 7; Boston Post, June 12, 1909.

Chapter 32

1. Kingston Gleaner, February 2, 1905.

2. Austin (MN) Herald, February 15; Kokomo Tribune, October 9; London Monitor and New Era, November 21, 1902; NY World, April 3; Racine Journal, April 11, 1903; Boston Post, January 24; NY Times, September 1, 1904; James L. Dickerson, Yellow Fever (New York: Prometheus Books, 2006), 180–181.

3. "The Panama Canal," http://www.cdc.gov/malaria/about/history/panama_canal.html.
4. *Marysville* (OH) *Tribune*, September 24, 1904, May 7, 1908; *NY Times*, January 28, 1905, July 22, 1906; *Boston Post*, August 19; *Syracuse Herald*, October 28, 1906; *Narka* (KS) *News*, March 6; *Ogden* (UT) *Standard*, March 24, 1908; *Kingston Gleaner*, February 2, 1905, November 13, 1906, June 25, 1907, September 1, 1908; Dickerson, *Yellow Fever*, 182–183.
5. *Washington Post*, August 22; *Boston Post*, August 23, 1915.

Chapter 33

1. *Ogden* (UT) *Standard*, August 14, 1915.
2. *Winslow* (IN) *Dispatch*, August 6, 1909.
3. *Atchison* (KS) *Globe*, June 14; *Laredo* (TX) *Times*, July 23; *Fremont* (IN) *Eagle*, December 28, 1916.
4. *Havana Post*, February 3; *Bar Harbor* (ME) *Times*, February 17; *Ardmore* (OK) *Ardmoreite*, July 2; *Boston Post*, December 12, 1917; *San Antonio News*, November 25, 1918; *Connersville* (IN) *Examiner*, September 13; *New York Times*, September 25; *Boston Globe*, October 6; *Galveston News*, November 27; *Indianapolis Star*, November 29; *Akron* (IA) *Tribune*, December 4, 1919; *Washington Post*, June 29, 1920; James Dickerson, *Yellow Fever*, 184–185; "Yellow Fever in South America and the Failure of the Noguchi Vaccine," http://exhibits.hsl.virginia.edu/hanson/yellow-fever-in-south-america-and-the-failure-of-the-Noguchi-vaccine.htm.
5. *Oakland Tribune*, January 1; *Kokomo Tribune*, February 24; *Tokyo Japan Advertiser*, April 18; *Boston Post*, May 1; *Kingston Gleaner*, June 23; *Syracuse Herald*, July 4, 1920.
6. "The West Africa Yellow Fever Commission, 1925–1934." http://exhibits.hsl.virginia.edu/hanson/the-west-africa-yellow-fever-commission-1925-1934.htm; "The Yellow Fever Vaccine: A History." http://www.ncbi.nlm.nih.gov/pmc/articles/PMC2892770; "Yellow Fever in South America and the Failure of the Noguchi Vaccine"; *Appleton* (WI) *Post Crescent*, December 2, 1927; *Reno Gazette*, May 22, 1928.
7. *Salt Lake Tribune*, October 2, 1934; "The Yellow Fever Vaccine: A History," http://www.ncbi.nlm.nih.gov/pmc/articles/PMC28992770; "Yellow Fever Work in North America and a New Vaccine," http://exhibits.hsl.virginia.edu/hanson/yellow-fever-work-in-north-america-and-a-new-vaccine.
8. *San Antonio Express*, April 23, 1931, May 11, 1932; *New Castle* (PA) *News*, May 12, 1932; *Newark* (OH) *Advocate*, December 11, 1936; *Joplin* (MO) *Globe*, March 23, 1938; "Yellow Fever Vaccine: A History"; "Yellow Fever Work in North America and a New Vaccine."
9. James Dickerson, *Yellow Fever*, 187–196; "The History of Biological Warfare," http:www.ncbi.nlm.nih.gov/pmc/articles/PMC1326439.
10. *Oakland Tribune*, December 6, 1940; *Panama City* (FL) *News Herald*, December 29, 1940; *Berkley* (CA) *Gazette*, March 8, 1941; *Annapolis* (MD) *Capital*, February 20; *Olean* (NY) *Times Herald*, April 6; *Ogden Standard Examiner*, July 24; *Adrian* (MI) *Telegram*, July 28, 1942; "Yellow Fever Vaccine"; "Yellow Fever Vaccine-Associated Hepatitis Epidemic During World War II: Follow-up More Than 40 Years Later," http://www.ncbi.nlm.nih.gov/books/NBK234464; John D. Grabenstein, Phillip R. Pittman, John T. Greenwood, and Renata J. Engler. *Immunization to Protect the U.S. Armed Forces: Heritage, Current Practice, Prospects* (Ft. Belvoir: Defense Technical Information Center, 2005).
11. "CBRNE—Biological Warfare Agents," http://emedicine.medscape.com/article/829613-overview; "United States biological weapons program, http://en.wikipedia.org/wiki/United_States_biological_weapons_program; "Introduction to Biological Weapons," http:///www.fas.org/programs/ssp/bio/resource/introtobw.html, Federation of American Scientists official site, 2009; James Dickerson, "Yellow Fever," 187–193; "History of Biological Warfare," http://www.ncbi.nlm.nih.gov/pmc/articles/PMC1326439/; "Germ Warfare/Biological Weapons," http://uic.edu/classes/osci/osci590/7_Germ%20Warfare%20Biological%20Weapons; "Weapons of Mass Destruction," http://www.hampshire.edu/pawss/weapons-of-mass-destruction; U.S. State Department Report on WMD, http://www.state.gov/t/vci/rls/rpt/51977.htm; *Indiana* (PA) *Gazette*, May 19; *Frederick* (MD) *News*, Nov 29, 1947.

Chapter 34

1. *St. Louis Post-Dispatch*, November 30, 2015 (bold type added).
2. Mark D. Gershman, "For the Record: A History of Yellow Fever Vaccine Requirements," http://wwwnc.cdc.gov/travel/yellowbook/2016/infectious-diseases-related-to-travel; "Yellow Fever Vaccination," http://wwwdc.cdc.gov/vaccines/vpd-vac/yf/default.htm.
3. *NY Times*, February 12, 1956; "The Yellow Fever Vaccine: A History"; "Yellow Fever Vaccine: Recommendations of the Advisory Committee on Immunization Practices (ACIP)," http://www.cdc.gov/mmwr/preview/mmwrhtml/rr5907a.htm; "Yellow Fever Work in North America and a New Vaccine," http://exhibits.hsl.virginia.edu/hanson/yellow-fever-work-in-north-america-and-a-new-vaccine; "Yellow Fever Vaccination Recommendations of the Advisory Committee on Immunization Practices, 2002," http://www.cdc.gov/mmwr/preview/mmwrhtml/rr5117a1.htm.
4. *Keokuk* (IA) *Gate City*, March 5, 1964.
5. "Yellow Fever," http://www.who.int/mediacentre/factsheets/fs100/en; "The Yellow Fever Initiative: providing an opportunity of a lifetime," http://www.who.int/csr/disease/yellowfev/brochure/en/; "Yellow Fever Vaccination to start," http://who.int/mediacentre/news/release/2009/yellow_fever_20091117/en/; "Yellow Fever Burden Estimation: Summary"; "Impact of Yellow Fever on the Developing World"; "Yellow Fever: The Recurring Plague"; "Emergency Preparedness, Response, Yellow Fever," all from http://who.int/csr/disease/yellowfev/en/; "Yellow fever Vaccination," http://www.cdc.gov/vaccines/vpd-vac/yf/default.htm; James Dickerson, "Yellow Fever," 230–233.

Glossary

1. Donald Venes, *Taber's Cyclopedic Medical Dictionary* (Philadelphia: F.A. Davis, 2005), 42.

2. *Little Rock* (AK) *Gazette,* May 7, 1866, from the *New York Tribune.*
3. *Gentleman's Magazine,* February 1, 1765.
4. *NY Times,* December 24, 1884.
5. J.M. Powell, *Bring Out Your Dead* (Philadelphia: University of Pennsylvania Press, 1993), 37.
6. Venes, 882.
7. "The History Dish: Pearlash, the First Chemical Leavening," www.fourpoundsofflour.com.
8. "Wild Pepper Grass," www.naturalmedicinalherbs.net/lepidium-virginicum=wild-pepper-grass.php.
9. Venes, 1646.
10. Ibid., 1647.
11. "Krameria," http://en.wikipedia.org/wiki/Krameria.

Bibliography

"Aaron Burr takes everyone to the bank." http://todayshistorylesson.wordpress.com/tag/manhattan-company/.

Anderson, James. *A few Facts and Observations on the Yellow Fever of the West Indies.* London: Robinsons, 1798.

Augustin, George. *History of Yellow Fever.* New Orleans: Searcy & Pfaff, 1909.

Bancroft, Edward Nathaniel. "An Essay on the disease called Yellow fever, with observations concerning Febrile Contagion." London: Printed for T. Cadell and W. Davis, 1811.

Barrett, A. D. T., and S. Higgs. 2007. "Yellow Fever: A Disease That Has Yet to Be Conquered." *Annual Review of Entomology.* 52: 209–230.

Beaver, Philip. *African Memoranda: Relative to an Attempt to Establish a British Settlement on the Island of Bulama, on the Western Coast of Africa, in the Year of 1792.* Westport, CT: Negro Universities Press, 1970.

Berry, Leonidas H. "Black Men and Malignant Fevers." *Journal of the National Medical Association* 56, no. 1 (January 1984), 43–47. http://www.ncbi.nlm.nih.gov/pmc/articles/pmc2610872/pdf/jnma00545-0047.pdf.

"Biological Warfare Agents—CBRNE." http://emedicine.medscape.com/article/829613-overview.

Blake, John B. "Yellow Fever in Eighteenth Century America." *Bull NY Acd Med* 44, no. 6 (June 1968). http://www.ncbi.nlm.nih.gov/pmc/articles/pmc1750737/pdf/bullnyacadmed00243-0085.pdf.

Blanco, Richard L. "Medicine in the Continental Army, 1775–1781." *Bull NY Acd Med* 57, no. 8 (October 1981).

Blane, Gilbert. *Observations on the Diseases Incident to Seamen.* London: Murray, 1785.

Boyce, Rupert, "Discussion of Yellow Fever." *Journal of Tropical Medicine and Hygiene* 14 (February 1, 1911): 42.

Bres, P. L. "A Century of Progress in combating yellow fever." *Bulletin of the World Health Organization* 64, no. 6 (1996).

Bryson, Alexander, M.D. *An Account of the Origin, Spread, and Decline of the Epidemic Fevers of Sierra Leone: With Observations on Sir W. Pym's Review of the "Report on the Climate and Diseases of the African Station."* London, 1849.

"Building the Panama Canal." http://history.state.gov/milestones/1899–1913/panema-canal.

"Carlos Finlay." http://en.wikipedia.org/wiki/Carlos _Finlay.

"Carlos Juan Finlay." http://yellowfever.lib.virginia.edu/reed/finlay.html.

Carroll, James. "Yellow Fever: A Popular Lecture." United States Congressional Serial Set, U.S. Government Printing Office, 1911, reprinted from *American Medicine* 9, no 22 (June 3, 1905).

"Chemical and Biological Weapons: Possession and Programs Past and Present." http://cns.miis.edu/cbw/possess.htm.

Choppin, Samuel. "History of the Importation of Yellow Fever Into the United States, from 1693–1878." Pub Health Pap Rep. 1878; 4. http://ncbi.nlm.nih.gov/pmc/articles/pmc2272343/pdf/publichealthpap00025-0197.pdf

"Cock Lane Ghost." www.localmythsandlegends.com

Coggins, Clemency Chase. "Medical Articles in Eighteenth Century American Magazines." *Bull Med Lib Ass* 53 no. 3 (July 1965). http://www.ncbi.nlm.nih.gov/pmc/articles/pmc198299/pmc/mlab00180–0136.

College of Physicians, Philadelphia. *Facts and Observations Relative to the Nature and Origin of the Pestilential Fever, which Prevailed in the City of Philadelphia, in 1793, 1797, and 1798.* 8 Vol. Philadelphia: Reprinted by Phillips in London, 1799.

"Colonial Diseases." http://mayflowerfamilies.com.

Crosby, Molly Caldwell. *The American Plague.* New York: Berkley Books, 2006.

"Cuban War of Independence." http://en.wikipedia.org/wiki/Cuban_War_of_Independence.

Currie, James. *Medical Reports, on the Effects of Water, Cold and Warm, as a Remedy in Fever and Febrile Diseases, Whether Applied to the*

Surface of the Body, or Used Internally. 4th ed. Liverpool: Cadell and Davies, 1806.

Currie, William. "A Description of the Malignant Infectious Fever Prevailing at Present in Philadelphia; with an Account of the Means to Prevent Infection, and the Remedies and Method of Treatment, Which Have Been Found Most Successful." Philadelphia: Thomas Dobson, 1793.

___. "An Enquiry into the Causes of the Insalubrity of Flat and Marshy Situations; and Directions for Preventing or Correcting the Effects Thereof." From the Transactions of the American Philosophical Society. Philadelphia, 1800.

___. "A Sketch of the Rise and Progress of the Yellow Fever, and of the Proceedings of the Board of Health, in Philadelphia, in the Year 1799; to Which Is Added, a Collection of Facts and Observations Respecting the Origin of the Yellow Fever in this Country; and a Review of the Different Modes of Treating It." American Philosophical Society. Philadelphia, 1800.

Danisi, Thomas C. *Uncovering the Truth About Meriwether Lewis*. New York: Prometheus, 2012.

Davis, N.S., ed. *Journal of the American Medical Association*. Chicago: Review, 1884.

Denney, Robert E. *Civil War Medicine: Care AND Comfort of the Wounded*. New York: Sterling, 1994.

Dickerson, James L. *Yellow Fever: A Deadly Disease Poised to Kill Again*. Amherst, NY: Prometheus, 2006.

Dire, Daniel J. "CBRNE—Biological Warfare Agents." http://emedicine.medscape.com/article/829613-overview.

"Dr. Thomas Young." http://www.christiandeistfellowship.com/dryoung/htm.

Duffy, John. "Yellow Fever in the Continental United States During the Nineteenth Century." *Bull NY Med* 44, no. 6 (June 1968). http://www.ncbi.nlm.nih.gov/pmc/articles/pmc1750233/pdf/bullnyacadmed00243-0099.

Edinburgh Medical Journal 27, no. 2 (January–June 1882). Edinburgh, 1882.

Fellowes, James. *Reports of Pestilential Disorder of Andalusia Which Appeared at Cadiz in the Years 1800, 1804, 1810 and 1813; with a Detailed Account of That Fatal Epidemic as It Prevailed at Gibraltar During the Autumnal Months of 1804; Also Observation on the Remitting and Interesting Fever, Made in the Military Hospitals at Colchester After the Return of the Troops from the Expedition to Zealand in 1809*. London: Printed by A. Strahan for Longman, Hurst, Rees, Orme, and Brown, 1815.

Fordyce, George. *A Fourth Dissertation on Fever: Containing the History of and Remedies to Be Employed in Irregular Intermitting Fevers*. London: Johnson, 1802.

Fothergill, A. "Friendly Cautions on the Prevention of Pestilential Contagion, and of Premature Interment; Drawn Up During the Ravages Occasioned by the Yellow Fever in Philadelphia, New York, &c. in the Epidemic of 1805; and Submitted to the Serious Consideration of the Inhabitants." Philadelphia: American Philosophical Society, 1806.

Frierson, J. Gordon. "The Yellow Fever Vaccine: A History." http://www.ncbi.nlm.nih.gov/pmc/articles/PMC2892770/.

Frischknecht, Friedrich. "The History of Biological Warfare." http://www.ncbi.nlm.nih.gov/pmc/articles/PMC1326439.

Fulton, John S. "Quarantine: The Delirum Ferox of American Sanitation." *Pub Health Pap Rep* 31, no. 1 (1905). www.http://www.ncbi.nlm.nih.gov/pmc/articles/pmc2222524/pdf/publichealthpap00000-0257.

Gaskell, E. "Early American Translations of European medical Works." *Med His* 14, no. 3 (July 1970). http://www.ncbi.nlm.nih.gov/pmc/articles/pmc1034062/pdf/medhist00134-0092.

Gaston, J. McFadden. "Present Status of Inoculation Against Yellow Fever." *Journal of the American Medical Association* 29. Chicago: AMA Press, 1897.

Gayarre, Charles. *History of Louisiana and Spanish Domination*. New York: William J. Widdleton, 1867.

"Germ Warfare/Biological Weapons." http://www.uic.edu/classes/osci/osci590/7_1Germ%20Warfare%20Biological%20Weapons.

Gorgas, W. C. "Recent Experiences of the United States Army with Regard to Sanitation of Yellow Fever in the Tropics." *Journal of Tropical Medicine* 6 (February 2, 1903): 49.

Grabenstein, John, and Phillip Pitman. "Immunization to Protect the U.S. Armed Forces: Heritage, Current Practice, Prospects." http://www.vaccines.mil.

"Hamilton and Burr Together for the Last Time." http://todayshistorylesson.wordpress.com/2010/02/22/hamilton-and-burr-together-for-the-last-time/.

Hardie, J. *Account of the Malignant Fever Lately Prevalent in the City of New York*. New York, 1798.

Hargis, R.B.S. "The Pensacola Yellow Fever Epidemic of 1882." *Pub Health Pap 1883* 9. ncbi: nlm.nih.gov/pmc/articles/PMC2272478/pdf/publichealthpap00020-031.pdf.

"The Havana Commission and Finlay's Theory. http://exhibits.hsl.virginia.edu/yellowfever/yellow-fever-research-end-19th-century/.

Heaton, Claude Edwin. "Yellow Fever in New York City." *Bull Med Library Assoc*. 34, no. 2 (April 1946). www.http://www.ncbi.nlm.nih.gov/pmc/articles/pmc194570/pdf/mlab00256-0013.pdf.

"History of the Panama Canal." http://en.wikipedia.org/History_of_the_panama_canal.

Hooper, Robert. *Lexicon Medicum; or, Medical Dictionary*. New York: Harper, 1842.

Horsman, Reginald. *Josiah Nott of Mobile*. Baton Rouge: Louisiana State University Press, 1987.

Hosack, Alexander, Jr. *History of the Yellow Fever, as It Appeared in the City of New York in 1795*. 8 vol. Philadelphia: Dobson, 1797.

Hosack, David, and John W. Francis. "Account of the Yellow Fever Which Prevailed in Virginia in the Years 1737, 1741 and 1742, in a Letter to the Late Cadwallader Colden, Esq. of New-York, from the Late John Mitchell, M.D. F.R.S. of Virginia." *American Medical and Philosophical Register*. New York: C.S. Van Winkle, 1814.

Humphreys, Margaret. *Yellow Fever and the South*. Baltimore: Johns Hopkins Press 1992.

Hunter, John. *Observations on the Diseases of the Army in Jamaica; and on the Best Means of Preserving the Health of Europeans in that Climate*. London: Nicol, 1788.

"Impact of the U.S. Army Yellow Fever Commission's Findings." http://exhibits.hsl.virginia.edu/yellowfever/impact.

Jackson, Robert. *An Outline of the History and Cure of Fever, Endemic and Contagious; More Expressly the Contagious Fever of Jails, Ships, and Hospitals; the Concentrated Endemic, Vulgarly the Yellow Fever of the West Indies*. 8 vol. Longman and Rees, 1798.

Jones, Absalom, and Richard Allen. *A Narrative of the Proceedings of the Black People, During the Late Awful Calamity in Philadelphia, in the Year 1793*. Philadelphia: William W. Woodward, 1794.

"Juan Carlos Finlay (1833–1915)." http://yellowfever.lib/virginia.edu/reed/finlay.html.

Kobres, Bob. "A Nickel Pickle," http://abob.libs.uga.edu/bobk/nica.html.

Kotar, S.L., and J.E. Gessler. *Ballooning: A History, 1782–1900*. Jefferson, NC: McFarland, 2011.

_____ and _____. *Cholera: A Worldwide History*. Jefferson, NC: McFarland, 2014.

_____ and _____. *The Rise of the American Circus, 1716–1899*. Jefferson, NC: McFarland, 2011.

_____ and _____. *Smallpox: A History*. Jefferson, NC: McFarland, 2013.

_____ and _____. *The Steamboat Era: A History of Fulton's Folly on American Rivers*. Jefferson, NC: McFarland, 2009.

Lambert, John. *Travels Through Canada, and the United States of North America, in the Years 1806, 1807, and 1808*. London: Cradock and Joy, 1813.

"Laveran and the Discovery of the Malaria Parasite." http://www.cdc.gov/malaria/about/history/laveran.html.

Lawrence, Vera Brodsky. *Strong on Music: The New York Music Scene in the Days of George Templeton Strong*. Chicago: University of Chicago Press, 1995.

Lempriere, William. *Practical Observations on the Diseases of the Army in Jamaica, as They Occurred Between the Years 1792 and 1797; on the Situation, Climate, and Diseases of That Island; and on the Most Probable Means of lessening Mortality Among the Troops, and Among Europeans in Tropical Climates*. 8 vol. London: Longman and Rees, 1799.

Ligon, Richard. *A True and Exact History of the Island of Barbadoes*. London: Peter Parker, 1657.

Lind, Dr. "Observations on the Diseases Which Attack Strangers in North America." London, 1768.

"Manhattan Company." http://en.wikipedia.org/wiki/The_Manhattan_Company.

Maxwell, Samuel, "E.H. Rogers." University of Nebraska, Lincoln. http://digitalcommons.unl.edu/cgi/viewcontent.cgi?article=1017&context=nebhisttrans).

McCandless, Peter, "Revolutionary Fever: Disease and War in the Lower South, 1776–1783." Trans Am Clin Climatol Assoc. 2007.

McClachlin, Edward. "Prison Life." *Stevens Point (WI) Journal*, March 14, 1885.

McCullough, David. "Mosquitoes, Malaria, and the Panama Canal." http://www.ralphmag.org/panema.html.

McGrew, Roderick E., and Margaret P. McGrew. *Encyclopedia of Medical History*. London: Macmillan, 1985.

McLean, Hector. *An Enquiry into the Nature and Causes of the Great Mortality Among the Troops at St. Domingo*. London: Cadell jun. and Davies, 1797.

Mertens, Charles de. *An Account of the Plague Which Raged at Moscow in 1771*. Translated from the French with notes. 8 vol. London: Rivingtons, 1799.

Michael, Jerrold M. "The National Board of Health: 1879–1883." http://www.ncbi.nlm.nih.gov/articles/PMC3001811/.

"Mosquitoes: Finding the Yellow Fever Vector through Experiments in Cuba." http://exhibits.hsl.virginia.edu/yellowfever/mosquitoes.

"National Board of Health: 1879–1883." http://www.ncbi.nih.gov/pmc/articles/PMC3001811/.

Neidhard, Charles. *On the Efficacy of Crotalus Horridus in Yellow Fever: Also in Malignant, Bilious, and Remittent Fevers*." New York: William Radde, 1860.

Nelson, Wolfred. *Five Years at Panama*. New York: Belford-Clarke, 1891.

_____. "Yellow Fever." *Journal of the American Medical Association* 13. Chicago: Printed at the Offices of the Association, 1889.

"New Strategies Work: Mosquito Eradication Vs.

Sanitation and Quarantine." http://exhibits.hsl.virginia.edu/yellowfever/new_strategies/.

Nuwer, Deanne Stephens. *Plague Among the Magnolias*. Tuscaloosa: University of Alabama Press, 2009.

Oswald, F.L. "Fever Factories." *Popular Science Monthly*. New York: D. Appleton, December 1878.

Padmanabhan, Sampath A. "Molecular targets for flavivirus drug discovery." *Antiviral Res* 81, no. 1 (January 2009).

"Panama Canal Zone." http://en.wikipedia.org/wiki/Panama_Canal_Zone.

"Patrick Manson." http://en.wikipedia.org/wiki/Patrick_Manson.

"Patrick Nelson." http://en.wikipedia.org/wiki/Patrick_Nelson.

Perkins, Benjamin Douglas. *The Influence of Metallic Tractors on the Human Body*. London, 1798.

Perkins, Elisha. *Certificates of the Efficacy of Doctor Perkins' Patent Medicine Instruments*. New-London. S. Green's, 1796.

"Politics of the Spanish-American War." http://exhibits.hsl.virginia.edu/yellowfever/politics/.

Powell, J.M. *Bring Out Your Dead: The Great Plague of Yellow Fever in Philadelphia in 1793*. Philadelphia: University of Pennsylvania Press, 1949, reprinted 1993.

Quarterly Journal of Science, Literature and Art 23 (January–June 1827). London: Henry Colburn, 1827.

Reed, Laura. "Weapons of Mass Destruction." http://www.hamphire.edu/pawss/weapons-of-mass-destruction.

Reports of Cases Argued and Defended in the Supreme Court of Louisiana, 1875. Vol. 27. New Orleans: Printed at the Republic Office, 1876.

"A Revolution in Haiti." http://scholar.library.miami.edu/slaves/san_domingo_revolution/revolution.html.

"Roots of Informed Consent: Case 5." https://highschoolbioethics.georgetown.edu/units/cases/unit3_5.html.

Rush, Benjamin. *An Account of the Bilious Remitting Yellow Fever, as It Appeared in the City of Philadelphia in the Year 1793*. 8 vol. Philadelphia: 1794.

___. *Medical Inquiries and Observations, Containing an Account of the Yellow Fever as It Appeared in Philadelphia in 1797, and Observations Upon the Nature and Cure of the Gout and Hydrophobia*. Vol. 5. Philadelphia: Mawman, 1801.

___. *Observations Upon the Origin of the Malignant, Bilious, or Yellow Fever, in Philadelphia, and Upon the Means of Preventing It*. Philadelphia: Dobson, 1799.

Senn, Nicholas. "The Qualification and Duties of the Military Surgeon." *Journal of the American Medical Association* (September 1898).

"Separation of Panama from Colombia." http://en.wikipedia.org/wiki/Separation_of_Panama_from_Columbia.

Shattuck, George B., ed. *Boston Medical and Surgical Journal* 3 (July–December 1884). Boston: Houghton, Mifflin, 1884.

"The Slave Rebellion in Haiti," http://www.latinamericanstudies.org/haiti/slave-rebellion/rebellion.htm.

Spann, Edward K. *The New Metropolis: New York City, 1840–1857*. New York: Columbia University Press, 1981.

Sternberg, George M. "The Transmission of Yellow Fever by Mosquitoes" *Popular Science Monthly*, July 1901.

Stevens, William. *Observations on the Healthy and Diseased Properties of the Blood*. London: John Murray, 1832.

Sullivan, John. *Diseases of Tropical Climates, with their Treatment*. London: J. & A. Churchill, 1877.

"Thomas Young." http://www.gilderlehrman.org/history-by-era/war-for-independence/timeline-terms/thomas-young.

Tracy, Roger S. "Yellow Fever." *The Popular Science Monthly*, October 1878.

Unicef. "Financial Threat to Global Supply of Vaccine Puts 120 Million at Risk of Yellow Fever." www.unicef.org/media/media_53980.html.

"United States Biological Weapons Program." http://en.wikipedia.org/wiki/United_States_biological_weapons_program.

"U.S. Army Commission Experiments." http://exhibits.hsl.virginia.edu/yellowfever/mosquitoes.

Van der Eijk, Philip. "An Episode in the Historiography of Malaria in the Ancient World," in *Medicine and Healing in the Ancient Mediterranean*. Philadelphia: Oxbow Books, 2014

Venes, Donald. *Taber's Cyclopedic Medical Dictionary*, Ed. 20. Philadelphia: F.A. Davis, 2005.

"Walter Reed Yellow Fever Commission in Cuba." http://exhibits.hsl.virginia.edu/yellowfever/commission.

Watts, Sheldon. "Yellow Fever Immunities in West Africa and the Americas in the Age of Slavery and Beyond: A Reappraisal." *Journal of Social History*, Summer 2001.

"William C. Gorgas." http://en.wikipedia.org/wiki/William_C._Gorgas.**

"William C. Gorgas." http://www.nnbd.com/people/522/000203910/.

Williams, John, and Parker Bennet. "Essays on the bilious fever: containing the different opinions of those eminent physicians John Williams and Parker Bennet, of Jamaica; which was the cause of a duel, and terminated in the death of both." London: T. Waller, 1752, reprinted by Ecco.

Willich, Anthony Florian Madinger, and James

Mease. *The Domestic Encyclopaedia; or, A Dictionary of Facts and Useful Knowledge.* Philadelphia: William Young Birch and Abraham Small, 1804.

Wills, Christopher. *Yellow Fever: Black Goddess.* Reading, MA: Addison-Wesley.

Wood, George Bacon, and Franklin Bache. *The Dispensatory of the United States.* Philadelphia: Grigg & Elliot, 1845.

"World War One and Wilsonian Diplomacy." http://history.state.gov/milestones/1914-1920.

"Yellow Fever," *British Medical Journal* 1, no. 1, London: January 5, 1907.

"Yellow Fever." http://en.wikipedia.org/wiki/Yellow_fever.

"Yellow Fever." *Journal of Tropical Medicine* IV (January 1–December 16, 1901). London: John Bale, Sons & Danielsson, 1901.

"Yellow Fever." Louisiana Office of Public Health, Infectious Disease Epidemiology Section. Annual Report, 1934: dhh.louisiana.gov.

"Yellow Fever." PubMedHealth. http://www.ncbi.nlm.hih.gov/pubmedhealth/PMH0002341/.

"Yellow Fever Deaths in New Orleans." http://nutrias.org/facts/feverdeaths.htm.

"Yellow Fever in Cuba during the Spanish-American War." http://exhibits.hsl.virginia.edu/yellowfever/cuba.

"Yellow Fever Vaccine-Associated Hepatitis Epidemic During World War II: Follow-up More than 40 Years Later." http://www.ncbi.nlm.hih.gov/books/NBK234464/.

"Yellow Fever Work in North America and a New Vaccine." http://exhibits.hsl.virginia.edu/hanson/yellow-fever-work-in-north-america-and-a-new-vaccine/.

World Health Organization (WHO)

"Emergencies Preparedness, Response: Yellow Fever." www.who.int/csr/disease/yellowfev/en.

"Impact of Yellow Fever on the Developing World." www.who.int/yellowfever.

"Yellow Fever." www.who.int.mediacentre/factsheets/fs100/en.

"Yellow Fever Biorisk Reduction." www.who.int/csr/bioriskreduction/en.

"Yellow Fever: Emergency Preparedness, Response." www.who.int/csr/disease/yellowfev/brochure/en.

"Yellow Fever: Global Alert and Response (GAR)." www.who.int/csr/disease/yellowfev/en/.

"Yellow Fever: The Recurring Plague." www.who.int/yellowfever.

"Yellow Fever Vaccination Campaign to Start." who.int/mediccentre/news/releases/2009/yellow_fever_20091117/en/index.html.

Centers for Disease Control and Prevention

"Frequently Asked Questions." http://www.cdc.gov/yellowfever/qa/index.html.

Gershman, Mark D. "For the Record: A History of Yellow Fever Vaccine Requirements." http://wwwnc.cdc.gov/travel/yellowbook/2016/infectious-diseases-related-to-travel.

"Laveran and the Discovery of the Malaria Parasite." http://www.cdc.gov/malaria/about/history/laveran.html. "The Panama Canal." http://www.cdc.gov/malaria/about/history/panama_canal.

"Prevention of Yellow Fever" cdc.gov/yellowfever/prevention/index.html.

"Symptoms and Treatment." cdc.gov/yellowfever/symptoms/index.html.

"Transmission of Yellow Fever Virus." cdc.gov/yellowfever/transmission/index.html.

"Yellow Fever Cavvination" http://www.cdc.gov/vaccines/vpd-vac/yf/default.htm.

"Yellow Fever Maps." cdc.gov/yellowfever/maps/index.html. "Yellow Fever Vaccination Recommendations of the Advisory Committee on Immunization Practices," 2002. http://www.cdc.gov/mmrw/preview/mmwrhtml/rr5907a 1.htm.

"Yellow Fever Vaccine." cdc.gov/yellowfever/vaccine/index.html.

University of Virginia Articles

"A Brief History of the Rockefeller Foundation's International Health Commission." http://exhibits.hsl.virginia.edu/hanson/a-brief-history-of-the-rockefeller-foundations-international-health-commission/.

"The Havana Commission and Finlay's Theor.," https://exhibits.hsl.virginia.edu/yellowfever/yellow-fever-research-end-19th-century/.

"Henry Hanson, M.D.: Biographical Essay of a Yellow Fever Fighter." http://exhibits.hsl.virginia.edu/hanson/henry-hanson-m-d-a-biographical-essay/.

"Impact of the U.S. Army Yellow Fever Commission's Findings." http://exhibits.hsl.virginia.edu/yellowfwver/impact/.

"Mosquitoes: Finding the Yellow Fever Vector Through Experiments in Cuba." http://exhibits.hsl.virginia.edu/yellowfever/mosquitoes.

"New Strategies Work: Mosquito Eradication vs. Sanitation and Quarantine." http://exhibits.hsl.virginia.edu/yellowfever/new_strategies/.

"Politics of the Spanish-American War." http://exhibits.hsl.virginia.edu/yellowfever/politics/.

"The U.S. Army Commission Experiments." http://exhibits.hsl.virginia.edu/yellowfever/mosquitoes.

"The Walter Reed Yellow Fever Commission in Cuba." http://exhibits.hsl.virginia.edu/yellowfever/commission/.

"West Africa Yellow Fever Commission, 1925–

1934." http://exhibits.hsl.virginia.edu/hanson/the-west-africa-yellow-fever-commission-1925-1934.

"Yellow Fever in Cuba During the Spanish-American War." http://exhibits.hsl.virginia.edu/yellowfever/cuba/.

"Yellow Fever in South America and the Failure of the Noguchi Vaccine." http://exhibits.hsl.virginia.edu/hanson/yellow-fever-in-south-america-and-the-failure-of-the-noguchi-vaccine.

Newspapers and Magazines

Ackley (IA) *World*
Adams Centinel/Adams Sentinel (PA)
Adrian (MI) *Telegram*
Akron (IA) *Tribune*
Albany (NY) *Log Cabin*
Albion (IN) *New Era*
Algona (IA) *Republican*
Alton (IL) *Telegraph and Democratic Review*
Alton (IL) *Weekly Courier*
Alton (IL) *Weekly Telegraph*
American Freeman (WI)
American Medical and Philosophical Register
American Register (London)
American Settler (London)
Ames (IA) *Intelligencer*
Anglo-American Times (London)
Annapolis (MD) *Capital*
Annual Register (London)
Annual Register on a View of the History, Politics, and Literature of the Year 1798 (London)
Antigallican Monitor and Anti-Corsican Chronicle (London)
Anti-Jacobin Review and Magazine (London)
Appleton (WI) *Motor*
Appleton (WI) *Post Crescent*
Ardmore (OK) *Ardmoreite*
Argus and Democrat, Weekly (WI)
Arkansas Weekly Gazette
Atchison (KS) *Globe*
Athens (OH) *Messenger*
Atlanta (GA) *Constitution*
Atlantic (IA) *Telegraph*
Atlas (London)
Aurora (IN) *Commercial*
Aurora (IN) *Spectator*
Austin (MN) *Daily Herald*
Australian Mail (London)
Baldwin's Weekly Journal (London)
Bangor (ME) *Daily Whig and Courier*
Bar Harbor (ME) *Times*
Baraboo (WI) *Republic*
Bell's Life of London and Sporting Chronicle
Bell's Weekly Messenger
Benton (IN) *Tribune*
Berkley (CA) *Gazette*

Berkshire County (MA) *Eagle*
Bessemer (MI) *Herald*
Biddeford (ME) *Journal*
Bloomington (IL) *Daily Leader*
Bloomington (IL) *Weekly Pantagraph*
Bluefield (WV) *Telegraph*
Boston Globe
Boston Medical and Surgical Journal, 1844
Boston Post
Brandon Sun (Manitoba)
British Banner (London)
British Critic (London)
British Mail
British Medical Journal
British Press (London)
British Spy; or, The Universal London Weekly Journal
British Standard (London)
British Statesman (London)
Brownstown (IN) *Banner*
Brownsville (TX) *Herald*
Bryan (TX) *Eagle*
Burlington (IA) *Gazette*
Burlington (IA) *Hawk-Eye*
Butte (MT) *Miner*
Calhoun County (MI) *Patriot*
Cambridge (OH) *Jeffersonian*
Camden (ME) *Herald*
Cannelton (IN) *Register*
Carlton Chronicle (London)
Carroll County (GA) *Times*
Cedar Rapids (IA) *Evening Gazette*
Central Press (London)
Centralia (IL) *Sentinel*
Centralia (WI) *Enterprise and Tribune*
Champion: A London Weekly Journal
Chariton (IA) *Patriot*
Chester (PA) *Daily Times*
Christian Cabinet (London)
Chronicle and Register, Weekly (London)
Church and State Gazette (London)
Church Weekly (London)
Civilian and Galveston (TX) *Gazette*
Claypoole's American Daily Advertiser (Philadelphia)
Cleave's Penny Gazette of Variety (London)
Colonial Gazette (London)
Colorado Springs Daily Gazette
Columbus (IN) *Times*
Connersville (IN) *Examiner*
Corona (CA) *Courier*
Corydon (IN) *Democrat*
Coshocton (OH) *Age*
Coshocton (OH) *Semi-Weekly Age*
Covina (CA) *Argus*
Crown Point (IN) *Register*
Cumberland (MD) *Daily Times*
Cynthiana (IN) *Argus*
Daily Derrick (PA)

Daily Evening News (IN)
Daily Free Press (WI)
Daily Herald (WI)
Daily Journal (IN)
Daily Ledger-Standard (IN)
Daily Patriot (WI)
Daily Sanduskian (OH)
Daily Sentinel and Gazette (WI)
Daily Washington (DC) *National Intelligencer*
Daily Wisconsin Patriot
Danville (IN) *Advertiser*
Davenport (IA) *Daily Gazette*
Dawson's Daily Times and Union (IN)
Dearborn (IN) *Independent*
Decatur (IL) *Daily Republican*
Decatur (IL) *Democrat*
Decatur (IN) *Eagle*
Defiance (OH) *Democrat*
Delaware State Reporter
Delphi (IN) *Weekly Times*
Democratic Banner (IA)
Democratic Expounder (MI)
Democratic Pharos (IA)
Des Moines (IA) *News*
Dixon (IL) *Daily Telegraph*
Drakard's Paper: A London Weekly Journal
Dublin Journal
Dublin Post and General Advertiser
Dubuque (IN) *Herald*
Dunkirk (NY) *Observer*
Dunlap's American Daily Advertiser
East Liverpool (OH) *News*
East Liverpool (OH) *Saturday Review*
Eau Claire (WI) *Daily Free Press*
Eau Claire (WI) *News*
Edinburgh Advertiser
Edinburgh Evening Courant
Edinburgh Medical Journal
Edinburgh Weekly Journal
El Paso Herald
Elkhart (IN) *Democrat*
Elkhart (IN) *Weekly Truth*
Elyria (OH) *Chronicle*
Eufaula (OK) *Indian Journal*
European Magazine (London)
Evans and Ruffy's Farmers' Journal (London)
Evansville (IA) *Daily Enquirer*
Evening Gazette (NY)
Evening News (IN)
Farmer and Mechanic (IN)
Ferdinand (IN) *News*
Fitchburg (MA) *Daily Sentinel*
Flake's Daily Galveston Bulletin
Flake's Semi-Weekly Galveston Bulletin
Fond du Lac (WI) *Whig*
Fort Atkinson (WI) *Standard*
Fort Wayne (IN) *Daily Democrat*
Fort Wayne (IN) *Daily Gazette*
Fort Wayne (IN) *Daily Sentinel*
Fort Wayne (IN) *Daily Times*
Fort Wayne (IN) *News*
Fort Wayne Times and People's Press
Frederick (MD) *Age*
Frederick (MD) *Herald*
Frederick (MD) *News*
Free Democrat, Daily (WI)
Free-Mason's Magazine (London)
Freeport (IL) *Daily Bulletin*
Freeport (IL) *Journal*
Freeport (PA) *Daily Bulletin*
Fremont (IN) *Eagle*
Galveston (TX) *Bulletin, Daily*
Galveston (TX) *Daily News*
Galveston (TX) *Evening Tribune*
Galveston (TX) *Weekly News*
Galveston Tri-Weekly Civilian
Gazette of the United States
Gazetteer and London Daily Advertiser
Gazetteer and London New Daily Advertiser
Gentleman's Magazine (London)
Gentleman's Magazine and Historical Chronicle (London)
Gettysburg (PA) *Star and Sentinel*
Goodland (IN) *Herald*
Goshen (IN) *Democrat*
Goshen (IN) *Independent*
Goshen (IN) *Times*
Grand Magazine of Magazines; or, London Universal Register
Grand Traverse (MI) *Herald*
Grant County (WI) *Herald*
Green Bay (WI) *Advocate*
Greencastle (IN) *Press*
Greenleaf's New York Journal
Greensburg (IN) *Standard*
Greenville (PA) *Advance*
Greenville (PA) *Advance Argus*
Greenville (PA) *Argus*
Guernsey (OH) *Jeffersonian*
Hagerstown (IN) *Exponent*
Hagerstown (MD) *Mail*
Hammond Like County (IN) *Times*
Havana (Cuba) *Post*
Helena (MT) *Independent*
Hillsdale (MI) *Whig Standard*
Home League (WI)
Hornellsville (NY) *Tribune*
Hull Advertiser (England)
Humeston (IA) *New Era*
Huntingdon (PA) *Journal*
Hutchinson (KS) *Daily News*
Illinois Weekly Courier
Indepencia Medica: Therapeutic Gazette (Britain)
Independent (IN)
Independent American and General Advertiser (WI)
Indiana (PA) *Democrat*
Indiana (PA) *Gazette*

Indiana (PA) *Progress*
Indiana County (PA) *Gazette*
Indiana Daily Journal
Indiana Democrat
Indiana Palladium
Indiana State Sentinel
Indianapolis Evening Journal
Indianapolis Journal
Indianapolis Sun
Iola (KS) *Register*
Iowa Liberal
Iowa State Register
Iowa State Reporter
Jackson (IA) *Sentinel*
Jackson County (IN) *Democrat*
Janesville (WI) *Daily Gazette*
Janesville (WI) *Morning Gazette*
Joplin (MO) *Globe*
Journal of Social History
Journal of Tropical Medicine and Hygiene (London)
Kane (PA)
Kennebec (ME) *Daily Journal*
Kenosha (WI) *Democrat*
Kenosha (WI) *Telegraph*
Kenosha (WI) *Times*
Keokuk (IA) *Gate City*
Kingston (Jamaica) *Gleaner*
Kokomo (IN) *Tribune*
La Crosse (WI) *Independent Republican*
Lamars (IA) *Sentinel*
Laredo (TX) *Times*
Lawrence (KS) *Gazette*
Lawrence (KS) *Journal World*
Lebanon (IN) *Patriot*
Lebanon (PA) *Daily News*
Lebanon (PA) *News*
Lemars (IA) *Semi-Weekly Sentinel*
Ligonier (IN) *Ledger*
Lions (IA)
Lloyd's Evening-Post (London)
Lockhart (TX) *Post*
Logansport (IN) *Critic*
Logansport (IN) *Daily Journal*
Logansport (IN) *Herald*
Logansport (IN) *Pharos Tribune*
Logansport (IN) *Telegraph*
Logansport (IN) *Weekly Journal*
London Age
London Albion and Evening Advertiser
London American Register
London and China Telegraph
London Argus
London Correspondent
London Courier
London Courier and Evening Gazette
London Daily Advertiser
London Daily News
London Daily Post

London Day
London Echo
London Evening Herald
London Evening Mail
London Evening Star
London Evening-Post
London Express
London Gazette
London General Advertiser
London Illustrated Times
London Magnet
London Man of the World
London Mid-Surrey Times
London Monitor and New Era
London Monthly Magazine
London Monthly Mirror
London Monthly Review; or, Literary Journal
London Morning Chronicle
London Morning Journal
London Morning Post
London Morning Post and Fashionable World
London Morning Post and Gazetteer
London Nautical Standard
London New Review
London New Times
London Nonconformist
London Observer
London Observer of the Times
London Patriot
London Philanthropic Gazette
London Public Advertiser; or, Political and Literary Diary
London St. James Gazette
London Standard
London Star
London Sun and Central Press
London Times
London True Briton
London True Sun
London Watchman and Wesleyan Advertiser
London Weekly Chronicle and Register
London Weekly News and Chronicle
London Weekly Paper and the Organ of the Middle Class
London Weekly Register
London Week's News
Loogootee Martin County (IN) *Tribune*
Lorain County (OH) *Argus*
Lowell (MA) *Weekly Sun*
Madison (IN) *Dollar Weekly Courier*
Madison (IN) *Herald*
Madison (IN) *Weekly Courier*
Malvern (IA) *Republic Leader*
Manchester (England) *Guardian*
Manitoba (Canada) *Free Press*
Manitowoc Lake Shore (WI) *Times*
Marion (OH) *Daily Star*
Marshall (MI) *Statesman*
Marshfield (WI) *Times*

Marysville (OH) *Tribune*
Massachusetts Magazine
Massillon (OH) *Independent*
McKean County (PA) *Miner*
Miami County (IN) *Sentinel*
Middletown (NY) *Argus*
Middletown (NY) *Press*
Milwaukee Daily Sentinel
Milwaukee (WI) *Daily American*
Milwaukee (WI) *Daily News*
Moberly (MO) *Monitor*
Monmouth (IL) *Gazette*
Monmouth (IL) *Republican Atlas*
Monroe (WI) *Sentinel*
Monroe's Iron-Clad Age (IN)
Monticello (IA) *Express*
Monticello (IN) *Express*
Morning Advocate
Mount Carmel (IL) *Register*
Mountain (CA) *Democrat*
Narka (KS) *News*
National (IN) *Democrat*
New Albany (IN) *Daily Commercial*
New Albany (IN) *Daily Ledger*
New Albany (IN) *Daily Standard*
New Albany (IN) *Daily Tribune*
New Albany (IN) *Public Press*
New Annual Register (London)
New Annual Register and General Repository of History, Politics and Literature (London), 1804
New Brunswick (NJ) *Daily Times*
New Castle (IN) *Courier*
New Castle (PA) *News*
New Harmony (IN) *Register*
New North (WI)
New Orleans Bee
New Philadelphia (OH) *Times*
New York Commercial Advertiser
New York Gazette
New York Herald
New York News
New York Sun
New York Times
New York True American
New York Weekly Museum
New York World
Newark (OH) *Daily Advocate*
Newport (RI) *Daily News*
Newport (RI) *Mercury*
Norristown (IA) *Herald*
North Manchester (IN) *Journal*
North-West (IL)
Oakland (CA) *Tribune*
Ogden (UT) *Standard Examiner*
Olean (NY) *Democrat*
Olean (NY) *Times Herald*
Oregonian (Portland), *Morning*
Orrville (OH) *Crescent*
Oshkosh (WI) *Daily Courier*

Oshkosh (WI) *Daily Northwestern*
Panama City (FL) *News Herald*
Pennsylvania Journal
People (IN)
People's Press (PA)
Perry (IA) *Chief*
Petersburg (VA) *Index-Appeal*
Philadelphia Federal Gazette
Philadelphia Gazette
Philadelphia Independent Gazetteer
Philadelphia Press
Philosophical Magazine (London)
Piqua (OH) *Miami Helmet*
Piqua (OH) *Morning Call*
Popular Science Monthly
Port Jervis (NY) *Evening Gazette*
Postville (IA) *Review*
Potosi (WI) *Republican*
Quarterly Journal of Science, Literature and Art (London)
Racine (WI) *Daily Advocate*
Racine (WI) *Daily Journal*
Read's Weekly Journal; or, British Gazetteer (London)
Reno Gazette and Stockman
Reno (NV) *Evening Gazette*
Renwick (IA) *Times*
Repertory of Arts and Manufactures (London)
Republic City (KS)
Republican Compiler (PA)
Republican Daily Journal (KS)
Richland County (WI) *Observer*
Ripley County (IN) *Journal*
Rochester (IN) *Republican*
Rockingham (Harrisonburg, VA) *Register*
Rockport (IN) *Democrat*
Rushville (IN) *Republican*
St. James Gazette (London)
St. James's Chronicle; or, British Evening-Post (London)
St. Louis Post-Dispatch
Salem (OH) *Daily News*
Salt Lake City Desert News
Salt Lake Daily Tribune
San Antonio Daily Express
San Antonio Light
San Antonio News
Sandusky (OH) *Clarion*
Scientific Magazine and Freemasons' Repository
Scots Magazine (Edinburgh)
Scots Magazine and Edinburgh Literary Miscellany
Semi-Weekly Wisconsin
Seymour (IN) *Times*
Sheboygan Lake (WI) *Journal*
Sioux County (IN) *Herald*
Southport (WI) *American*
Southport (WI) *Telegraph*
Spectator (New York)
Spirit Lake (IA) *Beacon*
Sprig of Liberty (PA)

Star (IN)
Star and Banner (PA)
Steubenville (OH) *Herald Star*
Stevens Point (WI) *Daily Journal*
Stratford Times, Bow and Bromley News and South Sussex Gazette (England)
Sullivan County (IN) *Union*
Sullivan (IN) *Democrat*
Supplementary Number to the Monthly Magazine
Surrey, Southwark, Sussex Gazette
Syracuse (NY) *Daily Courier and Union*
Syracuse (NY) *Daily Standard*
Syracuse (NY) *Herald*
Tallis's London Weekly Paper
Thomasville (GA) *Southern Enterprise*
Thomasville (GA) *Times Enterprise*
Tioga (PA) *Eagle*
Tioga County (PA) *Agitator*
Titusville (PA) *Herald*
Titusville (PA) *Morning Herald*
Tokyo Japan Advertiser
Torch Light and Public Advertiser (MD)
Ukiah (CA) *City Press*
Universal Gazette (Philadelphia)
Van Wert (OH) *Weekly Bulletin*
Wabash (IN) *Daily Express*
Warren (IN) *Republican*
Warren (PA) *Mirror*
Warrick (IA) *Democrat*

Washington (DC) *Post*
Washington (DC) *Globe*
Washington (IN) *Telegraph*
Washington Journal
Waterloo (IA) *Courier*
Waupaca (WI) *Spirit*
Wautoma (WI) *Journal*
Wayne (IN) *Citizen*
Weekly Cedar Rapids (IA) *Times*
Weekly Gazette and Free Press (WI)
Weekly Standard (NC)
Weekly Wisconsin
Wellsboro (PA) *Agitator*
Wellsville (NY) *Daily Reporter*
West Eau Claire (WI) *Argus*
Western Mirror (IN)
Westville (IN) *Indicator*
White River (IN) *Gazette*
White River (IN) *Standard*
Whitehall Evening-Post; or, London Intelligencer
Williamsport (IN) *Warren Republican*
Winslow (IN) *Dispatch*
Wisconsin Democrat
Wisconsin Free Democrat
Wisconsin State Journal
Wisconsin Tribune
Wyoming Post Herald
Yates County (NY) *Chronicle*
Zanesville (OH) *Daily Courier*

Index

Aaron, Mrs. C.B. 338
Academy of Sciences, Paris, France 162, 165, 384
Act of 1774 50
Adams, Abigail 55
Adams, Dr. 148
The Adams Centinel 119
The Adams (MA) *Sentinel* 189
Addison, Dr. Thomas 253
Addison's fever 253
Adgate, Andrew 70, 72
Aedes (mosquito genus) 5, 7, 175
Aedes aegypti 5, 7, 41, 358, 369, 385, 393, 395, 396
Aedes africanus 7
Aedes albopictus 5, 204, 374
African American 2, 61, 62, 63, 81, 272
African fever/disease 232, 256
Agamemnon (ship) 237
Agnes (steamship) 270
Agramonte, Dr. Aristides 355, 357, 363, 369
agues and fevers 21, 40, 41, 97
air balloon 55
Akerman, Amos T. 272
Alabama 204, 215, 223, 279
Alaska 340
Albany, New York 17, 60, 65, 66, 87, 92, 101, 102, 120, 182, 221, 222
The Albany (NY) *Log Cabin* 182
Alden, Surgeon General 351
Alexandre La Valley (ship) 375
Alexandria, Ohio 124
Alexandria, Virginia 210
Alger, Secretary of War 347, 352, 354
Algeria 325, 386
Algesira, Spain 154
Algiers, Algeria 201
Ali, Mehemet 191
Alicant, Spain 112, 129, 130, 131
Allen, Gov. Richard 58
Allen, Dr. Richard 61, 62, 63, 76, 93, 94

Alliancia (ship) 373
allopathic 235, 302
Almonte, General 189
amber 72
Amelia 157
Amelia (sloop) 49
American Eagle (ship) 85
American Public Health Association (APHA) 301, 358
ammonia 43, 60, 180, 315, 323
ammoniac 34
Amoy, China 324
Andalusia, Spain 126, 128, 149
Anderson, Dr. James 101, 341
Andersonville, Georgia 241
Andouard, Dr. 152
Andrews, Miss 207
The Anglo-American Times 349
Ann (ship) 49, 144
Annan 70, 73
Anopheles 325
Antequea 113
anthrax 318, 386, 390, 391
antibiotics 7, 36
Antigua, West Indies 12, 22, 46, 139, 179, 312
Antilles 12, 44, 139, 317
Antiphlogiston 58
Antoinette (ship) 83
APHA 301
Aptommas 209
Arabia/Arabian 276, 317, 335
Arbovirus 6
Argonauta (ship) 350
Argus 169
Arkansas 174, 215, 246, 279, 295, 319, 328
Arkansas City, Kansas 295
Armour, Phil D. (Pork King) 310, 327
Arran, J.M. 277
arrhythmia 7
arsenic 34, 56, 235
Arzillo 108
Asia 6, 11, 99, 167, 393, 396
Asia (ship) 134

Asiatic cholera 296
Asiatic fever 241
Asibi strain 381, 383, 384
Aspinwall (Colon) 333, 334
Aspinwall, Mr. G. 144
The Athens (OH) *Messenger* 284
Atlanta, Georgia 246, 339
The Atlanta Constitution 283, 284
The Atlanta New Era 246
Atrato (ship) 259
Augusta, Georgia 175, 204, 272, 285
Augustin, George 173, 297
Aurora 92
Auspicious (ship) 151
Austin, Dr. W.G. 291
Austin, Texas 313
Australia/Australians 256, 287, 396
Austria 14, 16, 17, 76, 87, 216
Aux Cayes 78
Ayamonte, Spain 113
Azores 228

Back-Stair Island 14
backbone fever 250
bacterial warfare 388
Bahamas 307
Bahia, Brazil 228
Bailly (Bally) Dr. 152
Baldwin, Mr. 124
Balize, Louisiana 183
Balm of Gilead 104
Balsam of Life 21
Baltimore (steamship) 312
Baltimore, Maryland 2, 82, 86, 91, 113, 114, 143, 144, 153, 158, 160, 167, 207, 209, 211, 212, 215, 219, 245, 284, 285, 304, 312, 328, 367
Baltimore American 207, 211
The Baltimore Gazette 304
Baltimore Patriot 211
Bancroft, Dr. Edward Nathaniel 108, 111, 148, 149

433

INDEX

The Bangor (Maine) *Courier* 189
The Bangor Maine Daily Whig & Courier 189
Barbados 11, 12, 18, 20, 25, 36, 46, 49, 84, 116, 138, 231, 339
Barbastro, Spain 151
Barcelona, Spain 106, 111, 126, 150, 151, 152, 153, 162, 287, 288
Barceloneta, Spain 111, 150, 151, 152
Barclay, John 58
Barclay, Rev. W.M. 105
Bard, Dr. John 84
Bard, Dr. Samuel 84
barley water 60, 67
Barnes, Surgeon General 281
Barnet, Major General 110
Barracouta (ship) 260
Barrett, Minister 373
Barrios, General 332
Barthelmess, Dr. 320
Bartie, Mr. 139
Barton, Clara 351
Barton, Dr. E.H. 190
Barton, Prof. Dr. Benjamin Smith 61, 123
Bastareche, Dr. Senor 234
Bates, Dr. 303
Baton Rouge, Louisiana 184, 195, 275
Baun (British sloop of war) 162
Bay of St. Louis, Mississippi 185
Bay Ridge, New York 221
Bayley, Dr. Richard 88
The Bayou Sara Ledger 202
Beach, H.L. 351
Beal, Mr. 165
Beal's Hotel 165
Beard, Mr. 21
Beau Soleil, Point-a-Petre 139
Beaufort, South Carolilna 240, 241
Beauregard, de Chevalier Feureau 165, 166
Beauregard, Gen. Pierce G.T. 241, 310
Beaver, Philip 46
Beaz Island (Boaz), Bermuda 232
Becket, Thomas 160
Beeuwkes, Dr. Henry 381
Belgium 216, 261, 378, 386
Belgravia, London 300
Belize 237, 259
Bell, Dr. 221
Bellinzaghi, Dr. Angel 363
Bell's Life in London 329
Bell's Weekly Messenger 126
Bellvue, New York 83
Bellvue College, New York 263
Bellvue Hospital, New York 86, 87, 88, 95, 114, 116, 304, 372
Bemis, Dr. Samuel M. 302, 308
Benge, Samuel 70

Benjamin Franklin (steamer) 207
Bennet, Dr. Parker 22, 23, 25
Benson, Egbert 216
Berchtold, Leopold Count 124
Berlin, Germany 125, 128, 323, 356, 368
Bermuda 41, 139, 231, 232, 242, 243, 244, 306, 327
Bernardi 209
Bernhardt, Sarah 315
Berwick's Bay, Louisiana 267
Bether, Emanuel 85
Beyer, Professor 365
Bibby, Captain 16
bicarbonate of soda 263
Bierce, Ambrose 348
Bill of Mortality 63
Billings, Dr. John 301
Biloxi, Mississippi 13, 185, 335
biological warfare (BW) 1, 243, 367, 377, 386, 388, 389, 390, 391
biological weapons 311, 386, 389, 390, 391
bioterrorism 242
Bird, Capt. Fredrick 83
Bird, Mr. 147
Black Beard Island 314
black death 3, 258
black flag 65
Blackburn, Dr. C.C. 246
Blackburn, Gov. Dr. Luke P. 186, 202, 243, 244, 245, 246, 251, 277, 293, 309, 311
Blackburn, John 246
Blackburn, Robert Bruce 246
Blackburne, Dr. W. 123
Blackburnsborough, Scotland 246
BlackVomit, Dr. 246
Blackwood's 339
Blaine, James G. 340
Blair, Dr. Daniel 286
Blanchard, Jean-Pierre Francois 55
Blanchard, M. 47
Blanche, Michael 85
Blanco, Gov.-Gen. Ramón 346, 355
Blane, Sir Dr. Gilbert 27, 37, 158, 162, 164
bleeding 7, 8, 21
Bliss, Colonel 195
blood letting 15, 16, 23, 26, 28, 29, 38, 60, 63, 67, 68, 73, 82, 84, 101, 118, 120, 125, 191, 209, 234, 235
Bogota, Colombia 132, 180
Bolama, Bissagos Island, West Africa 45, 405
Boldo leaves 303
Bolivia 6, 7
Bond, MD 18

Bonnetta (ship) 178
Bonny, Nigeria 257
Booth, John Wilkes 242, 250
Borbier 331
Boston (cruiser) 373
Boston, Massachusetts 2, 12, 17, 38, 39, 92, 94, 95, 143, 145, 176, 200, 219, 225, 239, 241, 245, 284, 285, 306, 327
The Boston Daily Advertiser 176
The Boston Gazette 114
The Boston Globe 209, 280, 300, 333, 342, 347, 348
The Boston Journal 290, 302
The Boston Post 39, 344
Boston Tea Party 58
The Boston Transcript 165
botulism 391
Boyce, Rupert 368
Boyd, Mayor 301
Boy's World 323
Bradley, Captain 242
Brandon, Mississippi 235
Brandreth Pills 193
Brazil 1, 6, 11, 227, 228, 261, 289, 300, 307, 310, 318, 319, 337, 341, 363, 368, 378, 379, 385, 386, 387, 393, 394
Brazoria County, Texas 249
Brett, Miss 48
Brimstone/Sulfur 33, 34, 110
Bristow, Mr. 281
The British Courier 161
The British Guardian 288
The British Medical Journal 300
The British Press 155
The British Standard 288
Brodum, Dr. 105
broken bone fever (break bone fever) 161, 175, 194, 250
bronze (the color) 210
bronze jack 277
bronze john 5, 252, 298
Brooklyn, New York 117, 159, 210, 212, 213, 214, 218, 221, 265, 267, 268
Brown, Capt. William 21
Brown, E. 131
Brown, Dr. Harvey E. 274
Browne, Dr. Joseph 90, 91
Browne, Dr. Pat 21
Brownsville, Texas 313
Brunner, Dr. W.F. 345
Brussels, Belgium 128, 386
Bryce, Dr. James 78, 79
Bryson, Alexander 192
Buchanan, Dr. 259
Buchanan, Pres. James 240
Buenos Ayres, Argentina 289
bulam fever 148, 178, 192
Bull, Captain 77
Burr, Aaron 90, 91
Burrough, L. 218

Index

Busbridge (ship) 78
Busck, August 375
Bush, Pres. George W. 391
Bush-Hill Hospital, Philadelphia 55, 58, 62, 70, 72, 73, 74
Butler, Gen. Benjamin 3, 240, 269, 271, 346
Butte, Dr. 141
Buzzard (ship) 178

cabbage 160
Cabell, Dr. James L. 301
Cabeuello, Dr. Don 286
Cadiz, Spain 19, 106, 107, 108, 109, 110, 113, 128, 131, 132, 134, 135, 136, 137, 148, 150, 153, 164, 165
Cady, Lieutenant 190
Cagliari, Italy 261
Cairo, Illinois 276
Caldas, Dr. 363, 364
Caldwell, Dr. Charles 59
Caldwell, J.F. 251
California 187, 228, 292, 303, 314, 387, 389
Callaway, Dr. J.M. 273, 274
calomel (Hg2Cl2) 58, 69, 73, 78, 82, 84, 89, 101, 121, 127, 180, 234, 235, 265, 290, 291
Cambridge, Massachusetts 322
Cameron, Mr. 165
Cameron, Mr. M.C. 245
Cameron, Mr. Simon 282
Cameron, Senator 343
camomile 60, 106
Camp E.A. Perry, Florida 35, 337
camp fever 67, 73
Camp Lazear 224, 357, 360, 361
Campbell, Lt. Gen. Colin 131
camphor 34, 50, 52, 59, 60, 66, 69, 199, 245, 291
Canada 12, 36, 183, 243, 244, 245, 246, 311, 335, 339, 340, 396
Canary Islands 117, 138
Canby, Mayor-General 252
cane juice 328
Canovas, Senor 345
Canton, China 232
Canvane, Dr. Peter 28, 29
Caraccas, Venezela 139
Carbally, Dr. 315
carbolic acid 279, 293, 295, 301, 308, 315, 371
carbon tetrachloride 385
Cardo, Col. Pedro 350
Carey, Matthew 62, 70
Carlisle Bay, Barbados 339
The Carlisle (PA) *Gazette* 70
Carmona y Valle, Dr. 320, 337
Carnochan, J.M. 267
Caroline (brig) 83, 162
Carpenter, Dr. William B. 233
Carregeot, Madame 231

Carrington, Dr. 305
Carroll, Dr. James 355, 356, 357, 358, 361, 363, 366, 380, 381
Carroll, Matthew 220
Carrollton, Missouri 201
Carson, John 51
Cartagena (Carthagena), Panama 14, 333
Carter, Dr. Henry R. 358, 373
Carter, Pres. Jimmy 376
Carteret (ship) 77
Carter's Spanish Mixture 235
Carthage, Missouri 322
Carthagena, Spain 129, 130, 131, 132, 333
Cascarilla bark 34
Caselee, Mr. 145
castile soap 106, 125, 126
The Castle (Indiana) *Courier* 242
Castleton Village, New York 213, 220, 221
Castor (ship) 138
castor oil 28, 29, 43, 265
Cathrall (Cathavel, Catharal, Cathral), Dr. Isaac 48, 70, 73
Catlin, George 262
cats 108, 121, 233
Catskill, New York 114
cattle 233, 275, 323
Cayenne, Guiana 228, 229
The Cedar Rapids Gazette 242
Central America 2, 6, 44, 234, 330, 332, 334, 338, 340, 370, 381, 396
Chabert, Dr. 180
Chagres Fever 332
Chaille, Dr. Stanford E. 193, 312, 315
chalk 303
chalybeate waters 18
Chandler, Commodore 265
charcoal 33, 60, 181, 309
Charenton, Louisiana 249
The Charleston News 142, 189, 272
Charles-Town (Charleston, SC) 39, 40, 41, 42
Charlestown (Charleston, SC) 115
The Charlestown Mercury 175
Chattanooga, Tennessee 315, 335
Chebucto, Halifax, Nova Scotia 17
Cheraw Hill Hospital 41
Chervin, Dr. Nicolas 162, 191, 193
Chester, New Jersey 92, 93
Chevot, Dr. 50
Chicago, Illinois 277, 298, 302, 323, 327, 371
The Chicago Times 282
The Chicago Tribune 353, 388
Chickahominy, Virginia 242
chicken pox 84

chikungunya 7
Childers, Mr. 287
Chile 303
Chille, Dr. 292
chimpanzees 367, 368
China 232, 259, 304, 316, 378, 392
Chinese 304, 324, 390
Chisholm, Dr. 119, 120, 121, 148, 158
chloride of lime 167, 168, 196, 211, 241, 308
chloride of soda 167, 168
Choppin, Dr. Samuel 241, 294, 302, 303, 307
Christlausen, Mr. 339
Cicella, Mayor 277
Cienfuegos, Cuba 273, 369
Cincinnati, Ohio 169, 197, 200, 294, 295, 298, 315, 328
The Cincinnati Enquirer 294, 302
The Cincinnati Israelite 249
The Cincinnati News 186
cinnamon 27, 60, 66, 84, 303
citronella 396
The Civilian 189
Claiborne, William Charles Cole 115
Clanny, Dr. 179, 180
Clapp, Reverend 182
Clark, Lt. Col. Alured 40
Clark, Dr. James 79, 89
Clarke, Herbert E. 336
Clarkson, Mayor Matthew 49, 50, 51, 53, 54, 55, 58, 61, 63, 70, 73
cleanliness 9, 32, 51, 82, 113, 212, 230, 254, 281, 286, 318, 354
Cleary, W.W. 245
Clendenin, Miss 355
Cleveland, Ohio 123, 316
Cleveland, Pres. Grover 323
climate change 8
Clinton, George 65
Clinton, Sir Henry 39, 40, 41
Clott, Dr. (Clot) (Clot-Bey) 191
cloves 60
coal 220, 295, 338
Coan, Dr. 298
Cochran, Professor 279
Cock Lane Ghost 56, 57
coffee 49, 50, 52, 54, 56, 57, 64, 74, 78, 83, 89, 92, 139, 143, 158, 162, 202, 231, 267, 268, 310
cold air-drinks-bath 36, 58, 66, 67, 68, 73, 82, 84, 85, 101, 111, 123, 125, 126, 129, 179, 192, 209, 216, 341
Cole, Francis 85, 86
Cole, William Charles 115
Colima, Mexico 320
College of Philadelphia 36
College of Physicians and Surgeons, New York 356, 357

Index

Colley, George 85, 86
Collineau, Dr. 162
Colnett, Captain 80
Colon, Panama 333, 334, 370, 371, 374, 378
Columbia 6
Columbia, South Carolina 241, 242
Columbia Barracks, Cuba 357, 358, 360, 369
Columbia (ship) 175
Columbus, Mississippi 253
Coma 7, 8, 26, 28
commercial 21, 38, 44, 53, 108, 143, 146, 155, 158, 207, 212, 223, 254, 257, 260, 281, 289, 290, 303, 307, 314, 327, 385
The Commercial (NY) *Journal* 345
Concha, Gov. Don Jose de la 234
Concordia Intelligencer 165
Coney Island, New York 218
Congo, Africa 394
Congreve, Henry 181
Connecticut 14, 18, 88, 93, 97, 98, 216
Connelly, John 70
Conner, Dr. M.E. 379
Constantine, Algeria 325
Constantinople, Turkey 233, 368
Constitution (steamer) 174
Cook, Captain 80
Copeland, Mr. 147
Copenhagen, Denmark 97, 112, 273
Corcoran, Dennis 186, 187
Cordoba (Cordova) 112
cordon 112, 130, 134, 135, 150, 151, 152, 154, 161, 180, 191, 236
Corlaer's Hook 89
Cornhill Magazine 292
Cornwallis, Gov. Edward (Nova Scotia) 17, 40, 41
Corpus Christi, Texas 189, 249, 373
Costa Rica 332, 394
cotton 20, 60, 83, 133, 134, 195, 211, 223, 226, 260, 268, 275, 284, 285, 286, 290, 294, 295, 327
Cottrell, Capt. Fredrick 138
Covington, Mississippi 298
Coxe, Dr. John 69, 123
Cragin, Captain 240
Crawford House (Norfolk, Virginia) 210
Creech, William 78
cremation 3, 303
Creole 100, 132, 169, 179, 210, 224, 232, 294, 332
creosote 193
Crescent City (New Orleans) 5, 171, 199, 267, 269, 295, 328

Crescent City (steamer) 198, 211, 212, 224, 225
criminals 105, 123, 165, 229, 304, 320, 385
Crispell, Dr. 241
Croakers 249
Crocker, Captain 144
La Cronica 234
Cronstadt, Russia 261
Crosby, W.J. 333
Croswell, Captain 211
Crotalus Horridus 234
Cruikshank, Mr. 148
Cuerno, Count de 332
Culex 324, 326, 358, 359
Cullen, Dr. William 8, 17, 104, 148
Cumming, J.P. 220
Cunningham, P. 180
Currie, Dr. James 125
Currie, Dr. William 51, 59, 60, 61, 84, 119, 120, 158
Cutler, Dr. 323

Daiquiri, Senegal 350
Dakar 383
Dalhousie, Earl 144
Dalrymple, Henry Hew 46
Darling, Dr. Samuel T. 370, 372
Darwin, Charles 289, 330
Dauntless (ship) 231
Davis, Dr. Charles 189
Davis, Gov. George 373, 375
Davis, Jefferson 243, 245, 300, 311
Davis, Jefferson, Jr. 300
Davis, John 116
Davis, Mr. 303
Dayton, Ohio 268
Dean, Private William 358
Dearborn, Indiana 306
The Dearborn (IN) *Independent* 306
de Arejula, Don Juan Manuel 126
DeBow, Professor 197
DeForest, Charles 220
Deforest, Henry 70
de'Lardenoy, Lieutenant-General 139
Delaware 47, 92, 98, 99, 216
de Lesseps, Ferdinand 330, 331
Delestra, Dr. M. 111
Delgado, Dr. Claudio 326, 333, 341
Demerara, Guiana 77, 178, 229, 286
de Mertens, Charles 30
dengue fever 1, 6, 7, 175, 194, 317, 353, 380, 390, 393, 396
Denmark/Danish 97, 112, 150, 183, 216, 228, 232, 261
Dennie (Denny), Richard 49
Dennie (Denny) Mrs. Richard 49
Denver, Colorado 306, 348

The Denver Tribune 306
The Des Moines Register 246
Dessaix (ship) 110
DesSonges 331
Detroit, Michigan 303
Deveze, Dr. Jean 73
Diana (frigate) 113
Dick, Senator 366
Dickens, Charles 57
Dickerson, James 396
Didier, Mr. 332
Dills, Dr. T.J. 292
Dingler, Jules 332
Dinmore, Dr. Richard 123, 124
Diocles 180
Dispatch (Despatch) (steamer) 281
dock fever 5, 100
Dr. Angelis' Four Herb Pill 95, 105
Dr. Crary's Anti-Septic Family Physic 128
Dr. James Fever Powder 21, 22
Dr. Norris's Fever Drops 79
Dr. Warburg's Vegetable Fever Drops 180
Dr. W.T. Owen's Pills 206
dogs 1, 55, 108, 233
Dolphin (ship) 106, 178
Dominica, West Indies 46, 79, 89, 178
Don (steamer) 265
Don, George 134, 154
Dongan, Gov. Thomas (NY) 12
Donnell, Mr. 235
Donnelly, Samuel B. 375
Doria, Sr. Menezes 319
Dornford, Daniel Clark 77
Dorsey, Nathan 51
Doty, Alvah H. 341
Doty, Dr. Alvah P. 355
Doughty, Edward 148
Douglas, Sen. Stephen A. 227
Douglass, Dr. Isaac S. 87, 88
Dowell, Dr. Greenville 297
Drake, Dr. 233
Draugod 205
Dreesen, Dr. W.C. 385
Dry Tortugas, Florida 250, 347
Dublin, Ireland 14, 49, 78
Ducker, Dr. 351
Duffield, Dr. Benjamin 57
Duffield, Dr. Samuel 51, 58, 93, 94
Dundas, General 178
Dunham, Dr. Herbert E. 363
Dunlap's American Daily Advertiser 56
Dupuytren, M. 162
Dusseau 331
dysentery 28, 79, 84, 101, 102, 114, 120, 148, 278, 290, 317, 345, 353, 370

Index

East Indies 67, 125
Eaton, General 304
Ebola 396
Ecuador 6, 378, 379
Edgar (ship) 34
Edinburgh, Scotland 22, 38, 66, 67, 84, 265, 356
The Edinburg Review 237
Edison, A. Thomas 337
Edson, Dr. Cyrus 349
Edwin Flye (ship) 203
Egypt 87, 125, 167, 191, 261, 315
Ehrenberg, Christian Gottfried 192
Ehrlich, Dr. 325
El Caney, Cuba 350, 351
El Paso, Texas 389
The El Paso Herald Post 389
elephantiasis 318, 324, 325
Ellis, Captain 16
Emily Souder (steamship) 298
Empire (steamer) 204
encephalitis 6, 383, 386, 396
endemic 6, 44, 80, 82, 101, 205, 215, 236, 300, 314, 323, 391, 392, 393, 395, 396
Esk (Royal mail steamer) 339
Etinene 331
Etna (ship) 178
Eucalyptus Globulus 303
Eustis, Senator 302
The Evening Telegram 319
The Excellent British Fever Pill 21
Experiment (ship) 174

Faget, Dr. C. 337
Fair American (ship) 78
Falcon (steamer) 222, 239
Falconer, Dr. Nathaniel 50, 53, 58, 98
Falkland Islands 266
famine fever 258
Farquhar, A.B. 302
Fayette, Mississippi 200, 278
Fayssoux, Peter 40
febris continua/recurrens (continued fever) 8
febris nervosa)(nervous fever 17
The Federal Gazette 68
Fegan, Dr. 314
Fellowes, Dr. Sir James 113, 148, 149
Fellows, A.S. 127
Fell's Point, Maryland 143
Fergusson, William (Ferguson) 161
Fernandina, Florida 293
fever tree 303
Fiddes, Alexander 265
La Fievre Matelotte (yellow fever) 25
Finland/Finish 261

Finlay, Dr. Charles 376
Finlay y Barres, Dr. Juan Carlos 325, 326, 327, 341, 358, 360, 363, 368
Firmeza, Cuba 351
Firth, M.D. 16
Fish, Hamilton, Jr. 352
Fisher, Dr. Edward 62
Fisher, L.C. 306
Flavivirus 6, 390
fleas 8, 390
Fletcher, Dr. 303
Flexner, Simon 383
Florence, Italy 166
Florence, South Carolina 272
Flores, Montevideo 341
Florida 14, 34, 35, 39, 41, 100, 158, 175, 240, 241, 250, 278, 285, 293, 303, 308, 321, 335, 337, 342, 346, 350
Florida (steamship) 204
Foeltzer, Lou 352
Foo, Hong Chin 304
Foo, Dr. Wow Chin 304
Forbes, Sir John 235
Ford, MD 76
Fordyce, Dr. George 119
Formosa, China 324
Forrester (ship) 178
Fort Adams 200
Fort Brown, Texas 372
Fort Detrick (Camp) (Maryland) 390
Fort George, Africa 256
Fort Hamilton 213, 214
Fort Jefferson, Dry Tortugas 250
Fort Louisbourg 17
Fort Monroe, Virginia 210
Fort Royal 46
Fort Sumter, South Carolina 240
Fort Wayne, Indiana 272, 311, 323
The Fort Wayne (IN) *Gazette* 272
The Fort Wayne (IN) *Sentinel* 272, 311
Forte (frigate) 177
Forwood, Arthur B. 254
Fothergill, Dr. A. 124
four thieves 59, 60
Fowler, Dr. 121, 235
France 6, 11, 12, 14, 16, 17, 34, 46, 55, 76, 78, 86, 87, 151, 165, 183, 216, 224, 227, 229, 230, 261, 316, 320, 332, 334, 335, 384
Francis Leland (ship) 237
Francois, Dr. 152
Frankfort, Germany 141
Frankfort, Kentucky 169
frankincense 72
Franklin, Benjamin 14, 16, 58
Frazer, Captain 257
Frazer, James 79
Frederick County, PA 160, 209
Frederick Hospital, Denmark 97

The Frederick (MD) *News Post* 388
The Frederick (MD) *Post* 388
Fredericksburg, Virginia 210, 346
Freedom (ship) 174
Freire (Frieze, Freise, Friez), Dr. Domingos (Domingo) 318, 319, 322, 333, 336, 337, 341
French & Indian War 12, 14, 16, 17, 19, 34
The French Moniteur 229
French National Academy of Science 236
Frith's Elixir 45
frogs, dried 59
Fulton, Louisiana 202
fumigate/fumigation 31, 33, 34, 72, 77, 93, 110, 118, 124, 132, 133, 155, 159, 164, 167, 211, 212, 213, 219, 239, 259, 261, 274, 280, 295, 301, 306, 362, 365, 372, 373
Fun (London magazine) 348
Fusileer (ship) 172
Fyen (bark) 268

Galt, John 117, 194
Galveston, Texas 119, 175, 187, 204, 235, 247, 247, 249, 251, 252, 262, 263, 265, 267, 268, 270, 271, 275, 276, 279, 281, 285, 287, 289, 297, 306, 310, 313, 353, 368
The Galveston Daily News 252, 265, 269, 270, 271, 281, 289
Gamgee, Prof. John 306, 307
gangrenous 9, 52
Garfield, Pres. James 322
Garland, Senator (Arkansas) 328
Garrett, Thomas 229
Garrigues, Edward 95
Gaston, Dr. J. McF 319, 322, 323
Gate, Gen. Horatio 41
Gayarre, Charles 292
Gazette de France 151
Gazette of the United States 96
Geddings, Dr. 357
Genoa, Italy 288
George, King 14, 16, 381
George Law (steamer) 238
George Washington University 367
Georgetown 40, 41
Georgia 14, 35, 39, 40, 115, 141, 204, 206, 215, 223, 226, 242, 246, 293, 301, 319, 347
The Georgia Daily Constitution 301
Gerard (Girard), Stephen 70
germ theory 36, 317, 323, 324
Germany/German 11, 47, 72, 87, 183, 205, 206, 216, 224, 226, 228, 234, 258, 276, 289, 316, 330, 339, 345, 378, 386, 389, 390

438   INDEX

Geronimo 335
Ghana, Africa 381
Gibbons, John 51
Gibier, Dr. Paul 337
Gibraltar, Spain 106, 108, 109, 110, 112, 129, 130, 131, 132, 134, 135, 151, 154, 155
Gibson, R.L. 302
Gilbert, Dr. M. 122
Gillkrest, Dr. James 236
Gilpin, Sir Joseph 158
Girand, Dr. John J. 125
Girerd, Dr. 327, 332, 333
Girerd, Dr. L. 320
Gladiola (steamer) 275
Glasgow, Scotland 82, 181
Glauber's Salts 43, 84
goat 152, 225, 277, 355
God 12, 23, 37, 38, 62, 63, 83, 111, 125, 143, 176, 183, 192, 205, 207, 210, 226, 244, 269, 311, 335, 354
Godfrey, Dr. 335
Goldberg, Dr. 366
Golden Rule (steamer) 328
Gomez, Bernandino Antonio 132, 133, 134
Gorgas, Dr. Gen. William Crawford (Gorges) 343, 354, 363, 364, 368, 371, 372, 374, 375, 378, 379, 380, 381
Gorgas Hospital 20
The Goshen (IN) *Times* 246, 311, 375
Gosport (man of war) 16
Gosport, Virginia 207, 209
Governor's Island (New York) 65, 268, 270
Graham, James 73
Grand Gulf, Mississippi 200
Granite Peak, Utah 390
Granizo, Dr. 320
Grant, Pres. U.S. 272
The Grant County Herald 165
Grantham (ship) 77
Gravesend Bay, NewYork 213, 218, 239
Gray, William 62
Greeley, Horace 245
Green, Dr. Samuel A. 302
Green Bush, Rensselaer County, New York 66
green fever 292
green tea 27
Greene, Gen. Nathanael 42
Greenleaf's New York Journal 87, 97
Greenwich, Connecticut 116, 144
Gregg, Ralph E. 361
Gregory, Professor 84
Grenada, West Indies 46, 77, 109, 119, 134, 135, 178, 295, 298
Grey Eagle (slave ship) 232

Griffitts, Dr. Samuel Powel 51, 52, 59
Griscom, Dr. 221
Guadaloupe 115, 139, 178, 187, 312
guaiacum wood 72
Guantanamo Bay, Cuba 350
Guardian of the Poor 54, 55, 58, 70
Guatemala 332, 379, 394
Guayaquil, Equador 189, 334, 378, 379
Guaymas, Mexico 314
Guiana, West Indies 178, 228
guinea pigs 319, 336, 355, 381
Guiteras, Dr. John (Juan Guiteras) 312, 337, 351, 354, 361, 363, 379
Gulf of Mexico 177, 261, 271, 274, 307
gun powder 34, 52
Gunn, Dr. A.H. 239
Guthrin, Dr. 221

Haagen, Eugene 384
Hagerstown, Maryland 279
The Hagerstown (MD) *Mail* 297
The Hague 291
Hahnemann's system 235
hair ghouls 314, 315
Haiti 46, 78, 340
Hale, Reverend Dr. 31, 33
Halifax, Nova Scotia 17, 144, 177, 243, 244, 245, 335
Hall, Edwin J. 245
Hall, Mayor George 214, 216
Hall, Dr. James 94, 303
Hallock, Grace T. 356
Hamilton, Alexander 65, 66, 90, 91, 92
Hamilton, Adm. Charles Powel 145
Hamilton, Surg.-Gen. John B. 313, 314, 332, 333, 337
Hamilton, William 55
Hamilton, Montana 387
Hamilton County, Illinois 355
Hamilton Hotel, Bermuda 243
Hammond, Gov. James (SC) 226
Hanger, Maj. George 41
Hankey (ship) 46
Hanson, Dr. Henry 379
Hard Times (ship) 185
Hardacre, Mr. 145, 146, 147
Hardcastle, Mr. 146, 147
Hardee, Dr. Col. T.S. (L.S.) 302, 303
Hardie, T.S. 88, 312
Hargis, Dr. B.S. 278
Harmony, Captain 306
Harper's Weekly 32, 81, 216, 230, 298, 342, 352
Harris, Dr. Elisha 221
Harris, J.O. 201

Harris, J.W. 245
Harris, Senator 307, 308
Harrison, Pres. Benjamin 340, 341
Harrison, Thomas 70, 72
Harvard, Major 363
Harvard, Boston, Massachusetts 290, 383
Hasell, Bentley D. 272
Hastings, Samuel 291
Havanna (Havannah), Cuba 5, 77, 139, 159, 255, 305
Hayes, Pres. Rutherford B. 302
Haygarth, Dr. 98
The H.D. Bacon (steamboat) 200
headache 1, 7, 29, 258, 263, 320, 322, 326, 350
Heamogogus 5
Heard, T.J. 247
Hearst, William Randolph 345
Hebrew Benevolent Society 249
Hecla (bark) 259
Hector (ship) 79
Hektoen, Dr. Ludvig 366
Helm, Peter 70, 72
Helsingfors, Russia 261
hemorrhage 7, 9, 26, 166
Henderson, Dr. Stewart 126
Henriques, Dr. A. 235
hepatitis B 389
hepatotrophic 390
Herald of Health 337
Higgon, Mr. 146, 147
High Hills Hospital of Santee 41
Highprice, Dr. 266
Hill, Colonel 140
Hill, H.W. 197
Hillard, Dr. E.D. 277
Hillary, Dr. Williman 25, 26, 28, 98
Hilton Head, South Carolina 241
Hincks, Mayor J. 211
Hines, Dr. L.L. 343
Hines, Dr. William 294
Hippocrates 23, 27, 37, 50, 60, 158
Hispaniola, West Indies 17, 78
Hitchcock, Captain 203
Hitler, Adolf 388
Hodges, Dr. 50
Hodgson, Dr. S.H. 363
Hoffman, Frederick 76
Hoffman, Mr. 265
Hoffman Island, New York 364
hogs 233, 277
Holland, Sir Henry 192, 193
Holland, Netherlands 77, 109, 216, 261
Hollingsworth, P. 95
Holstein, J. 249
Holt, Dr. Joseph 323, 335
Home Journal 117, 194
Honduras 16, 139, 256, 332, 394

Hood, John 242
Hood, Gen. John B. 268, 310
Hooker, General 302
hookworm 378, 379
Hooper, Dr. P.O. 319
Hooper. Dr. Robert 9
Hoover, Pres. Herbert 383
Hopkins, Dr. T.S. 286
horehound 60
Horn Island, Mississippi 390
horses 55, 90, 108, 309, 343, 355
Horsman, Reginald 192
Hosack, Dr. Alexander (David's brother) 84
Hosack, Dr. David 84, 147, 148, 158
hospital fever 67
Houston, Texas 175, 241, 248, 249, 265, 268, 273, 287, 303
The Houston Intelligencer 175
The Houston Telegraph 250
Howard, Dr. Leland O. 367
Howard Association 196, 197, 198, 199, 200, 201, 202, 207, 209, 210, 214, 224, 225, 226, 248, 249, 250, 251, 268, 275, 276, 277, 284, 285, 294, 298, 335
Huaco plant (Guaco plant) 180
Hubbard, Dr. S.P. 290
The Hudson (Catskill NY) *Bee* 114
Humboldt, Dr. G. 234, 265, 340
Humboldt, Dr. William Lambert de 234
Hunter, General 241
Hunter, Dr. John 37, 44, 45
Huntsville (ship) 241
Huskisson, Mr. 164
Hutchinson, Dr. James 50, 51, 53, 54, 58, 59, 60, 61
Hutson, Richard 39
Hutton, Dr. W.H.H. 337
Hyams, Godfrey Joseph 244
hydropathic 235, 303
hydrophobia 121, 316, 339, 366
Hygeian Vegetable Universal Medicine 180

Icarus (ship) 259
ignes fatui (deceptive or deluding) 19
Illinois 216, 276, 353, 355
Illinois (hospital ship) 252
Imaum (ship) 260
immune 2, 63, 81, 200, 280, 319, 346, 347, 348, 349, 351, 353, 357, 371, 372, 383, 384, 385, 394
immunes 347, 348, 350, 351
immunity 8, 10, 11, 36, 61, 81, 246, 271, 280, 304, 323, 346, 361, 364, 383, 385
immunization 10, 363, 367, 382, 384, 387, 389, 395, 396

India 303, 315, 316, 368, 371, 381, 387
Indiana 146, 193, 208, 216, 242, 275, 302, 305, 349, 361, 364, 390
The Indiana Herald 242
Indianola, Texas 249, 269
Indianapolis, Indiana 243, 324, 330, 358
The Indianapolis (IN) *Journal* 243, 324, 330
Indians 12, 16, 17, 118, 249, 251, 314, 315, 323, 330, 335; Iroquois 14
indigent class 135
influenza 52, 84, 120, 122, 191, 229, 387
informed consent 360, 361
Ingram, Dr. Dale 21
Inman, S.M. 285
inoculation 4, 16, 36, 43, 206, 234, 286, 318, 319, 320, 322, 323, 326, 327, 329, 336, 337, 339, 340, 341, 359, 387, 388
Inskeep, Joseph 70, 72
Inspector of Strangers 135
Intoxication Stage (Stage 3) 8
The Iola 27
Iowa 200, 332
ipecacuanha (tartar emetic) 15, 67, 404
Iran 392
Ireland 6, 76, 139, 140, 182, 183, 203, 205, 206, 216, 224, 226, 276, 277, 316, 318
Iroquois 14
Irving, Allan 209
Ishii, Shiro (Japanese) 390
Islay, Peru 256
Isle of Leon, Spain 134, 135, 136, 150, 178, 192, 395
Isle of Majorca, Spain 153
Israel 70, 392
Isthmus of Panama 135, 256, 287, 332, 333, 334, 370, 372, 374, 375, 378
Isthmus of Tehuantepec, Mexico 330
Italy/Italian 6, 8, 87, 95, 112, 183, 216, 224, 289, 316, 325, 341

J. Titus (brig) 244
Jackson, Gen. Andrew 140
Jackson, Dr. Robert 40, 82, 120, 121, 149, 151
Jackson, William 94
The Jackson Sentinel 280
Jacksonville, Florida 241, 278, 293, 301, 303, 335, 342
jail fever 99
jalap 58, 61, 69, 73, 78, 84, 127, 235
Jamaica 13, 14, 19, 20, 21, 22, 23, 44, 76, 77, 78, 80, 93, 94, 121, 126, 129, 140, 148, 177, 219, 231, 260, 265, 300, 303, 314, 328, 332, 333, 334, 371
The Jamaica Gleaner 265
James, Mr. 128
Jameson, Dr. Henry 324
Jane, Betsy 250
Jane, Eliza 159
Janesville (WI) 288
The Janesville (WI) *Gazette* 288
Japan 241, 379, 387, 390
Japanese Encephalitis 6
jaundice 5, 7, 8, 9, 23, 45, 105, 128, 161, 326, 350, 353, 359, 380, 386, 388, 389, 391
Jay, Gov. John (NY) 83, 90
Jay, Monsieur 109
Jefferson, Thomas 181
Jefferson City (Missouri) 201
Jellenghaus, William 220
Jenkins, Robert 14
Jerome, Dr. J.H. 239
Jew/Jewish 109, 124, 249, 327
John B. Gibson (bark) 338
John Hopkins Hospital, Massachusetts 322, 355, 356, 381, 389
John Potter (bark) 238
johnny vomito 227
Johnson, Pres. Andrew 245, 246
Johnson, Samuel 56
Johnson, William 17
Johnston, Thomas 181
Jones, Dr. Absalom 61, 62, 63
Jones, Captain 94
Jones, Dr. Joseph 320
Jorawur (British ship) 312
Jouett, Adm. James 333
Journal de Leon (Spain) 150
Journal of American Medicine 353
Journal of Commerce (FL) 175, 189
Journal of Commerce (NY) 274, 308
Journal of Health 290
Journal of Immunology 390
Journal of New Orleans Medical and Surgical 192
Journal of the American Medical Association 319, 388
Journal of the American Medical Sciences 191
Journal of the Philadelphia Medical and Physical 123, 359
Journal of the Philadelphia School of Pharmacy 168
jungle fever 385
juniper, leaves and berries 72

kalmus, root 72
Kansas 27, 81, 310
Kansas City 355

Kanso, Russia 261
Kate (ship) 241
Kean, Maj. Jefferson Randolph 368
Keith, George 13
Keith, Lord 108
Kelley, Dr. 287
Kendrick, Mr. 174
Kenning, Dr. 109
Kent, William 56
Kent-Lynes, Elizabeth 56
Kent-Lynes, Fanny 56
Kentucky 169, 215, 243, 246, 293, 298, 309, 311
Kerr, Jas 70
Key West, FL 187, 203, 240, 241, 273, 275, 281, 282, 308, 335, 350, 352
Kibbee, Dr. 303
King, Gov. John A. (NY) 218, 220
King George 16, 38
King James II 12
King of Terror 336
King Pedro II 229
King William 12
King's College, NY 36
King's Hospital (Haslar) 19
King's Hospital (London) 28, 131
Kingston, Jamaica 19, 22, 23, 76, 94, 123, 148, 220, 265
Kingston, NY 187
Kinyon, Dr. 337
Kissinger, John R. 361, 362, 366
Klek, Prof. Edwin 364
Koch, Robert 386
Koch, Dr. Rudolph 323, 336
krameric acid 166
Ku Klux Klan 272
Kuhn, Dr. Adam 51, 66, 67
Kyasanur Forest 390

la peste 106, 210
La Mancha, Spain 135
Labarraque, M. 167
Lacailel, Dr. 323
Lackey, Oscar F. 355
Lafayette, Louisiana 183, 276, 309
The Lafayette Advertiser 276
Lagos, Nigeria 381
LaGuayra (Guaira), Venezuela 139
Laidlaw, Dr. 180
L'Aigret, Dr. Jean (Laigret) 383, 384
Lake Champlain Vermont 92
Lamar, Sen. Albert R. 246, 283, 302
Lambert, John 127
Lamborn, Dr. Robert H. 338
Lancaster, Pennsylvania 21, 80
Lane, Dr. H.M. 322
Langstaff, Dr. 299
Laredo, Texas 313

LaRoche, Dr. Rene 233, 354
Larrey, Dominique-Jean 42
Las Guasimas, Cuba 350
Latrobe, Benjamin Henry 142
Latrobe, Henry Sellon Boneval 142
laudanum 60, 66, 303
lavender 60, 66, 111
Laveran, Alphonse 325
Lawrence, Dr. 299
lazaretto (quarantine warehouse) 33, 53, 86, 109, 110, 129, 130, 135, 143, 150, 151, 162, 167, 191, 268, 286
Lazear, Dr. Jesse W. 355, 356, 357, 358, 359, 366
Leadbutter 18
Lebby, Dr. Robert 301
Lebrija, Spain 153
LeCompte, M. 266
leeches 69
Leeward Islands, Caribbean Islands 14, 22, 76, 138
Leghorn, Spain 112, 125, 166, 261
Leith, Sir James 139
lemon(s), juice 27, 84, 155, 189, 210, 249
Lempriere, Dr. 80, 121
Lenox, Colonel 76
Leon, Ponce de 270
LePrince, Mr. Joseph Agustine 371
Lerida, Spain 151
Leslie, Frank 321
Leslie, Prof. John 167
Letcher, Mr. 236
Letchworth, John 70
Levant, Eastern Mediterranean 261, 99, 113, 261
Lewis, Captain 77
Lewis, Paul A. 386
Lewis & Clark Expedition 69
Lexicon Medicum 8, 69, 397
Libby Prison, Richmond, VA 242
Liberia 334, 395
Liberty Mills, Indiana 361
Libya 392
Lieb, Dr. 73
Ligon, Richard 6
Lima, Peru 256, 379
lime(s) 60, 69, 189, 247, 249, 260, 289, 343
lime, chloride of 167, 196, 211, 241, 308, 309
lime, phosohate of 22
lime, quick 74, 332
lime, septate of 102
Limerick, Ireland 14
limestone 315
Lincoln, Pres. Abraham 242, 245, 246, 250, 311
Lincoln, Gen. Benjamin 40

Lind, Dr. James 19, 28, 34, 39, 106, 123
Lingendes, Gov. M. Vidal de 228
Lister, Dr. 323
Little, Richard 86
Little, William 85
Little Mud Island, Philadelphia 18, 58
Little War (1879–1880) 340
Liverpool, England 53, 83, 84, 125, 126, 144, 145, 147, 203, 205, 220, 307, 363, 368
The Liverpool England School of Tropical Medicine 363, 368
Livingston, Brockholst 83
Llewellyn, Dr. 139
Lloyd, Dr. Bolivar J. 385
Lloyd's Evening Post 39, 80, 99, 105
Lloyd's London 39, 80, 99, 105, 237
Lo, Hin 324
Lobo, Dr. Manuel de Gamma 318
Logansport, Indiana 155, 200, 299
The Logansport Journal 155, 200, 299
The London Chronicle 38, 260, 345
The London Colonial Gazette 178
The London Daily News 232, 368
The London Evening Mail 80
The London Evening Post 39
The London Gazette 178
The London Herald 80
The London Intelligencer 20
The London Lancet 256
The London Monthly Review 22, 102
The London Nonconformist 199
The London Observer 92
The London Post 39, 262
The London Standard 240, 258, 288, 289
The London Times 229
Long Island, New York 13, 115, 153, 158
Louis XVI 76
Louisburg, North Carolina 19
Louisiana 34, 71, 141, 156, 157, 197, 202, 215, 223, 226, 252, 275, 291, 292, 295, 307, 308, 310, 323, 335, 340
The Louisianan 172
Louisville, Kentucky 174, 246, 298, 315
The Louisville Courier 299
The Louisville Kentucky Journal 183, 299
Lowell, Captain 58
Lownes, Caleb 70, 72

Lush, Thomas R. 218
Lynch, Dr. Jordan R. 180
Lyons, Dr. Robert 230

Maass, Miss Clara 230
Macacus rhesus 381
Maclean, Dr. Charles 120, 158
Macon, Georgia 226, 242
Madeira (near Africa) 138
Madeira wine 66, 73, 155
Madrid, Spain 132, 134, 135, 136, 151, 343, 345
Magdalena (ship) 231
Magdalena, Portugal 230
MaGee, Surg. Gen. James C. 388
Magoon, Gov. Charles (Cuba) 369
Mahaffy, Dr. Alexander F. 381
Mahan, Capt. Alfred 386
Mahaska (iron clad steamship) 251
Maine 201, 216
USS *Maine* (ship) 346, 347
Maitland, Gen. (Col.) John 40, 141
Major, Samuel 21
Majorca, Spain 153
mal de Siam 12
Malaga, Spain 106, 109, 110, 111, 112, 151, 153
Mallory, Colonel 347
Manchuria, China 368
Manatee, Florida 337
manna 23, 28, 67
Manson, Dr. Patrick 324, 325, 357
Manzini, Dr. 234
Maria Pla (steamer) 287
Marietta, Georgia 160
marjoram 60
Marmion (ship) 172
Marsh, Dr. Marjor Edward J.T. 346
marsh fever 193, 325
Marshall, Charles 43
Marshall, Christopher 43
Martinique 12, 46, 76, 77, 106, 139, 140, 231
Maryland 35, 39, 215, 356, 390
Mason, John 70
Massachusetts 5, 12, 39, 58, 94, 98, 353
Matamoras, Mexico 189, 313
Mathews, Frank 220
Mathis, Constant 383
Mauldew, Dr. 304
Mauritius, Africa 257
May, M.D. 16
Mayali, Francois 383
Mayan language 6
Mayo, Commander 175
Mazatlan, Mexico 314

McArthur, Maj. Archibald 41
McCandless, Peter 41
McCarthy Island, Africa 257
McClellan (transport ship) 355
McClellan guards 298
McCraven, William 265
McCreary, Gov. James (Kentucky) 293
McCubbin, Mrs. Ellen Leigh 291
McCubbin, Mr. William 291
McGill, Bishop R.C. 210
McGoldrick, Michael 351
McGregor, Mr. 125
McIlvaine, William 51
McKee, James A. 271
McKenzie, Major-General 131
McKinley, Pres. William 370
McLean, Dr. Hector 101
McNulty, Dr. 221
M'Culloch, John 70
Mease, Dr. James 58
measles 15, 37, 84, 120, 123, 124, 168, 270
The Medical and Hospital News Gazette 205, 234
Medical Gazette of Lisbon 230
Medicus 56, 57
Mediterranean 33, 100, 130, 151, 180, 237, 261, 287
Melklejohn, Secetary of War 354
Melville, Herman 57
Memphis, Tennessee 81, 174, 221, 247, 251, 268, 277, 278, 278, 280, 284, 285, 292, 295, 298, 299, 300, 302, 304, 309, 310, 314, 315, 328
The Memphis Appeal 277
The Memphis Post 251
The Mercantile Advertiser 169
Mercer, Dr. A. 294
Merchant, Traveller 339
Merck, George 390
mercury 59, 60, 61, 66, 68, 69, 79, 82, 89, 94, 125, 174, 180, 235, 274
Merriam, Mr. 210
Messrs. Parke, Davis & Co., Detroit 303
Metchnikoff, Elie 325
Metzger, Dr. 122
Mexico 2, 5, 161, 177, 180, 184, 189, 234, 275, 281, 282, 313, 314, 318, 320, 330, 337, 339, 340, 367, 380, 394
Mexico City, Mexico 177, 185, 231
Meyer, Dr. Karl F. 387
Meyrigna, Dr. 320
M'Gown, Mr. 66
M'Grigor, Sir James 158
miasma 3, 9, 15, 18, 44, 45, 47, 48, 49, 51, 87, 88, 118, 124, 132, 134, 136, 167, 180, 192, 232, 260, 278, 289, 290

miasmata 1, 34, 59, 82, 108, 119, 123, 152, 349
mice 383, 384
Michigan 353
Michigan (ship) 200
microcephaly 393
micrococcus of yellow fever 319
Micrococcus zantogenus 319
Mifflin, Gov. Thomas (Philadelphia) 50, 53, 54, 55, 57, 58
mikamia-guaco 234
Milford Haven, Wales 278
military fever 258, 316
Miller, Dr. Edward 116, 123
The Milwaukee (WI) *Sentinel* 338
Mississippi 13, 42, 195, 215, 223, 235, 243, 253, 278, 280, 295, 298, 308, 328, 339, 358, 390
Mississippi River 34, 155, 156, 183, 184, 186, 206, 223, 226, 235, 276, 277, 294, 298, 367
Missouri 155, 216, 322
Mitchell, Dr. 308
Mitchell, Dr. John 14, 15, 58, 102, 123, 149
Mitchell [Indiana] *Commercial* 146
Mobile, Alabama 14, 35, 161, 174, 175, 176, 185, 187, 191, 193, 194, 198, 201, 206, 208, 224, 233, 242, 243, 251, 270, 274, 281, 285
The Mobile Advertiser 176, 247
The Mobile (Alabama) *Journal* 176
The Mobile Register 176, 201, 276
Mohawk (steamer) 240, 251
molasses 17, 84, 202, 219, 268
mold (mould) 263, 341
Molina, Dr. Z.R. 355
Mongolian 304
monkey 6, 7, 289, 368, 381, 383, 384, 394
Monkey Hill burying ground, Panama 334
Monroe Doctrine 331
Montana 387
Montauk Point, New York 352, 354
Montevideo, Uruguay 111, 341
Montgomery, Alabama 204
The Montpelier Royal Cordial Drops 29
Moralis, Gen. A.F. 347
Moran, John J. 361, 362
Morgan, J.P. 91
Morland, John Martin 21
Morris, Dr. Merean 278
Morrison, George S. 370
Morveau, Guyton 60, 124, 132, 133, 134
Moscow, Russia 29, 30, 72, 258
Mosher, Dr. 274
mosquito eggs 6, 11, 121, 290, 326, 338, 358, 367, 385, 394

mosquito nets 9
mosquito theory 326, 357, 360, 373
Mozart (bark) 339
Mudd, Dr. Samuel 250
mule 295, 343, 347
Muller, Justice William 220
Munroe, Dr. 129
muscle aches (symptom of yellow fever) 7
mustard 210, 249, 303
Myers, Dr. 363
myrrh 72
myrtle 111

Naples, Italy 76, 87, 116, 261
Napoleon, Louis 87, 330
Napoleonic 55, 139, 332
Nashville, Tennessee 198
Nassau, Bermuda 106
Nassy, David 73
Natchez, Mississippi 156, 171, 173, 183, 184, 198, 200, 243, 267, 271, 304
National Academy of Science (NSA) 390
National Library of Medicine 10, 20, 32, 35, 71, 81, 107, 115, 122, 157, 163, 188, 212, 215, 224, 230, 255, 257, 290, 301, 311, 321, 331, 342, 352, 356, 359, 360, 364, 369, 373, 376, 380, 382
Native Americans (Indians) 170
Nayden (ship) 138
Nebraska 310
Needham, Henry Beach 375
negro (black) 106, 110, 152, 155, 255
Negroes 5, 11, 33, 47, 57, 61, 63, 77, 81, 82, 152, 155, 162, 170, 190, 206, 229, 240, 247, 249, 269, 276, 277, 284, 285, 292, 295, 298, 299, 309, 310, 332, 334, 340, 347, 349, 350, 353, 355, 371
Nelson, Admiral 113
Nelson, Dr. Wolford 333
Nervous Cordial and Botanical Syrup 105
nervous fever (first stage) 8, 16, 17, 29, 123
Nestor (ship) 171
Netherlands 11, 76
Nevis, West Indies 139
New Archangel, Russia 268
New Bedford, Massachusetts 219
New Hampshire 98, 241
New Haven, Connecticut 14, 219
New Jersey 16, 18, 36, 43, 88, 166, 214, 216, 218, 221, 267, 363, 371
New London, Connecticut 92, 93, 219
New Milford, Vermont 92

The New Orleans Bee 182, 196
The New Orleans Bulletin 171, 172, 185, 205, 224, 252, 265, 269
The New Orleans Chronicle 176
The New Orleans Commercial Bulletin 205, 252
The New Orleans Courier 170, 172, 185, 186
The New Orleans Crescent 190, 202
The New Orleans Delta 2, 184, 185, 186, 192, 195, 199, 206, 225, 235
The New Orleans Democrat 293
The New Orleans National 186
The New Orleans Picayune 173, 185, 202, 205, 225, 240, 251, 271, 293, 297, 365
The New Orleans Republican 183
The New Orleans Times 3, 182, 185, 186, 212, 251, 266, 267, 316
The New Orleans Tropic 189
The New Orleans True American 172
The New Orleans Union 171
New Providence, Rhode Island 115
New York Hospital 84
The New York Bulletin 308
New York Commercial Advertiser 96, 159
The New York Daily News 204, 237
The New York Evening Post 159, 198
The New York Gazette 41, 143, 159
The New York Herald 13, 189, 218, 221, 227, 267, 268, 270, 272, 289, 299
New York Journal 87, 97
New York Journal of Commerce 175, 189, 308
The New York Ledger 336
The New York Post 159, 189, 228
The New York Sun 5, 256, 327, 355
The New York Times 198, 204, 218, 219, 220, 221, 227, 239, 240, 255, 263, 271, 319, 320, 334, 359, 374, 381
The New York Tribune 198, 221, 244
The New York World 274, 275, 276, 280, 281, 286, 291, 292, 333, 334, 338, 340, 345, 346, 348, 351
New Zealand 256, 287
Newark, New Jersey 145
Newbern, North Carolina 242, 244, 245
Newburyport, Massachuttes 92, 94

Newport, Rhode Island 92
Niagara Falls, Canada 244, 245
Nicaragua 256, 330, 332, 334, 370, 394
Nicholson, Dr. Thomas 179
Nicolle, Prof. Charles 384
Nigeria 381, 382, 394
Nightingale, Florence 285, 288
nitre 22, 27, 54, 60, 67, 69, 82
Nixon, John 72
Nixon, Pres. Richard M. 391
Nobel Prize 325, 386
Noell, Thomas 13
Noguchi, Dr. Hideyo 379, 380, 381, 382
Noll, Dr. 298
non-immune 7, 361, 363, 365, 379
Nooth, Dr. 109, 110
Norfolk, Virginia 84, 85, 86, 113, 158, 160, 208, 209, 210, 211, 236, 244, 245, 284, 285, 298, 335, 352
Norfolk Eagle (ship) 86
Norfolk Naval Shipyard 207
North Carolina 41, 114, 117, 153, 215, 242, 244, 272
The North China Herald 213
Norwich, Connecticut 39, 97
Nott, Dr. Josiah Clark 191, 192, 193, 201, 208, 209, 274
Nova Scotia 12, 14, 17, 144, 183, 245
Numancia (ironclad ship) 274
Nunez, Dr. B.C. de Villavicencio 320
Nuremberg, Germany 320
Nyaden (ship) 138

Odessa, Russia 258
Offley, Daniel 72
Ogden, Joseph 72
The Ogden Standard 378
O'Hara, General 108
Ohio 123, 124, 155, 156, 160, 172, 216, 246, 268, 298, 339
The Ohio Item 351
The Ohio Star Herald 324
Okow-Bele, Dr. Jean-Marie 395
olive oil 124, 189
Olsen, John 273
Olyphant, Dr. David 40
Omsk hemorrhagic fever 390
"On the grunt" 250
O'Neil, Captain 352
Opelousas, Louisiana 156
opiate 27, 66, 74
Oporto, Portugal 228
Orange County, Indiana 18
oranges 106, 210, 242
Orfila, Mariquita 233
organ failure 8
origin of yellow fever 5, 89, 92, 102, 160, 191, 366

Index 443

Orwood, Mississippi 358
Osgood, Dr. Daniel 164
Oswald, Dr. Felix Leopold 302
Ottoman Empire 87, 261
Owners Goodwill (ship) 21
oysters 142, 233

Paddock, Senator 302
Palestine 25
Pall Mall British Gazette 336
Palma, Spain 153
palmae christi (olive oil) 28, 29
Palmetto, Florida 337
Panama 4, 256, 262, 287, 300, 314, 320, 327, 330, 331, 332, 333, 334, 370, 371, 372, 373, 374, 375, 376, 379, 387, 394
Panama Canal, Panama 1, 4, 6, 257, 330, 333, 372, 375, 376, 378, 396
Papilland, Dr. Lucien 234
Para, Brazil 228
Paracelsus, physician 37
Paris, France 38, 162, 163, 167, 202, 231, 291, 325, 330, 333, 341, 350, 356
Pariset, Dr. 152, 153, 162, 167, 168
Park, Sir Peter 39
Parke, Dr. Thomas 51
Parker, Dr. 365
Parkinson, Mrs. & Mr. 48, 49
Parodi, Teresa 209
Parson, William 56
Pascagoula, Mississippi 195
Pass Christian, Mississippi 185
Pasteur, Louis 318, 319, 323, 325, 336, 386
Pasteur Institute, Paris, France 325, 356, 383, 384
Paul, Dr. Constantine 316
pearlash (potassium carbonate) 235, 236
Pearson, Dr. 22, 69
Pedro, King II 229
Peete, Dr. George W. 270, 271
Pelleties, Mr. 291
Pendergast, James P. 273
Pennsylvania 43, 83, 98, 155, 193, 302, 339, 355
Pensacola, Florida 19, 35, 36, 39, 160, 175, 185, 275, 278, 281, 284, 313, 340
The Pensacola Gazette 175
peppermint 60, 66, 84
Pepperrell, Sir William 17
Perea, Dr. William 395
Perkins, Benjamin Douglas 98
Perkins, Dr. Elisha 97, 98
Perm, Russia 258
Pernambuco, Brazil 227, 228
Perry, Dr. 280
Perth Amboy, New Jersey 267

Peru 6, 22, 28, 166, 256, 300, 371, 379
Peruvian bark 28, 29, 69, 84, 180, 291, 394
la peste 106, 210
pesthouses (pest hole) 53, 62, 192, 207, 251, 290, 378
pestilential fever 15, 100, 101, 108, 111, 123, 148
pestilential infection 31
petechia (petechio) 8, 9
Peters, Thomas 70
Petersburg, Virginia 159, 236
Petropolis, Brazil 228
Pettenkoffer, Dr. 278
Pettus, Gov. John J. (Mississippi) 243
The Philadelphia Gazette 94, 96, 101
The Philadelphia Inquirer 244
The Philadelphia (PA) *Ledger* 235
The Philadelphia Press 246, 276, 283, 323
Phipps, Mr. J.L. 268
phlebotomy 26, 235
Physick, Dr. (Physis) 49, 70, 73
Pierce, Pres. Franklin 209
Pim, Capt. Bedfore R.N. 333
pimento 20, 231
Pinckard, Dr. 126
Pintard, John 116
Pisa, Italy 166
Plainfield, Connecticut 97
Plant City, Florida 337
The Plantation News 16, 17
Plaquemine Parish, Louisiana 308
La Plata (ship) 237
Plymouth (steamship) 306, 327
Poinsett (ship) 175
Point-a-Petre (Martinique) 139
Poland 183, 315, 378
polka fever 227
Pope, Dr. Lieutenant Colonel 351
Popham, Sir Home 140
Popular Science 302
Pork King 310, 327
The Port Arthur (TX) *News* 388
Port-au-Prince, Haiti 17, 76, 78, 83, 86, 115, 139, 231
Port Baltimore, Maryland 143, 153, 211
Port Boston, Massachusetts 219
Port Cartagena, Colombia 14
Port Catalonia 153
Port Charleston, South Carolina 273
Port Eads, Mississippi 298
Port Gibson, Mississippi 200
Port Guayaquil, Ecuador 278
Port Havana, Cuba 141
Port Honduras 16
Port Key West, Florida 241, 273

Port Kingston, New York 187
Port Louis 285
Port Mahon, Spain 261
Port Majorca 153
Port Malaga 153
Port New Bedford, Massachusetts 219
Port New Haven, Connecticut 219
Port New London, Connecticut 219
Port New Orleans, Louisiana 282
Port New York 32
Port Newport, Rhode Island 219
Port of Marseilles 153
Port Orotava, Canary Islands 138
Port Perth Amboy, New Jersey 267
Port Portland, Maine 219
Port Portsmouth 219
Port Providence, Rhode Island 219
Port Royal, Georgia 293
Port Royal, Jamaica 123, 314
Port Royal, Nova Scotia 12
Port St. Mary, Spain 137, 153
Port Vera Cruz, Mexico 5, 141
Portabello 129
portabello mushroom 129
Porter, Captain 370
Portland Oregon 92
Portland, Duke of 108
Portland, Maine 201, 287
Portsmouth, Virginia 19, 86, 92, 114, 205, 206, 207, 209, 210, 211, 335
Portugal 6, 11, 46, 76, 77, 87, 113, 132, 153, 228, 229, 231, 261
potatoes 67, 160, 391
Pothier, Dr. 365, 366
Poughkeepsie, New York 158
Powel, Samuel 57
Powell, J.M. 69
Powell, Mayor (Brooklyn, NY) 221
Powell, Mrs. 94
Powers, Hiram 117, 194
Powers, Weightman, Rosengarten & Son 290, 291
President Fillmore (ship) 238
President's Island, New Orleans 251
Prevost, Gen. Augustine 40
primates 5, 7
Prince Edward (ship) 19
Prince's Bay, New York 218
Prior, Thomas 129
Providence (ship) 111
Providence, Rhode Island 17, 86, 92, 113, 115, 117, 125, 219
The Providence (RI) *Journal* 305
Prussia 16, 124, 183, 216, 258, 261, 288

Public Health Reports 300
Puerto Barrios, Guatemala 394
Puerto Rico (Porto Rico) 256, 387, 395
Pulitzer, Joseph 345
Pym, Dr. Sir William 148, 149, 192
Pyne, Dr. 158
pyrethrum 385

Q-fever (biological weapon) 391
Quebec, Canada 12, 36, 244
Quemados, Cuba 357, 361
quinine 35, 73, 180, 192, 234, 235, 255, 258, 260, 265, 290, 291, 295, 349, 372

rabbits 319, 336
Radway's Ready Relief and Regulators 235
Raleigh (ship) 229
The Raleigh (NC) *Register* 240
Ramirez, Dr. 320
Ramsay, David 40
Ramsey, Dr. William T. 299
Rand, Dr. Isaac 88
Random, Rodrick 104
Ranger (ship) 370
ratanhia (Krameria triandra) 166
Raven (ship) 178
Reamy, Dr. 294
Rebourgeon, Dr. 320
receptor-mediated endocytosis 7
Reclus, Armand 331
Rector Street epidemic 158
Red Hook, New York 222
Redman, Dr. John Coxe 51, 61, 66, 69
Reed, Dr. Maj. Walter 354, 355, 356, 357, 358, 360, 363, 366, 380
Reichenbach, Dr. 193
Reilly, Dr. Frank W. 278
Remington, Jesse 167
Remission Stage (Stage 2) 7
remittent fever 44, 67, 69, 79, 109, 124, 128, 149, 161, 234, 258
Rev. WM. Barclay's Patent Antibilious Pills 105
Reynolds, James Bronson 375
Rhenish wine 167, 181
rheumatism 21, 84, 105, 254, 349
Rhode Island 86, 98, 113, 216
rhubarb 27, 28, 67, 84
Richards, Dr. T.G. 323
Richmond (ship) 172
Richmond, Virginia 210, 213, 215, 221, 252, 298, 300
The Richmond Enquirer 207
Ricinus Americanus major (castor oil) 29
Ricketts, John Bill 47, 54, 55
Rio de Janeiro 5, 227, 256, 312, 320, 322, 323, 335, 336, 364, 393
Ripley, Dr. T.S. 193
Ritchie, Samuel J. 307
Rivas, Nicaragua 256
Robert Fulton (ship) 156
Roberts, Gov. Oran (Texas) 313
Robeson, Mr. Tar 282
Robinson, Capt. Edward 229
Rochelle salt 180
Rock, Edward 79
Rockefeller Foundation 378, 379, 380, 381, 382, 383, 384, 385, 386, 387, 390, 394
Rodney, Adm. Sir George 37, 183
Rogers, E.H. 322
Rome, Georgia 242, 347
Rome, Italy 199
Rontgen, Wilhelm 343
Roosevelt, Pres. Franklin D. 389, 390
Roosevelt, Pres. Theodore 366, 368, 369, 370, 371, 374, 375
rosemary 60, 111
Rosenau, Dr. 366
Ross, Andrew 51
Ross, Dr. John 373
Ross, General 131
Ross, Ronald 325, 357
Rotterdam, Netherlands 261
Roux, Professor 341
Royal Oak (ship) 164
Royal Patent Medicinal Snuff 21
Royal Towns, Vermont 92
Ruby (steamboat) 275
Rush, Dr. Benjamin 2, 16, 18, 49, 50, 51, 52, 55, 56, 57, 58, 59, 60, 61, 62, 66, 67, 68, 73, 74, 82, 89, 99, 100, 101, 121, 158, 193, 346
Rush, Julia 59
Rush's Thunderbolts 69
Rush's Thunderclappers 69
Rushville, Indiana 307
The Rushville (IN) *Republican* 307
Russell, Dr. Frederick 383
Russell, Dr. P. 149, 158, 271
Russia 29, 87, 216, 258, 261, 381, 391, 392
Ruston, Dr. Thomas 67, 122
Ryan, Dr. J. Murry 277

Sabine Pass, Texas 241
saffron jack 277
saffron john 320
St. Augustine 161, 175
St. Bartholomew 139
St. Christopher 14
St. Croix 66, 74, 257
St. Ferdinand 135, 330
St. George 242, 244, 381
St. Helena Sound, South Carolina 241
St. John's 22, 179, 270
St. Joseph 178
St. Kitts, Trinidad 11, 46, 139, 312
St. Lawrence (ship) 241
St. Louis, Missouri 183, 185, 185, 187, 197, 200, 223, 233, 244, 268, 270, 298, 309, 324, 337, 368, 380
The St. Louis Globe Democrat 326
The St. Louis Hard Times 185, 200
St. Louis (MO) *Post-Dispatch* 1, 346
The St. Louis Republican 184
The St. Louis Reveille 186
St. Lucia 76, 85
St. Mary, Spain 137, 153, 201
The St. Paul (MN) *Herald* 339
St. Petersburg, Russia 258, 369
St. Thomas, Virgin Islands 12, 37, 138, 207, 220, 231, 232, 233, 254, 255, 259, 260
St. Vincent, West Indies 46
Sainte-Croix deTeneriffe 257
Saleratus (baking soda) 236
Saleta (ship) 313
salt peter (petre) 72, 367
Salta, Peru 300
Salva, Don Francisco 126
Samaritan Society 201, 209
Sampson, Adm. William T. 350
Sampson (ship) 78
Samuel Major's Imperial Phoenix Snuff 21
San Antonio, Texas 313, 335, 343
The San Antonio Light 346
San Domingo (Santo) 5, 46, 61, 77, 78, 85, 101, 110, 115, 120, 122, 140, 340, 348
San Fernando, Isle of Leon 136
San Francisco, California 201, 256, 287, 314
San Juan de Uilon (Mexican prison) 320
San Lucar, Spain 106, 153
San Pedro Sula 394
San Roque 154
San Salvador 332
Sanarelli, Dr. Guiseppe 341, 342, 355, 356, 357, 363
Sandy Hook, New Jersey 214, 216, 218, 221, 239
Sanitary Magazine 315
Sansom, William 58
Santa Cruz, Canary Island 117, 138, 306
Santa Maria, Spain 107, 136
Santiago de Cuba 212, 255, 256, 343, 350, 351, 352, 354, 355
Santo Domingo, Haiti 46, 340
Santos, Mr. 109
Saratoga, New York 17, 18, 214

Index

Sardinia Island 19, 261
Saunders, William 127
Savannah, Georgia 40, 47, 159, 199, 203, 204, 219, 242, 252, 272, 291, 292, 303
The Savannah Advertiser 283
The Savannah News 283, 284, 285, 286, 292
Savery, Thomas 70
Sawyer, Dr. Wilber A. 383, 384
Say, Dr. Benjamin 51
Scalpel (ship) 263
scarlet fever (scarlatina) 84, 120, 123, 191, 243, 270, 278, 317, 339
Scarlett, Mr. 145
Schiedam Aromatic Schnapps 290
Schooley's Mountain Springs, New Jersey 18
Schoolfield, Dr. 207
Schuyler, Brant 13
Schuylkill River 18, 58, 91, 94
The Science 341
Scientific American 278
scorpion 265
Scotland 79, 183, 246
Scots Magazine 80
Scott, Gen. Winfield 185, 189
Scout (ship) 178
Seaman, Dr. Valentine 84, 88
Sedillot, Dr. 162
Seguine's Point, New York 218
Seguranca (steamship) 340
Seine (ship) 259
seizures 7, 8
Seldon, Lt. Gov. Henry R. 218
Selkirk, J.M. 272
Sellards, Andrew Watson 381, 383
Semmes, Dr. 284
Senegal 6, 318, 382, 383
Senn, Lt.-Col. Nicholas 353
Serbia 378
Seville, Spain 108, 109, 134, 135, 136, 137
Seward, William H. 246, 251
Shafter, Gen. William 350, 351, 352, 357
Shakespear, E.O. 355
Shandy, Tristram 104
Sharswood (Sharfwood), James 70
sheep 83, 233, 234, 298, 345
The Shelbyville (Indiana) *National Democrat* 208, 302, 305
Sheridan, Maj.-Gen. Phil 248, 251
ship fever 5, 185, 207
Shippen, William 51, 52
Shreveport, Louisiana 275, 276, 277, 279, 280
Siboney, Cuba 350, 351, 352, 360
Sicily, Italy 113, 183

Siede, Julius 209
Sienna, Italy 166
Sierra Leone, Africa 6, 162
Simmons, L.R. 276
Simmon's Liver Regulator 303
Singapore 387
slave ship 5, 33, 232, 349
slave trade 5, 11, 46, 61, 232, 240, 380
slaves 11, 15, 17, 40, 46, 81, 172, 177, 190, 226, 232, 234
slow fever 21, 23
smallpox 8, 11, 15, 31, 32, 33, 34, 36, 40, 41, 43, 56, 80, 84, 103, 123, 124, 220, 234, 243, 254, 255, 256, 267, 270, 279, 292, 316, 339, 366, 371, 384, 391
Smith, A.P. 333, 334
Smith, Captain 244
Smith, Dr. Charles G. 371
Smith, Hugh 384, 385, 386
Smith, J.C. 365
Smith, John 164
Smollett, Tobias 104
snake-root 15, 28, 84, 349
sodium salicylate 318
Solomon, Dr. S. 104
Sonora, Mexico 177
Soper, Dr. Fred L. 394
South Carolina 12, 14, 16, 17, 21, 35, 41, 82, 141, 215, 226, 240, 241, 242, 246, 272
The South Side (VA) *Democrat* 334
Southampton, England 231, 237, 259
Spain 4, 6, 11, 16, 34, 76, 106, 107, 108, 112, 113, 125, 129, 130, 131, 132, 134, 135, 140, 149, 150, 151, 152, 153, 155, 161, 162, 164, 183, 216, 261, 311, 340, 341, 342, 343, 345, 346, 348, 350, 354
Sphinx (ship) 17
Spinner, General 251
Spirit of Spruce (turpentine concoction) 78
spotted fever 112, 258
Spring Hill, Alabama 208
Spring Hill Hospital (VA) 208
Sproat, the Rev. James 61
Srakosch, Amalia Patti 209
Srakosch, Maurice 209
Stafford Springs, Connecticut 18
stagnant water 18, 53, 83, 88, 89, 181, 223, 304, 349
Stall, Dr. John 69
Staten Island, New York 39, 187, 204, 213, 216, 218, 219, 220, 221, 252
Steep, Thomas W. 351
Steers, Edward, Jr. 245
Stegomyia fasciata 362, 368
Stephens, Dr. 291

Sternberg, Dr. George Miller 308, 312, 324, 337, 341, 346, 354, 355, 357, 358, 367
Sterne, Lawrence 104
The Steubenville (OH) *Herald* 324
Stevens, Dr. Alexander H. 221, 222
Stevens, Dr. Edward 66
Stevens, John Frank 374
Stevens, Dr. William 179, 180
Stevens Island, Cuba 177
Stewart, Dr. D.F. 126, 148
Stimson, Henry L 387, 388, 389, 390
Stockholm, Sweeden 260
Stokes, Adrian 381, 382
Stone, Dr. Warren 210, 251, 263, 274
"Straight-back Dick" 247
Straits of Magellan 256, 330
stranger's fever 5
Stratton, George Fredrick 145, 147
Stubbs, Mayor Simon S. (Norfolk,VA) 209
Sullivan, Dr. John 300
Sullivan's Island, Charlestown, SC 141
sulphur 34, 69, 72, 265, 299, 349, 362, 367
sulphuric acid 16, 120, 133, 265, 303, 308
sulphurous chalybeate waters 18
Sumter, Gen. Thomas 41
Sunderland, England 178, 229, 315
Superb (ship) 151
Susquehanna (steamer) 219
Swaine (Swain), James 70
swamp fever 283
Swan, Edward C. 243, 244
Swansea, Wales 259, 349
Swanson Rheumatic Cure Company 349
Swanwick, John 72
Sweden 183, 216, 261
Switzerland 183, 216
Sylvatic (jungle) yellow fever 7, 385
symptoms of yellow fever 3, 5, 7, 9, 25, 83, 234, 320, 338, 341
synocha (inflammatory fever) 8, 258
synochus icteroides 51
Syracuse, New York 13, 207
Syracuse (NY) *Herald* 13
Syria 392

Tacna, Peru 256
Talmy, Dr. 318
tamarinds 28, 67
Tampa, Florida 337

Tampico, Mexico 177
Tangier 108, 112
tar water 129
Tarleton, Lt. Col. Banastre 41
Tartar (ship) 19
Tasmanian (ship) 259
Taunton, Massachusetts 290
Taylor, Gen. Zachary 189, 195
Taylor, Mississippi 358
Temple, Texas 353
The Temple (TX) *Tribune* 353
ten-and-ten 58
Tenner, Dr. D.P. 276, 279
Tennessee 197, 215, 246, 268, 295, 298, 309
Tennessee (flagship) 333
Terre Haute, Indiana 390
Texas 175, 177, 189, 206, 241, 246, 249, 263, 269, 275, 276, 292, 295, 297, 307, 310, 313, 315, 323, 366, 367, 372, 373
Thacher, James 42
Thames (convict ship) 232
Thayer, Dr. A.E. 366
Theiler, Dr. Max 381, 383, 384, 386
Thetis (ship) 138
Thomas, Wolferstan H. 368
Thomas Wilson (ship) 93, 94
Thomasville, Georgia 286
Thompson, Mrs. Elizabeth 302, 307
Thompson, Jake 246, 246
Thompson, John C. 220
Thompson, Dr. R.H. 211, 213, 218, 219, 220
Thone, Frank 388
Thorburn, Grant 117, 194
Thornton, Dr. Robert John 123
Thorton, Sir Edward 307
Thurston, D. 246
The Titusville Herald 273
tobacco 34, 85, 108, 127, 155, 238, 268, 342, 349, 362
Tobago 46, 115, 178
Tombs, New York 304
Tomkins, Jacob, Jr. 58
Tomkins, Gov. Ray (New York) 213, 220
Tompkinsville, New York 213
Toner, Dr. J.M. 278
Tonyn, Patrick 41
Toronto, Canada 244
The Toronto Ledger 246
transmission cycle 6
Treat, Dr. Malachi 83
Treaty of Aix-la-Chapelle 17
Treaty of Campo Formio 87
Treaty of Paris 350
Treaty of Ryswick 12
Treaty of Utecht 14
Trebla, Mrs. 304
Trebla, Gen. Yos 304

Trenton, New Jersey 92, 166
Trigge, Sir Thomas 109
Trinidad 46, 178, 180, 379
tropical disease 6, 14, 80, 100, 175, 232, 300, 325, 370, 387
Truner, Mr. 291, 308
tuberculosis 9, 36
tularemia (biological weapon) 391
Tunis 383, 384
Turkey 33, 261, 368
Turner, Dr.C.E. 356
turpentine 43, 78
Turtle, Maj. James 373
Tuscany, Italy 76, 166
Tuthill, Dr. 221
typhoid fever 40, 230, 258, 263, 270, 316, 353, 353, 355, 381

umbrella cage 367
Union (ship) 110
University of Aberdeen (Scotland) 324
University of California 387
University of Cornel Medical College 375
University of Louisiana 252
University of Maryland 356
University of New York 148
University of Texas 366
University of the South 372
University of Virginia 355
urban yellow fever 7
US Mail Steamship 238
Utah 390

vaccination 9, 10, 37, 234, 319, 320, 334, 336, 381, 384, 385, 387, 388, 389, 393, 394, 395
Valentin, Dr. Louis 166
Valetta, Malta 131
Vallance, Mr. 167
Valparaiso (bark) 277
Vance, Dr. R.Y. 129, 130
Vanda (schooner) 187
Vanderbilt, Jacob 220
Vanderpoel, Dr. 274, 280, 290, 311
Vanhovenburg, Dr. 187
VanSlooten, William 314
Varick, Mayor Richard (NYC) 64, 90
Venezuela 139, 378, 379
Vera Cruz, Mexico 5, 17, 132, 139, 141, 161, 177, 180, 189, 190, 234, 269, 275, 314, 318, 320, 322, 365
Vermont 92, 98, 216
vervain leaves 291
Vicksburg, Louisiana 183, 198, 200, 205, 206, 223, 235, 241, 278, 295, 298, 302
The Vicksburg Herald 280
Victoria (brig) 273

Victoria, Queen of England 243
Vienna 67
Vincent, George E. 379, 381
Vincenzo Accame (ship) 313
vinegar 28, 33, 34, 50, 52, 59, 60, 80, 84, 107, 132, 152, 166
viral hemorrhagic 5, 390
Virginia 14, 15, 35, 40, 41, 42, 58, 66, 84, 86, 153, 159, 206, 207, 209, 215, 242, 244, 295, 353
Virginiana (ship) 28
Vis Medicatrix 37
vital air (pure air) 60
vomito negro (black vomit) 106, 110, 255
Von Humboldt, Alexander 330
Vulcan (British ship) 312

Wainwright 23
Wakeman, Maurice 386
Walker, Dr. 148
Walker, Rear Admiral 370, 373, 375
Wall, Dr. John P. 337
Wallace, John F. 372, 374
Waller, T 22
Walling, Captain 218
Ward, Artemus 250, 339
Warren, Dr. 14, 25, 26, 27, 84
Warren, Dr. John 88, 120, 149
Warren, Sir Peter 17
Warrentown 200
Warrior (ship) 164
Warsaw, Poland 386
Wasdin, Dr. 357
Washington, Pres. George 36, 42, 47, 66, 97, 248, 272, 367
The Washington Chronicle 323
Washington Daily National Intelligencer 164, 166, 180, 208
The Washington (DC) *Globe* 172, 182, 189, 196
The Washington (DC) *Union* 189
Watson, Dr. 366
Weaver, Jacob 70
Webb, Miss 48
Webster, Noah 12, 84, 88, 118, 121, 139
Weed, Thurlow 218
The Weekly News Chronicle 237
Wegg, Dr. John A. 300
Welch, Dr. S.M. 273, 274
Wemyss, Major 40
Wendell, Mr. 238
West, E.B. 191
West, Dr. Jacob S. 310
West Africa 6, 11, 46, 381, 383, 387
West Indies 18, 19, 35, 44, 74, 78, 79, 80, 85, 92, 100, 126, 147, 164, 177, 178, 180, 190, 232, 252, 254, 300, 312, 352

Index

West Nile Fever 396
Westfield, NY 218
Westville, Indiana 348
The Westville (IN) *Indicator* 348
Wetherill, Samuel 70
Weyler, Capt.-Gen. Valeriano 343, 345, 346
Wheeler, Sir Francis 12
The Wheeling Times 172
White, Dr. C.B. 305
White, General 76
White, Dr. Joseph H. 379
White, Dr. W. 127
white flag 74
"White Man's Grave" 380
Whitehall, England 83, 145
Whitehall Evening Post 20
The Whitehall Post 20
The Whitesboro (TX) *News* 104
Whiting, Dr. 187
whooping cough (hooping cough) 84, 270
Wildfire (slave ship) 240
Wiley, John 211
William Agnew (ship) 237
William of Orange 12
William (ship) 83
Williams, Attorney General 275
Williams, Dr. C.L. 385
Willich, Dr. 105
Wilmington, Delaware 92, 114, 194
Wilmington, North Carolina 241, 272
The Wilmington (NC) *Journal* 241
Wilson, Dr. 191
Wilson, Dr. Bruce 383
Wilson, James 58, 70
Windsor, Vermont 92
Winship, Captain 172
Wipprecht, R. 235
The Wisconsin Weekly 184, 185
Wise, John 210
Wistar, Dr. Casper Jun. 51, 66
Wistar, Thomas 70, 72
Wolfe, Udolpho 290
Wood, Gov.-Gen. Leonard 354, 355, 360, 364, 368
Wood, Mayor Fernando 211
Woodsworth, Dr. John W. 295, 289, 302
World Health Organization (WHO) 10, 284, 393
World War I 379, 386, 387, 388
World War II 390, 391, 393
wormwood 27, 60, 338, 349
Worrell, Mr. 241
Worthless, Dr. 266
Wright, Dr. 120, 158
Wuchereria Bancrofti 324
Wyman, Surg. Gen. Walter 365, 366

Xeres de la Fontera, Spain 108, 153

Yaba, Nigeria 381
Yazoo Pass, Mississippi 223
yeast 77
Yeats, Samuel 20
yellow fever plot 242, 243
yellow fever virus 6, 7, 376, 384, 390, 396
yellow flag 177, 232, 237, 247, 259, 274, 353
Yellow Hook, New York 213, 219
yellow jack 5, 204, 232, 240, 250, 265, 271, 277, 278, 283, 294, 336, 345, 379, 385
yellow jacket 5
yellow journalism 345
yellow plague 5
Yellow Rainer 5
yellow skin, eyes 7, 236
Yorktown, Virginia 42
Young, Mr. 139
Young, Dr. Thomas 58
Young, William 382, 386
Young Nicholas (ship) 110
Youth's Companion 336
Ypres, Belgium 386
Yucatan, Mexico 11, 313, 380

Zadkiel 315
The Zanesville (Ohio) *Courier* 2
Zeilin & Co., Detroit, Michigan 303
Zeimbraske 331
Zepher (brig) 83
Zika virus 393
Zimmerman, Mr. 332
zymotic 265, 270, 318, 327

www.ingramcontent.com/pod-product-compliance
Ingram Content Group UK Ltd.
Pitfield, Milton Keynes, MK11 3LW, UK
UKHW050544150426
5217IPUK00026B/2068